Series Editors:
Steven F. Warren, Ph.D.
Marc E. Fey, Ph.D.

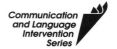

Communication
and Language
Intervention
Series

Treatment of Language Disorders in Children

Also in the *Communication
and Language Intervention Series:*

*Autism Spectrum Disorders:
A Transactional
Developmental Perspective*
edited by Amy M. Wetherby, Ph.D.,
and Barry M. Prizant, Ph.D.

*Promoting Social Communication:
Children with Developmental
Disabilities from Birth to Adolescence*
edited by Howard Goldstein, Ph.D.,
Louise A. Kaczmarek, Ph.D., and
Kristina M. English, Ph.D.

*Dual Language Development
and Disorders:
A Handbook on Bilingualism
and Second Language Learning*
Fred Genesee, Ph.D.,
Johanne Paradis, Ph.D., and
Martha B. Crago, Ph.D.

*Phonological Disorders in Children:
Clinical Decision Making in
Assessment and Intervention*
Alan G. Kamhi, Ph.D., and
Karen E. Pollock, Ph.D.

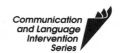

Communication
and Language
Intervention
Series

Treatment of Language Disorders in Children

edited by

Rebecca J. McCauley, Ph.D.
Professor
Department of Communication Sciences
University of Vermont
Burlington, Vermont

and

Marc E. Fey, Ph.D.
Professor
Hearing and Speech Department
University of Kansas Medical Center
Kansas City, Kansas

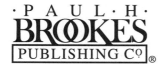
·PAUL·H·
BROOKES
PUBLISHING CO.®

Baltimore • London • Sydney

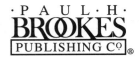

Paul H. Brookes Publishing Co.
Post Office Box 10624
Baltimore, Maryland 21285-0624

www.brookespublishing.com

Typeset by Integrated Publishing Solutions, Grand Rapids, Michigan.
Manufactured in the United States of America
by The Maple-Vail Book Manufacturing Group, York, Pennsylvania.

Video finishing and DVD authoring by Harley W. Blake III, Readsboro/Burlington, Vermont.

The individuals described in this book are based on the authors' experiences and are composites or real people whose situations have been masked. Names and identifying details have been changed to protect confidentiality.

The accompanying DVD contains a videotaped segment for most of the interventions discussed in *Treatment of Language Disorders in Children* (see the DVD icons in the table of contents). The video clips were supplied by the chapter authors, and permission was obtained for all individuals shown in footage contained in the DVD.

Third printing, September 2009.

Library of Congress Cataloging-in-Publication Data

Treatment of language disorders in children / edited by Rebecca J. McCauley
and Marc E. Fey.
      p.   cm.—(Communication and language intervention series)
  Includes index.
  ISBN-13: 978-1-55766-688-8 (pbk.)
  ISBN-10: 1-55766-688-1 (pbk.)
  1. Language disorders in children.   2. Language disorders in children—Treatment.
  I. McCauley, Rebecca Joan, 1952–   II. Fey, Marc E., 1952–   III. Series.
  RJ496.L35T74   2006
  618.92'855—dc22
                                              2005030769

British Library Cataloguing in Publication data are available from the British Library.

Contents

Series Preface

The purpose of the *Communication and Language Intervention Series* is to provide meaningful foundations for the application of sound intervention designs to enhance the development of communication skills across the life span. We are endeavoring to achieve this purpose by providing readers with presentations of state-of-the-art theory, research, and practice.

In selecting topics, editors, and authors, we are not attempting to limit the contents of this series to viewpoints with which we agree or that we find most promising. We are assisted in our efforts to develop the series by an editorial advisory board consisting of prominent scholars representative of the range of issues and perspectives to be incorporated in the series.

Well-conceived theory and research on development and intervention are vitally important for researchers, educators, and clinicians committed to the development of optimal approaches to communication and language intervention. The content of each volume reflects our view of the symbiotic relationship between intervention and research: Demonstrations of what may work in intervention should lead to analysis of promising discoveries and insights from developmental work that may in turn fuel further refinement by intervention researchers. We trust that the careful reader will find much that is of great value in this volume.

An inherent goal of this series is to enhance the long-term development of the field by systematically furthering the dissemination of theoretically and empirically based scholarship and research. We promise the reader an opportunity to participate in the development of this field through debates and discussions that occur throughout the pages of the *Communication and Language Intervention Series.*

Editorial Advisory Board

About the Editors

Rebecca J. McCauley, Ph.D., Professor, Department of Communication Sciences, University of Vermont, 489 Main Street, Burlington, Vermont 05405

Dr. McCauley is a Board-Recognized Specialist in Child Language, and an associate editor of the *American Journal of Speech-Language Pathology.* She received a master of arts degree in social sciences and a doctorate in behavioral sciences from The University of Chicago and did her postdoctoral training in speech-language pathology at The University of Arizona and The Johns Hopkins University. Although her primary interests lie in assessment of communication disorders in children (especially children with severe speech sound disorders), Dr. McCauley's growing interest in the challenges associated with developing and proving the value of interventions and in making such information accessible to the many parties led her enthusiastically to the current project. She has previously authored *Assessment of Language Disorders in Children* (Lawrence Erlbaum and Associates, 2001) and edited *Language, Speech, and Reading Disorders in Children: Neuropsychological Studies* (Little, Brown, 1988), by Rachel E. Stark and Paula Tallal.

Marc E. Fey, Ph.D., Professor, Hearing and Speech Department, University of Kansas Medical Center, 3901 Rainbow Boulevard, Kansas City, Kansas 66160

Dr. Fey's research and clinical interests include the role of input on children's speech and language acquisition, the relationship between oral and written language, and the efficacy and effectiveness of speech and language intervention for children. Dr. Fey was editor of the *American Journal of Speech-Language Pathology* from 1996 to 1998 and was chair of the American Speech-Language-Hearing Association Publications Board from 2003 to 2005. Along with his many publications, including articles, chapters, and software programs, he has published two other books on language intervention, *Language Intervention with Young Children* (Allyn & Bacon, 1986), and *Language Intervention: Preschool Through the Elementary Years* (co-edited with Jennifer Windsor & Steven F. Warren; Paul H. Brookes Publishing Co., 1995).

Contributors

Melissa M. Agocs, B.A.
Research Associate
Scientific Learning Corporation
300 Ogawa Plaza, Suite 600
Oakland, California 94612

Andrea Barton, M.A.
Speech-Language Pathologist
Children's Healthcare of Atlanta
4850 Sugarloaf Parkway, Suite 500
Lawrenceville, Georgia 30084

Nancy C. Brady, Ph.D.
Associate Research Professor
University of Kansas
Schiefelbusch Institute for Life Span
    Studies
1052 Dole, 1000 Sunnyside Drive
Lawrence, Kansas 66045

Shelley L. Bredin-Oja, M.A., CCC-SLP
Speech-Language Pathologist
University of Kansas Medical Center
3901 Rainbow Boulevard
Kansas City, Kansas 66160

Martha S. Burns, Ph.D., CCC-SLP
Adjunct Associate Professor
Northwestern University
Director, Clinical Specialists
Scientific Learning Corporation
300 Ogawa Plaza, Suite 600
Oakland, California 94612

Barbara M. Calhoun, Ph.D.
Director of Research
Scientific Learning Corporation
300 Ogawa Plaza, Suite 600
Oakland, California 94612

Stephen M. Camarata, Ph.D.
Director, Program in Communication
    and Learning
John F. Kennedy Center for Research
    on Development and Disabilities
Director, Scottish Rite Child Language
    Disorders Clinic
Professor
Department of Hearing and Speech
    Sciences
Vanderbilt University School of Medicine
230 Appleton Place
Peabody Box 40
Nashville, Tennessee 37203

Sharon A. Cermak, Ed.D., OTR/L, FAOTA
Professor of Occupational Therapy
Boston University, Sargent College
635 Commonwealth Avenue
Boston, Massachusetts 02215

Marjorie H. Charlop-Christy, Ph.D.
Professor of Psychology
Director, The Claremont Autism Center
850 Columbia Avenue
Claremont McKenna College
Claremont, California 91711

Melissa Cheslock, M.A.
Speech-Language Pathologist/
    Research Coordinator
Department of Communication
Georgia State University
Post Office Box 4000
Atlanta, Georgia 30302

Kevin N. Cole, Ph.D.
Senior Researcher
Washington Research Institute
150 Nickerson Street, Suite 305
Seattle, Washington 98109

James W. Cunningham, Ph.D.
Professor Emeritus of Education
University of North Carolina
    at Chapel Hill
Chapel Hill, North Carolina 27599

Logan E. De Ley, M.A., M.S.
Research Associate
Scientific Learning Corporation
300 Ogawa Plaza, Suite 600
Oakland, California 94612

Susan Ellis Weismer, Ph.D.
Professor and Chair, Department of
    Communicative Disorders
University of Wisconsin–Madison
1975 Willow Drive
Madison, Wisconsin 53706

Karen A. Erickson, Ph.D.
Associate Professor
Director, Center for Literacy and
    Disability Studies
CB #7335
University of North Carolina
    at Chapel Hill
Chapel Hill, North Carolina 27599

**Martha Fairchild Escalante, M.S.,
    CCC-SLP**
Clinical Educator
Appalachian State University
Post Office Box 2746
Boone, North Carolina 28607

Lizbeth H. Finestack, M.A.
Doctoral Student
Hearing & Speech Department
University of Kansas Medical Center
3901 Rainbow Boulevard
Kansas City, Kansas 66160

Gail T. Gillon, Ph.D.
Professor
Department of Communication Disorders
University of Canterbury
Private Bag 4800
Christchurch, 8005
New Zealand

Luigi Girolametto, Ph.D.
Associate Professor
Department of Speech-Language
    Pathology
University of Toronto
160-500 University Avenue
Toronto, Ontario M5G 1V7
Canada

James W. Halle, Ph.D.
Professor
Department of Special Education
University of Illinois
1310 South Sixth Street
Champaign, Illinois 61820

Terry B. Hancock, Ph.D.
Research Assistant Professor
Box 328 Peabody College
Vanderbilt University
Nashville, Tennessee 37203

Mary Louise Hemmeter, Ph.D.
Associate Professor
Box 328 Peabody College
Vanderbilt University
Nashville, Tennessee 37203

Paul R. Hoffman, Ph.D.
Professor
Department of Communication Sciences
    and Disorders
Louisiana State University
63 Hatcher Hall
Baton Rouge, Louisiana 70803

Cathleen Jones, Ph.D.
Educational and Behavioral Consultant
Southeastern Regional Education Service
    Center
29 Commerce Drive
Bedford, New Hampshire 03110

Ann P. Kaiser, Ph.D.
Professor
Department of Special Education,
    Psychology and Human Development
Box 328 Peabody College
Vanderbilt University
Nashville, Tennessee 37203

David A. Koppenhaver, Ph.D.
Associate Professor
Language, Reading, and Exceptionalities
    Department
Appalachian State University
Reich College of Education
124 Edwin Duncan Hall
Boone, North Carolina 28608

Young Sook Lim, Ph.D.
Senior Researcher
Washington Research Institute
150 Nickerson Street, Suite 305
Seattle, Washington 98109

Mary E. Maddox, M.Ed.
President
Washington Learning Systems

2212 Queen Anne Avenue North, #726
Seattle, Washington 98109

Steven L. Miller, Ph.D.
Senior Vice President, Outcomes
  Research
Scientific Learning Corporation
300 Ogawa Plaza, Suite 600
Oakland, California 94612

Tracy W. Mitchell, M.S., OTR/L
Lehigh Valley Hospital
Post Office Box 689
Allentown, Pennsylvania 18105

Keith E. Nelson, Ph.D.
Professor
Penn State University
414 Moore Building
University Park, Pennsylvania 16802

Nickola Wolf Nelson, Ph.D.
Charles Van Riper Professor
Department of Speech Pathology
  and Audiology
Director, Ph.D. Program in
  Interdisciplinary Health Studies
College of Health and Human Services
Western Michigan University
1903 West Michigan
Kalamazoo, Michigan 49008

Janet A. Norris, Ph.D.
Professor
Department of Communication Sciences
  and Disorders
Louisiana State University
63 Hatcher Hall
Baton Rouge, Louisiana 70803

Michaelene M. Ostrosky, Ph.D.
Associate Professor
University of Illinois at
  Urbana–Champaign
1310 South Sixth Street
Champaign, Illinois 61820

Shari Robertson, Ph.D.
Associate Professor of Speech-Language
  Pathology

Indiana University of Pennsylvania
570 S. Eleventh Street, 203 Davis Hall
Indiana, Pennsylvania 15701

MaryAnn Romski, Ph.D.
Associate Dean for Social and Behavioral
  Sciences
College of Arts and Sciences
Professor of Communication and
  Psychology
Georgia State University
Post Office Box 4000
Atlanta, Georgia 30302

Rose A. Sevcik, Ph.D.
Associate Professor
Department of Psychology
Georgia State University
Post Office Box 5010
Atlanta, Georgia 30302

Adelia M. Van Meter, M.S.
Clinic Coordinator and Faculty
  Specialist II
Department of Speech Pathology and
  Audiology
Western Michigan University
1903 West Michigan
Kalamazoo, Michigan 49008

Steven F. Warren, Ph.D.
Director, Schiefelbusch Institute for
  Life Span Studies
Director, Kansas Mental Retardation
  and Developmental Disabilities
  Research Center
Professor of Applied Behavioral
  Science
University of Kansas
1052 Dole Building
1000 SunnySide Avenue
Lawrence, Kansas 66045

Elaine Weitzman, M.Ed.
Executive Director
The Hanen Centre
1075 Bay Street, Suite 515
Toronto, Ontario, M5S 2B1
Canada

Foreword

In 1982, the Boys Town Institute on Communication Disorders in Children and the American Speech-Language-Hearing Association cosponsored a national conference to examine the historical roots, present characteristics, and future course of language intervention for various clinical populations. Jon Miller, David Yoder, and Richard Schiefelbusch (1983) edited a conference proceedings titled *Contemporary Issues in Language Intervention.* The final section of the book was a charge to clinicians who provide language intervention services. Rees's chapter urged clinicians to broaden their perspectives on language intervention and to produce new ideas and expectations about language intervention in light of recent research results in areas such as information processing, cognitive development, social development, and literacy. Rees wanted the language clinicians of her day to "…find a way to integrate the available information about language and language related factors and incorporate it into professional roles and practices" (1983, p. 311).

Rees raised a number of questions about issues that posed special challenges to clinicians. One question was, "What are the proper goals of language intervention with children?" Rees noted that too often, the clinical goals she saw on therapy plans were tied to language skills that were directly assessed by items on published tests. In their zeal for accountability, clinicians may have selected therapy targets that could be measured easily. Rees charged clinicians with targeting language structures that are pertinent to children's language communities and then helping children use those structures in socialization, problem solving, and learning contexts.

Rees's second question was, "What are the limits of language intervention?" She was aware of the growing literature on the relationships between oral and written language, and she challenged clinicians to work on reading and to incorporate writing or other augmentative systems into language intervention. Rees also encouraged clinicians to extend the limits of language intervention to include sociolinguistic and pragmatic factors that affect language use in everyday circumstances.

Rees's third question was, "Where does cognition fit in?" Rees believed that research on cognitive prerequisites to language development and evidence of an interactive relationship between cognition and language were pertinent to language intervention. She charged clinicians with finding ways to integrate cognition and language into language intervention with children at all levels of development, from prelinguistic communication to the production of complex texts.

Finally, Rees asked, "Where does perception fit in?" Rees was dubious about the existence or importance of a separable auditory processing factor that could be measured and remediated in language intervention programs. She emphasized that processing spoken language involves operations on acoustic, phonetic, phonological, lexical, semantic, syntactic, and pragmatic levels. Her challenge to clinicians was to determine the role of auditory processing in the larger context of teaching and learning functional language.

Treatment of Language Disorders in Children provides ample evidence that there has been a great deal of progress on each of Rees's charges in the past 23 years. The book presents readers with critical information about 15 treatments that directly or indirectly affect language development in children with language disorders. Each chapter is authored by individuals who had a critical role in developing and studying the treatment about which they are writing. The authors describe the treatment in detail, advise readers about the kinds of children who are likely to derive the most benefit from the treatment, discuss the theoretical bases of the treatment, summarize the scientific evidence for the treatment, propose methods for assessing treatment effectiveness, and provide a sample of therapeutic interaction. There is also an accompanying DVD that contains a 3-minute video of 14 of the treatments.

Recall that Rees (1983) was concerned that the clinical goals of her day were often tied to nonfunctional skills that were easily assessed. She will be delighted to see that nearly all of the treatments that are summarized in this text include strategies for supporting the development of language form, content, and use in functional contexts such as play, parent–child and teacher–child bookreading, and within classroom interactions. In addition, a number of the treatments include parent education components in order to facilitate functional communication at home. Finally, each chapter provides specific suggestions for making the treatment pertinent to children from a variety of social and linguistic communities.

Rees charged clinicians with expanding the limits of language intervention to include prelinguistic cognition, literacy, augmentative communication, and sociolinguistic behaviors. Responsivity education/prelinguistic milieu teaching (Chapter 3) summarizes effective treatments for prelinguistic communication behaviors such as following the child's attentional lead, building social routines, and increasing the frequency of nonverbal vocalizations. Treatments that foster literacy development include phonological awareness intervention (Chapter 12), visual strategies to facilitate written language development (Chapter 14), and the writing lab approach for building language, literacy, and communication (Chapter 15). There are also three chapters that present augmentative communication strategies for children at a variety of developmental levels: the Picture Exchange Communication System (Chapter 5) for children with minimal functional communication, the System for Augmenting Language (Chapter 6) for children with beginning intentional communication skills, and balanced reading intervention and assessment (Chapter 13) for school-age children with severe speech and physical impairments. It is clear from the treatments summarized in this book that the field has expanded the limits of language intervention in precisely the directions that Rees suggested.

Rees's third charge to clinicians was to integrate cognition and language into language intervention with children at all levels of development, from prelinguistic communication to the production of complex texts. One important similarity across the treatments in this book is that all are based on transactional models of language and cognition that involve reciprocal (bi-directional) relationships between language, experience, and cognition. A number of authors emphasize the importance of information processing abilities (i.e., working memory, speed of processing, attentional mechanisms, and speech perception) in the learning process. Finally, most authors explain the neurolinguistic bases that underlie their treatments. For example, Nelson and Van Meter (Chapter 15) indicate that the writing lab approach for building language, literacy, and communication was designed to promote improved coordination and connectivity among brain centers that are responsible for higher-level cognitive-linguistic functions such as discourse comprehension. Cermak and Mitchell (Chapter 17) tie sensory integration therapy to neural plasticity research, and Agocs and her colleagues (Chapter 18) cite research on cortical reorganization as the basis for Fast ForWord treatment. The sections of each chapter that concern the theoretical bases of the interventions suggest strongly that clinicians and clinical scientists have given careful thought to the research on the relationships between language and cognition and have incorporated critical concepts from this research base into their treatments.

Finally, Rees challenged clinicians to think carefully about the role of perception in language intervention. *Treatment of Language Disorders in Children* contains two chapters that focus on perception-based treatments: sensory integration (Chapter 17) and Fast ForWord (Chapter 18). Both treatments reflect multidimensional models of perception. Occupational therapists use sensory integration activities to help children improve their ability to process and use auditory, visual, and haptic input in daily activities. Fast ForWord was designed to help children process phonemes, syllables, words, and sentences with greater speed and precision. The evidence for the benefits of each of these treatments is equivocal. However, research on new treatments such as sensory integration and Fast ForWord will help clinicians meet Rees's charge to gain a clearer understanding of the function of perception in language disorders and language intervention.

Rees ended her chapter in *Contemporary Issues in Language Intervention* with the following statement: "In a sense, what I have been saying is that knowledge is a burden, but I hope you will agree that the burden is exciting and stimulating, and a welcome substitute for the bliss of ignorance" (1983, p. 316). Clinicians and clinical scientists who read *Treatment of Lan-*

guage Disorders in Children will see that the authors have given careful consideration to new knowledge in multiple fields of inquiry, and have incorporated that knowledge into the language intervention activities for infants, toddlers, preschoolers, and school-age children. The treatments that are summarized in this book show the considerable breadth of our current perspectives on language intervention and the extent to which thoughtful clinicians have lived up to the challenge of incorporating new knowledge into language treatment protocols. Children with language disorders are the direct beneficiaries of the progress that has been made.

Ronald B. Gillam, Ph.D.
Professor
Department of Communication
Sciences and Disorders
The University of Texas at Austin

REFERENCES

Miller, J., Yoder, D.E., & Schiefelbusch, R. (Eds.). (1983). *Contemporary issues in language intervention* Rockville, MD: American Speech-Language-Hearing Association.

Rees, N.S. (1983). Language intervention with children. In J. Miller, D.E. Yoder, & R. Schiefelbusch (Eds.), *Contemporary issues in language intervention* (pp. 309–316). Rockville, MD: American Speech-Language-Hearing Association.

Acknowledgments

The volume editors are deeply grateful to each of the authors who contributed to this book. They worked diligently to bring their interventions to life while conforming to the organizational structure set out for them. They were collegial, generally patient of their colleagues' varied paces of work, and in some cases, courageous, given the personal circumstances through which they worked and produced their chapters.

There are many people connected with Paul H. Brookes Publishing Co. to whom the editors owe thanks. Chief among these are Elaine Niefeld and the editorial board for the *Communication and Language Intervention Series*. Elaine provided guidance from the acquisition process through most of the book's preparation. Her laughter and optimism were always sources of comfort. The editorial board made numerous suggestions at the beginning of the project that helped us to move the project forward. Astrid Zuckerman, who took over the project for Elaine in recent months, helped get the book to its final destination. Finally, Jan Krejci has been one of the most thorough and tactful production editors with whom the editors have had the opportunity to work.

In Burlington, Rebecca has benefited greatly from the encouragement and support provided by her friend and University of Vermont colleague Barry Guitar. His generous counsel and comments on drafts of her contributions were especially helpful. She has also benefited from the wisdom of Brenda Bennett, a gifted school-based speech-language pathologist who thrives on her work with children with language problems. In addition, Harley Blake, the technical wizard behind the DVD included with the book, was the soul of patience and we are grateful for his expertise.

In Kansas City, Marc would like to thank Steve Warren for his collegiality and friendship and for his role in getting Marc involved in the *Communication and Language Intervention Series* at Brookes and in this book. He also thanks Shelley Bredin-Oja, Liza Finestack, and Shari Sokol, three doctoral students who were a continuing source of motivation and support for the entire period over which this book took shape.

Finally, we wish to thank the children and families who continually inspire us to learn more and work harder.

To my sisters, Ruth McCauley and Mary McCauley Doerksen

—RJM

To my friend and father, Bill Fey

—MEF

1

Introduction to *Treatment of Language Disorders in Children*

REBECCA J. MCCAULEY AND MARC E. FEY

THE PURPOSE OF THIS BOOK

Challenged by the number and diversity of available treatments, professionals and family members can be bewildered in their efforts to determine the potential value of a particular intervention for a child with a language disorder. Although personal testimonials and clinical endorsements of treatments abound, the premise of this volume is that stronger bases than these should be used to select a treatment approach. These bases include theoretical arguments (often grounded in developmental or physiological data) suggesting that a treatment *should* work and, far stronger still, empirical demonstrations that it actually *does* work for children with problems and characteristics similar to those of the child for whom treatment is sought. Indeed, even when empirical data are available, differences can be found in the quality of evidence they provide in support of an intervention's efficacy. This book is designed to provide an up-close and personal look at 15 contemporary language interventions presented by authors who have contributed to the development of the approaches. This view will include an introduction to the children whom the approaches are designed to benefit, the conditions in which the interventions are (or are not) likely to have their desired effects, and the evidence available to support claims of efficacy.

Authors in this book have closely followed a template they were given for presenting the details of their approach. Having interventions described by experts who have participated directly in their development allows for a particularly rich and detailed assessment of strengths and weaknesses. However, the use of a standard template is designed to minimize any undervaluing of *less* flattering and overvaluing of *more* flattering information that might creep in to even the best-intentioned review of one's own work. In addition, by their willingness to participate in this project and their responsiveness to editorial comments, authors in this volume have demonstrated an openness to the critical examination of the treatment approach about which they have written. It is their hope (and ours) that this process will both foster the most appropriate application of these interventions in the present and lead to their future improvement by paving the way for additional research designed to widen and deepen knowledge about for whom and to what extent the treatments can be used effectively.

The 15 treatments described in this volume fall naturally into three sections, including interventions that target 1) prelinguistic communication and early language, 2) advanced language and literacy, and 3) multiple levels of language and/or nonlanguage goals. Across the three groupings, the interventions illustrate a wide range of treatment goals, settings, therapeutic agents, and technological sophistication. Many attempt to modify specific language or communication forms, such as words, grammatical structures, or analysis of words into phonemes. Others seek much broader changes, such as increases in the frequency of language use or longer and more coherent written narratives. Finally, a small number target nonlanguage goals, such as improved auditory processing or better attentional focus, with the idea that these represent prerequisites to further communication development. Whereas most of the interventions represented here require little in the way of technological support, others take advantage of modern technology to affect the nature of input the child is receiving or to facilitate the child's communication output. Some interventions are implemented by individual clinicians or parents; others, by interdisciplinary teams. Thus, the treatments included here illustrate many of the variables manipulated in contemporary interventions for the diverse population of children with language disorders.

Despite the authors' careful descriptions of the components of their interventions, it is difficult to convey in words alone the essence of any language treatment. Therefore, the authors have provided a brief video example of the intervention they have presented for the accompanying DVD. These brief segments cannot transmit the full richness and organizational complexity of the treatments, but we believe they capture some of the core procedures found in each approach and provide examples of the types of children for whom the interventions may be appropriate. This should help readers to better understand each intervention and, therefore, to make better comparisons across approaches.

HOW TREATMENTS ARE DESCRIBED IN THIS BOOK

To encourage greater uniformity in presentation across treatment chapters, a template was used by authors to introduce readers to their intervention. Embodied within this template is a mix of information that is meant to allow readers to determine 1) the treatment's feasibility within their setting, 2) its appropriateness to the individual(s) for whom it is being considered, and 3) most especially, the evidence base on which it rests. Table 1.1 lists the title

Table 1.1.   Content specifications of the template followed within each chapter

Section	Content
Abstract	A summary indicating the population for whom the approach is recommended, the target of treatment, the strongest argument favoring the treatment's use, and a very brief description of its methods
Target Populations and Assessments for Determining Treatment Relevance and Goals	Target populations including both those for whom the intervention is primarily designed as well as secondary populations, when there is 1) empirical support or 2) theoretical support for use and methods used to identify them and determine goals
Theoretical Basis	Outline of the theoretical explanation or rationale for the treatment approach, including the nature of deficit/compensation being targeted and the language or nonlanguage area that is the focus of intervention
Empirical Basis	Detailed discussion of research supporting the effectiveness of a treatment with the target population(s)
Practical Requirements	Summary of resources needed to implement the treatment, including time demands, personnel needs, training required for personnel, and any materials that are required
Key Components	A description of the approach that may include discussion of treatment stages, procedures, goals, and the involvement of participants other than the primary clinician (e.g., parents, peers, other professionals)
Assessment Methods to Support Ongoing Decision Making	Description of methods to be followed by the clinician adopting the treatment to ensure that it is actually effective for the child and to guide revisions in treatment needed to improve effectiveness
Considerations for Children from Culturally and Linguistically Diverse Backgrounds	Descriptions of the applicability of the treatment to children from linguistically or culturally diverse backgrounds and ways in which it might be modified to be more appropriate for such children
Application to an Individual Child	A real or hypothetical case illustrating the selection of the treatment approach, its implementation, and its effectiveness
Future Directions	Description of research needed to support and extend existing claims of treatment effectiveness for the current population as well as those for whom it has suspected, but untried, value
Recommended Readings	A small group of references directing readers to pertinent additional information about the intervention

and content for each of the major sections that authors were asked to include in their treatment descriptions.

Following an abstract and an introduction, the first section of each chapter addresses Target Populations and Assessments for Determining Treatment Relevance and Goals. Here, the focus is on the population or populations of children for whom the intervention has been intended. The population may be described in terms of age, developmental level, and diagnosis. Treatment-specific assessment procedures that can be used to help confirm the appropriateness of the intervention to a particular child and the point at which to begin treatment are also described in this section.

The next section, Theoretical Basis, describes the theoretical explanations or rationales for the structure and content of the treatment, often drawing on ideas about the underlying nature of the child's language disorder or on factors seen as facilitating communication development more generally. This section almost always includes an explanation for the nature of outcomes that serve as targets of the intervention. Therefore, this section should help the reader judge whether the treatment is expected to address an underlying deficit or functional limitation directly or, instead, to address the social skill, activity, or social role restrictions that result from it (World Health Organization, 1980, 2001).

The third major section of each chapter, Empirical Basis, provides a summary of evidence supporting the value of the intervention for the population of children for whom it has been most studied. Authors were encouraged to describe studies in terms of three categories within the continuum discussed below by Fey (2002, 2004). This includes *exploratory studies,* in which important variables that might be exploited in an intervention are studied in a preliminary way; *efficacy studies,* in which interventions are studied under ideal conditions; or *effectiveness studies,* in which interventions are studied under the rough-and-tumble conditions of settings, clinicians, and children who are more like those encountered in everyday practice than those included within efficacy studies. Information regarding the magnitude of differences between treatment and control groups (i.e., effect sizes) generally is presented, although readers will see that this information is missing from many accounts—often because the original data were not reported in such a way as to make that possible. Nonetheless, this section presents the best scientific information the authors could assemble to provide support for use of their intervention.

The next three sections of each chapter—Practical Requirements, Key Components, and Assessment Methods to Support Ongoing Decision Making, are designed to illustrate in detail how the intervention is implemented. These sections and the DVD clips that accompany the book also should help clinicians to judge the feasibility of the intervention for their particular setting and practice conditions and assist them in drawing some initial impressions of the face validity of the method. Although the details of an intervention that can be provided within a book are limited, our intent is to make the interventions come alive so that experienced clinicians might actually be able to put them into practice, based on the descriptions provided.

The section on Practical Requirements called for authors to paint the larger picture of resources required to carry out the intervention in terms of personnel, the training needed for participants, time demands, and materials important for the treatment's implementation. In the section on Key Components, authors describe the structure of the treatment in greater detail, including the roles of all important participants and the temporal structure within individual sessions and across multiple sessions. In addition, more information is provided about the nature of treatment goals. The section entitled Assessment Methods Used to Support Ongoing Decision Making highlights the important component of recurring assessment used to make decisions about goal attainment and sequencing as well as about changes needed in activities and procedures over the duration of treatment.

Each chapter contains a section entitled Considerations for Children from Culturally and Linguistically Diverse Backgrounds. This section allows chapter authors to share their own general recommendations for adapting the intervention based on knowledge of cultural differences in parenting, language use with children, and attitudes toward literacy, as well as specific adaptations developed during the course of research or clinical use.

The section describing the treatment's application to an individual child supplements the information provided in other sections describing intervention methodology through the use of an extended example. The greater specificity and personal focus of this section may help some readers develop a clearer sense of what the treatment "feels like." Although this type of information adds little scientific weight to the process of choosing a particular treatment based on evidence of its efficacy, it may nonetheless prove helpful to readers as they assess a treatment's fit with their client families' values and clinician preferences.

In Future Directions, authors were encouraged to share their vision of the additional research needed to advance and broaden the efficacy and effectiveness claims that can be made on behalf of their intervention. In addition to promoting research by other investigators, this section should provide additional insight into the strengths and limitations of the existing evidence base for an intervention. Recommended Readings are designed to point readers to a small number of particularly valuable and often more comprehensive descriptions of the intervention.

As a last contribution to the clarity with which treatments are described, authors were asked to contribute a number of terms for inclusion in the glossary that appears at the end of this book.

For the DVD accompanying the book, authors were asked to contribute a 3-minute clip illustrating what they considered to be representative, significant, or visually memorable elements of the treatment approach. As was the case for the application section of the chapter text, these brief glimpses are expected to contribute to the reader's sense of an intervention in a way that is difficult to convey through text.

A STRUCTURAL MODEL OF INTERVENTION

In this section, we present a model that identifies components that must be addressed explicitly or implicitly in the development of a language intervention approach. Authors of the chapters were not instructed to use this model in their description of their interventions. Nevertheless, we present this model because it can help readers to deconstruct a single intervention into its constituent parts and make comparisons and contrasts across interventions. It can

also help with planning systematic modifications to an existing intervention—
either for purposes of advancing research designed to improve it or for purposes of meeting the clinical needs of an individual child for whom it is a close,
but imperfect, fit as currently specified. The model, represented graphically
in Figure 1.1, is based on work by Fey and colleagues over almost 20 years
(Fey, 1986, 1990, 1992; Fey, Catts, & Larrivee, 1995; Fey & Cleave, 1990). This
version of the model differs from earlier presentations principally in only two
ways. First, it explicitly incorporates a component concerned with the dosage,
or intensity, of treatment. Second, it identifies the clinical evaluation of treatment effectiveness as a component in its own right. In earlier descriptions of
this model, initial and ongoing assessment of the child's learning had been included within other components, but here it is singled out for more focused
attention.

Because the model focuses on the structure of intervention, the same
components can be used to describe interventions based on different theo-

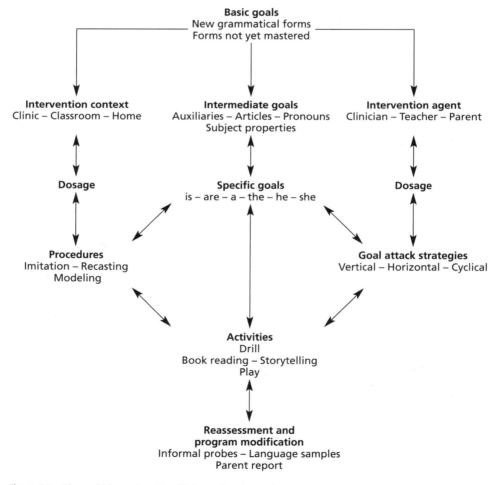

Figure 1.1. The multidimensionality of intervention focused on grammar.

ries of the nature of the problem being addressed and on different hypotheses regarding the mechanisms by which intervention can effect improvement or compensation. Its use by readers may facilitate an appreciation of not only how basic theoretical differences lead to greater elaboration of some components than others, but also of how different theoretical perspectives can converge on common structural components. In succeeding subsections, each of these components is described briefly.

Intervention Goals

Intervention goals are described within a hierarchy of increasing specificity, with four levels: basic goals, intermediate goals, specific goals, and subgoals (Fey, 1992). The use of *four* levels is somewhat arbitrary, but four are represented here to convey the general process by which a clinician can begin with more global or functional aspirations for a child's learning and work toward planning the individual steps by which those aspirations are to be reached. The chain from the highest to the lowest goal in the hierarchy ensures that at every step of the intervention, the clinician is ultimately emphasizing functional objectives that should make notable changes in the child's communication abilities and quality of life.

Basic goals are the most general type. They identify the areas of a child's communication system or related domains on which the treatment will center. These areas are selected because they represent areas of the greatest importance from the standpoint of functionality or severity of deficit. For example, in a preschool child who is demonstrating little verbal output, the primary basic goal may be an increase in the frequency of linguistic productions (e.g., words and multiword combinations). The same child may have a basic goal of increasing the length and complexity of multiword constructions and/or increasing intelligibility. Alternatively, in a child of school age whose written discourse is structurally deficient, a basic goal might be greater use of standard structural components in writing products.

Intermediate goals provide greater specification of areas within one or more basic goals, which will be addressed during treatment. Intermediate goals can be seen as representing choices about the clinician's theoretical view of how information can be organized within the domain represented in the basic goal. Often, there are numerous levels of intermediate goals associated with a single basic goal. Because they are written at a level that is still broader than goals considered to be *specific*, we regard them all as intermediate. For the preschooler with little verbal output and the basic goals of increasing verbalizations and increasing the length and complexity of multiword combinations, an intermediate goal might include increased use of words and multiword combinations that serve to request objects and services and/or to protest. For an individual child with few verbalizations of any kind, a clinician might reason that this goal should take precedence over the production of words that serve a commenting or other more purely social function. For example, it is relatively easy for the clinician to help the child to learn and use target words and multiword constructions to obtain objects and services the child clearly desires. In this way, the clinician can focus on the instrumental function of early word and phrase production. In fact, the clinician might hypothesize that if the intermediate objective of increasing the frequency of verbal requests is reached, the child might also increase productions of comments and other acts of joint attention without the clinician placing clinical attention directly on these nonrequestive speech acts. Furthermore, if the child increases word usage to perform requests, this might facilitate the child's use of new speech sounds, thus improving intelligibility. From the outset, then, the clinician may decide to target requests. If resulting increases in word usage are limited to requests, or if anticipated changes in the child's speech sound system do not arise, the clinician would raise the priority of other intermediate goals associated with joint attention and intelligibility and target them more directly,

For the school-age child with deficient written discourse, an intermediate goal might be increased use of standard story grammar elements in retold oral narratives. If resulting increases in story grammar elements within student compositions are limited to personal narratives and fail to extend to informative narratives as well, the clinician may switch focus toward intermediate goals related to prompted or spontaneous use of planning or editing process procedures.

Specific goals target specific exemplars of the language forms (e.g., words, grammatical forms, story structure), content (e.g., semantic relations, elements of story plot), or use (e.g., communication acts, aspects of topic management) that have been identified as intermediate goals. For example, specific goals for the preschooler used in our ongoing example might focus on increased use of specific nouns to make requests to get things during a specific routine, such as mealtime (e.g., *milk, banana, juice*). At least in the early stages, specific goals might include mostly nouns, but a focus on verbs and social words would be necessary if the child did not begin to use some of these forms spontaneously. Similarly, the goals for the school-age child might focus on increased inclusion or elaboration of setting, characters, and problem in written narratives. Because of the hierarchical organization of intervention goals, specific goals imply more general goals, even when general goals are unstated (Fey & Cleave, 1990); that is, specific goals are never ultimate goals themselves. Rather, they are important steps along a path to their broader and more functional superordinate objectives. Selection of specific goals implies the clinician's assumption that the child will progress more rapidly on intermediate and basic goals if the intervention provides some type of focus on the specific targets. Consequently, the clinician must develop activities that will provide high concentrations of models and/or opportunities for use of the specific goal being targeted. This logic is clearly reflected in several treatments described in this book, such as responsivity education/prelinguistic milieu teaching (Chapter 3), focused stimulation (Chapter 8), and conversational recasting (Chapter 10). Other interventions place a higher priority on communication and meaning at the level of basic and intermediate goals, assuming that if communication and meaning are always targeted first, gains on specific goals (especially language forms such as sounds, words, and grammatical constructions) arise naturally as a consequence of increased participation and interaction with competent language users. This logic can be found in chapters on It Takes Two to Talk—The Hanen Program for Parents (Chapter 4) and the Language is the Key approach (Chapter 7). In these programs, although the thematic nature of selected activities may enable some focus on specific language targets, no special emphasis is placed on the child's acquisition and use of any particular language form or communication act.

In some intervention approaches, specific goals also imply *subgoals*, a carefully constructed set of measurable steps by which specific goals are achieved. Subgoals often incorporate operational measures of achievement that relate more to the activities used in treatment than to the overall functional outcomes that represent the larger aspirations represented at more abstract levels of goal planning. In fact, subgoals are usually developed after choices are made about other components of the intervention, such as goal attack strategies and particular procedures (Fey et al., 1995). Thus, an early subgoal for our preschool child with limited verbal communication might be *three to five uses of target words during a snack activity with a verbal prompt, or even an imitative stimulus*. As the child begins more consistent use of this type of word production with prompts, the prompts would be faded until the same words are used spontaneously to request common objects. At this point, the specific goal would have been reached, and other subgoals, requiring progressively more independence from the child may be developed, where necessary. Similarly, a specific subgoal for an older child with limited skills at constructing adequate written discourse might be increased inclusion of standard story grammar elements on the retelling in writing of a simple narrative from pictures. As the child becomes more proficient at including standard elements, the visual cue provided by the pictures could be faded until the child is able to construct a structurally complete narrative that is spontaneously generated, thereby meeting the specific goal. These types of objectives are more likely to be developed in some approaches developed in this book (e.g., Chapter 9, enhanced milieu teaching, or Chapter 19, functional communication training) than others (e.g., Chapter 4, It Takes Two to Talk, and Chapter 7, Language is the Key), and they are one of many components that clearly distinguish these interventions.

Goal Attack Strategies

Goal attack strategies offer methods for managing multiple specific goals within a child's intervention. Three general such strategies have been described (Fey, 1986, 1990, 1992), although there are many possible variations of each. *Vertical strategies* involve a progression from one goal to another, and advancement to the next goal is based on the child's attainment of a predetermined level of performance on an outcome variable. *Horizontal strategies* involve simultaneous attention to multiple specific goals, often within a single session. Within this strategy, goals and, therefore, progress on goals are viewed independently so that progress on one goal does not influence decision making about another. *Cyclical strategies* involve clinical focus on one set of goals for a period of time, followed by movement to another set of goals without reference to progress made on the first set of goals. This strategy is based on the assumption that the child will continue learning, even when a goal is no longer serving as a focus of treatment (Hodson & Paden, 1991). The strategy is considered cyclical because previously addressed goals may be returned to in a cyclic fashion (or "recycled") if learning related to a particular goal has not reached criterion levels during periods when it is not being targeted directly.

Procedures and Activities

Procedures consist of all of the acts performed by the intervention agent that are expected to lead the child directly to the intervention goals. They make up the active ingredients of the intervention and include acts, such as modeling the child's target, giving the child structured practice with the target, reinforcement of the child's use of target behaviors, systematic responses to child utterances or actions, and even explicit description of the target (Fey, 1990).

Activities create the social and physical conditions within which the intervention agent may apply the procedures. They fall along a continuum that moves from a high level of adult intrusiveness toward less structure and greater similarity to the child's life outside of treatment (Fey et al., 1995). The most intrusive activities tend to be some form of drill. In the middle of the continuum, we include game-like interactions that are selected or are structured to provide some emphasis on the child's specific goals. The least intrusive activities are those that occur outside the context of therapy, including play, bath time, and snack time for younger children and art class, group writing assignments, or even reading group for school-age children. Although the activity is virtually the same as the procedure in some cases, such as drill, it is fruitful to keep these constructs distinct. For example, a child may gain no special language or communication benefit from dinnertime or play during the bath. The same activity, however, may provide multiple opportunities for the intervention agent to model the target, for the child to attempt it, and for the adult to respond to the child's attempts. Language intervention takes place only when special procedures, designed to instruct and provide opportunities for use and mastery, are applied during the course of activities, which may in turn require the adult to intrude to varying degrees on the child's agenda.

Activities are the most obvious aspect of treatment because they are the part that can easily be described by an observer with little knowledge of the intervention. Lay observers, and at times even beginning clinicians, can sometimes confuse an activity with an intervention as a whole. That is, the observer recognizes the activity but fails to take note of the procedural steps taken by the interventionist. Selecting or creating the appropriate activity, however, requires considerable skill. It is not easy to create activities that are meaningful and motivating for the child yet provide many opportunities for the application of intervention procedures directed toward specific goals. In fact, successful activity planning requires attention to many other elements of intervention, including the goals of the intervention (at all levels), the assumed mechanism by which learning will take place most efficiently, and the availability of particular agents and materials.

Dosage

Dosage applies both to the frequency with which treatment sessions are held as well as to the frequency with which targeted goals are addressed within a given treatment session. Anyone who has pursued the acquisition of an unfamiliar skill as an adult, such as playing the piano or learning to golf, has probably developed the suspicion that at least, in general, more attempts at learning result in "better" learning than do fewer efforts: practice makes perfect, after all. On the firmer basis of literatures addressing various forms of human learning (e.g., Schmidt & Wrisberg, 2000), we can further infer that dosage may have huge effects on outcomes. There is a broad literature indicating that learning based on trials that are spaced over time is better, in the sense of more lasting and more likely to generalize, than learning that occurs with massed trials (e.g., Magill, 1993). This literature makes clear that more may not always be better. However, although dosage differences have been raised as an explanation for the better results of some treatment approaches than others (Kamhi, 1999; Law & Conti-Ramsden, 2000), there has been almost no systematic study of this aspect of treatment among children with language disorders. In clinical practice, scheduling the frequency of treatment sessions is often guided by no stronger a principle than that children with more severe impairments are generally seen more frequently than those with less severe impairments. Still, clinicians who use the results of published studies to support their intervention choices must attend closely to dosage. They should be concerned whenever they choose or are forced to select a treatment intensity that differs significantly from that used in published research reports.

Intervention Agents

Typically, intervention agents are individuals who interact with the child for the purpose of realizing treatment goals. Clinicians, parents, other caregivers, teachers, paraprofessionals, and, less frequently, peers can act as agents in interventions proposed for children with communication disorders. Although clinicians are typically the most active in planning details of an intervention, the actual implementation of the intervention may rest in the hands of other competent communicators who are taught to carry out activities and use procedures deemed helpful to the child's attainment of intervention goals. Parents, in particular, should also be quite actively involved in the selection of intervention goals, especially basic goals, as part of the special education process within the United States (Donahue-Kilburg, 1992).

Even for interventions that incorporate intensive involvement with a computer program as the central element of a child's treatment, human agents remain vital to the intervention process. When computerized stimuli are a focus of the child's attention in treatment, human agents may not be as active in providing direct models of targets, prompts for child behaviors, or feedback on the child's moment-to-moment performance; nonetheless, they almost certainly continue to play important roles in decision making and in monitoring and facilitating the child's overall level of effort (Veale, 1999).

Intervention Context(s)

Contexts are the social and physical environments in which interventions take place. Physical contexts include the child's home, classroom, or clinic room. Contexts in which interventions are carried out may be selected on theoretical grounds because of their functional value to the child (Bronfenbrenner & Morris, 1998) or because of increased expectations of generalization and maintenance of behaviors. Contexts are often selected on practical grounds; for example, participation by parents is often only feasible, or at least is more convenient, in some settings rather than others. When the context is forced by such circumstances, there are often ramifications in other components of intervention. For example, it may be possible to utilize certain procedures, such as recasts (Chapter 10), within the typical classroom setting or when children are working in small in-class groups. It may not be possible, however, to implement certain procedures, such as imitative drill or observational modeling, in a discreet manner within the classroom setting.

Comprehensive Assessment of the Intervention

Within the structural model of intervention described thus far, the child's achievement of subgoals represents an integrated and handy method by which the effects of the intervention can begin to be gauged for an individual child. In general, performance-related goals that are low in the hierarchy are easier to measure than higher level goals. There is an inherent danger here, however. Because subgoals are so highly particular to specific procedures and outcomes, progress on subgoals may or may not lead to predictable achievement on the higher level goals that prompted intervention in the first place (Fey & Cleave, 1990). Because the intent of intervention is to effect positive change in a child's life, it is important to determine that goals lower in the hierarchy (e.g., subgoals/specific goals) are having the desired effect of helping the child to attain higher level goals (e.g., intermediate/basic goals). Ultimately, attainment of basic goals should lead to meaningful changes in the child's life, and those changes should be (but rarely are) carefully measured (Bain & Dollaghan, 1991; Kazdin, 1999, 2001; McCauley, 2001).

EVIDENCE-BASED PRACTICE AND TREATMENT OF CHILDREN WITH LANGUAGE DISORDERS

Evidence-based practice (EBP) can be defined by adopting the definition given for its predecessor *evidence-based medicine* (EBM), "the integration of best research evidence with clinical expertise and patient values" (Sackett, Straus, Richardson, Rosenberg, & Haynes, 2000, p. 1). In medicine, this approach to clinical practice has pervaded all subdisciplines and has led to numerous professional initiatives intended to help increase clinicians' access to and effective use of existing research. In fact, in the United Kingdom and Canada, where it began, EBM has had far-reaching effects on research and clinical funding and governmental policy formation (Guyatt & Rennie, 2002). Despite the smaller research base in speech-language pathology, EBP is seen by many in the profession as sharing a similar potential to improve the research base and clinicians' access to and use of scientific information in clinical decision making (e.g., American Speech-Language-Hearing Association [ASHA], 2004; Bothe, 2004; Dollaghan, 2004; Justice & Fey, 2004; Meline & Paradiso, 2003; Yorkston et al., 2001). Ultimately, the effects of EBP will be extended to related funding and policy matters (ASHA, 2004; Gillam, Johnston, & Ehren, 2004).

Table 1.2 offers an overview of the steps recommended in an EBP approach to treatment selection (McCauley & Hargrove, 2004; McKibbon, 1999; Sackett et al., 2000). A detailed elaboration of each of the steps displayed in Table 1.2 is beyond the scope of this book, but we wish to make two crucial points here. First, steps 1 and 4 require clinicians to carefully consider the individual child, the child's family, and their interests, desires, and values in making decisions regarding intervention options. Clinicians must also con-

Table 1.2.   Steps involved in an evidence-based practice approach to treatment selection

Step 1. Formulating the clinical question: treatment selection

Step 2. Finding relevant evidence

Step 3. Evaluating and synthesizing the evidence

Step 4. Integrating research evidence with client- and clinician-specific information and values to make and implement the treatment selection decision

Step 5. Evaluating the process

sider their own experience, expertise, and preferences in the decision-making process. Although we do not examine these crucial elements in detail in this volume, attempts to exclude them from treatment decisions are not likely to be successful and do not represent sincere efforts to practice EBP. Second, we believe this volume can be useful in beginning the processes found in steps 2 and 3 of the EBP treatment selection process: finding, synthesizing, and evaluating the evidence.

Before we provide our recommendations for using this volume as part of EBP, it should be noted that some advocates of EBP see textbooks as vehicles for the perpetuation of unattested or repudiated traditional clinical methods that fail to promote newer, more appropriate methods. In fact, Sackett et al. (2000, p. 30) implore their readers to "Burn your (traditional) textbooks!" in favor of peer-reviewed journals containing original efficacy and effectiveness studies and/or systematic reviews and meta-analyses of treatment studies. Nonetheless, even in fields such as medicine, in which far more clinical experiments are produced and change occurs at a rate far faster than it does in speech-language pathology, books still retain their value in providing information about more basic concepts, in introducing specific skills with a presumed longer shelf-life, and in providing a historic context for a broad area of study. In addition, they can provide a more detailed account of theoretical underpinnings and clinical procedures than is often possible in other types of publications. All of these potential advantages of textbook descriptions of child language interventions can be found in the chapters represented in this volume. Furthermore, despite their strong negative views on traditional textbooks, Sackett and his colleagues acknowledge that some textbooks are organized with an eye toward clinical use and that much of the information they contain will actually be current because newer, contradictory information has not yet appeared. To minimize their potential weaknesses, however, Sackett and colleagues recommend that textbooks be revised frequently, be heavily referenced with regard to clinical recommendations so that outdated information can be more readily spotted, and be constructed with an eye to explicit principles of evidence.

The present volume has been constructed as much as possible to approach the ideals mapped out by Sackett and colleagues (2000). For example, numerous references are provided to establish the time frame of particular ideas and pieces of information. Through the use of the standard template described earlier in this chapter, authors were encouraged to discuss the quality of the evidence they provided and to do so in a comprehensive manner. In addition, because EBP calls for clinicians to use the highest level of evidence possible for a specific topic, it is not inconceivable that for some topics, a book chapter or book may provide the highest quality available.

Nonetheless, readers are cautioned that this volume is more likely to remain a useful resource for a reasonable period of time if viewed as a preliminary, rather than exhaustive, source of information and if its chapters are recognized as narrative reviews written by advocates of the approaches they describe rather than as systematic reviews, meta-analyses, or practice guidelines. With these essential caveats in mind, we have five broad recommendations for clinicians considering any intervention represented in the volume or wishing to compare potential outcomes from one of the represented interventions with another treatment option. First, consider the information in the Target Populations and Assessments for Determining Treatment Relevance and Goals and the Empirical Basis sections of each chapter as an initial, possibly biased, and almost certainly nonexhaustive survey of the available research literature. Second, from this skeptical perspective, determine whether evidence presented in these same sections is applicable to a specific child you are considering as a potential candidate for the treatment. If it is not, is there any theoretical reason that would make the intervention more or less effective with the target child? Third, based on the information in the Practical Requirements, Key Components, and Application to an Individual Child sections, and from an examination of the clips on the DVD, is the approach feasible for the target child under existing circumstances? Do you have the resources to implement the approach at an intensity level close enough to that observed in studies cited to make a successful outcome likely? Fourth, identify at least one of the articles used by the authors as strong support for the methods they describe and critically examine the original research report. Does the evidence presented in the research report support a decision to attempt the technique with the target child in the manner and to the degree anticipated based on the conclusions of the chapter authors? Fifth, do an additional computer-based search for at least one article that is more recent than the literature cited in the article and potentially relevant for the target child. If such an article is identified, read and evaluate the study critically. Are the results of this study consistent with a decision to use the approach or to try some alternative?

The types of critical evaluations associated with our fourth and fifth recommendations are referred to as critically appraised topics (or CATs) by Sackett and colleagues (2000). Minimally, the clinician should address each of the following questions as part of this critical evaluation: 1) Does the research report include children like the one being considered for treatment? 2) Does the study report gains that are substantial and clinically meaningful? 3) Does the study apply adequate controls over maturation and the effects of other nonintervention factors? This could include multiple baselines for treated *and* nontreated goals in single subject experiments, or the use of a control group in a group design. If a group design is used, were subjects assigned randomly to groups? 4) Does the study employ methods to limit experimenter bias, such as steps to keep the testers or coders blind to the groups to which the children were assigned?

It is not our intention to present the information or provide the experience needed to instruct readers to perform these types of critical evaluations, but we believe efforts to teach these skills should be part of the curricula for every graduate program in speech-language pathology. Furthermore, students and clinicians attempting to use the information presented in the intervention descriptions found in this book will be most richly rewarded when they apply both their existing clinical experience and expertise along with their knowledge and skills as critical consumers of research every step of the way.

CONCLUDING COMMENTS

To contribute to the tutorial value of this book, we have included three additional chapters—Chapters 2, 11, and 16—as overviews of the chapters representing each section. In these chapters, the nature of interventions contained in the section and its theoretical and empirical supports will be reviewed. In its totality, therefore, this book will help readers learn about 15 important treatments, some of which are viewed today as relatively traditional and others of which are surrounded by considerable controversy. The descriptions provided should make it possible for experienced clinicians or well-supervised students to faithfully apply most approaches, where it is deemed appropriate to use one. Secondarily, however, we trust that this book will also help readers become admirers of, and potentially more robust participants in, the ongoing difficult work represented in the treatment research and development process described throughout the volume.

REFERENCES

American Speech-Language-Hearing Association. (2004). *Evidence-based practice in communication disorders: An introduction.* Technical report. Retrieved June 16, 2005, from http://www.asha.org/members/deskref-journals/deskref/DRVol4.htm (login required)

Bain, B.A., & Dollaghan, C. (1991). The notion of clinically significant change. *Language, Speech, and Hearing Services in Schools, 22,* 264–270.

Bothe, A. (Ed.). (2004). *Evidence-based treatment of stuttering: Empirical bases and clinical applications.* Mahwah, NJ: Lawrence Erlbaum Associates.

Bronfenbrenner, U., & Morris, P. (1998). The ecology of developmental processes. In W. Damon & R.M. Lerner (Eds.), *Handbook of child psychology, Vol. 1: Theoretical models of human development* (5th ed., pp. 993–1028). New York: John Wiley & Sons.

Dollaghan, C. (2004). Evidence-based practice myths and realities. *ASHA Leader, 9*(7), 4.

Donahue-Kilburg, G. (1992). *Family-centered early intervention for communication disorders: Prevention and treatment.* Gaithersburg, MD: Aspen.

Fey, M.E. (1986). *Language intervention with children.* Boston: Allyn & Bacon.

Fey, M.E. (1990). Understanding and narrowing the gap between treatment research and clinical practice with language impaired children. *ASHA Reports, 20,* 31–40.

Fey, M.E. (1992). Articulation and phonology: An addendum. *Language, Speech, and Hearing Services in Schools, 23,* 277–282.

Fey, M.E. (2002, March). *Intervention research in child language disorders: Some problems and solutions.* 32nd annual Mid-South Conference on Communicative Disorders, Memphis, TN.

Fey, M.E. (2004). *EBP in child language intervention: Some background and some food for thought.* Working group on EBP in Child Language Disorders, May 20, 2004, Austin, TX.

Fey, M.E., Catts, H.W., & Larrivee, L.S. (1995). Preparing preschoolers for the academic and social challenges of school. In S.F. Warren & J. Reichle (Series Eds.) & M.E. Fey, J. Windsor, & S.F. Warren (Vol. Eds.), *Communication and language intervention series: Vol. 5. Language intervention: Preschool through the elementary years* (pp. 3–37). Baltimore: Paul H. Brookes Publishing Co.

Fey, M.E., & Cleave, P.L. (1990). Efficacy of intervention in speech-language pathology: Early language disorders. *Seminars in Speech and Language, 11,* 165–182.

Gillam, R., Johnston, J., & Ehren, B. (2004). *Meeting summary: Evidence-based practice.* Child Language Disorders Working Group. Unpublished manuscript. Retrieved June 16, 2005, from http://www.bamford-lahey.org/meetingsummary.html

Guyatt, G., & Rennie, D. (2002). *Users' guides to the medical literature: Essentials of evidence-based clinical practice.* Chicago: American Medical Association Press.

Hodson, B., & Paden, E. (1991). *Targeting intelligible speech: A phonological approach to remediation.* Austin, TX: PRO-ED.

Justice, L.M., & Fey, M.E. (2004, September 21). Evidence-based practice in schools: Integrating craft and theory with science and data. *ASHA Leader*, pp. 4–5, 30–32.

Kamhi, A.G. (1999). To use or not to use: Factors that influence the selection of new treatment approaches. *Language, Speech, and Hearing Services in Schools, 30,* 92–98.

Kazdin, A.E. (1999). The meanings and measurement of clinical significance. *Journal of Consulting and Clinical Psychology, 67,* 332–339.

Kazdin, A.E. (2001). Almost clinically significant ($p < .10$), Current measures may only approach clinical significance. *Clinical Psychology: Science and Practice, 8*(4), 455–462.

Law, J., & Conti-Ramsden, G. (2000). Treating children with speech and language impairments: Six hours of therapy is not enough. *British Medical Journal, 321,* 908–909.

Magill, R.A. (1993). *Motor learning: Concepts and applications* (4th ed.). Madison, WI: WCB Brown & Benchmark Publishers.

McCauley, R.J. (2001). *Assessment of language disorders in children.* Mahwah, NJ: Lawrence Erlbaum Associates.

McCauley, R.J., & Hargrove, P. (2004). A clinician's introduction to systematic reviews in communication disorders: The course review paper with muscle. *Contemporary Issues in Communication Science and Disorders, 31,* 173–181.

McKibbon, A. (1999). Introduction. In A. McKibbon, with A. Eady & S. Marks (Eds.), *PDQ evidence-based principles and practice* (pp. 1–31). Hamilton, Ontario: BC Decker.

Meline, T., & Paradiso, T. (2003). Evidence-based practice in schools: Evaluating research and reducing barriers. *Language, Speech, and Hearing Services in Schools, 34,* 273–283.

Sackett, D.L., Straus, S.E., Richardson, W.S., Rosenberg, W., & Haynes, R.B. (2000). *Evidence-based medicine: How to practice and teach EBM* (2nd ed.). New York: Churchill Livingstone.

Schmidt, R.A., & Wrisberg, C.A. (2000). *Motor learning and performance* (2nd ed.). Champaign, IL: Human Kinetics Publishers.

Veale, T.K. (1999). Targeting temporal processing deficits through Fast ForWord®: Language therapy with a new twist. *Language, Speech, and Hearing Services in Schools, 30,* 353–362.

World Health Organization. (1980). *ICIDH: International classification of impairments, disabilities, and handicaps.* Geneva: Author.

World Health Organization. (2001). *ICF: International classification of functioning, disability and health.* Geneva: Author.

Yorkston, K.M., Spencer, K., Duffy, J., Beukelman, D., Golper, L.A., Strand, E., & Sullivan, M. (2001). Evidence-based medicine and practice guidelines: Application to the field of speech-language pathology. *Journal of Medical Speech-Language Pathology, 9*(4), 243–256.

I

Interventions Targeting Prelinguistic Communication

2

Overview of Section I

Interventions Targeting Prelinguistic Communication Through Developing Language

REBECCA J. MCCAULEY AND MARC E. FEY

Interventions featured within Section I have as their basic goals children's communication development from the earliest establishment of nonverbal routines through the elaboration of language form, content, and use characteristic of the early school-age years (see Table 2.1). Although not all approaches represented in this section target oral language (e.g., see responsivity education/prelinguistic milieu teaching [RE/PMT], Chapter 3; Picture Exchange Communication System [PECS], Chapter 5; and the System for Augmenting Language [SAL], Chapter 6), they all address children's primary communication systems rather than written language. Research and clinical innovations in this area have been plentiful, leading to several highly developed and often historically related intervention approaches—all meriting attention. Consequently, it is not surprising that this is the longest section in the book, comprising eight chapters.

Basic and intermediate goals within these interventions include both foundational nonverbal communication goals (RE/PMT, Chapter 3) as well as goals directed toward more advanced language forms (e.g., focused stimulation, Chapter 8; conversational recasting, Chapter 10). In addition, several interventions identify parents as supplemental (responsivity education, Chapter 3) or primary intervention agents (It Takes Two to Talk—The Hanen Program for Parents, Chapter 4; enhanced milieu teaching [EMT], Chapter 9). Those interventions that train parents to act as language facilitators in the home and elsewhere are intended to capitalize on parents' potential to be exceptional interventionists because of their unique knowledge of, access to, and commitment to their children. Two of the interventions in this section feature augmentative and alternative communication (AAC) strategies (PECS, Chapter 5, and the SAL, Chapter 6). Nonetheless, with the exception of the Hanen Program, which depends on access to video equipment, and the SAL, which makes intensive use of voice output communication aids (VOCAs), interventions in this section make little use of technology.

Table 2.1. Characteristics of interventions featured in Section I

Treatment	Responsivity education/prelinguistic milieu teaching (RE/PMT)	It Takes Two to Talk—The Hanen Program for Parents	Picture Exchange Communication System (PECS)	System for Augmenting Language (SAL)	Language is the Key (LIK)
Chapter	3	4	5	6	7
Client age (chronological or developmental)	Children who are functioning developmentally between approximately 9 and 15 months (often at the chronological age of 2 or 3 years)	Toddlers and preschool-age children	Children across a wide age range	Children across a wide age range, many with significant developmental delays	Children who are functioning developmentally below approximately the 4-year level
Primary client populations	Children with developmental delays who are not using gestures and vocalizations at a frequency and in a manner consistent with the onset of language use	Children who are late-talkers and preschoolers with cognitive and developmental delays	Children with autism spectrum disorders and others with minimal functional communication	Children with moderate to severe cognitive disabilities who demonstrate at least beginning intentional communication skills as well as toddlers and preschoolers with developmental delays	Children with unmet communication needs and children with limited English proficiency
General characterization of methods	Combined use of a clinician-implemented intervention and parent training in techniques designed to facilitate nonverbal communication development	Parent training in methods designed to facilitate communication development in natural contexts with special attention paid to goals identified for individual children	A visually based AAC method used in conjunction with behavioral teaching techniques	An integrated language and AAC approach implemented using a collaborative service-delivery model in which a speech-generating device is used in everyday contexts and symbol use is modeled by communicative partners	Use of and/or teaching others about common language facilitation techniques that can be implemented within contexts such as play and book reading (e.g., use of open-ended questions and expansion of children's utterances)

Nature of goals	Increase the frequency and complexity of intentional nonverbal communication as a precursor for language and increase the parents' ability to support this development	Increase parents' use of general interaction strategies taught within the program as a means of facilitating the child's communication	Increased use, especially spontaneous use of communication, beginning with picture-mediated requests and progressing toward more advanced communications, such as comments	Facilitation of language development and use within everyday environments, particularly at school and at home	Facilitation of advances in form, content, and use of early language forms
Intervention agents	SLPs and parents	Parents supported by SLPs	A trainer and assistant with training in PECS	SLPs, teachers, and family members	Professionals (including SLPs, teachers, and librarians), paraprofessionals (including child care providers), and family members
Nature of sessions	Individual sessions	Small-group parent-training sessions, preceded by individual assessment sessions and followed by individual videotaped feedback sessions	Individual sessions	Individual sessions and as a part of everyday interactions across settings	Direct individual sessions conducted by SLP or by significant others who have been trained to use the targeted facilitation techniques
Demands for technology	None	Video equipment for use in recording parent–child interactions for purposes of providing feedback	None	Intensive use of voice output communication aids (VOCAs)	None

(continued)

23

Table 2.1. (continued)

Treatment	Focused stimulation approach to language intervention	Enhanced milieu teaching (EMT)	Conversational recast intervention
Chapter	8	9	10
Client age (chronological or developmental)	Toddlers through early elementary school-age children	Preschool children as well as older children with early language development	Toddlers and preschoolers, as well as children who are functioning at the preschool level developmentally
Primary client populations	Late-talking toddlers, children with specific language impairments, and children with mental retardation,	Children in early stages of language development, including those with mental retardation, specific language impairments, or severe disabilities	Children with specific language impairments, mental retardation, hearing impairment, or autism spectrum disorders
General characterization of methods	Exposure of the child to multiple exemplars of specific linguistic forms, content, or use within meaningful contexts, followed by optional elicitation of spontaneous productions of the targeted form within the context of a contextually based service delivery model	Use of environmental arrangement, responsive interaction strategies (including contingent feedback, modeling language targets, expansions, and balanced turn taking), and milieu teaching procedures to prompt language production	A procedure that may be used as part of individual or small-group treatment approaches in which children's productions are responded to using recasts (language models that are somewhat more complex than the original productions)
Nature of goals	Improvement of vocabulary and early grammatical skills	Promotion of functional use of productive language skills in naturalistic interactions	Increased use of any linguistic form, including phonemes, words, grammatical morphemes, grammar, and/or complex sentences
Intervention agents	Clinicians and/or parents	Parents who are trained in the method by clinicians	Clinician or others trained in the procedure
Nature of sessions	Individual clinician-directed sessions supplemented by parent application within the home	Individual	Individual
Demands for technology	None	None	None

Despite the differences between approaches highlighted above, the treatments in this section show considerable overlap. Readers will see numerous similarities in rationales, procedures, and goals across interventions, reflecting common theoretical roots. Several of these approaches are among the most well studied of those included in this volume. Nonetheless, while continuing through this section, pay particular attention to the specifics of rationale, goals, procedures, and activities as well as the populations for which the evidence base is strongest for each intervention. Considering these factors should lead to clearer decisions about which, if any, of the interventions may be appropriate for the very specific needs, interests, and resources of individual children and families.

RESPONSIVITY EDUCATION/ PRELINGUISTIC MILIEU TEACHING (CHAPTER 3)

In their chapter, Warren, Bredin-Oja, Fairchild, Finestack, Fey, and Brady describe RE/PMT, an intervention comprising two components; one, a parent intervention intended to increase parents' abilities to respond effectively to their children's communications (RE), and the other, a direct intervention with the child (PMT). Because RE/PMT is intended to foster children's development of nonverbal gestures and vocalizations used to comment and request as part of early communicative exchanges, the target population for this intervention is children with developmental delays. Specifically excluded are children who demonstrate emerging language, such as consistent use and recognition of words. These children are excluded because of evidence suggesting that this intervention is unlikely to be as effective for these children as it is for children at earlier stages of development and that it should therefore be passed over in favor of interventions targeting vocabulary and other early language forms (Yoder & Warren, 2002). As readers will see, RE/PMT shares much in common with one designed for somewhat more advanced learners—enhanced milieu teaching (EMT) (Chapter 9).

RE/PMT is theoretically based on a transactional model of social communication development that has been studied both in children who are typically developing and those whose development is delayed (e.g., Hart & Risley, 1995; Prizant & Wetherby, 1990; Yoder & Warren, 2002). The two-pronged structure of RE/PMT reflects two assumptions of the model about how to optimize the communication and language learning environment for children with significant developmental delays. First, Warren and his colleagues have learned that these children can benefit from the clinician's use of a set of procedures designed to facilitate children's use of acts of joint attention and requesting. Second, they assume that the parents of children with delays may initially or eventually respond differently to their children's later emerging efforts to engage in nonverbal communications and therefore may benefit from instruction designed to help them respond in an alternative, more facilitative fashion (Yoder, Warren, McCathren, & Leew, 1998).

According to Warren and his colleagues, PMT, the clinician-administered component of this intervention, requires from a few weeks to more than 6 months to help the child acquire the intended communication skills and be ready for interventions targeting vocabulary acquisition. PMT is closely related to milieu teaching (MT; Warren & Bambara, 1989) but differs in that nonverbal communication is targeted rather than early language. The techniques used in PMT include the arrangement of what are described as *enabling contexts.* These are situations in which the clinician creates the conditions for communication (e.g., by following the child's lead in the choice of activities and by placing desired objects just out of reach) and uses specific teaching techniques (e.g., linguistic mapping, or supplying a verbal label for an object the child shows or gives to the adult). Through the arrangement of enabling contexts, the child is enticed to initiate communication to achieve access to a desired object or activity. In addition to linguistic mapping, prompts, models, and providing natural consequences for communicative attempts are the major procedures applied within these situations, often as part of social routines. Children who initiate interactions at low rates are seen as especially appropriate recipients of this intervention.

The parent-directed intervention, RE, involves teaching parents techniques that differ somewhat from those in PMT and can even involve use of materials developed for the Hanen Program (Chapter 4). Methods described within RE include teaching parents to follow the child's lead and engage in linguistic mapping or otherwise respond positively to child acts in ways that do not require the child to produce a response. This intervention is used for a shorter period of time than PMT, with the expectation that parents' deliberate use of taught strategies will be replaced by a naturally responsive interaction style as the child's communications become more complex.

Initial assessment methods for this intervention are principally designed to determine that the child's delays in language and communication are significant enough to warrant this intervention over others. The assessments combine the use of the Communication and Symbolic Behavior Scales (CSBS™; Wetherby & Prizant, 1993) and informal probes conducted in naturalistic settings. Repeated probes are also used to detect a decrease in the child's need for prompting and an increase in nonverbal and vocal communicative acts to two per minute—indicators that PCI may no longer be an appropriate intervention and those targeting vocabulary should be initiated.

Empirical support began with exploratory studies involving small numbers of participants. According to Warren and his coauthors in Chapter 3, these initial studies reported encouraging effects on rates and generalization of prelinguistic requesting when teachers and parents responded contingently to children's incipient nonverbal requests.

In a later, larger study, Yoder and Warren (1998, 2001) found that PMT was more beneficial for children whose mothers' pretreatment style was relatively more responsive. The key to the success of PMT, then, appeared to be the parents' ability to respond to children's developing communication skills.

This finding led Yoder and Warren (2002) to add the RE component to PMT. They observed good outcomes, but only for children without Down syndrome who started the intervention with limited joint attention and limited vocalization. Fey and colleagues (2004) replicated the Yoder and Warren (2002) study with modifications and produced modest but more uniformly positive findings that cut across the broad group of children included in their study. Although considerable work to evaluate RE/PMT and refine its delivery remains, the history of empirical investigation regarding this approach is a model for the development of other interventions.

IT TAKES TWO TO TALK—
THE HANEN PROGRAM FOR PARENTS (CHAPTER 4)

It Takes Two to Talk is one of a series of programs comprising the Hanen Program. This program targets children who have expressive or receptive language disorders, or both. Other Hanen interventions are intended for use with parents of children with autism spectrum disorders, parents of children with developmental delays, and teachers of children without identified disorders in a preschool setting. It Takes Two to Talk is one of the most widely known and most researched of those included in the book, with beginnings dating back to the early 1970s (Manolson, 1974). Whereas RE/PMT involves parents as complementary intervention agents, It Takes Two to Talk involves parents as primary intervention agents. Intervention procedures are delivered using adult teaching techniques in a highly structured, small-group training conducted by a speech-language pathologist (SLP). Although the SLP works with the parents and child in a consultative role even after formal training sessions have ended, the principal communication facilitation is performed by the parents. Individual interaction and early language skills are targeted by parents using specific strategies designed to place the child at the center of the interaction, to promote interaction, and to model language.

The philosophical bases of the Hanen Program are family- and child-centeredness as well as the use of naturalistic activities, routines, interaction partners, and consequences within everyday surroundings. It also finds theoretical support in social interactionist models of language acquisition in which emphasis is placed on structuring adult language so that it is just in advance of the child's current level of functioning and is responsive to the child's processing capacities and focus. The program entails parent education about language learning, instruction and practice for parents in the use of specific strategies, and the provision of parent support over six to eight sessions.

Children who are candidates for It Takes Two to Talk are seen for an assessment in which natural communication exchanges with their primary caregiver are video-recorded to serve as a baseline for later comparisons. Formal testing may also be conducted using developmentally appropriate measures of language and communication. After parental preferences are identified, treatment planning is conducted jointly with the SLP and parent(s) serving as equal partners. Goals for the child may be lexical, morphological, or syntactic and are matched with parent goals intended to promote achievement of the child's goals (e.g., modeling of specific forms by the parent). Later assessment methods include three individual feedback sessions in which videotapes made by the parents at home are brought in for discussion with the SLP.

The empirical studies of It Takes Two to Talk highlighted in this chapter by Girolametto and Weitzman deal with two versions—one dating from 1982 to 1996 and the other used since that time. In the earlier version, parents were only taught to use general stimulation techniques; in the later version, they were also taught to use focused stimulation strategy to address specific communication goals. The focused stimulation strategy includes the use of multiple repetitions of a form by the parent which is sometimes followed first by repetition of the pattern minus the targeted form, then by waiting for the child's participation. (Compare this technique with focused stimulation as it is described in Chapter 8.)

Girolametto and Weitzman describe two randomized controlled trials of the earlier general stimulation version of the intervention (Girolametto, 1988; Tannock & Girolametto, 1992)—both of which involved children with developmental and language delays, but relatively heterogeneous etiologies. The later of these studies modified methods from the earlier study by including additional outcome measures, a follow-up component to look for later-occurring effects of treatment, and subject selection allowing for comparison of effects on children who were more or less advanced developmentally (developmental age older or younger than 16 months). The results of these studies were similar, however, with respect to parent variables. Specifically, they suggested clear improvements in interaction variables for the parents (e.g., increased use of child-centered strategies and language modeling). In contrast, whereas Girolametto (1988) observed significant and consistent effects on child interactional performance (e.g., increased participation), these positive effects on child performance were not replicated in the Tannock et al. study. Neither study reported evidence for positive effects on standardized language measures. These results have led the authors to add specific language targets and a focused stimulation component to the intervention, when the basic goals for a child address early language forms as much as or more than basic communication patterns.

For the more recent version of It Takes Two to Talk, which includes focused stimulation of specific language forms, Girolametto and Weitzman describe three randomized controlled trials (Girolametto, Pearce, & Weitzman, 1996a, 1996b, 1997; Girolametto, Weitzman, & Clements-Baartman, 1998). Whereas participants in the first two of these studies were late-talking toddlers without broader developmental delays, participants in the third study were children with Down syndrome. These studies documented positive effects on mothers' interaction styles (consistency in their use of behaviors targeted in their training) but also demonstrated improved language outcomes for the child participants. The authors note that these studies offer somewhat stronger evidence for the effectiveness of the intervention for late talkers than for the children with Down syndrome.

Thus, it has been well established that It Takes Two to Talk has the capability of changing parent behaviors as they interact with their children. Effects of these parent changes on children are less clear-cut, however. The general stimulation version has had mixed results in two studies, and the more recent focused stimulation version appears to have somewhat stronger effects on children with rather mild delays specific to speech and language as compared with children with Down syndrome. The variation in findings across studies and with different populations of children demonstrates the importance of replication and programmatic research in the study of language intervention.

PICTURE EXCHANGE COMMUNICATION SYSTEM (CHAPTER 5)

PECS is in far earlier stages of development than either RE/PMT or the Hanen Program; however, its rationale and many of its methods derive from AAC strategies and behavioral approaches to intervention that are far more well established. It is a picture-based system intended for use with children with autism spectrum disorders or other conditions resulting in severe social communication deficits. In the beginning stages, PECS involves the child's selection of a picture of a desired object followed by an exchange of the picture for the object. PECS incorporates behavioral methods to help children learn to initiate and use early communicative forms to serve early emerging functions and, with advancing skills, potentially early and later linguistic forms as well. Although PECS was first developed by Bondy and Frost (Bondy & Frost, 1994; Frost & Bondy, 1994), Charlop-Christy and Jones, who describe it in this chapter, have been active in the accumulation of evidence about it and thus can be considered important contributors to the development of the approach.

Charlop-Christy and Jones propose that PECS represents a potentially important tool to help children with autism acquire communication skills, including through spoken language. Although they acknowledge that concerns have been expressed that the initial nonverbal nature of PECS may prove counterproductive if speech is the goal, they counter with a number of reports suggesting that spontaneous speech may increase subsequent to PECS training (e.g., Charlop-Christy, Carpenter, Le, Leblanc, & Kellet, 2002). Furthermore, they emphasize that PECS should be used in combination with methods designed to encourage speech production (Charlop-Christy et al., 2002). Prerequisite behaviors are few and are limited to the child's demonstration of the attentional and physical skills required to select a picture stimulus from a small array and give it to a communication partner.

Charlop-Christy and Jones acknowledge that PECS grew out of pragmatic attempts to devise an AAC strategy other than sign language, which they indicated had been the most commonly used method for children with autism. The use of pictures allowed for an iconic rather than a symbolic relationship between label and referent and thus was thought to lend itself to a focus on requests (mands) as early emerging forms in communication development. It was further reasoned that this system would avoid the need for eye contact that may prove particularly problematic for some children with this diagnosis. The theoretical rationale proposed by Charlop-Christy and Jones particularly highlights processing of static visual stimuli as a relative strength in children with autism, citing a large number of studies supporting this view.

PECS makes use of a binder that contains Velcro strips to which the child can attach cards including ones containing carrier phrases (e.g., *I want*) and small black-and-white photographs that represent preferred items, as determined through a preference test. These are used initially to teach mands through prompting. The intervention proceeds with the use of behavioral strategies such as prompt fading and increasing demands associated with the task (e.g., by increasing the distance the child has to move in order to reach the trainer to relinquish the picture card). Intermediate phases include steps taken to ensure that the child distinguishes between pictures as more pictures are added. Later phases teach the child to use phrases, answer direct questions, and comment.

Empirical support for the PECS consists of evidence included in the PECS manual and other informational reports that have described positive outcomes for increased speech use, increased PECS use, and decreased problem behaviors. Four studies, each using a multiple baseline across participants design, are also described by the authors. With one exception, these have been presented as conference papers and are being prepared for journal submission. In Charlop-Christy and colleagues (2002), the baseline for each of three children consisted of the continuation of previous interventions, and dependent measures included frequency of speech, social behaviors, and maladaptive behaviors. Desired outcomes were obtained within less than 200 minutes of intervention with PECS across three children.

The authors of this chapter acknowledge that the study of PECS outcomes is in the early stages. Studies with stronger research designs and involving more participants are needed to further document the efficacy of the approach and to test its limits with children with varying communication and cognitive profiles. Further study will also be needed to clarify indicators that may suggest how to optimize facilitation of oral as well as nonverbal communications and to predict which children will most benefit from this intervention.

THE SYSTEM FOR AUGMENTING LANGUAGE (CHAPTER 6)

Romski, Sevcik, Cheslock, and Barton describe a system designed both to augment current communication efforts and to foster continuing language development among children with moderate to severe cognitive disabilities. The SAL is designed for children who demonstrate at least beginning intentional communication, little or no spoken vocabulary, and at least gross pointing skills. It is similar in these regards to RE/PMT (Chapter 3). Unlike RE/PMT, however, although the SAL has recently been used with children below school age who demonstrate these characteristics, it was originally designed for school-age children. Diagnoses found among these children include Down syndrome, pervasive developmental disorder, autism spectrum disorders, cerebral palsy, and deafblindness. The authors avoid detailed specification of prerequisite cognitive skills because of evidence supporting the success of AAC among individuals who lack many ostensible prerequisites (e.g., Reichle & Yoder, 1985).

The SAL is described as a system because of its complexity. It depends on a multicomponent collaborative service delivery model structured so as to embed intervention within all aspects of the child's day. Intervention is intended to achieve numerous intermediate and basic goals through a range of activities performed by numerous intervention agents in everyday contexts. This embedded quality represents a key strategy for circumventing problems in generalization that are common among interventions for this population. Key components of the SAL include the selection of visual graphic symbols for use on a VOCA (voice output communication aid), modeling of the use of the VOCA by adult communication partners, and ongoing support for communication throughout the child's day.

To achieve the desired degree of integration of intervention into the child's everyday activities, primary communication partners such as parents and teachers receive extensive instruction prior to the child's exposure to the SAL and subsequent ongoing support so that they can serve as intervention agents. These individuals ultimately need to manage the practicalities of the complex system, including maintenance, troubleshooting, and ongoing refinement of materials used in connection with the VOCA. In addition, however, they need to balance their roles as effective listeners and active modelers of desired child behaviors. Thus, this intervention requires close attention to two groups of learners—children and their communication partners—as is the case with several of the interventions described in this section.

Romski et al. provide considerable detail on procedures designed to help children gain access to VOCAs and to involve them in the complicated process of symbol/icon selection. They provide less detail regarding the teaching methods used within the natural communicative exchanges that form the contexts for the SAL intervention. The authors, however, acknowledge the controversial nature of these teaching methods in an approach that places special emphasis on development of skills that are not specific to the training context.

The SAL's theoretical underpinnings rest on understanding how children who are typically developing acquire speech and language as well as how AAC strategies can be used to compensate for severe deficits in speech and language. Romski and her coauthors see reduced ability to access developmentally appropriate experiences in communication and receptive and expressive language as missing ingredients for speech and language development among children with severe cognitive limitations. They note that although historical approaches to AAC have focused on physical, and especially motoric, limitations to access, cognitive limitations may also be addressed through AAC. The authors' expanded view of the possible role of AAC not only includes its use to facilitate existing speech and language *output*, then, but *input* as well, emphasizing its promise for use in teaching. The choice of VOCAs as the primary augmentative strategy within this intervention stems from the way in which such devices provide the child with a multimodal (visual and auditory) means of expression while facilitating comprehension through access to the visual modality.

The research basis for the SAL began with studies involving school-age children with severe cognitive disabilities and later was enlarged to include studies focused on younger children. Romski and Sevcik (1996) examined the effects of the SAL on the speech and language development of 13 children with a mean age of 12 years, 8 months. In particular, communication use and vocabulary growth were examined across the child's use of VOCAs, gestures, and vocalizations. Children were matched in pairs based on age, receptive vocabulary, cognitive level, and school placement level; then, one member of each pair was randomly assigned to receive either home- or school-based instruction in year 1, followed by use in both contexts for both groups in year 2. Although participants varied in the extent of their achievements, the authors were confident that overall changes exceeded those typically reported for other interventions used with population. Still, they acknowledged that the nature of their control groups did not directly support this interpretation.

Additional studies of the same 13 participants after 5 or more years of experience with the SAL focused on their communication with unfamiliar communication partners as a long-term indicator of treatment effects. Romski, Sevcik, and Adamson (1999) found continuing benefits from use of VOCAs during communication with unfamiliar partners through a comparison of conversational appropriateness, ambiguity, and specificity of information provided by the child under conditions in which they did or did not have access to the aid (Romski et al., 1999). In addition, Romski, Sevcik, Adamson, and Bakeman (2005) found performance below that of speaking children with similar cognitive deficits but surpassing that of nonspeaking children with similar cognitive deficits who had not been exposed to the SAL.

The process of extending the application of the SAL to younger children is ongoing, with a project involving 60 children with severe developmental delays and fewer than 10 spoken words, a randomized control design, and the use of two interventions in addition to the SAL. One of these interventions focuses solely on "augmented communication production" (Chapter 6, p. 132) and the other on verbal communication only—thus, these two interventions omit the focus on input that is a central aspect of the SAL. In addition to the continuation of this work, the authors describe the following as major next steps in the development of the SAL: the development of parent training protocols, extension of this work to new populations (e.g., children with autism spectrum disorders and children with severe physical disabilities), and the development of language and communication assessments that can successfully reflect the functional impact of such interventions.

LANGUAGE IS THE KEY (CHAPTER 7)

Cole, Maddox, and Lim describe an intervention intended for children at a somewhat higher developmental level than those described in the preceding four chapters. Specifically, Language is the Key (LIK) is meant for use with children who are functioning below approximately the 4-year level and have unmet communication needs, including children who have limited English proficiency with a language other than English as their home language. The main prerequisite for participation is the child's interest in interaction with the adult around a targeted activity (book reading or play). There are two versions of LIK, one that uses book reading as the intervention activity and another that uses play. These activities serve as contexts in which adults can be taught to apply techniques directed toward intermediate and basic goals of the facilitation of language form, content, and use. The book-reading version of LIK serves as the focus of this chapter.

As was the case in the interventions described in the preceding chapters, LIK employs a variety of intervention agents. In fact, of those interventions considered in this volume, LIK is perhaps the widest ranging intervention in this respect: within this approach, SLPs are encouraged to provide training not just to parents and teachers, but also to child care providers, older siblings, volunteers, and librarians—in fact, to any individual who may have contact with children with unmet language needs.

There are at least two reasons why book reading is considered appropriate for children from many diagnostic categories, and even those who are typically developing, as an activity within which LIK procedures can be implemented. First, the principal techniques taught to adult intervention agents, such as the use of open-ended questions and expansions of children's utterances, are naturally used by parents of children with typical development and can be used in shared book-reading activities just as well as in play. Second, these techniques have been found to be helpful for children with broader developmental delays as well as for those with the more circumscribed delays associated with specific language impairment.

LIK is implemented through training programs that make use of written materials, videotapes, and, most recently, access to streaming video on the Internet. Training of parents and others may be carried out in child care facilities and homes, as well as in speech-language clinics. Training can be individual or group-based. After parents have received training in the techniques and are given reminder handouts that describe each technique, they are encouraged to engage in book-reading sessions of about 15 minutes each day. Education is provided for the use of LIK techniques in both play and book reading, with book reading usually presented first unless the child comes from a culture in which reading is less common. The chief strategies parents are taught to use more frequently include 1) commenting and waiting for the child's response, 2) asking questions and providing other input appropriate to the child's developmental level, and 3) responding by expanding the child's utterance. Parents are also encouraged to use strategies that facilitate the home's heritage language.

Assessment information provided by Cole and his colleagues highlights measures obtained from language samples for use in tracking children's progress (e.g., mean length of utterance [MLU], rate of utterances, vocabulary diversity) rather than specific norm-referenced tools that might be used for initial diagnostic purposes. These language sample methods provide information on the child's oral language performance, which can then serve as the basis for measuring clinical progress.

Empirical support for LIK comes largely from work on dialogic reading, which is the principal component of LIK intervention. Dialogic reading differs from a simple reading of text to a child or use of picture books to prompt storytelling in that the adult employs strategies such as asking open-ended and "what" questions, expanding the child's utterances, and responding to answers with questions. In their review of this literature, Cole, Maddox, and Lim focus on the work of Whitehurst and his colleagues, researchers who explored the value of dialogic reading in typically developing children from families of differing levels of socioeconomic status (Lonigan & Whitehurst, 1998; Whitehurst, Arnold, et al., 1994; Whitehurst, Falco, et al., 1988) and on the work of Dale and his colleagues, who examined its effects for children with varying degrees of language impairment (Crain-Thoreson & Dale, 1999; Dale, Crain-Thoreson, Notari, & Cole, 1996). Positive effects on expressive language were noted independent of the identity of the reader but seemed to be best when parents were involved. Both short-term and long-term gains were noted. Other studies cited by Cole et al. looked at efficacy of dialogic reading practices for children from other cultures, including children from Mexican (Valdez-Menchaca & Whitehurst, 1992) and Asian families (Lim & Cole, 2002, 2003). An important feature of many of the reviewed studies was the correlation of parents' implementation of suggested strategies and children's advances in language with findings indicating that it was the specific intervention that resulted in positive outcomes.

Cole and his coauthors plan to continue to add refinements to the current LIK training programs and to the support provided to families during and after training. Despite the sound rationale for these changes, newer versions of the LIK model must be tested with the children and for the purposes for which it was originally intended. In addition, Cole and his colleagues wish to test the approach for the prevention of later literacy difficulties and with different age groups and populations (e.g., children with pervasive developmental disability or autism spectrum disorders, children with hearing loss, and children with severe developmental delays).

FOCUSED STIMULATION APPROACH TO LANGUAGE INTERVENTION (CHAPTER 8)

Ellis Weismer and Robertson describe an approach that may be incorporated into broader intervention packages (e.g., the Hanen Program, Chapter 4) or may itself incorporate other procedures found in this volume (e.g., conversational recasting, Chapter 10). Focused stimulation is intended for use with children who are late talkers, as well as with preschoolers and early school-age children who exhibit specific language impairment or developmental delays and for whom specific language goals are selected. It consists of providing the child with exposure to multiple examples of specific words, grammatical constructions, or speech sounds within meaningful interactions so that their content, form, and use are as transparent as possible. Focused stimulation can be administered by clinicians, parents, or both within a contextually based service delivery model implemented in the home or small playgroups as well as in group and individual treatment settings.

According to Ellis Weismer and Robertson, prerequisite skills for this approach are the child's capacity for joint and sustained attention, as well as at least a minimal level of social engagement. Once conventional assessment methods are used to establish the need for intervention, language sampling is used to choose potential targets. During the intervention itself, the authors urge data collection about the frequency with which a form is modeled by the adult facilitator, and they provide examples of how such data may be collected efficiently. They note that although 10 times per session may represent a reasonable number of models for vocabulary targets, grammatical constructions may require a greater number of exposures to optimize the child's learning.

The natural conversational contexts used in this intervention are modified to increase the salience of the target form; for example, by providing multiple replicas of each referent for a vocabulary item so that modeling can occur more naturally and with less obvious repetitiveness. In the version of focused stimulation in which no response is expected of the child, spontaneous use is nonetheless acknowledged positively by the facilitator. Additionally, in the form of focused stimulation in which the child is prompted by a direct request for labeling of an object or event, the naturalness of that activity is promoted by increasing the likelihood that a naming game might naturally arise; for example, by hiding objects that can be found and then labeled as part of a play routine between the facilitator and child.

Focused stimulation was originally named and proposed by Leonard (1981) as an alternative to more general stimulation techniques. Ellis Weismer and Robertson suggest that it represents a hybrid intervention (Fey, 1986) in which the clinician's active role in choosing stimuli and manipulating input is intertwined with the child's active role in interacting with a natural context and guiding the moment-to-moment focus of intervention through displays of interest (and noninterest). They also contend that its theoretical support comes from a convergence of numerous perspectives suggesting that children's language learning can be facilitated within a social context by enhancing the quality of linguistic input they receive.

Ellis Weismer and Robertson describe a range of studies providing empirical support for the use of focused stimulation. Although most of these studies were conducted under more highly controlled conditions focused on often less functional and shorter term outcomes (efficacy studies), some were conducted under more typical conditions focused on more functional and long-term outcomes (effectiveness studies). Still others were exploratory in nature. In their discussion, the authors separate studies in which clinicians versus parents function as facilitators. They also consider studies that suggest the value of this intervention in a variety of contexts and for a variety of language goals.

Ellis Weismer and Robertson consider evidence on the use of focused stimulation in both monolingual and bilingual children (Thordardottir, Ellis Weismer, & Smith, 1997), when emphatic stress is added as a component of the intervention (e.g., Robertson & Ellis Weismer, 1999), and with or without the active elicitation of the child's productions (Culatta & Horn, 1982; Leonard et al., 1981). They consider evidence supporting the parent implementation of focused stimulation as somewhat weaker than that supporting clinician implementation, but note that the approach has yielded significant gains in vocabulary, grammar, and speech sound production with late talkers (Lederer, 2001), children with specific language impairment or with mild cognitive delays (Culatta & Horn, 1982; Fey, Cleave, Long, & Hughes, 1993), as well as children with more significant cognitive delays, such as Down syndrome (Cheseldine & McConkey, 1979; Girolametto et al., 1998). As a whole, the studies marshaled by Ellis Weismer and Robertson represent a particularly rich research base for this intervention when offered across a range of goals, settings, facilitators, and children.

In their concluding discussion of future directions for research on focused stimulation, Ellis Weismer and Robertson call for more efficacy studies for children with developmental delays, such as those with Down syndrome, as well as for more studies to examine child characteristics that may help predict the value of focused stimulation for children varying in age, cognitive abilities, and linguistic/cultural background. In addition, they call for further comparisons of parent versus clinician implementation of this intervention and for effectiveness studies to examine outcomes affecting the child's social, academic, and familial functioning.

ENHANCED MILIEU TEACHING (CHAPTER 9)

As with focused stimulation, EMT represents a well-studied parent-implemented intervention for children in the early stages of language development. It bears a close relationship to other interventions discussed in this section (compare with RE/PMT, Chapter 3). EMT differs from parent-administered versions of focused stimulation (Chapter 8) most significantly in its use of prompts requiring the child to imitate the target language form and in its extensive parent education component, which is required to support the detailed teaching requirements of the approach. Elements of EMT have been under study for almost 30 years (Hart & Rogers-Warren, 1978). It is composed of environmental arrangement (or "enabling conditions," as in RE/PMT, Chapter 3), responsiveness interactions (as in RE/PMT and It Takes Two to Talk, Chapter 4 and most other chapters in this section), and MT. Hancock and Kaiser consider it most effective for children who are verbally imitative, have an MLU of 1–3.5 morphemes, and have at least 10 productive words. In other words, it appears to be appropriate for children who exceed the ceiling requirements for RE/PMT and who demonstrate early use of words and semantic relations. Its use has been studied in children who have cognitive and language delays or autism spectrum disorders, and in children who come from high-risk, low-income families.

Within EMT, parents are taught to use environmental arrangement, responsive interaction strategies, and MT techniques over 24–36 sessions within a period of about 3–5 months. After obtaining a high level of skill in implementing these methods (usually by about the twentieth session), they are observed and coached as they work with their child. During parent training, the clinician not only shares information with parents about methods but also works with the parents to review progress on their and their child's behaviors, role-play specific strategies, and reviewing videotaped interactions. Data collection is primarily performed by the clinician for both parent and child behaviors. Sessions are conducted in the child's home approximately two times per week for 45 minutes to 1 hour each time. Joint planning of homework activities is also included.

In their chapter, Hancock and Kaiser review skills required of the clinician for successful parent training. They acknowledge that parents who are committed to the level of participation required by EMT are possibly different from parents as an overall group. However, they contend that they have seen no relationship between success in learning EMT and variables such as parents' age, gender, education, or socioeconomic status, with the exception that higher levels of stress encountered by parents of low socioeconomic status may be somewhat predictive of less successful participation for that subgroup.

Environmental arrangement, the first component of EMT, consists of methods designed to select, arrange, and manage toys and the environment to optimize opportunities for communication. *Responsive interaction strategies,* which make up the second component, are used to foster interaction patterns that facilitate the child's active participation. Hancock and Kaiser identify communication strategies and linguistic strategies falling within this component. Communication strategies consist of those that facilitate turn taking through responsiveness to the child's apparent and communicated interests and include strategies such as following the child's lead and matching and extending the child's topic. Linguistic strategies consist of matching the child's linguistic level, imitating or expanding the child's productions, and describing ongoing activities.

The third component of EMT, *milieu teaching,* entails the use of prompts to facilitate more elaborate communicative responses. This component is described as episodic in nature and embedded within the overall context created by the other components of EMT. MT comprises four specific procedures: 1) modeling, 2) mand-model, 3) time delay, and 4) incidental teaching. Modeling consists of the parent's use of a verbal label related to the child's interest. Correctly produced imitations are met with positive reinforcements such as expansions and allowing the child access to desired objects, whereas partial, unintelligible, or otherwise inaccurate models are followed by a second model. At that point, a correct imitation is rewarded and an incorrect one or a no-response is followed by the parent's repetition of the model and provision of the desired object. The mand-model procedure is similar to the modeling technique, but it includes a question providing choices to the child or an instruction (mand) to get the child to produce a part of the target response. Thus, for example, in this procedure a child might be asked, "What do you want?" "Do you want juice or milk?" or "Tell me what you want." Time delays are used to encourage verbal initiations by the child when verbal requests from the child seem likely (e.g., the child seems to need assistance or to desire an object). Time delay is especially useful to facilitate child-initiated communication when the child knows an appropriate communicative form. Incidental teaching consists of the parent's setting up a situation in which the child is likely to verbalize, and then using one of the other three techniques to support the child's production of a well-formed request.

As with several of the more established and more researched interventions in this section, the empirical support for EMT comes primarily from a large set of studies addressing specific and earlier versions of components of the intervention (e.g., MT), with a smaller body of research focusing on EMT per se. In the course of their description of this body of evidence, Hancock and Kaiser also describe *blended EMT* and *behavior intervention,* a modified version of EMT that is intended to address the needs of children whose language problems are exacerbated by coexisting behavioral problems (see Chapter 19).

Hancock and Kaiser describe particularly strong support for the MT component of EMT in the form of 50 studies examining modeling, mand-model, time delay, and incidental teaching procedures (Alpert & Kaiser, 1992; Kaiser, Yoder, & Keetz, 1992). In studies to examine responsive interaction, Kaiser and her colleagues have included comparisons of that component with MT for use by teachers and parents (e.g., Kaiser et al., 1990).

Results suggesting that either responsive interaction strategies or MT can be effective for children with language disorders associated with numerous etiologies led to the development of EMT, which has been the focus of several efficacy studies (Hemmeter & Kaiser, 1994; Kaiser & Hancock, 2000). In the first of these (Hemmeter & Kaiser, 1994), positive effects of the intervention on children's use of targeted structures and on parent and child affect were shown using single-subject design methods. In the later study, Kaiser and Hancock (2002) compared three treatment conditions (responsive interaction strategies-parent implementation; EMT-parent implementation, EMT-clinician implementation) and a no-treatment condition. Positive effects accrued from each of the interventions.

Hancock and Kaiser suggest that a more direct examination of the effects of EMT on parent–child relationships represents an important avenue for further study because of incidental research findings suggesting that responsive interaction training may promote such indirect benefits for participating families. In addition, they suggest that possible effects of EMT on children's peer relationships warrant additional investigation, in part because of the socialization difficulties that are so common among children with developmental disabilities.

CONVERSATIONAL RECAST INTERVENTION WITH PRESCHOOL-AGE AND OLDER CHILDREN (CHAPTER 10)

Whereas other chapters in this section describe broad-based interventions containing many or all of the intervention components described in Chapter 1 (see Figure 1.1), in Chapter 10, Camarata and Nelson describe conversational recasting, a naturalistic speech and language procedure that is an important component of most of the approaches in this section. Recasts have been defined in many ways, but most generally they borrow the words and meaning from child utterances and add grammatical or semantic features, rendering the child's utterance more complete and adult-like. This intervention procedure has been used for targets related to grammar, vocabulary, and phonology and plays a central role in most applications of focused stimulation (see Chapters 4 and 8).

Conversational recasting has been studied for children with a wide range of diagnoses, including specific language impairment, mental retardation, hearing loss, and autism spectrum disorders. Although historically it has been used with children who are functioning at the prelinguistic or preschool language levels, Camarata and Nelson suggest that it may be useful for older children with more advanced language and perhaps for treatment of reading disorders. The techniques that constitute recasting may appear deceptively simple at first because, as previously stated, what is required is an adult model following a child's attempted production. However, there are many crucial decisions that clinicians must make to ensure that recasts are provided with sufficient frequency to facilitate children's language development. For example, clinicians must decide whether recasts will be applied generally to immature child utterances independent of their specific structure (e.g., as in the general stimulation version of It Takes Two to Talk) or whether specific speech and language targets will be selected (as in focused stimulation as described in Chapter 4 and Chapter 8). This decision has important implications regarding the clinician's preparation for intervention. General applications of recasting can occur during almost any type of activity the child enjoys. If specific goals are selected, however, the clinician must plan activities likely to generate frequent opportunities for recasts of the child's specific targets. Thus, here, as with other interventions, the selection of goals can have significant impact on the design of activities within which the clinical procedures can be implemented. Although recasting can be a part of interventions that differ in at least some of their underlying theoretical assumptions, there are two fundamental assumptions that all users of conversational recasts appear to accept. First, they assume that recasts provide ideal examples of target structures, because they are presented against a backdrop of child utterances in which the child has self-selected words and meanings. Second, it is assumed that by using recasts and, perhaps, increasing the frequency with which they occur, even children with language impairments are capable of increasing their rates of learning speech and language forms. Camarata and Nelson explicitly reject the assumption that efforts to influence children's general sensory profiles, their attention levels, or their auditory processing abilities (see Chapters 17 and 19) are essential to speed children's acquisition and development of lexical, grammatical, and phonological forms. They point out, however, that advances in speech processing may occur as a by-product of a period of successful use of recasting (Camarata & Yoder, 2002).

There is a rich empirical base of support for conversational recasting. For example, in a series of studies, Camarata and his colleagues (Camarata & Nelson, 1992; Camarata, Nelson, & Camarata, 1994; Nelson, Camarata, Welsh, Butkovsky, & Camarata, 1996) demonstrated that recasting implemented within natural conversational contexts was more effective than discrete trial interventions in which children were reinforced for correct imitations of target structures. Furthermore, Gillum, Camarata, Nelson, and Camarata (2003) observed that children who were poor imitators at the start of treatment performed particularly poorly on imitation treatment, whereas children who were relatively strong in imitation skills prior to treatment did not demonstrate higher gains in imitation treatment.

There is also some evidence that the *number* of recasts provided may be particularly important (Proctor-Williams, Fey, & Loeb, 2001) and that some grammatical targets may be more appropriate than others (Camarata & Nelson, 1992: Fey & Loeb, 2002). Camarata and Nelson also acknowledge that, although the role of recasts in aiding children's development is much more difficult to interpret when it is applied as one component in a multi-component intervention, there are numerous examples in which recasting has been a part of a successful intervention package (Delaney & Kaiser, 2001; Fey et al., 1993; Leonard, Camarata, Brown, & Camarata, 2004; Yoder, Camarata, & Gardner, 2005). In their anticipation of future research related to conversational recasting, Camarata and Yoder note that more information is needed about how to select goals and identify children who are most likely to benefit from the intervention and how to optimize parameters associated with its implementation (e.g., dosage, developmental level, and settings). They also call for studies designed to examine the physiological (neural) and psychological (cognitive) variables that mediate the effects of conversational recasting on children's productions and, possibly, on their receptive language as well.

SUMMARY

Given that they all focus on helping young children progress more quickly on the path to improved communication, the interventions represented in this first section overlap frequently in goals, in the activities used to engage children in learning (conversation, play, book reading), and in the people seen as most likely to be effective agents in the process (clinicians, parents, teachers). Nonetheless, the treatments vary considerably in complexity, in their degree of relatedness to other interventions, and in the specific procedures selected to highlight the information it is hoped the children will acquire.

This section includes the most thoroughly studied child language interventions, but it is important to note that none of the approaches can boast adequate documentation of their efficacy or, especially, their effectiveness. Notwithstanding this assessment, most of the approaches represented in this section have been subjected to experimental evaluations that support their use. Thus, these are the approaches most likely and commonly to be in practice. It is crucial for clinicians who use or are considering use of one of these approaches to be aware of the level and quality of evidence supporting the intervention, the consistency of findings, and, especially, the gaps in our knowledge about the effects, efficacy, and effectiveness of the clinical approach. The chapters in this section (and throughout the book) provide an excellent starting point for clinicians to gather evidence on the efficacy of treatments that address goals like those of the children they serve. Thus, these chapters offer an excellent introduction not simply into the specifics of interventions for children with language disorders, but also to the methods used by researchers to examine claims about whether and for whom an intervention is likely to prove useful.

REFERENCES

Alpert, C.L., & Kaiser, A. (1992). Training parents as milieu language teachers. *Journal of Early Intervention, 16*(1), 31–52.

Bondy, A., & Frost, L. (1994). The picture exchange communication system. *Focus on Autistic Behavior, 9,* 1–19.

Camarata, S., & Nelson, K. (1992). Treatment efficiency as a function of target selection in the remediation of child language. *Clinical Linguistics and Phonetics, 6,* 167–178.

Camarata, S., Nelson, K., & Camarata, M. (1994). A comparison of conversation based to imitation based procedures for training grammatically structures in specifically language impaired children. *Journal of Speech and Hearing Research, 37,* 1414–1423.

Camarata, S., & Yoder, P. (2002). Language transactions during development and intervention: Theoretical implications for developmental neuroscience. *International Journal of Developmental Neuroscience, 20*(3–5), 459–465.

Charlop-Christy, M.H., Carpenter, M., Le, L., LeBlanc, L, & Kellet, K. (2002). Using the Picture Exchange Communication System (PECS) with children with autism: Assessment of PECS acquisition, speech, social-communicative behavior, and problem behaviors. *Journal of Applied Behavior Analysis, 35,* 213–231.

Cheseldine, S., & McConkey, R. (1979). Parental speech to young Down's syndrome children: An intervention study. *American Journal of Mental Deficiency, 83,* 612–620.

Crain-Thoreson, C., & Dale, P. (1999). Enhancing linguistic performance: Parents and teachers as book reading partners for children with language delays. *Topics in Early Childhood Special Education, 19,* 28–39.

Culatta, B., & Horn, D. (1982). A program for achieving generalization of grammatical rules to spontaneous discourse. *Journal of Speech and Hearing Disorders, 47,* 174–180.

Dale, P., Crain-Thoreson, C., Notari, A., & Cole, K. (1996). Parent-child storybook reading as an intervention technique for young children with language delays. *Topics in Early Childhood Special Education, 16,* 213–235.

Delaney, E.M., & Kaiser, A.P. (2001). The effects of teaching parents blended communication and behavior support strategies. *Behavioral Disorders, 26*(2), 93–116.

Fey, M.E. (1986). *Language intervention with young children.* Needham Heights, MA: Allyn & Bacon.

Fey, M.E., Cleave, P., Long, S., & Hughes, D. (1993). Two approaches to the facilitation of grammar in children with language impairment. *Journal of Speech and Hearing Research, 36,* 141–157.

Fey, M.E., & Loeb, D.F. (2002). An evaluation of the facilitative effects of inverted yes-no questions on the acquisition of auxiliary verbs. *Journal of Speech-Language-Hearing Research, 45,* 160–174.

Fey, M.E., Warren, S.F., Brady, N.C., Finestack, L., Bredin-Oja, S., Sokol, S., & Fairchild, M. (2004, November). *Early effects of parent responsive education/prelinguistic milieu teaching.* Poster presented at the American Speech-Language-Hearing Association annual convention, Philadelphia.

Frost, L.A., & Bondy, A.S. (1994). *The Picture Exchange Communication System training manual.* Cherry Hill, NJ: Pyramid Educational Consultants.

Gillum, H., Camarata, S., Nelson, K.E., & Camarata, M. (2003). Pre-intervention imitation skills as a predictor of treatment effects in children with specific language impairment. *Journal of Positive Behavior Intervention, 5*(3), 171–178.

Girolametto, L. (1988). Improving the social-conversational skills of developmentally delayed children: An intervention study. *Journal of Speech and Hearing Disorders, 53*, 156–167.

Girolametto, L., Pearce, P., & Weitzman, E. (1996a). The effects of focused stimulation for promoting vocabulary in children with delays: A pilot study. *Journal of Childhood Communication Development, 17*, 39–49.

Girolametto, L., Pearce, P., & Weitzman, E. (1996b). Interactive focused stimulation for toddlers with expressive vocabulary delays. *Journal of Speech and Hearing Research, 39*, 1274–1283.

Girolametto, L., Pearce, P., & Weitzman, E. (1997). Effects of lexical intervention on the phonology of late talkers. *Journal of Speech, Language, and Hearing Research, 40*, 338–348.

Girolametto, L., Weitzman, E., & Clements-Baartman, J. (1998). Vocabulary intervention for children with Down syndrome: Parent training using focused stimulation. *Infant-Toddler Intervention, 8*, 109–125.

Hart, B., & Risley, T.R. (1995). *Meaningful differences in the everyday experience of young American children.* Baltimore: Paul H. Brookes Publishing Co.

Hart, B.M., & Rogers-Warren, A.K. (1978). Milieu teaching approaches. In R.L. Schiefelbusch (Ed.), *Bases of language intervention* (pp. 193–235). Baltimore: University Park Press.

Hemmeter, M.L., & Kaiser, A.P. (1994). Enhanced milieu teaching: Effects of parent-implemented language intervention. *Journal of Early Intervention, 18*, 269–289.

Kaiser, A.P., Alpert, C.L., Fischer, R., Hemmeter, M.L., Tiernan, M., & Ostrosky, M. (1990, October). *Analysis of the primary and generalized effects of milieu and responsive-interaction teaching by parents.* Paper presented at the annual meeting of the Division of Early Childhood, Albuquerque, NM.

Kaiser, A.P., & Hancock, T.B. (2000). *Supporting children's communication development through parent-implemented naturalistic interventions.* Presented at the 2nd annual Conference on Research Innovations in Early Intervention (CRIEI), San Diego.

Kaiser, A.P., & Hancock, T.B. (2002, March). *Four critical issues in naturalistic teaching.* Paper presented at Conference on Research Innovations in Early Intervention (CRIEI), San Diego.

Kaiser, A.P., Yoder, P.J., & Keetz, A. (1992). Evaluating milieu teaching. In S.F. Warren & J. Reichle (Series & Vol. Eds.), *Communication and language intervention series: Vol. 1. Causes and effects in communication and language intervention* (pp. 9–47). Baltimore: Paul H. Brookes Publishing Co.

Lederer, S.H. (2001). Efficacy of parent-child language group intervention for late-talking toddlers. *Infant-Todder Intervention, 11*, 223–235.

Leonard, L. (1981). Facilitating linguistic skills in children with specific language impairment. *Applied Psycholinguistics, 2*, 89–118.

Leonard, L.B., Schwartz, R.G., Chapman, K., Rowan, L.E., Prelock, P.A., Terrell, B., et al. (1981). Early lexical acquisition in children with specific language impairment. *Journal of Speech and Hearing Research, 25*, 554–564.

Leonard, L., Camarata, S., Brown, B., & Camarata, M. (2004). Tense and agreement in the speech of children with specific language impairment. *Journal of Speech, Language, and Hearing Research, 47*, 1363–1379.

Lim, Y.S., & Cole, K.N. (2002). Facilitating first language development in young Korean children through parent training in picture book interactions. *Bilingual Research Journal, 26*, 367–381.

Lim, Y.S., & Cole, K.N. (2003). *One-year follow-up of Korean parent training in picture book interactions.* Manuscript submitted for publication.

Lonigan, C.J., & Whitehurst, G.J. (1998). Relative efficacy of parent and teacher involvement in a shared-reading intervention for preschool children from low-income backgrounds. *Early Childhood Research Quarterly, 13*, 263–290.

Manolson, H.A. (1974). *It takes two to talk: A parent's guide to helping children communicate.* Toronto: The Hanen Centre.

Nelson, K.E., Camarata, S.M., Welsh, J., Butkovsky, L., & Camarata, M. (1996). Effects of imitative and conversational recasting treatment on the acquisition of grammar in children with specific language impairment and younger language-normal children. *Journal of Speech and Hearing Research, 39*, 850–859.

Prizant, B., & Wetherby, A.M. (1990). Toward an integrated view of early language and communication development and socioemotional development. *Topics in Language Disorders, 10*(4), 1–6.

Proctor-Williams, K., Fey, M.E., & Loeb, D.F. (2001). Parental recasts and production of copulas and articles by children with specific language impairment and typical language. *American Journal of Speech-Language Pathology, 10*, 155–168.

Reichle, J., & Yoder, D. (1985). Communication board use in severely handicapped learners. *Language, Speech, and Hearing Services in Schools, 16*, 146–157.

Robertson, S.B., & Ellis Weismer, S. (1999). Effects of treatment on linguistic and social skills in toddlers with delayed language development. *Journal of Speech, Language, and Hearing Research, 42*, 1234–1248.

Romski, M.A., & Sevcik, R.A. (1996). *Breaking the speech barrier: Language development through augmented means.* Baltimore: Paul H. Brookes Publishing Co.

Romski, M.A., Sevcik, R.A., & Adamson, L.B. (1999). Communication patterns of youth with mental retardation with and without their speech-output communication devices. *American Journal on Mental Retardation, 104*, 249–259.

Romski, M.A., Sevcik, R.A., Adamson, L.B., & Bakeman, R. (2005). Communication patterns of individuals with moderate or severe cognitive disabilities: Interactions with unfamiliar partners. *American Journal on Mental Retardation, 110*, 226–239.

Tannock, R., & Girolametto, L. (1992). Reassessing parent-focused language intervention programs. In S.F. Warren & J. Reichle (Series & Vol. Eds.), *Communication and language intervention series: Vol. 1. Causes and effects in communication and language intervention* (pp. 49–80). Baltimore: Paul H. Brookes Publishing Co.

Thordardottir, E.T., Ellis Weismer, S., & Smith, M.E. (1997). Vocabulary learning in bilingual and monolingual clinical intervention. *Child Language Teaching and Therapy, 13*, 215–227.

Valdez-Menchaca, M.C., & Whitehurst, G.J. (1992). Accelerating language development through picture book reading: A systematic extension to Mexican daycare. *Developmental Psychology, 28*, 1106–1114.

Warren, S.F., & Bambara, L.M. (1989). An experimental analysis of milieu language intervention: Teaching the action-object form. *Journal of Speech and Hearing Disorders, 54*(3), 448–461.

Wetherby, A.M., & Prizant, B. (1993). Profiling communication and symbolic abilities in young children. *Journal of Childhood Communication Disorders, 15*(1), 23–32.

Whitehurst, G.J., Arnold, D., Epstein, J.N., Angell, A.L., Smith, M., & Fischel, J.E. (1994). A picture book reading intervention in day care and home for children from low-income families. *Developmental Psychology, 30*, 679–689.

Whitehurst, G.J., Falco, F.L., Lonigan, C.J., Fischel, J.E., DeFarshe, B.D., Valdez-Menchaca, M.C., & Caufield, M. (1988). Accelerating language development through picture book reading. *Developmental Psychology, 24*, 552–558.

Yoder, P.J., Camarata, S., & Gardner, E. (2005). *Treatment effects and predictors of speech intelligibility and length of utterance in children with specific language and intelligibility impairments.* Manuscript submitted for publication.

Yoder, P., & Warren, S. (1998). Maternal responsivity predicts the prelinguistic communication intervention that facilitates generalized intentional communication. *Journal of Speech, Language, and Hearing Research, 41*(5), 1207–1219.

Yoder, P., & Warren, S. (2001). Relative treatment effects of two prelinguistic communication interventions on language development in toddlers with developmental delays vary by maternal characteristics. *Journal of Speech, Language, and Hearing Research, 44*(1), 224–237.

Yoder, P., & Warren, S.F. (2002). Effects of prelinguistic milieu teaching and parent responsivity education on dyads involving children with intellectual disabilities. *Journal of Speech, Language, and Hearing Research, 45*(6), 1158–1174.

Yoder, P., Warren, S.F., McCathren, R.B., & Leew, S. (1998). Does adult responsivity to child behavior facilitate communication development? In S.F. Warren & J. Reichle (Series Eds.) & A.M. Wetherby, S.F. Warren, & J. Reichle (Vol. Eds.), *Communication and language intervention series: Vol. 7. Transitions in prelinguistic communication* (pp. 39–58). Baltimore: Paul H. Brookes Publishing Co.

3

Responsivity Education/ Prelinguistic Milieu Teaching

STEVEN F. WARREN, SHELLEY L. BREDIN-OJA, MARTHA FAIRCHILD, LIZBETH H. FINESTACK, MARC E. FEY, AND NANCY C. BRADY

ABSTRACT

Responsivity education/prelinguistic milieu teaching (RE/PMT) is most appropriate for children who are functioning developmentally between the ages of approximately 9 and 15 months. Many children with developmental delays do not reach this developmental period until they are 2 or 3 years of age. RE/PMT consists of two components: prelinguistic milieu teaching (PMT), which is delivered by the clinician to the child, and responsivity education (RE), which is delivered by the clinician to the parents. PMT is designed to increase the frequency and complexity of intentional *nonverbal* communicative acts to set the stage for later language learning. Our approach assumes that many parents may not be optimally responsive to the nonverbal communicative bids of their children. Consequently, we provide the second component, RE. In this chapter, we describe the structure of our approach and its theoretical and empirical bases, and we present several issues that clinicians must consider to use the intervention effectively.

INTRODUCTION

Throughout the first year of life, the building blocks for language development are assembled. Auditory development accelerates, complex babbling emerges, social responsiveness and receptive language skills blossom, and with the onset of coordinated attention, intentional communication appears, first in only nonverbal forms (e.g., proto-declaratives such as pointing at

Support for much of the research reported in this chapter was provided by grants from the National Institute of Child Health and Human Development (R01 HD27594; R01 HD34520) and the Office of Special Education Programs of the U.S. Department of Education (H023C20152; H0324C990040). We would like to acknowledge the central role played by Paul Yoder in much of the research described here and also acknowledge the support for this research provided by the NICHD Mental Retardation Research Centers at the University of Kansas and Vanderbilt University.

a plane overhead to draw the parent's attention to it and thus create joint attention). These developmental breakthroughs typically occur by 9 or 10 months of age, well before children utter their first spontaneous words (Bates, Benigni, Bretherton, Camaioni, & Volterra, 1979). A significant delay in the emergence of these building blocks of communication is a strong indicator that the onset of productive language will also be delayed (McCathren, Warren, & Yoder, 1996). The basic premise of the two-component intervention (RE/PMT) approach we present in this chapter is that prelinguistic communication development establishes the foundation for later language development. We further assume that, when prelinguistic communication development is delayed or disordered, a carefully targeted and well-implemented treatment program can help to develop the critical intentional communication skills necessary for early language intervention to be maximally effective. In this chapter, we address issues related to identification of candidates for RE/PMT, discuss the theoretical and empirical bases for the approach, and describe the practical requirements for this intervention and its key components. We conclude by presenting our ideas on how children's progress with prelinguistic intervention can be monitored, how the procedures can be accommodated to a family's cultural and linguistic differences, and future directions in the development and use of the approach.

TARGET POPULATIONS AND ASSESSMENTS FOR DETERMINING TREATMENT RELEVANCE AND GOALS

RE/PMT is designed for young children who have not yet become frequent, clear prelinguistic communicators by approximately 12–18 months of age. By this age, and even earlier for children with severe developmental delays such as those with Down syndrome, speech-language pathologists (SLPs) can conclude that some form of intervention to facilitate communication development is likely to be beneficial, if not necessary. Research on RE/PMT has focused on children with a mental age of at least 9 months (Warren & Yoder, 1998; Yoder & Warren, 2001; Yoder, Warren, & Hull, 1995). However, the primary issue in assessment usually is not whether children are too delayed, but whether they are already too advanced. Applying the intervention with children for whom early *language,* rather than *communication* intervention is more appropriate would be a serious miscalculation (Yoder & Warren, 2002).

RE/PMT is appropriate for children who need to increase their frequency of gestures and vocalizations. Children who already are frequent communicators will not gain substantially from this approach. Consequently, if there is reliable evidence that a child uses more than 10 words or signs productively or understands more than 75 words, we would typically recommend that intervention focus on expressive vocabulary (using speech or an alternative communication system), regardless of the child's existing intentional communication repertoire. Additionally, RE/PMT is not appropriate for children who produce more than 1 or at most 2 spontaneous, intentional communication acts per minute in social play with an adult, especially if these acts typically include a canonical vocalization (i.e., a true consonant plus a vowel). These criteria for determining which children are too advanced for RE/PMT also serve as the guides for determining when it is time for them to move on into early language intervention. Yoder and Warren (2002) found that when RE/PMT was implemented with children who exceeded these criteria, the effects of intervention were minimal.

The Communication and Symbolic Behavior Scales (CSBS™) is an assessment instrument that has been developed specifically to describe the level of a child's prelinguistic communication skills (Wetherby & Prizant, 1993a, 1993b). This assessment has been independently shown to have very high reliability and predictive validity (McCathren, Yoder, & Warren, 1999, 2000; Wetherby, Allen, Cleary, Kublin, & Goldstein, 2002). Its primary drawback is the length of time it takes to apply and score all of the segments, which include assessments of comprehension and play skills. Obviously, if norm-referenced information is needed, especially for children who do not clearly have significant delays in communication development, administration of the entire test would be desirable (note that the CSBS is appropriate only up to 24 months developmentally). For our purpose of describing children's rate of communication and rates of different types of prelinguistic communication, we administer only the *communication temptations* and *sharing books* segments as part of our standard assessment. These two segments provide children with opportunities to request objects, request social interaction, comment about novel events, and repair communication breakdowns within a series of scripted play interactions. We videotape the interactions and later record and count the number of nonverbal requests (proto-imperatives) and comments (proto-declaratives) in order to determine whether a child is likely to benefit most from a RE/PMT (as opposed to a linguistically based intervention) and as a baseline for examining treatment outcomes.

THEORETICAL BASIS

The basic premises and hypotheses underlying RE/PMT stem from a transactional model of social communication development (McLean & Snyder-McLean, 1978; Sameroff & Chandler, 1975). This model presumes that early social and communication development are facilitated by bidirectional, reciprocal interactions between children and their environment. For example, a change in the child, such as the onset of intentional communication, may trigger a change in the social environment. Parents may be more inclined to repeat and expand the child's messages using words, a response we refer to as *linguistic mapping*. These changes then support further development in the child (e.g., increased communication and vocabulary) and subsequent changes in the caregivers input (e.g., more complex language interaction with the child). In this way both the child and the environment change over time and affect each other in reciprocal fashion as early achievements pave the way for subsequent development.

A transactional model may be particularly well suited to understanding social-communication development in young children because caregiver–child interaction can play such an important role in this process. The period of early development (from birth to approximately age 3 years) may represent a unique time during which transactional effects can have a substantial impact on development. Specifically, the young child's relatively restricted repertoire during this period may allow any changes in behavior to be especially salient and observable to caregivers. This in turn may allow adults to be more responsive to the developing skills of the child than is possible later in development when children's behavioral repertoires are far more expansive and complex. During this natural window of opportunity, the relationship represented by the transactional model may be employed by a clever practitioner to multiply the effects of relatively circumscribed interventions and perhaps alter the very course of the child's development in a significant way. However, the actions of the practitioner may need to be swift and intense, or they may be muted by the child's steadily accumulating history.

To appreciate the true potential of transactional effects, consider that an input difference in positive affect expressed by parents toward their child of 10 events per day (a difference of less than 1 event per waking hour on average) will result in a cumulative difference of 10,950 such events over a 3-year period. A child who experiences less positive affect may also experience cumulatively more negative affect (e.g., "Stop that," "Get out of there," "Shut your mouth up," "You're a bad baby"). It is easy to conceive of the combination of these qualitative and quantitative experiential differences contributing to deficits in attachment, exploratory behavior, self-concept, language development, later school achievement, and so forth.

What evidence do we have that such large cumulative deficits occur and/or that they play havoc with social and communication development? Although the evidence is mostly correlational, it is nevertheless compelling. There is substantial evidence that young, typically developing children experience large differences in terms of the quantity and quality of language input they receive, and these differences correlate with important indicators of development later in childhood (e.g., vocabulary size, IQ, reading ability, school achievement) (Feagans & Farran, 1982; Gottfried, 1984; Hart & Risley, 1992; Prizant & Wetherby, 1990; Walker, Greenwood, Hart, & Carta, 1994). Because young children with developmental delays or sensory disorders often display low rates of initiation and responsiveness (Rosenberg & Abbeduto, 1993; Yoder, Davies, & Bishop, 1994), they also may experience input that differs substantially in quantity and quality from the input that high achieving, typically developing children receive despite the best intentions and efforts of their caregivers (Brooks-Gunn & Lewis, 1984; Crawley & Spiker, 1983).

The challenges faced by young children who initiate infrequently may be further multiplied if their caregiver(s) are or learn to be relatively unresponsive to their children's communicative efforts (e.g., Hart & Risley, 1995; Saxon, Colombo, Robinson, & Frick, 2000; Tamis-LeMonda, Bornstein, Baumwell, & Melstein Damast, 1996).

Caregivers who are unresponsive to their young child's initiations and/or who often display depressed or negative affect toward the child may represent a risk factor in terms of the child's emotional, social, and communication development (Landry, Smith, Miller-Loncar, & Swank, 1997). Unresponsive caregivers often have children who are insecurely attached (Ainsworth, Blehar, Waters, & Wall, 1978), which is a risk factor for poor social-emotional development (Bornstein, 1989). Furthermore, there is evidence that caregivers with low rates of responsivity toward their infants can negate or minimize the positive transactional effects of early intervention efforts because they fail to respond to changes in their child's repertoire being generated by the intervention (Mahoney, Boyce, Fewell, Spiker, & Wheeden, 1998; Yoder & Warren, 1998). In short, the generation of transactional effects likely depends on sensitive, responsive caregivers who notice and nurture the child's growth.

The generation of strong transactional effects in which the growth of emotional, social, and communication skills is scaffolded by caregivers can have a multiplier effect in which a small dose of early intervention may lead to long-term effects. These effects are necessary when we consider that typical early intervention by a skilled clinician may represent only 1–2 hours per week of a young child's potential learning time (Bailey, Aytch, Odom, Symons, & Wolery, 1999). Even a relatively intense intervention of 5 hours per week of intensive interaction would represent just 5% of the child's available social and communication skill learning time if we assume the child is awake and learning 100 hours per week. Thus, unless direct intervention accounts for a large portion of a child's waking hours, transactional effects involving caregivers are necessary for early intervention efforts to achieve their potential.

In summary, RE/PMT is grounded in the assumption that prelinguistic skills form the foundation for later language skills. In addition, the transactional model of adult–child interaction serves as a mechanism by which enhanced prelinguistic development can serve as a scaffold for communication and language development. That is, if the child begins to produce more intentional communication acts and/or acts that are more complex (e.g., through PMT), parents should respond to those acts in ways that ultimately will encourage the child to reproduce and revise their acts. Some parents of children with developmental delays may develop patterns of responding to their children that are not optimal for their children's communicative development. Responsive interaction training may be useful to help them recognize and respond to even small changes in the topography of their children's communicative acts (Tannock, Girolametto, & Siegel, 1992). These interactions set the stage for more communicative interactions that are higher in quality and, ultimately, for functional communication using words or signs.

EMPIRICAL BASIS

The initial explorations of the effects of PMT, one of the two key components of RE/PMT, by Yoder and Warren and their colleagues focused on just a few children and used single-subject (multiple baseline) designs. These studies showed that increases in the children's frequency and clarity of prelinguistic requesting following intervention were correlated with increases in linguistic mapping by teachers and parents who were naïve as to the specific techniques and goals of the intervention (Warren, Yoder, Gazdag, Kim, & Jones, 1993; Yoder, Warren, Kim, & Gazdag, 1994). In other words, the teachers and parents of children who increased their use of nonverbal requests increased their use of contingent responses that repeated, rephrased, or otherwise incorporated the presumed meaning of the child's act. Furthermore, children's intentional requesting targeted in these studies was shown to generalize across people, settings, communication styles, and time.

Based on the promising results of these initial small intervention studies, Yoder and Warren (1998, 1999a, 1999b, 2001) conducted a relatively large ($N = 58$) longitudinal experimental study of the effects of PMT on the communication and language development of children with general delays in development. Fifty-eight children between the ages of 17 and 32 months (mean = 23; $SD = 4$) with developmental delays and their primary parent participated in the study. The children were recruited from three early intervention centers in Tennessee. Fifty-two of the children had no productive words at the outset of the study; the remaining six children had between one and five productive words. All children scored below the 10th percentile on the expressive scale of the MacArthur-Bates Communicative Development Inventories (CDIs) (Fenson et al., 1993) and fit the Tennessee definition of developmental delay (i.e., at least a 40% delay in at least one developmental domain, or at least a 25% delay in at least two developmental domains).

The children were randomly assigned to one of two treatment groups. Twenty-eight of the children received PMT; the other 30 children received an intervention termed *responsive small-group* (RSG). Treatment sessions for both groups were 20 minutes per day, 3 or 4 days per week, for 6 months. PMT represented an adaptation of milieu language teaching (Kaiser, Yoder, & Keetz, 1992) that aimed to teach the form and functions of requesting and commenting. It consisted of the following key components: 1) following the child's attentional lead; 2) building social play routines (e.g., turn-taking interactions such as rolling a ball back and forth); 3) using prompts, such as time delays (e.g., after rolling the ball back and forth, withholding it until the child initiated a request to roll it); as well as 4) natural consequences to the child's acts (e.g., giving the child the desired ball).

RSG represented an adaptation of the responsive interaction approach. The adult played with the children in a highly responsive manner and commented on what they were doing but never attempted to elicit or prompt any communication function or form directly. Caregivers were kept naïve as to the specific methods, measures, records of child progress, and child goals throughout the study. This allowed Yoder and Warren to investigate how change in the children's behavior as a result of the interventions might affect the behavior of the primary caretaker and how this, in turn, might affect the child's development later in time. Data were collected at five points in time for each dyad: at pretreatment, at posttreatment, and 6, 12, and 18 months after completion of the intervention.

Although there were no significant main effects of either PMT or RSG, both interventions had a range of effects on intentional communication development among subgroups of the children. The treatment that was most effective depended on the pretreatment maternal interaction style and the education level of the mother (Yoder & Warren, 1998, 2001). For children with highly responsive and relatively well-educated mothers (i.e., 3–4 years of college), PMT was effective in fostering generalized intentional communication development. However, for children with relatively unresponsive and less well-educated mothers, RSG was relatively more successful in fostering generalized intentional communication development.

The two interventions differed along a few important dimensions that provide a plausible explanation for these effects. PMT uses a child-centered play context in which verbal or time delay prompts for more advanced forms of communication are employed as well as social consequences for target responses, such as specific acknowledgment (e.g., "That's right") and compliance (e.g., immediately giving the child a toy he or she had requested). RSG emphasized following the child's attentional lead and being highly responsive to child initiations while avoiding the use of direct prompts for communication. Maternal interaction style may have influenced which intervention was most beneficial because children may develop expectations concerning interactions with adults (including teachers and clinicians) based on their history of interaction with their primary caretaker. Thus, children with consistently responsive parents may learn to persist in the face of communication breakdowns, such as might be occasioned by a direct prompt or time delay, because their history leads them to believe that their communication attempts will usually be successful. On the other hand, children without this history may cease communicating when their initial attempt fails. Thus, children of responsive mothers in the PMT group may have persisted when prompted and learned effectively in this context, whereas children with unresponsive parents may not have. In contrast, when provided with a highly responsive adult who virtually never prompted them over a 6-month period, children of unresponsive mothers showed greater gains than did children of responsive parents receiving the same treatment. For these children, exposure to a highly responsive adult was a novel experience that generated a high degree of initiation and responsiveness by them, apparently leading to the treatment response that was observed, which eventually washed out during the 12-month follow-up (Yoder & Warren, 2001).

The effects of maternal responsivity as a mediator and moderator of intervention effects rippled throughout the longitudinal follow-up period. Yoder and Warren demonstrated that children in the PMT group with relatively responsive mothers received increased amounts of responsive input from their mothers in direct response to the children's increased intentional communication (Yoder & Warren, 2001). Furthermore, the effects of the intervention with this group were found on the number of intentional communication acts (Yoder & Warren, 1998) and of requests and comments (Yoder & Warren, 1999b). These became greater with time and significantly affected measures of expressive (i.e., lexical density; expressive scores on the Reynell Developmental Language Scales [Reynell & Gruber, 1990]) and receptive language development (i.e., number of semantic relations understood; receptive scores on the Reynell Scales) 6 and 12 months after intervention ceased (Yoder & Warren, 1999a, 2001). This finding contrasts with the results of several early intervention studies in which the effects were reported to wash out over time (Farran, 2000).

Finally, two observations from the Yoder and Warren studies support the prediction of the transactional model that children's early intentional communication will elicit mothers' linguistic mapping, which in turn will facilitate children's vocabulary development. First, the amount of responsive input by the primary caregiver was partly responsible for the association between intentional communication increases and later language development (Yoder & Warren, 1999a). Second, there was a significant longitudinal relationship between maternal responsivity and expressive language development (Yoder & Warren, 2001).

The implications of the results achieved by the Yoder and Warren study (1998, 1999a, 1999b, 2001) are tempered by a more recent efficacy study (Yoder & Warren, 2002). This study involved 39 prelinguistic toddlers with developmental delays and their primary parent. As in the previous Yoder and Warren study, all children scored below the 10th percentile on the expressive scale of the CDIs (Fenson et al., 1993) and met the Tennessee definition for developmental delay. However, in this study 17 of the children (44% of the sample) had Down syndrome, whereas in the earlier Yoder and Warren study (1998) only 4 of 58 children had Down syndrome (7%). Half of the children were assigned randomly to a two-pronged treatment condition. In this condition, the children received PMT and the primary caretakers went through a training program intended to ensure that they used a highly responsive parenting style with their child. Results indicated that the parent-training component of the intervention did enhance parent responsivity.

However, the pattern of results in terms of various measures of child communication development varied by pretreatment characteristics, and on some measures the control group achieved growth superior to that of the intervention group. Although the exact reasons for these findings were unclear, post hoc analysis suggested that the criteria for entry into the study included children for whom the intervention may have targeted skills that were "too low." Specifically, the intervention accelerated growth in comments and lexical density if children began treatment with low frequencies on these measures, but it appeared to decelerate growth along these dimensions for children who began treatment with relatively high rates of comments and canonical vocal communication.

The most recent investigation of the effects of PMT and parent responsivity training has also produced the most positive results yet reported. Fey et al. (in press) systematically replicated the second Yoder and Warren study (Yoder & Warren, 2002) with 51 toddlers (average age 26 months at the start of the study) with developmental delays. Children were randomly assigned to either a combination of PMT and parent responsivity training or to receive only those services already provided by the community program in which they were enrolled. Twenty-six of the 51 participants had Down syndrome. Due to the ambiguous results obtained by Yoder and Warren (2002), three important procedural modifications were made. First, to be enrolled in the study, all children were required to have relatively low rates of prelinguistic commenting and canonical vocalizations because these characteristics were associated with the most positive outcomes in the second Yoder and Warren study (2002). Second, clinicians took special care to desist from persistent efforts to prompt requests when children were nonresponsive to such requests. Third, when a child produced a clearly intentional act, clinicians responded by complying with the request and by expanding it rather than modeling some additional behavior, such as a nonlinguistic vocalization.

Based on data collected at the end of 6 months of intervention, Fey et al. reported the first "main effect" of PMT plus parent responsivity training. Specifically, they reported a statistically significant increase in intentional communication relative to the community intervention group. The results obtained for comments and declaratives were not significant, but all adjusted means were greater for the intervention group. The positive effect on intentional communicative acts was also found to be statistically significant for the 13 subjects with Down syndrome when compared directly with the 13 Down syndrome subjects in the community intervention group. The clinical significance of this finding will ultimately depend largely on the extent to which these early gains are followed by later gains on verbal measures in this ongoing longitudinal investigation.

The initial longitudinal study by Yoder and Warren (1998, 2001) represents a relatively rare experimental example of children's influence on adults' use of behavior that in turn fosters the child's further development (Bell & Harper, 1977). It supports the potential power of the transactional model, at least during the early period of development when children's behavior repertoires are small and their developmental history relatively short. Furthermore, it suggests that RE/PMT can be highly effective with children under some conditions. Alternatively, the second longitudinal study by Yoder and Warren (2002) suggests that this approach may be ineffective with children who have already attained a relatively high level of prelinguistic development. The recent Fey et al. (in press) study used more conservative entry criteria to ensure that a prelinguistic intervention was truly appropriate for the children's communication levels and also included minor but perhaps important modifications in the PMT intervention procedures. The main effect on intentional communication resulting from the intervention implemented by Fey et. al. suggests that these modifications were highly functional. Consequently, we present these same recommendations below.

PRACTICAL REQUIREMENTS

As noted, the RE/PMT we have been using and testing involves two components. First, the interventionist (e.g., an SLP or teacher) must be able to work on a one-to-one basis directly with the child several times per week until the child has acquired the necessary skills to be a frequent, clear prelinguistic communicator. Depending on the child's developmental profile, this may take anywhere from a few weeks to more than 6 months. In our clinical and research experience, the average prelinguistic intervention takes several months until the child achieves the exit criteria and goals can be shifted to productive vocabulary.

The second component is RE for the child's parents. As discussed previously, a relatively high degree of parental responsivity appears necessary to ensure that the direct training of the child's prelinguistic skills has maximal impact. We have found It Takes Two to Talk—The Hanen Program for Parents (see Chapter 4; Manolson, 1992) serves as an excellent approach for helping parents from many backgrounds to establish more responsive interaction patterns with their children. In general, we do not advocate teaching parents to use PMT procedures. Although these procedures require the adult to follow the child's lead and to be sensitive to the form and content of the child's communicative efforts, they also involve consistent efforts to push the child to higher levels of communication frequency and complexity. Many parents are reluctant to take on this role of teacher. Those who do sometimes find it difficult to separate their direct instruction roles as teachers and their highly responsive roles as parents and communication facilitators. Furthermore, this intervention is only appropriate for a few months for most children. However, a highly responsive parenting style that will naturally evolve as children grow and develop is appropriate under most conditions and supports the child's development across a wide range of related domains (Landry, Smith, Swank, Assel, & Vellet, 2001).

KEY COMPONENTS

Situations termed *enabling contexts* help to provide an optimal environment for highly responsive caregiver–child interaction and/or the use of specific teaching techniques. These contexts are the same for interventionists using PMT and for parents who adopt the role of responsive communicator in RE. The principles that help to create enabling contexts are 1) arrange the environment to increase opportunities for communication, 2) follow the child's attentional lead, and 3) build social routines in which the child and adult play predictable roles. These principles are applied at all levels of the intervention to encourage a high degree of engagement by the child and to create frequent teaching interactions between the child and the adult. The basic formats for implementing these principles were developed for use in naturalistic early language intervention approaches such as milieu teaching (Warren, 1991) and responsive interaction training (Wilcox & Shannon, 1998).

Arranging the Environment

Children are most likely to initiate communicative acts about things they need, want, or find novel and interesting (Hart & Risley, 1968). Arranging the environment so that it naturally supports the need to communicate can increase the frequency of these states, thus giving the child more opportunities to communicate. This, in turn, gives the interventionist more opportunities to focus on the clarity and complexity of these acts. For example, adults can place desired items (e.g., food, toys) either out of reach of the child or in a context in which adult assistance is necessary to access them. This often happens quite naturally in homes and child care environments in which the child's interests and patterns of action are readily observable. The environment can then be arranged so that the child's expectations are challenged. In a classroom context, certain toys might be kept in clear plastic containers with lids on them that children cannot open without adult assistance (see DVD Clip 12). Crayons might be placed on the floor next to the adult where the child can see them but cannot easily reach them. Extra cupcakes might be placed in clear view but beyond the child's reach. Alternatively, containers and shelves that typically bear the child's toys and objects of interest can be emptied or filled with new, unanticipated items. Positioning should also be considered when trying to create enabling contexts. Positioning refers to how an adult places his or her body in relation to the child's body and a focal object. To the extent possible, the clinician should directly face the child and focal object at the child's eye level. With infants and toddlers, this may mean the adult will need to lie on the floor with the child or sit on the floor while the child sits on a couch or a chair (see DVD Clip 4). This type of close, face-to-face contact facilitates coordinated joint attention between the adult and child (MacDonald, 1989). Sitting behind or above the child makes this type of interaction more difficult.

Following the Child's Attentional Lead

Young children attend more closely to objects or events of their choosing, rather than to objects or events of an adult's choosing (Bruner, Roy, & Ratner, 1980). Furthermore, young children have difficulty deploying their attention on command for longer than very short periods (Goldberg, 1977). Thus, following the child's attentional lead, a universal tenet of virtually all naturalistic early communication and language intervention approaches (Fey, 1986; Hepting & Goldstein, 1996), is used to sustain the child's interest in activities and social interaction. In practice, this might mean that the adult plays with toys or engages in activities of interest to the child (typically selected by the child from an array of choices) in a manner similar to the child's play. Children who are passive and engage in low rates of action, or children who engage in repetitive behavior, can make it challenging to maintain this procedure. Adults can easily lapse into directive styles in which they dominate most interaction episodes with the child. Our experience suggests that if the goal is to build initiations, then it is far better to simply adapt one's behavior to the child's initiation rate even if it is low. This technique is easier to implement if the adult has made some effort to arrange the environment to increase the likelihood that the child will attend and react spontaneously to target stimuli in the intervention context.

Contingent motor imitation is a technique that can be quite helpful with a young child who seldom initiates (Gazdag & Warren, 2000). Contingent motor imitation is an exact, reduced, or slightly expanded imitation of the child's motor production that is performed by the adult immediately following the child's motor production. It represents a specific form of following the child's attentional lead. This simple technique may be used at the start of intervention to establish a basic form of turn taking between the child and adult that over time can be transformed into interaction and play routines. Contingent imitation may benefit children because it allows them to regulate the amount of social stimulation received, it increases the probability that adult input will be easily processed and understood (Dawson & Lewy, 1989), it may encourage children to imitate adult behavior on a broader scale (Snow, 1989), and it may result in more differentiated play schemes (Dawson & Adams, 1984).

Contingent vocal imitation offers many of the same advantages and benefits as contingent motor imitation. It occurs when adults follow children's nonverbal vocalizations that are independent of communicative content with a partial, exact, or modified vocal imitation. For example, a child might vocalize [ga] while holding a plastic ring by her face, making no obvious attempt to share the act with the adult. In this case, the adult might immediately imitate [ga], or [gaga], as a form of vocal play or turn taking (see DVD Clip 1). This type of vocal imitation (as with motor imitation) allows children to regulate the amount of social stimulation they receive and may encourage children to increase their rate of vocalization and to imitate adult vocalizations spontaneously (Gazdag & Warren, 2000).

Social Routine Building

Social routines are repetitive, predictable turn-taking games and rituals, such as Peekaboo and Pat-a-cake. Arranging the environment and following the child's attentional lead support the development of social routines. Social routines, in turn, provide an excellent context for facilitating social communication development. They can be established in the course of daily activities such as feeding, bathing, and dressing, as well as games and toy play. They can be unconventional and unique to a given child. The predictable structure of social routines may help children learn and remember new skills. Once children learn predictable roles in a routine, they can devote greater attention to analyzing adult models of new ways to communicate (Conti-Ramsden & Friel-Patti, 1986; Nelson, 1989). Additionally, the effectiveness of models may be enhanced because slight variations in the routine may create "moderately novel" situations that are particularly salient to young children (Piaget & Inhelder, 1969).

Research with children who are typically developing and with children who have intellectual impairments has shown that social routines are particularly powerful stimuli for linguistic (Snow, Perlmann, & Nathan, 1987; Yoder & Davies, 1992) and prelinguistic communication (Bakeman & Adamson, 1984). Once a social routine is well established with a child, adults can often elicit a high rate of requests and comments by interrupting or modifying the routine. Social routines also provide a natural context for modeling these communication functions and related skills such as turn taking.

Component 1: Prelinguistic Milieu Teaching

The overall goal of PMT is to help children establish and/or increase the frequency, clarity, and complexity of their nonverbal communicative acts. Although it is possible to categorize these acts in many ways, PMT focuses on two broad types of acts: requests and comments. *Requests* are instrumental acts in which the child seeks some object or action. In contrast, *comments* are more purely social acts that seek only to share observations and experiences with a partner.

In Table 3.1, we break down the basic goal of increasing the frequency, clarity, and complexity of the child's nonverbal communicative acts into five

Table 3.1.   Prelinguistic milieu teaching procedures

Intermediate goal	Specific techniques
1. Establish routines to serve as the context for communicative acts (see DVD Clip 1)	A. Imitate the child's motor acts B. Imitate the child's vocal acts C. Interrupt the child's established pattern of actions with an adult turn, and then wait for the child to take a turn D. Perform an action the child finds funny or interesting; pause, then repeat to get more laughter E. When the child produces one part of the routine, oblige by performing the act needed to complete it
2. Increase the frequency of nonverbal vocalizations (see DVD Clips 2–4)	A. Recast the child's nonverbal vocalization with a word if the child is focused on a clear referent B. During vocal play activities (i.e., when the vocalizations are not part of a communicative act), model vocalizations with sounds and word shapes known to be outside the child's repertoire C. Model a sound within the child's sound and word shape repertoire when the vocalizations are not part of a communicative act D. Imitate the child's spontaneous vocalizations with sounds and syllable shapes known to be within the child's repertoire when the vocalizations are not part of a communicative act E. Imitate the child's spontaneous vocalizations as precisely as possible when the vocalizations are not part of a communicative act
3. Increase the frequency and spontaneity of co-ordinated eye gaze (see DVD Clips 5–7)	Create a need for communication within a routine in which the child looks at the object, then: A. Provide the child with the desired object or action contingent on looking B. Verbally prompt for eye gaze C. Move the desired object to the adult's face to encourage a more explicit look D. Intersect the child's gaze by moving the adult's face into the child's line of regard E. Once the child complies, explicitly acknowledge the child's look with fun and well-pleased affect F. If, after using the methods above, the child fails to produce the targeted act, provide the child with the desired object or action
4. Increase the frequency, spontaneity, and range of conventional and non-conventional gestures (see DVD Clips 8–10)	Create a need for communication within a routine (e.g., by placing a desired object out of reach), then: A. Provide the child with the desired object or action contingent on the use of a gesture B. Pretend not to understand by looking and gesturing quizzically and saying "What?" or "What do you want?" C. Ask or tell the child to be more specific (e.g., "Show me which one!" "Which one do you want?") D. Tell the child, explicitly, to produce a particular gesture (e.g., "Show me!" "Give it to me!") E. Model an appropriate gesture

[handwritten note: May need to use hand-over-hand]

F. Once the child complies, verbally acknowledge child's gesture

G. If, after using the methods above, the child fails to produce the targeted act, provide the child with the desired object or action

5. Combine components of intentional communication acts. The three components of intentional communication acts are eye contact with partner, vocalization, and gesture (see DVD Clips 11–13)

A. If the child produces one or two components of a communication act, wait expectantly (i.e., use time delay) to prompt the second (or third) component

B. If the child produces one or two components of a communication act and does not add another component after the time delay:

- Ask, "what do you want?" or another general prompt and wait again

- Intersect the child's gaze or use the child's name to prompt eye gaze

- Model or help the child to produce a gesture

- If the child has produced a communicative act that is focused clearly on an object, attribute, or event, the clinician should recast the act by producing a word

- If the child produces components yielding a communicative act, the clinician should not produce a nonverbal model

- Immediately after the child produces the targeted component, provide the appropriate consequence and verbal feedback, as described under intermediate goals 1–4 above

- If, after using the methods above, the child fails to produce the targeted act, provide the child with the desired object or action

intermediate goals. The first intermediate goal is to establish and maintain social routines (as discussed in the preceding section). The next three intermediate goals are to increase the frequency and spontaneity of the three basic components of prelinguistic requesting and commenting acts. These basic components are nonlinguistic vocalizations, coordinated eye gaze, and conventional and unconventional gestures. *Nonlinguistic vocalizations* are defined as either canonical (syllables with a true consonant, e.g., [ba]) or noncanonical (syllables with only vowel-like sounds or glides, e.g., [a], [m:], [wa]). *Coordinated eye gaze* refers to a child's alternating attention between an object or event of interest and the adult. For example, a child might hear a noise outside, look toward the window, and then look toward the adult. *Unconventional gestures* are hand movements that are highly contextual. These include reaches, proximal points (touching an object with index finger extended), pantomiming an action, giving objects to an adult, and moving objects toward or away from an adult. *Conventional gestures* include intentionally communicative acts, such as a headshake or nod, a hand wave (e.g., *hi*), an upturned palm (e.g., *gimme*), or a point to a distal object. Finally, the fifth intermediate objective is to help the child combine these three nonlinguistic components into increasingly complex and clear requests and comments.

Three principle procedures are used to address all of the intermediate goals and, ultimately, the overall goal of clear, frequent, intentional communication (see Table 3.1). These are *prompts, models,* and *natural consequences.*

Prompts   Prompts are used to evoke intentional communication attempts by the child or to evoke specific components of intentional communication (i.e., vocalizations, coordinated eye gaze, gestures). They take the form of time delay, nonverbal prompts, and verbal prompts, all of which can be used to encourage more frequent and/or complex nonverbal communication attempts. A time delay for initiation is a type of nonverbal prompt that often functions as an interruption of an ongoing turn-taking routine. For example, if a child and adult were playing a tickling game, the adult might hold her hands away from the child to interrupt this routine, then look at the child expectantly until the child initiates a request to continue the routine (see DVD Clip 10). Examples of other nonverbal prompts include holding out an upturned palm (e.g., to get the child to give an object; see DVD Clip 8), moving an object of the child's interest near or directly in line with the adult's face (e.g., to get the child to look at the adult), or physically intersecting the child's line of regard in order for the child to look at the adult (see DVD Clip 6). Verbal prompts for communication can be open-ended questions (e.g., "What?" see DVD Clip 12) or direct commands (e.g., "Show/tell me") intended to elicit communication responses. Verbal prompts also can be used to elicit a specific component of communication. For example, when a young child makes a request without eye contact, the directive, "Look at me" or the child's name may be used to evoke eye contact. If a child does not respond to a prompt, or reacts aversively to a prompt, it is best not to persist with the interaction.

Models   Models are used to support and enhance the vocal and gestural topography of the child's intentional communication attempts. Vocal models of sounds that the adult has heard the child produce (e.g., [ba]) can be used during a motor act that is not focused on a clear referent or is not otherwise part of a child's communicative act. For example, while the child is banging a stick, the clinician might model [baba]. To ensure that the child does not misinterpret the adult's nonlinguistic vocalization as an actual label, it is important that nonlinguistic models are only given in the absence of clear referents. For example, if the adult models [bababa] while the child points to a dog, the child may be induced to think that the label for dog is [ba]. Gestural models are used to encourage the child to use and imitate gestures. For example, when an airplane passes overhead, the adult might point to it as a model for the child to use pointing as an element of commenting (see DVD Clips 9 and 10 for additional examples).

Providing Natural Consequences PMT is based on milieu teaching (MT), which is a form of language intervention for children learning words and early grammatical structures (Warren & Bambara, 1989). It differs most dramatically from MT in that the targeted behaviors for PMT are nonverbal acts; in contrast, in MT, the clinician will prompt and provide the child's desired consequences only for verbal acts. Thus, for PMT, nonverbal communication attempts that are appropriately clear and complex should be consequated in accordance with their intent: child requests should yield the desired objects and actions, and child comments should result in adult attention to the child's topic. Continued attention and interaction by the adult are assumed.

These natural consequences may be supplemented with specific acknowledgment and/or by a verbal recast of the child's meaning (i.e., linguistic mapping). Specific acknowledgment is provided by a smile and comment after the child produces a targeted intentional communication component. For example, when a child makes eye contact with a caregiver in the course of initiating a request, the caregiver might break into a big smile and comment, "You looked at me!" while responding to the child's request (see DVD Clips 5, 6, and 7). Frequent use of specific acknowledgment may disrupt the flow of interaction, and praise statements tend to lose their meaning for recipients if used too frequently. Therefore, these statements should be used primarily when a child is first acquiring a new behavior and infrequently thereafter.

Linguistic mapping occurs when the adult verbalizes the core meaning of the immediately preceding child communication act. For example, a child might point to a photo on a shelf for the adult to see (a comment), and the adult might respond, "Yes, that's Thomas" (see DVD Clip 9). Research with both typically and atypically developing children has indicated that linguistic mapping can be a powerful contributor to vocabulary development (Nelson, 1989). Therefore, we encourage the frequent use of linguistic mapping as part of adult responses to intentional communication attempts.

Teaching Intentional Communication The specific principles and procedures we have described should be embedded into ongoing interactions and used as dictated by the context and the child's current communication goals. Some specific techniques may be used quite frequently (e.g., linguistic mapping); others, only until the child begins to intentionally use the targeted skill (e.g., intersection of gaze). However, the enabling procedures of arranging the environment, following the child's attentional lead, and social routine building are to be used whenever possible and will continue to play an important role when efforts shift toward language goals (Warren, 1991).

It is important to remember that the frequency and quality of children's engagement with objects of interest and their conversational partners (i.e., their routines) will determine the occasions for the use of any specific technique. Prompts are used only when motivation to communicate is high (e.g., when the child is intently engaged in social interaction). Additional consequences can follow any intentional communication attempt. Specific teaching episodes should be brief, positive, and embedded in the ongoing stream of interaction. If a child is not responsive to a prompt, it is best to desist and move on with the interaction. The procedures outlined in Table 3.1 illustrate a kind of hierarchy, with the techniques requiring the most sophisticated child responses described first. Children who respond reliably to these high level techniques may not require the procedures that fall lower in the hierarchy. On the other hand, when a child does not respond to the higher-level procedures, the clinician must fall back to the lower steps, providing the child with more scaffolding. Once the child begins to respond reliably to this level of assistance, the clinician gradually adopts higher level procedures that place more responsibility on the child. This general method of utilizing the steps in Table 3.1 is exemplified in the case example later in this chapter.

Teaching Proto-imperatives   It is helpful to first establish social routines that involve turn taking between the adult and child (e.g., rolling a ball back and forth, dropping blocks into a container, or playing a musical instrument). Once an initial set of routines has been established and a particular instance of a given routine has gone on for at least two turns, the adult may stop the routine by withholding his or her turn and looking expectantly at the child (a time delay for initiation). A verbal prompt also might be given, such as "What?" (to start the activity) or "Do you want this?" (while maintaining eye contact and holding up an object the child needs to resume the activity). If there is not an appropriate response to the interruption of the routine, or if the child's response is incomplete (i.e., it is missing a component necessary to be considered intentional communication), then the adult may provide further assistance to the child. For example, if the child looks at a toy and reaches toward it or provides a vocalization, but does not make eye contact with the adult, then the adult might say, "Look at me," intersect the child's gaze, or move the toy near the adult's face. The adult also might provide a gestural model if needed to complete the communication act. Once the child begins to request across different routines intentionally, then prompts, models, and specific acknowledgments should be faded out. Linguistic mapping should continue as part of the adult's response to the requests, however.

Teaching Proto-declaratives   Proto-declaratives are taught in a decidedly different manner from proto-imperatives (Yoder & Warren, 1999b). The primary motivation for a proto-declarative is recruitment of another's attention and the sharing of an affective state. Our experience suggests that it is often necessary for young children to first develop a positive relationship with an adult before they will initiate proto-declaratives to the adult frequently. Of course, proto-declaratives may be modeled at any time.

Proto-declaratives are taught by modeling and by providing situations likely to stimulate their use, or in some contexts by directly prompting with physical assistance (e.g., prompting a distal point by physically assisting the child; see DVD Clip 9). One such situation is the introduction of novel events or objects. This can take many forms such as adding new toys or items within routines (which can be done frequently), taking advantage of occasional occurrences of silly or unusual events (planned or unplanned), a sabotaged routine, a walk, or a ride in the car. The clinician can model a proto-declarative by pointing to an object or novel event and directing the child to look. The clinician should also linguistically map the object or event as a part of this modeling technique. The clinician can model proto-declaratives concurrent with or just after the novel event of interest. On occasion, when something novel occurs, the adult may pretend not to notice. The intent in this case is to set up a situation in which the child feels the need to direct the adult's attention to the object or event. Yet another approach is to seed an area with interesting, novel objects and let the child have the run of the room for a few minutes, but with the adult clearly observing from a short distance away. As the child discovers novel items in this manner, the child may then comment to the adult. However, our clinical observation has been that, by far, the majority of proto-declaratives occur about an object or event that the child has reason to believe the adult is already attending to. That is, they occur in a context in which the child and adult are engaged in joint attention (Carpenter, Nagell, & Tomasello, 1998).

To summarize, it is important to remember that PMT procedures should be embedded into ongoing social and play routines that represent the enabling contexts described earlier. Furthermore, procedures should be goal-driven. Specific procedures may work well with some goals and poorly with others. Also, clinicians should carefully monitor for and avoid any tendency to use the procedures in a didactic or directive manner. The effectiveness of these procedures depends in part on having a high level of child engagement that is best maintained by following the child's attentional lead at all times.

Component 2: Responsive Interaction Training

There is considerable correlational evidence (Landry et al., 1997; Murray & Hornbaker, 1997; Smith, Landry, Miller-Loncar, & Swank, 1997) and some experimental evidence (Landry, Smith, & Swank, in press; Yoder, Warren, McCathren, & Leew, 1998) suggesting that an optimal style of parenting for promoting social and cognitive competence is one that fosters reciprocal interactions between parent and child. Such an interaction style allows the child to have some degree of control over the interaction. Responsive interaction techniques (see Chapter 4; Wilcox & Shannon, 1998) are intended to create just such an optimal style in caregivers. This approach is widely used in parent training. It Takes Two to Talk—The Hanen Program for Parents (Manolson, 1992) is an excellent example of such an approach. Its major goal is to increase the child's social communication skills by enhancing the quality of interaction between the adult and the child, and it has been shown to be effective in helping parents of children with developmental delays reach this goal (see Chapter 4).

Responsive interaction techniques also have been referred to as *interactive modeling* (Wilcox, Kouri, & Caswell, 1991). As with PMT, these techniques require the provision of *enabling contexts* (e.g., following the child's attention lead), described earlier in this chapter, to maximize their effectiveness. Linguistic mapping also is strongly encouraged. However, responsive interaction approaches generally discourage the direct elicitation of specific child responses via requests to imitate, or even in some cases the use of test questions (e.g., "What is that?"). Focused input is provided based on the child's attentional lead. This input may include models in the form of descriptive talk or linguistic mapping.

In our current research, parents receive 8–10 sessions of RE over a 6-month period. This training is provided by an SLP who has been trained to conduct The Hanen Parent Training Program. However, our approach represents an adaptation of The Hanen Program, not an attempt to directly replicate it. The training sessions are conducted in the parent's home. The initial goal for these sessions is to develop a sense of trust between the clinician and the parent. In our experience, if this trust is not established initially, it can be difficult for the parent to accept the information or apply it to his or her interactions with the child. The clinician and the parent spend some time just getting to know each other through conversation that does not necessarily focus on the child or the intervention. Self-disclosure on the clinician's part and listening to the parent regardless of the topic serve as effective tools to establish the environment for open and honest communication.

Once the clinician–parent relationship is established, the focus of the sessions moves to the direct teaching of responsive interaction techniques. In order to implement these techniques, it is imperative that the parent have a clear understanding of his or her child's intentional communication. To illustrate this point, the clinician may point out instances of intentional communication from videotaped PMT sessions with the child. Parents begin RIT with varied skill levels in terms of how they interact with their child. For example, some parents are proficient in following their child's lead but struggle with allowing their child adequate time to communicate. Other parents experience difficulty following their child's lead during play activities, whereas a few parents are proficient in most of the responsive interaction techniques before beginning the intervention and need just a little fine tuning. In our experience, the most difficult technique for many parents to apply is allowing their child adequate time to communicate. Videotaped sessions of the parent and child playing together are viewed so the clinician and parent can identify instances of high and low responsivity to child initiations. These viewings should be interaction and parent driven to the extent possible to maintain the team-based relationship rather than the teacher–student relationship. The clinician provides cues to direct the parent to specific instances of high or low responsivity.

ASSESSMENT METHODS TO SUPPORT ONGOING DECISION MAKING

Children's communication skills will advance to the point where PMT is no longer the appropriate intervention. To determine a child's readiness to move from PMT to an early language intervention such as MT, several factors must be considered. A decrease in the amount of prompting needed is often the first indication that a child may be ready for language intervention. In addition, the overall rate of intentional communication should be approaching 2 acts per minute in a social interaction play situation. This can be determined by watching the child interact with the parent or another adult and counting the number of intentional communication acts over a 5- or 10-minute period. These acts should include proto-declaratives as well as proto-imperatives. Most communicative acts should include all three components (gazes, gestures, and canonical vocalizations). Our impression is that children with high rates of gesture and mutual gaze are appropriate candidates for language intervention, even if their rates of canonical vocalization are very low. This observation is consistent with Yoder and Warren's (2002) finding that children who produced high rates of communication acts prior to intervention responded better without PMT than they did with it. For many such children with limited phonetic capabilities, this will be the appropriate time to make a decision whether an augmentative or alternative communication system would be best for the child and, if so, what kind of system would likely be most effective.

During the course of PMT, the clinician should also note an increase in the range of consonants and vowels in the child's phonetic inventory and the use of a large variety of gestures, including distal point, contact point, give, reach, wave, as well as other nonconventional gestures. These factors can be determined during the course of an intervention session as opposed to conducting a lengthy evaluation.

CONSIDERATIONS FOR CHILDREN FROM CULTURALLY AND LINGUISTICALLY DIVERSE BACKGROUNDS

RE/PMT and the two intervention components described earlier reflect a set of biases about social communication development and the appropriate roles of caregivers and practitioners. The acceptability of these procedures, and hence their ultimate effectiveness, may vary in some cases because of differences in cultural values and beliefs (Johnston & Wong, 2002; van Kleeck, 1994). Early social-communication intervention may be even more susceptible to problems associated with cultural differences than other forms of intervention for two reasons. First, it often takes place within the family context and carries an expectation that the caregivers will play an active role and even adopt a style of interaction with their child that may directly violate some of their views of appropriate parent–child interaction (Bornstein, 1989). Second, the focus on communication and language development and differences is inherently one of the most sensitive areas for cross-cultural discourse. A range of basic SES and ethnic differences is frequently manifested in language differences (Heath, 1986). Furthermore, even a basic goal such as *increase the child's rate of communicative initiations* can be problematic. For example, in her study of the Inuit in northern Canada, Crago (1990) found that "talkativeness" by young children was considered a sign of a "learning problem" by their parents and was discouraged.

We presume that many if not most potential sources of bias can be limited or at least identified through the careful collection and consideration of information on individual family values, beliefs, and desires. This information then can be used to modify intervention strategies to enhance their acceptability and thus their ultimate effectiveness. For example, in the Inuit culture mentioned previously, it may be most appropriate to involve older siblings or other caregivers in RE rather than parents. Older youths to whom children might be expected to speak frequently also might be trained to perform PMT under an SLP's supervision. A thorough consideration of individual family differences should be a given with all families, irrespective of their cultural or ethnic background. Thus, embracing this perspective should place no additional burden on practitioners. It is in fact completely congruent with the notion of individualizing efforts to meet the unique needs of the family and child, a widely held tenet of early intervention practices in many countries and cultures (Odom & McLean, 1996).

APPLICATION TO AN INDIVIDUAL CHILD

Bonnie, age 27 months, was born 14 weeks prematurely. Her cognitive skills were at the 13-month level as determined by the Bayley Scales of Infant Development (Bayley, 1993). Bonnie's motor skills were also delayed; she was unable to walk but sat unassisted. She grasped objects in either hand and transferred objects from one hand to the other. During the initial communication assessment, Bonnie produced an average of 1 vocalization per minute; however, these vocalizations were not directed to an adult and typically were judged to be noncanonical syllables because they did not contain a true consonant. Her rate of canonical vocalizations was 0.51 per minute. Bonnie's gestures included holding up her arms to request being lifted by an adult and reaching for objects. When she could not reach an object she wanted, she vocalized in protest but did not look to an adult for assistance. She averaged 0.21 proto-declaratives and 0.76 proto-imperatives per minute.

Bonnie was enrolled in PMT for four 20-minute sessions weekly. RE was also provided to her mother 1–2 times per month. The first intermediate goal for Bonnie was to establish turn-taking routines to serve as a context for communication (see intermediate goal 1, Table 3.1). Bonnie enjoyed shaking and patting musical instruments, so the clinician began by imitating Bonnie's actions (specific technique 1A, Table 3.1). The clinician continued this activity with a variety of toys until Bonnie noticed the clinician's actions and began to vary her own actions more frequently. The clinician then introduced turn taking by only having one toy available; the clinician played with the toy in a way she had seen Bonnie play with it, then immediately moved the toy to lie within her range of grasp. Once Bonnie had played with the toy for several seconds, the clinician took the toy and played with it for a few seconds. The clinician then placed the toy near Bonnie again (specific technique 1C, Table 3.1).

Once this routine was firmly established, the clinician moved on to intermediate goals 2–4 (see Table 3.1), which address the individual components of proto-imperatives (i.e., requesting) and proto-declaratives (i.e., commenting). Bonnie did not use alternating gaze yet, so intermediate goal 3 was targeted first. The clinician lifted a desired toy close to her face so that Bonnie did not have to look far to make eye contact (specific technique 3C, Table 3.1). It was often necessary to intersect Bonnie's line of vision as well (specific technique 3D, Table 3.1). As soon as Bonnie alternated her gaze from the toy to the clinician, the clinician praised her for looking and gave her the toy (specific technique 3E, Table 3.1). Eventually the clinician was able to hold the toy farther away from her face, requiring Bonnie to look from the toy back to the adult.

Although alternating eye gaze (i.e., intermediate goal 3, Table 3.1) was targeted during the initial few sessions, once predictable routines had been established, intermediate goals 2–4 were addressed concurrently during each successive session. Different established routines allowed for elicitation of different individual components. To encourage canonical vocalizations (i.e., intermediate goal 2, Table 3.1), the clinician began by imitating Bonnie's vocalizations, often while she held a toy, such as a Slinky or a tube, up to her face (specific technique 2E, Table 3.1). This use of the toy made the vocal play activity more of a game and directed Bonnie's attention to the clinician's mouth. The clinician vocalized into the Slinky, stacking ring, or cup, then handed the toy back to Bonnie for her to take a turn. In later sessions, the clinician followed Bonnie's vocalization with one or more syllables that differed from Bonnie's by adding consonant sounds. At first, these sounds were those Bonnie sometimes used (specific technique 3C, Table 3.1). Later, new sounds not yet in Bonnie's babbling repertoire were added (specific technique 3B, Table 3.1). To address intermediate goal 4 (i.e., use of gestures), the clinician employed the enabling context of arranging the environment so that desired toys were in sight but out of reach. The clinician then modeled both contact points and distal points and encouraged Bonnie to produce these to request the toys (specific technique 4E, Table 3.1). Proto-declaratives were also targeted in this way by having a toy perform an unexpected action. The clinician then modeled a distal point and said, "Look." To encourage the gesture of a give, toys were placed in clear bags or jars that were difficult to open. It was often necessary for the clinician to prompt for a give by extending her hands and asking Bonnie if she needed help (specific technique 4E, Table 3.1). After 2 months, the clinician no longer needed to model a gesture; she simply asked Bonnie to show her which toy she wanted (specific technique 4C, Table 3.1).

Once Bonnie began to readily produce each individual component of an intentional communication act, the clinician moved on to intermediate goal 5 (see Table 3.1). For example, when Bonnie alternated her gaze from a desired toy to the clinician, the clinician prompted for a canonical vocalization by saying "What?" As soon as Bonnie produced a canonical vocalization, the clinician gave her what she wanted and labeled the object ("Oh, you want the Slinky"). Similarly, if Bonnie used a contact point to request an object, the clinician called her name to prompt for an alternating gaze to accompany the gesture. The object was supplied only after Bonnie looked up at the clinician.

After 6 months of PMT, Bonnie was producing intentional communication acts at a rate of 2.0 per minute to make both proto-imperatives and proto-declaratives. The number of prompts that were required and the length of time for waiting during the time-delay technique had decreased greatly. Bonnie's rate of canonical vocalizations increased to 1.3 per minute. At this time, it was determined that she met the criteria to move into language intervention, and her goals shifted to productive word acquisition and use.

FUTURE DIRECTIONS

Relative to early language intervention, very little research has been conducted on RE/PMT. Furthermore, although this approach clearly holds great potential, we do not yet know its true value or what type of children benefit the most from it.

We are presently conducting a longitudinal experimental study to determine whether RE/PMT generates a great enough impact on long-term development of young children with developmental delays to warrant its widespread clinical and educational application. In this study, we are comparing two groups of 2-year-olds with developmental disabilities. In one group, the children receive 6 months of PMT and the parents receive RE. The other group receives no treatment through our project. Twelve months after entry into our program, all children receive 6 months of milieu language intervention to supplement what they get through the schools. We are interested in comparing the performance of children in these two groups at each 6-month interval in terms of their rates of communication acts and, at the later time points, their language abilities. We will have the results of this research in 2006. Meanwhile, Paul Yoder is conducting an analysis of the effects of RE/PMT with young children with autism. These studies should go a long way toward indicating the potential of RE/PMT in general. However, there is already clear evidence of its efficacy for at least some individuals, most notably those that do not communicate very frequently at the outset and who have highly responsive parents.

Most of the research on RE/PMT has been conducted by only a handful of individuals in a few locations. Reliable knowledge of the effects and effectiveness of RE/PMT as well as the development of a full range of specific intervention procedures will require an expanded effort conducted by additional investigators in different settings with varied populations. Finally, the question of whether increasing the intensity of RE/PMT will generate substantial increases in its effects remains to be answered. The prelinguistic intervention we have described in this chapter involves 60–80 minutes per week of the clinician actually working one on one with the child. The minimal intensity of this intervention should be obvious. A recent report by a committee of the National Research Council (2001) suggests that young children with autism receive 25 hours of direct intervention per week to achieve maximal effects. We have no idea what the optimal intensity of RE/PMT for children with developmental delays might be, but surely it is more than 80 minutes per week. Consequently, in 2005 we (Warren, Fey, and Yoder) began a 5-year longitudinal experimental intervention study of RE/PMT with random assignment to high-intensity (5 hours of direct intervention per week) and low-intensity (1 hour per week) conditions with the support of the National Institute of Deafness and Other Communicative Disorders.

RECOMMENDED READING

Wetherby, A.M., Warren, S.F., & Reichle, J. (Vol. Eds.). (1998). In S.F. Warren & J. Reichle (Series Eds.), *Communication and language intervention series: Vol. 7. Transitions in prelinguistic communication.* Baltimore: Paul H. Brookes Publishing Co.

REFERENCES

Ainsworth, M.S., Blehar, M.C., Waters, E., & Wall, S. (1978). *Patterns of attachment: A psychological study of the strange situation.* Hillsdale, NJ: Lawrence Erlbaum Associates.

Bailey, D.B., Aytch, L.S., Odom, S.L., Symons, F., & Wolery, M. (1999). Early intervention as we know it. *Mental Retardation and Developmental Disabilities Research Reviews, 5*, 11–20.

Bakeman, R., & Adamson, L.B. (1984). Coordinating attention to people and objects in mother-infant and peer-infant interaction. *Child Development, 55*(4), 1278–1289.

Bates, E., Benigni, L., Bretherton, I., Camaioni, L., & Volterra, V. (1979). *The emergence of symbols: Cognition and communication in infancy.* New York: Academic Press.

Bayley, N. (1993). *Bayley Scales of Infant Development* (2nd ed.). San Antonio, TX: Harcourt Assessment.

Bell, R., & Harper, L. (1977). *Child effects on adults.* Hillsdale, NJ: Lawrence Erlbaum Associates.

Bornstein, M.H. (1989). *Maternal responsiveness: Characteristics and consequences. New directions for child development.* San Francisco: Jossey-Bass.

Brooks-Gunn, J., & Lewis, M.H. (1984). The development of early visual self-recognition. *Development Review, 4*(3), 215–239.

Bruner, J.S., Roy, C., & Ratner, R. (1980). The beginnings of request. In K.E. Nelson (Ed.), *Children's language* (Vol. 3, pp. 91–138). New York: Gardner Press.

Carpenter, M., Nagell, K., & Tomasello, M. (1998). Social cognition, joint attention, and communicative competence from 9–15 months of age. *Monographs of the Society for Research in Child Development, 63*(4), v–174.

Conti-Ramsden, G., & Friel-Patti, S. (1986). Mother-child dialogues: Considerations of cognitive complexity for young language learning children. *British Journal of Disorders of Communication, 21*(2), 245–255.

Crago, M. (1990). Development of communicative competence in Inuit children: Implications for speech-language pathology. *Journal of Childhood Communication Disorders, 13*, 73–83.

Crawley, S.B., & Spiker, D. (1983). Mother-child interactions involving two-year olds with Down syndrome: A look at individual differences. *Child Development, 54*(5), 1312–1323.

Dawson, G., & Adams, A. (1984). Imitation and social responsiveness in autistic children. *Journal of Abnormal Child Psychology, 12*(2), 209–225.

Dawson, G., & Lewy, A. (1989). Arousal, attention and the socioemotional impairments of individuals with autism. In G. Dawson (Ed.), *Autism: Nature, diagnosis, and treatment* (pp. 49–74). New York: Guilford Press.

Farran, D. (2000). Another decade of intervention for children who are low income or disabled: What do we know now? In J. Shonkoff & S. Meisels (Eds.), *Handbook of early childhood intervention* (2nd ed., pp. 510–548). Cambridge, England: Cambridge University Press.

Feagans, L., & Farran, D.C. (1982). *The language of children reared in poverty: Implications for evaluation and intervention.* New York: Academic Press.

Fenson, L., Dale, P., Reznick, S., Thal, D., Bates, E., Hartung, J., Pethick, S., & Reilly, J. (1993). *The MacArthur-Bates Communicative Development Inventories: User's guide and technical manual.* Baltimore: Paul H. Brookes Publishing Co.

Fey, M. (1986). *Language intervention with young children.* Austin, TX: PRO-ED.

Fey, M.E., Warren, S.F., Brady, N.C., Finestack, L., Bredin-Oja, S., Sokol, S., Fairchild, M., & Yoder, P.J. (in press). Early effects of prelinguistic milieu teaching and responsivity education for children with developmental delays and their parents. *Journal of Speech, Language, and Hearing Research.*

Gazdag, G.A., & Warren, S.F. (2000). Effects of adult contingent imitation on development of young children's vocal imitation. *Journal of Early Intervention, 23*, 24–35.

Goldberg, S. (1977). Social competence in infancy: A model of parent-infant interactions. *Merrill-Palmer Quarterly, 23*, 163–177.

Gottfried, A.W. (1984). Home environment and early cognitive development: Integration, meta-analyses, and conclusions. In A.W. Gottfried (Ed.), *Home environment and early cognitive development: Longitudinal research* (pp. 329–342). New York: Academic Press.

Hart, B., & Risley, T. (1968). Establishing use of descriptive adjectives in the spontaneous speech of disadvantaged preschool children. *Journal of Applied Behavior Analysis, 1*(2), 109–120.

Hart, B., & Risley, T. (1992). American parenting of language-learning children: Persisting differences in family child interactions observed in natural home environments. *Developmental Psychology, 28*(6), 1096–1105.

Hart, B., & Risley, T. (1995). *Meaningful differences in the everyday experience of young American children.* Baltimore: Paul H. Brookes Publishing Co.

Heath, S.B. (1986). Taking a cross-cultural look at narratives. *Topics in Language Disorders, 7*(1), 84–94.

Hepting, N.H., & Goldstein, H. (1996). What's "natural" about naturalistic language intervention? *Journal of Early Intervention, 20,* 250–265.

Johnston, J.R., & Wong, M. (2002). Cultural differences in beliefs and practices concerning talk to children. *Journal of Speech, Language, and Hearing Research, 45*(5), 916–926.

Kaiser, A.P., Yoder, P.J., & Keetz, A. (1992). Evaluating milieu teaching. In S.F. Warren & J. Reichle (Series & Vol. Eds.), *Communication and language intervention series: Vol. 1. Causes and effects in communication and language intervention* (pp. 9–48). Baltimore: Paul H. Brookes Publishing Co.

Landry, S.H., Smith, K.E., Miller-Loncar, C.L., & Swank, P.R. (1997). Predicting cognitive-language and social growth curves from early maternal behaviors in children at varying degrees of biological risk. *Developmental Psychology, 33*(6), 1040–1053.

Landry, S.H., Smith, K.E., & Swank, P.R. (in press). Responsive social contexts: The origins of early communication and independent problem solving. *Developmental Psychology.*

Landry, S.H., Smith, K.E., Swank, P.R., Assel, M.A., & Vellet, S. (2001). Does early responsive parenting have a special importance for children's development or is consistency across early childhood necessary? *Developmental Psychology, 37*(3), 387–403.

MacDonald, J. (1989). *Becoming partners with children: From play to conversation.* San Antonio, TX: Special Press.

Mahoney, G., Boyce, G., Fewell, R.R., Spiker, D., & Wheeden, C.A. (1998). The relationship of parent-child interactions to the effectiveness of early intervention services for at-risk children and children with disabilities. *Topics in Early Childhood Special Education, 18*(1), 5–17.

Manolson, A. (1992). *It Takes Two to Talk.* Toronto: The Hanen Centre.

McCathren, R.B., Warren, S.F., & Yoder, P.J. (1996). Prelinguistic predictors of later language development. In S.F. Warren & J. Reichle (Series Eds.) & K.N. Cole, P.S. Dale, & D.J. Thal (Vol. Eds.), *Communication and language intervention series: Vol. 6. Advances in assessment of communication and language* (pp. 57–76). Baltimore: Paul H. Brookes Publishing Co.

McCathren, R.B., Yoder, P.J., & Warren, S.F. (1999). Prelinguistic pragmatic functions as predictors of later expressive vocabulary. *Journal of Early Intervention, 22,* 205–216.

McCathren, R.B., Yoder, P.J., & Warren, S.F. (2000). Testing predictive validity of the communication composite of the Communication and Symbolic Behavior Scales. *Journal of Early Intervention, 23,* 36–46.

McLean, J.E., & Snyder-McLean, L. (1978). *A transactional approach to early language training.* Columbus, OH: Charles E. Merrill.

Murray, A.D., & Hornbaker, A.V. (1997). Maternal directive and facilitative interaction styles: Associations with language and cognitive development of low risk and high risk toddlers. *Development and Psychopathology, 9*(3), 507–516.

National Research Council. (2001). *Educating children with autism.* Committee on Educational Interventions for Children with Autism. Division of Behavioral Social Sciences and Education. Washington, DC: National Academy Press.

Nelson, K.E. (1989). Strategies for first language teaching. In M.L. Rice & R.L. Schiefelbusch (Eds.), *The teachability of language* (pp. 263–310). Baltimore: Paul H. Brookes Publishing Co.

Odom, S.L., & McLean, M.E. (1996). *Early intervention/early childhood special education recommended practices.* Austin, TX: PRO-ED.

Piaget, J., & Inhelder, B. (1969). *The psychology of the child.* New York: Basic Books.

Prizant, B., & Wetherby, A.M. (1990). Toward an integrated view of early language and communication development and socioemotional development. *Topics in Language Disorders, 10*(4), 1–16.

Reynell, J.K., & Gruber, C.P. (1990). *The Reynell Developmental Language Scales, U.S. Edition.* Los Angeles: Western Psychological Services.

Rosenberg, S., & Abbeduto, L. (1993). *Language and communication in mental retardation: Development, processes, and intervention.* Hillsdale, NJ: Lawrence Erlbaum Associates.

Sameroff, A.J., & Chandler, M.J. (1975). Reproductive risk and the continuum of caretaking casualty. In F.D. Horowitz, E. Hetherington, S. Scarr-Salapatek, & G. Siegel (Eds.), *Review of child development research* (Vol. 4, pp. 187–244). Chicago: University of Chicago Press.

Saxon, T., Colombo, J., Robinson, E.L., & Frick, J.E. (2000). Dyadic interaction profiles in infancy and preschool intelligence. *Journal of School Psychology, 38*, 9–25.

Smith, K.E., Landry, S.H., Miller-Loncar, C.L., & Swank, P.R. (1997). Characteristics that help mothers maintain their infants' focus of attention. *Journal of Applied Developmental Psychology, 18*(4), 587–601.

Snow, C.E. (1989). Imitativeness: A trait or a skill? In G.E. Speidel & K.E. Nelson (Eds.), *The many faces of imitation in language learning.* New York: Springer-Verlag.

Snow, C.E., Perlmann, R., & Nathan, D. (1987). Why routines are different: Towards a multiple factors model of the relation between input and language acquisition. In K.E. Nelson & A. van Kleeck (Eds.), *Child language* (Vol. 6, pp. 65–97). Hillsdale, NJ: Lawrence Erlbaum Associates.

Tamis-LeMonda, C.S., Bornstein, M.H., Baumwell, L., & Melstein Damast, A. (1996). Responsive parenting in the second year: Specific influences on children's language and play. *Early Development and Parenting, 5*(4), 173–183.

Tannock, R., Girolametto, L., & Siegel, L.S. (1992). Language intervention with children who have developmental delays: Effects of an interactive approach. *American Journal on Mental Retardation, 97*, 145–160.

van Kleeck, A. (1994). Potential cultural bias in training parents as conversational partners with their children who have delays in language development. *American Journal of Speech-Language Pathology, 31*, 67–78.

Walker, D., Greenwood, C., Hart, B., & Carta, J. (1994). Prediction of school outcomes based on early language production and socioeconomic factors. *Child Development, 65*(2 Spec No), 606–621.

Warren, S.F. (1991). Enhancing communication and language development with milieu teaching procedures. In E. Cipani (Ed.), *A guide for developing language competence in preschool children with severe and moderate handicaps* (pp. 68–93). Springfield, IL: Charles C Thomas.

Warren, S.F., & Bambara, L.M. (1989). An experimental analysis of milieu language intervention: Teaching the action-object form. *Journal of Speech and Hearing Disorders, 54*(3), 448–461.

Warren, S.F., & Yoder, P.J. (1998). Facilitating the transition to intentional communication. In S.F. Warren & J. Reichle (Series Eds.) & A.M. Wetherby, S.F., Warren, & J. Reichle (Vol. Eds.), *Communication and language intervention series: Vol. 7. Transitions in prelinguistic communication* (pp. 365–385). Baltimore: Paul H. Brookes Publishing Co.

Warren, S.F., Yoder, P.J., Gazdag, G.E., Kim, K., & Jones, H.A. (1993). Facilitating prelinguistic communication skills in young children with developmental delay. *Journal of Speech and Hearing Research, 36*(1), 83–97.

Wetherby, A., Allen, L., Cleary, J., Kublin, K., & Goldstein, H. (2002). Validity and reliability of the communication and symbolic behavior scales developmental profile with very young children. *Journal of Speech, Language, and Hearing Research, 45*(6), 1202–1218.

Wetherby, A.M., & Prizant, B.M. (1993a). *Communication and Symbolic Behavior Scales™ (CSBS)*. Baltimore: Paul H. Brookes Publishing Co.

Wetherby, A.M., & Prizant, B.M. (1993b). Profiling communication and symbolic abilities in young children. *Journal of Childhood Communication Disorders, 15*(1), 23–32.

Wilcox, M., Kouri, T., & Caswell, S. (1991). Early language intervention: A comparison of classroom and individual treatment. *American Journal of Speech-Language Pathology, 1*, 49–62.

Wilcox, M., & Shannon, M. (1998). Facilitating the transition from prelinguistic to linguistic communication. In S.F. Warren & J. Reichle (Series Eds.) & A.M. Wetherby, S.F. Warren, & J. Reichle (Vol. Eds.), *Communication and language intervention series: Vol. 7. Transitions in prelinguistic communication* (pp. 385–416). Baltimore: Paul H. Brookes Publishing Co.

Yoder, P.J., & Davies, B. (1992). Do children with developmental delays use more frequent and diverse language in verbal routines? *American Journal on Mental Retardation, 97*(2), 197–208.

Yoder, P.J., Davies, B., & Bishop, K. (1994). Reciprocal sequential relations in conversations between parents and children with developmental delays. *Journal of Early Intervention, 18*(4), 362–379.

Yoder, P.J., & Warren, S.F. (1998). Maternal responsivity predicts the extent to which prelinguistic intervention facilitates generalized intentional communication. *Journal of Speech, Language, and Hearing Research, 41*(5), 1207–1219.

Yoder, P.J., & Warren, S.F. (1999a). Maternal responsivity mediates the relationship between prelinguistic intentional communication and later language. *Journal of Early Intervention, 22*, 126–136.

Yoder, P.J., & Warren, S.F. (1999b). Self-initiated proto-declaratives and proto-imperatives can be facilitated in prelinguistic children with developmental disabilities. *Journal of Early Intervention, 22*, 337–354.

Yoder, P.J., & Warren, S.F. (2001). Relative treatment effects of two prelinguistic communication interventions on language development in toddlers with developmental delays vary by maternal characteristics. *Journal of Speech, Language, and Hearing Research, 44*(1), 224–237.

Yoder, P.J., & Warren, S.F. (2002). Effects of prelinguistic milieu teaching and parent responsivity education on dyads involving children with intellectual disabilities. *Journal of Speech, Language, and Hearing Research, 45*(6), 1158–1174.

Yoder, P.J., Warren, S.F., & Hull, L. (1995). Predicting children's response to prelinguistic communication intervention. *Journal of Early Intervention, 19*(1), 74–84.

Yoder, P.J., Warren, S.F., Kim, K., & Gazdag, G.E. (1994). Facilitating prelinguistic communication skills in young children with developmental delay. II: Systematic replication and extension. *Journal of Speech and Hearing Research, 37*(4), 841–851.

Yoder, P.J., Warren, S.F., McCathren, R.B., & Leew, S. (1998). Does adult responsivity to child behavior facilitate communication development? In S.F. Warren & J. Reichle (Series Eds.) & A.M. Wetherby, S.F. Warren, & J. Reichle (Vol. Eds.), *Communication and language intervention series: Vol. 7. Transitions in prelinguistic communication* (pp. 39–58). Baltimore: Paul H. Brookes Publishing Co.

4

It Takes Two to Talk—
The Hanen Program for Parents

*Early Language Intervention
Through Caregiver Training*

LUIGI GIROLAMETTO AND ELAINE WEITZMAN

ABSTRACT

It Takes Two to Talk—The Hanen Program for Parents is a well-known parent-focused model of language intervention for toddlers and preschoolers with language disorders. The program is an indirect service delivery model that empowers parents to facilitate language development in naturalistic contexts, thereby maximizing daily opportunities for communication development. It Takes Two to Talk is offered by a speech-language pathologist (SLP) to groups of eight families and consists of a preprogram assessment, a minimum of 16 hours of group training for parents, and three video feedback sessions. Parents are taught to use 1) child-centered strategies (e.g., follow the child's lead), 2) interaction promoting strategies (e.g., ask questions that continue the conversation, wait for your child to take a turn), and 3) language modeling strategies (e.g., label, expand, comment). In addition to learning general language facilitation strategies, parents also target specific interaction and communication goals (e.g., prelinguistic skills, vocabulary, two-word phrases) that are selected jointly by the family and the SLP. This intervention program has been used effectively with late-talking toddlers and preschool-age children with developmental delays (e.g., Down syndrome). Its use with children who have expressive and receptive language disorders is beginning to be explored.

INTRODUCTION

It Takes Two to Talk—The Hanen Program for Parents, which was founded by Ayala Manolson in 1974, is one of the four mediator programs that The Hanen Centre offers for caregivers of young children. Three of these four programs are designed for parents of children with language disorders. It Takes Two to Talk is for parents of children with expressive and/or receptive disorders in communication development; More Than Words is for parents of children with autism spectrum disorders, and the Target Word Program is for parents of late-talking toddlers. In addition, there is an in-service training program for early childhood educators/preschool teachers, Learning Language and Loving It, that focuses on general language facilitation strategies and early literacy for children in preschool settings. Each program has specific materials, content, and teaching format (e.g., number of group sessions, video feedback sessions).

The content of It Takes Two to Talk is derived from studies of parent–child interaction that identify language facilitation strategies associated with the optimal development of communication skills in typically developing infants, toddlers, and young children (e.g., Bruner, 1983; Cross, 1981; Snow & Ferguson, 1978). Consequently, the primary objective of this program is to promote adult behaviors that are thought to influence children's developmental progress in prelinguistic aspects of communication (e.g., joint attention/action, intentional communication acts), vocabulary, and early word combinations (including early morphological development).

TARGET POPULATIONS AND ASSESSMENTS FOR DETERMINING TREATMENT RELEVANCE AND GOALS

Target Populations

Participants in empirical reports of this intervention program have included late-talking toddlers between 18 and 30 months of age (Girolametto, Pearce, & Weitzman, 1996a, 1996b) and preschool-age children with cognitive and developmental delays (Girolametto, Weitzman, & Clements-Baartman, 1998; Tannock, Girolametto, & Siegel, 1992). Clinically, the program has also been offered to parents of preschoolers with specific language impairment.

Because parents are the direct recipients of the SLP's efforts, a description of parental characteristics is equally important to an appreciation of the populations for whom it is relevant. In empirical studies of this intervention, the participants have generally been well-educated, middle-income families who are English speaking and self-refer to the program in response to recommendations by professionals or physicians. However, extensive clinical experience over 25 years has indicated that most parents are successful participants if they are motivated to help their child, have resources for child care and transportation, attend all (or most of) the sessions, and are willing to share their experiences with other families in the group. It has been possible to adapt the program for families of children at risk who come from diverse socioeconomic circumstances and have diverse educational and linguistic backgrounds (e.g., Manolson, Ward, & Dodington, 1995; Watson, 1995).

Assessment

The preprogram assessment normally includes one session of approximately 1.5 hours and may be conducted during a clinic or home visit. Following a brief case history, the mother–child and father–child interaction is videotaped for approximately 5 minutes during free play using toys available in the child's environment. During the play sessions, the SLP records an informal inventory of speech sounds, obtains information about the child's level of play, identifies parents' interaction strategies that facilitate the child's communication, and keeps a record of the child's communication abilities. These observations form an informal baseline of child and parent behaviors that may be targeted in the program. Following the videotaped play sessions, the clinician may administer the Preschool Language Scale–3 (Zimmerman, Steiner, & Pond, 1992) or a similar assessment instrument that is suitable for the child's age and developmental level, such as the Rossetti Infant–Toddler Scale (Rossetti, 1990) or the MacArthur-Bates Communicative Development Inventories (CDIs; Fenson et al., 1993). Finally, the SLP introduces the topic of communication goals for the child to the parents, who are asked about their goals for their child. The SLP then provides some direction regarding broad communication goals, based on the assessment results and the preferences of the parents. These goals are refined as the program progresses.

The assessment information is used in the first video feedback session during which the clinician and parents jointly continue to determine program goals. Basic goals may be stated in broad terms to include strategies that parents will use to help the child achieve the goal. Examples include 1) *I will pause and wait expectantly so my child will take a turn in a social routine by using a gesture,* and 2) *I will observe and wait for my child to start an interaction using a single word.* If a child needs specific language goals, the parent and clinician may jointly select lexical, morphological, or syntactic targets. Examples include 1) *I will model the word bubbles* at least 5 times during a social routine in which I blow bubbles for him, and 2) *I will model the use of the word* more *in two-word phrases when my child wants more of something.* Consistent with the emphasis on the caregivers' behaviors, the overall objectives of selecting intervention goals for the parent–child dyad are to 1) facilitate positive, reciprocal interactions and 2) encourage parents to use responsive language input that is well matched to their child's level of communication development.

THEORETICAL BASIS

Philosophical Foundation

The philosophical foundation reflects the underlying values and approach, derived from best practices, for when and how intervention should occur. It Takes Two to Talk reflects a family-centered model of intervention, focusing on the child within the family context. This philosophical orientation recognizes the family as a dynamic social system in which individual family members are so interrelated that any action or experience affecting one member of the family unit will affect them all (Brown, Thurman, & Pearl, 1993; Donahue-Kilburg, 1992). The importance of viewing *the family* as the client and of involving parents in their children's intervention is widely recognized. According to Bronfenbrenner (1974), active involvement by families in a child's intervention program is critical and without such family involvement, intervention is unlikely to be successful and any short-term effects are unlikely to be long-lasting. In addition, Rossetti (2001) noted that the earlier parents of children with disabilities are involved in their children's intervention programs, the better the outcomes for the children.

The ultimate goal of family-centered intervention is to empower families and to enhance their sense of competence and self-worth (Dunst, Trivette, & Deal, 1988). It Takes Two to Talk is philosophically compatible with family-centered approaches to early intervention in that it recognizes the family as the constant and most important element in a child's life. Moreover, the program includes parents, as well as siblings, other caregivers, and members of the extended family, should they wish to be involved. It Takes Two to Talk also involves a collaborative, respectful partnership with parents, in which parents are acknowledged as knowing their child best. For example, when parents and the SLP collaborate on goal selection, parents identify what they want their child to learn as well as the contexts they consider most conducive for the learning to take place. The clinician listens carefully to parents' ideas and priorities and provides support and guidance as needed, primarily in relation to the selection of realistic goals for the child. It Takes Two to Talk's family-centered orientation is also reflected in its format, which includes group sessions for parents. These sessions provide opportunities for social support, which is thought to contribute significantly to the well-being of both parent and child (Crnic & Stormshak, 1997). Social support is also provided from the parents' ongoing and personal relationship with the SLP, whose role extends beyond that of instructor to both coach and counselor. The ultimate goal of any family-centered service is to enable parents to feel competent and confident in their ability to play a central role in their child's intervention. In the case of It Takes Two to Talk, the goal is for parents to feel empowered to become their child's primary language facilitator.

In addition to its family-centered focus, It Takes Two to Talk reflects a naturalistic approach to intervention, which involves "strategies that identify and use opportunities for learning that occur throughout the child's natural activities, routines, and interactions; follow the child's lead; and use natural consequences" (Sheldon & Rush, 2001, p. 2). In a review of 56 intervention studies, McLean and Woods-Cripe (1997) concluded that interventions that were naturalistic resulted in improved skills for young children at early stages of communication development, confirming the value of this approach. Natural environments include three dimensions: the setting, the type of activity, and the practitioner (Dunst, Trivette, Humphries, Raab, & Roper, 2001). The optimal setting is one that provides the child with contextualized learning opportunities, such as those that involve interactions with parents and significant others in real-life everyday situations and that foster acquisition of "socially adaptive and culturally meaningful behavior" (Dunst et al., 2001, p. 51). An optimal setting also provides a multitude of opportunities for the child to practice existing skills and learn new ones. Parents who attend It Takes Two to Talk learn to facilitate their child's language learning in naturally occurring situations during the child's daily routines, play activities, and everyday conversations. In addition, parents learn that any real-life activity has the potential for fostering interaction and communication—unlocking a door and hanging up the key, paying bus fare and riding on the bus, filling the bathtub and having a bath, and watching the mailman deliver the mail are just a few examples of everyday settings that are rich in their potential for social conversation and language learning.

The *type of activity* dimension refers to the extent to which the activity is child initiated or adult directed. The notion of child-centeredness, which is at the core of It Takes Two to Talk, is of critical importance because child-initiated activities and conversational topics are inherently more motivating and engaging for the child than adult-directed ones. When a child's initiations are acknowledged and responded to by his or her caregivers, it promotes a sense of competence and self-determination, thereby increasing the child's intrinsic motivation to continue the interaction, as well as to try to communicate in more conventional ways.

The final dimension of the natural environment, the *practitioner* dimension, reflects whether it is the clinician or the parent who is implementing the intervention. In It Takes Two to Talk, the parent is clearly responsible for providing the child with ongoing opportunities to engage in extended, meaningful interactions within which language learning can take place, thereby maximizing the natural learning environment. The naturalistic approach espoused in It Takes Two to Talk also serves to promote generalization of skills, because these skills are learned through repeated interactions that occur naturally in the child's environments.

Theoretical Foundation

The theoretical foundation describes the theory of language acquisition to which an intervention approach ascribes. It Takes Two to Talk adheres to social interactionist perspectives of language acquisition, which maintain that the simplified language input provided by caregivers helps children make comparisons between the nonlinguistic and linguistic contexts and induce the relationships between objects, actions, external events, and words (Bohannon & Bonvillian, 1997). The social interactionist perspective contains two alternative but compatible explanations of the relationship between adult language input and child language development. The first explanation is the *structural* hypothesis in which it is believed that adult language input that is grammatically one step ahead of the child may facilitate development because it provides models within the child's zone of proximal development (Vygotsky, 1978). This hypothesis focuses on structural features of the language input (e.g., length of utterances, grammatical complexity) and is derived from social interactionist accounts of language development in which the adult's input to typical children is characterized as short, syntactically simple, redundant, and slower in tempo (e.g., Cross, 1977; Snow & Ferguson, 1978). Thus, in interventions arising from this perspective, parents are taught to reduce the structural complexity of their speech by using shorter utterances, a slower rate of speech, and fewer utterances. Use of these strategies assumes that structural simplifications of maternal input are crucial for facilitating child language learning.

The second, complementary explanation, the *responsivity hypothesis*, focuses on the contingency between child's utterances and the adult's responses (e.g., imitation, expansion) and explains the facilitatory effect as a match between the child's processing mechanisms and responsive input. In this model, language input that is responsive to the child's plan-of-the-moment reduces contextual ambiguities, provides redundancy, and increases the saliency of the input. Thus, responsive language input is more easily processed and permits the child to redirect more cognitive resources for language learning (e.g., Rocissano & Yatchmink, 1983). Empirically, this model is supported by studies that have identified significant positive correlations between maternal semantic contingency and variation in child language development (e.g., Cross, 1981). The social interactive model of language intervention has also adopted these features of linguistic input. In this model, parents are taught to match their semantic content to the child's attentional focus (e.g., responsive labeling) and ensure that their input is contingent on the child's vocalizations (e.g., imitation, interpretation) or verbalizations (e.g., expansions). Table 4.1 outlines three clusters of responsive interaction strategies that are associated with this model: child-oriented strategies (designed to foster frequent episodes of joint activity around the child's interests), interaction promoting strategies (designed to foster balanced turn taking and reciprocal interaction), and language modeling strategies (that assist the child to induce relationships between language content, form, and use).

Unfortunately, the underlying theoretical framework of the social interactionist model is somewhat debatable because the precise impact of responsive language input on the children's lexical, morphological, and syntactic development has been difficult to demonstrate consistently. In fact, some researchers have concluded that there is little evidence to support the claim that structural and contingent features of parental input have any direct or long-lasting influence on child language development (for reviews see Pine,

Table 4.1. Strategies of the social interactionist model of language intervention

Child centered	Interaction promoting	Language modeling
Follow the child's lead	Take one turn at a time	Imitate
Wait for the child to initiate	Wait with anticipation	Interpret child's message
Enter the child's world by being at the child's physical level, maintaining face-to-face interaction, being animated	Ask questions that encourage turns on topic	Responsive labeling
	Use routines, games, songs to engage children in interactions	Expand child's utterances
		Extend the topic of child's utterances
		Use parallel talk, self-talk

1994; Richards, 1994). Despite this contention, clinicians and researchers continue to view this intervention model as a viable option for young children with language disorders (e.g., Conti-Ramsden, 1994). Moreover, empirical evidence for its efficacy has been provided by a series of experimentally controlled studies that document concomitant changes in both adult language input and child language development (e.g., Girolametto et al., 1996a, 1996b; Tannock et al., 1992; Weistuch & Lewis, 1986). Although the precise mechanisms are unclear, the social interactionist model of intervention appears to have a facilitative effect on the language development of children with language disorders. One reason for this finding may be that children with language disorders are much more dependent on external environmental support for optimal language learning than are typically developing children (Snow, 1994). Indeed, a critical rationale for this intervention model is that the language environment of children with language disorders can be optimized to influence their communication behaviors.

EMPIRICAL BASIS

There are two distinct versions of It Takes Two to Talk. From 1982 to 1996, the *general stimulation version* of It Takes Two to Talk was used. This version trained parents to follow the child's lead in terms of topic and activity and to provide models of language content and form that are contingent on the child's focus. There were no specific language goals for the children. The objective of the general stimulation version was to produce successful joint interactions, and the outcomes were measured in terms of length of engagement, participation in interaction, or number of conversational turns.

Since 1996, a *focused stimulation strategy* has been added to the language modeling strategies. (The focused stimulation strategy is included in a newly revised edition of *It Takes Two to Talk* [Pepper & Weitzman, 2004].) In this version of It Takes Two to Talk, the clinician and parents jointly select communication goals and parents use focused repetition (i.e., three to five repetitions of a communication pattern) to make these goals salient during naturalistic interactions. They learn to set up obligatory contexts for the goal (e.g., routines where the word *go* may be modeled), to use fillers to encourage the word's use (e.g., "Ready, set, ___"), and to pause and wait expectantly for a response. They do not use explicit prompts to elicit child productions, however, and if the child does not respond, the parent continues the interaction. Parents also use the same strategies listed in Table 4.1 that are taught in the general stimulation version. Studies employing both versions of It Takes Two to Talk have been completed and are discussed in the following sections.

Efficacy of General Stimulation

Two randomized controlled trials of the general stimulation version of It Takes Two to Talk have been conducted. The first study randomly assigned 20 families of children with developmental and language disorders to experimental and delayed treatment control groups (Girolametto, 1988). The participants were between 22 and 62 months of age, their etiologies were mixed (e.g., Down syndrome, chromosomal abnormalities, mild cerebral palsy, general delays in development), and their language levels ranged from prelinguistic, intentional communication to the single-word stage. Following intervention, mothers in the experimental group used fewer turns, a more balanced turn-taking ratio, and maintained longer conversational exchanges (number of turns taken on topic) than mothers in the control group. In addition, the mothers who received training were more responsive and less directive than those in the control group. At posttest, the children in the experimental group exhibited greater responsiveness and assertiveness, were more verbal, and used a more diverse vocabulary than children in the control group. Their increased participation and verbal productivity in interaction is an important finding relative to the theoretical underpinning of the model because it is assumed that children who use language assertively elicit more responsive language input from their caregivers. However, whereas children's changes in communication ability were positive, the changes could not be interpreted as unequivocal evidence of the *acquisition* of new linguistic structures. For example, it was possible that the children in the experimental group simply used more of what they already knew (i.e., they demonstrated greater productivity). The lack of impact on measures of language acquisition may have reflected a slower rate of learning for children with developmental delays and suggested that a lagged treatment effect might be observed at a later point in time.

A subsequent randomized controlled trial involving 32 families of children with developmental delays and language disorders extended the previous findings by including 1) multiple measures and sources of outcome data, 2) follow-up measures to assess a lagged treatment effect, and 3) stratification for developmental level (i.e., mental age [MA] younger than 16 months and MA equal to or older than 16 months) (Tannock et al., 1992). The children in the low MA group were 14–30 months of age and were intentional but preverbal; a few children had vocabularies of between one and eight single words. Those in the high MA group were 21–60 months of age and had vocabularies of between 10 and 100 words; many of these children used two-word phrases. Their etiologies were comparable to those reported for the previous study. Following intervention, mothers in the experimental group used more child-centered strategies, interaction promoting strategies, and language modeling strategies than mothers in the control group. Furthermore, mothers in the experimental group maintained their gains at follow-up, 4 months later. Secondary treatment effects on family functioning were also found. Mothers in the intervention group reported less depression on a measure of parenting stress in comparison with the control group (Tannock & Girolametto, 1992), suggesting that the parent program may have an unexpected, indirect effect on aspects of family functioning. Additionally, subjective data derived from parent questionnaires documented changes in other areas of child and family functioning which were untapped by formal measures, including positive changes in child behavior, increased child cooperation, and improvements in the parent–child affective relationship (Girolametto, Tannock, & Siegel, 1993).

Unfortunately, as in the first study, there were no effects of treatment on measures of the children's language acquisition. In comparison with the control group, children in the experimental group increased their use of vocal turn taking in interaction but did not differ on any other measures of turn taking, socio-interactional skills, language productivity, or development. Moreover, there were no differential gains according to developmental level (e.g., high versus low). In contrast to these findings, other social interactionist models of language intervention have reported more favorable findings for children with language disorders (and no cognitive disorders), including increased mean length of utterance (MLU) relative to controls (e.g., Weistuch & Brown, 1987; Weistuch, Lewis, & Sullivan, 1991). Future research using the general stimulation version of It Takes Two to Talk with families of children without cognitive or developmental delays is needed to determine whether this model of intervention can similarly accelerate language development.

Efficacy of Focused Stimulation

Empirical evidence for the focused stimulation version of It Takes Two to Talk is derived from three randomized controlled trials. In the first study (Girolametto et al., 1996a; Pearce, Girolametto, & Weitzman, 1996), 16 families with late-talking children were randomly assigned to experimental and delayed treatment control groups. The children were between 2 and 3;6 years of age and at the single-word stage of language development. Following treatment, mothers in the experimental group reduced their MLU, used focused stimulation more frequently, and became less directive than mothers in the control group. The children in the experimental group acquired more target words than the control group, although they did not differ on total vocabulary size as measured by the CDIs. Finally, mothers of children in the experimental group reported an improvement in early gestures on the CDIs and a reduction in aggressive/destructive behaviors as measured by the Child Behavior Checklist (Achenbach & Edelbrock, 1983). In summary, this study demonstrated primary effects on the parents' use of program strategies and the children's acquisition of target words and secondary effects on early gestures and behavior.

A follow-up study was designed to replicate the findings of the pilot study using a larger sample size, multiple outcome measures, and a more cohesive group of late-talking children (Girolametto et al., 1996b). In this study, 25 mothers and their late-talking toddlers were randomly assigned to treatment and delayed-treatment (control) groups. The children were between 23 and 35 months of age and all scored below the 5th percentile on the CDIs. The intervention program was identical to the one used for the pilot study and included responsive input strategies as well as the focused stimulation strategy. Following treatment, the experimental mothers' language input was slower, less complex, and included more focused stimulation when compared with mothers in the control group. Concomitantly, their children used more target words in a structured play task and a more diverse vocabulary in free play, and were reported to have larger lexicons overall as measured by parent report on the CDIs. In addition, the treatment had an unequivocal effect on their language development—the children in the experimental group used more multiword combinations and early morphemes than did the control group. Finally, the children in the experimental group also experienced secondary gains in speech sound development (i.e., phonetic inventory, syllable shape) (Girolametto et al., 1996b) and symbolic play behavior (Girolametto, Sparks, Weitzman, & Pearce, 2003) although these areas were not directly targeted by the intervention.

The focused stimulation version of It Takes Two to Talk also yielded positive results for children with Down syndrome who had disorders in both cognitive and language development (Girolametto et al., 1998). In a third study, 12 families of children with Down syndrome were randomly assigned to experimental and delayed-treatment control groups. The children were between 29 and 46 months of age and communicated using single words or signs. None of the children used word or sign combinations. Following intervention, mothers in the experimental group reduced their rate of speech and used more target labels and more focused stimulation of target words than mothers in the control group. At posttest, their children used twice as many targets as the control group based on a parent questionnaire. Consistent with parent report, children in the experimental group also used a greater number of signed or spoken target words during free play with their mothers when compared with the control group dyads. However, there were no differences between the two groups on a standardized vocabulary measure (i.e., CDIs). Although these findings are less robust than those for late talkers in the previous study, they provide preliminary evidence in support of the focused stimulation version of It Takes Two to Talk for children with cognitive and language disorders.

PRACTICAL REQUIREMENTS

It Takes Two to Talk is led by SLPs who have completed a Hanen Certification Workshop (see www.hanen.org for information on Hanen workshops), which provides training in the principles of adult education, how to lead groups, and how to provide effective feedback on videotaped parent–child interactions. When leading It Takes Two to Talk, the SLP uses a parent guidebook, *It Takes Two to Talk* (Pepper & Weitzman, 2004), which is typically provided to each family; a leader's guide, *Making Hanen Happen* (Pepper, Weitzman, & McDade, 2004); a teaching videotape that provides selected video examples for each session of the program; and videotaping equipment (camera, VCR, and TV).

The time commitment involved for an SLP to lead It Takes Two to Talk includes time to plan each group session. Planning activities include familiarizing oneself with program content, examples from the teaching video (used to demonstrate session content), session activities, and the logistics of facilitating each activity. As familiarity with program content, format, and logistics increases, less time is required to plan group sessions. There are no group sessions during the weeks when video feedback sessions are conducted. During these weeks, the SLP schedules sessions that are 1–2 hours long with each family, depending on whether one or both parents are participating in the program. These sessions include videotaping a short segment of parent–child interaction, followed by a review and discussion of the videotaped interaction. They may be conducted in the home or clinic.

KEY COMPONENTS

It Takes Two to Talk has three primary objectives that are addressed throughout the program in an integrated manner. The first objective is parent education. Over the course of It Takes Two to Talk, parents learn some basic concepts about communication and language that may be unfamiliar to them but are essential to increasing their understanding of their child's needs. Concepts such as the sequence of communication development, the importance of nonverbal communication, and the difference between receptive and expressive language are fundamental to enhancing parents' understanding of their children's stage of development and to enabling them to set realistic goals. This knowledge also helps parents become more responsive to their children's communicative attempts, setting the stage for more frequent, extended interactions.

The second objective of It Takes Two to Talk is early language intervention. During the course of the program, parents learn many strategies to facilitate their children's communication development. They may already be using some of these strategies, in which case increasing their self-awareness serves to increase the frequency of strategy use. If the language facilitation strategies are new to parents, they need to learn to apply and integrate them into their daily interactions with their children. Application of new strategies begins during group sessions, when strategies are introduced, illustrated, and practiced in a simulated situation. It continues when parents practice at home and during videotaping and feedback sessions. The SLP helps parents apply program strategies flexibly and spontaneously in a variety of daily routines and contexts, so that intervention becomes a continual process that continues throughout the day.

The third objective of It Takes Two to Talk is social support, which has been found to have a direct, positive influence on the well-being of the child and the family when a child has a disability (Crnic & Stormshak, 1997). Parents receive both formal and informal social support when they participate in It Takes Two to Talk. The support provided by the SLP constitutes formal support, whereas the support and kinship offered by the other group members during and outside of group sessions constitutes an informal support network. When parents meet other parents in It Takes Two to Talk, they have a context within which to share their successes, frustrations, and concerns as well as to learn from one another and share ideas, thereby gaining a sense of community. The value parents place on the support component of It Takes Two to Talk has been demonstrated in a study of consumer satisfaction by Girolametto et al. (1993), in which group sharing was evaluated as a highly important activity.

Program Content and Schedule

It Takes Two to Talk has the following four components: 1) an orientation meeting, 2) a preprogram assessment for each child, 3) a series of group sessions for parents, and 4) three individual video feedback sessions. The total time commitment expected from parents' attendance at these sessions is approximately 30 hours. Prior to the start of the program, parents are invited to attend an orientation meeting where they can obtain information about It Takes Two to Talk, the commitment involved, and their role in the intervention process. At this meeting, an introductory videotape is shown, in which parents talk about their participation in It Takes Two to Talk, demonstrate the strategies they learned, and describe the program's impact on their children's communication development. After attending the orientation meeting, parents decide whether they wish to enroll in the program.

If parents decide to enroll in It Takes Two to Talk, they are then scheduled for a preprogram assessment with the SLP (discussed previously). After the preprogram assessments have been completed, the group sessions begin. It Takes Two to Talk consists of a series of six to eight group sessions for up to eight families. Parents may choose to attend the program with a spouse, partner, family member, or close friend, or to come alone. It Takes Two to Talk programs must provide parents with at least 16 hours of group training. Each group session lasts approximately 2.5 hours and includes a combination of interactive presentation, group discussion, videotape analysis, and opportunities to practice (see SLP as Adult Educator). Each group session includes 1) review and discussion of home activities, including the child's responses; 2) review of information from previous session(s); 3) presentation of new information, including new strategies; 4) opportunities to practice strategies, with feedback and discussion; 5) refreshment break (and opportunities for parents to circulate and talk to one another); and 6) planning for application of strategies at home. The program content and schedule is outlined in the Appendix.

During the course of It Takes Two to Talk, each parent receives three individual video feedback sessions from the SLP. Although the SLP may choose to conduct videotaping and feedback sessions in the clinic for practical reasons, there are advantages to having these sessions take place in the child's natural environment. Being in the family home gives the SLP an opportunity to understand each family's unique culture, dynamics, and approach to child rearing. Home-based visits also facilitate generalization of newly learned skills to this context. The purpose of the video feedback session is for parents to practice program strategies in real-life contexts, with coaching and feedback from the SLP, to review and revise the child's goals, and to discuss any concerns they may have in relation to their child and the program. Table 4.2 outlines the steps a clinician may follow in conducting video feedback sessions.

Role of the Speech-Language Pathologist

The role of the SLP as group leader in It Takes Two to Talk is a complex and multifaceted one. Whereas It Takes Two to Talk is designed to provide early language intervention for the child, the fact that the intervention is implemented by parents requires that the SLP expands the traditional role of service provider to include the roles of early language interventionist, adult educator, and coach/counselor. The SLP's first role is that of *early language interventionist.* In order to teach parents the language facilitation strategies in It Takes Two to Talk, the SLP must be able to implement these strategies so that they can be modeled for parents when necessary. In addition, the SLP's mastery of these strategies is crucial when he or she is called on to evaluate which strategies may be most effective with individual children and

Table 4.2. Steps for conducting a video feedback session

Step	Action
Step 1	The clinician briefly reviews with the parent the strategies he or she has been practicing and the child's goals.
Step 2	The clinician asks permission to coach the parent during the interaction, if necessary.
Step 3	The clinician videotapes approximately 5 minutes of the parent–child interaction during a daily routine or play activity, coaching as necessary to facilitate successful application of program strategies.
Step 4	Immediately following the videotaping, parent and clinician review the videotape from beginning to end with little discussion. They then watch it again, pausing to discuss aspects of the interaction, with the clinician facilitating the parent's self-evaluation. The discussion focuses primarily on instances in which the parent successfully applied strategies and the consequent positive effect on the child. In addition, instances are identified where the parent had difficulty applying the strategies or missed an opportunity to do so, followed by collaborative problem solving around how to address this in the future.
Step 5	The clinician and parent review and revise the child's goals, as necessary.
Step 6	The clinician summarizes the strategies the parent will focus on for the next week and in which contexts.
Step 7	The parent raises any concerns related to the child and the program.

to troubleshoot with parents when a strategy is not working or is difficult to apply (Kaiser & Hancock, 2003).

The second and less familiar role of the SLP is that of *adult educator.* When faced with a group of parents (i.e., typically eight families), the clinician has the challenging task of helping a diverse group of adult learners acquire new knowledge and skills. An important part of meeting the diverse needs of adult learners involves adapting teaching methods to accommodate their varying learning styles. For example, interesting presentations may accommodate learners who like to obtain information by listening to the "expert," experiential learning activities may be more suitable for parents who enjoy learning by doing, and opportunities for discussion and brainstorming may be most appreciated by parents who enjoy developing their own solutions (McCarthy, 1987). This model of teaching utilized in It Takes Two to Talk recognizes the unique characteristics of adult learners, accommodates their different learning styles, and provides a comprehensive learning experience.

In order to facilitate adult learning, the SLP uses a series of activities, each of which has a specific purpose. First, the SLP utilizes a concrete, experiential activity, which activates parents' background knowledge and draws on their prior experience (e.g., an analysis of a simulated interaction between adults, developing solutions to a hypothetical problem, or role playing an imaginary situation). The purpose of the experiential activity is to engage parents by drawing on their life experiences to make connections between old and new knowledge. These activities are usually conducted in small groups or pairs to ensure that each parent has the opportunity to participate and interact.

The next set of activities is utilized to teach the rationale and method for implementing a program strategy. The SLP uses a variety of media to present this information in an interesting and engaging manner, including flip charts, PowerPoint slides, props (e.g., toys, children's books), and many videotaped examples. To make these presentations dynamic and interactive, group discussions are frequently integrated. For example, after presenting information on a new strategy, parents may watch a videotaped example and then, in small groups, identify specific instances of the adult's use of a strategy and the child's response. Learning theory has demonstrated that adults learn well from their peers, making small-group activities an obvious way of drawing on the expertise and experience of all group members (Dinmore, 1997).

Once the SLP has introduced and demonstrated a new strategy, parents are provided with opportunities to practice and experiment with its application. Practice occurs in simulated contexts during group sessions and in real-life contexts in the home. Practice activities within the group session may involve simulating an everyday situation, such as having a snack with a child or playing a familiar game. Parents have an opportunity to role play with partners, attempting to apply the strategy they have just learned. Parents may also practice by evaluating videotaped parent–child interactions. During practice activities, metacognitive strategies are promoted to help parents "remember to remember," which can be challenging when they try to apply the strategies at home. In-class practice activities are summarized as *action plans,* which parents complete during the session so that they have a predetermined plan for trying out the strategies at home with their children.

In the role of adult educator, the SLP forgoes the role of expert and assumes the role of facilitator of learning. This role changes as the group forms and establishes its own identity. At first, the SLP's major focus is on creating opportunities for parents to get to know one another. As parents become more comfortable with the new endeavor, the focus changes to fostering group cohesion by setting up learning activities that encourage discussion and sharing of ideas. Over time, as parents come to rely on one another as sources of support and information, the SLP's role is adjusted so that it fosters more autonomy on the part of the parent group. Activities are set up so parents can lead some of their own group activities and can take more responsibility for their own learning, with the SLP providing a supportive role. The role of adult educator in It Takes Two to Talk is a dynamic one, constantly drawing on the skills, creativity, and flexibility of the SLP.

The final role of the SLP is that of coach and counselor. The role of coach implies collaboration with parents, which represents a reciprocal process. Such a process involves both parties sharing their skills, knowledge, and expertise with the ultimate goal of fostering parents' mastery of the program strategies. The role of counselor comes into play when helping parents deal with the emotions and stresses that arise from having a child with a communication problem. A child's language disorder may make it more difficult for the parent to establish and maintain interactions with the child and can result in fewer mutually satisfying interactions. Parents may share their grief and their frustrations with the SLP, who needs to exhibit several characteristics identified by Rogers (1961) as being critical to the counseling process. These include authenticity, acceptance, empathetic understanding, and unconditional positive regard. Listening to parents without interruption and reflecting an understanding of what they are expressing will communicate acceptance, enabling parents to develop a sense of trust and openness to the learning process.

Coaching, in the traditional sense, is utilized by the SLP while videotaping the parent and child in a video feedback session. In this situation, the parent may need specific, concise feedback so that corrective action can be taken. For example, if a parent is dominating the interaction and not following the child's lead, the SLP might coach by saying, "Wait for Jacob to send you a message. As soon as he does, respond." The result of such coaching is usually a change in the parent's behavior, an improved response from the child, and a more successful interaction for the SLP and parent to review on videotape.

When reviewing the videotape together with the parent, the SLP's role of coach becomes one of supporting the parent to blend new skills with existing skills and to promote self-observation, self-evaluation, and self-reflection. Parents should leave the video feedback session with an increased sense of competence and with the ability to implement new strategies successfully. It is important for the SLP to listen carefully to parents' self-evaluation while watching the videotape because the parent's level of self-awareness determines the approach the SLP takes in the discussion that follows. For example, despite being coached to use a specific interactive behavior, a parent may still be unaware of exactly what was different after being coached. In this case, it is helpful for the SLP to juxtapose the two segments of the videotape and to facilitate a detailed analysis of the differences, with a focus on the differential impact on the child. The SLP pauses the videotape frequently, using a process of questioning and reflective listening to facilitate learning. When parents can clearly see the difference in the children's responsiveness and communication as a result of their own interactive behavior, their motivation to apply the strategy is far stronger. Sometimes, however, longstanding patterns of behavior are hard to change and parents express their frustration at how difficult it is to replace old habits with new ones. To help parents self-monitor their interactive behavior, the SLP explores with them the use of metacognitive strategies. These strategies, used as mental reminders, are designed to help parents monitor and adapt their interactive behavior. For example, a parent may decide to use the mental reminder, "Turn a question into a comment" to use comments instead of test questions. The SLP and parents then plan how the parents will remember to use this strategy and how to evaluate whether the strategy was used successfully. It is important for parents to be given the opportunity to identify instances of successful application of the strategies on the videotape so use of the strategy can be reinforced. Seeing the pleasure their child derives from interaction within a simple social routine or how repeated use of labeling enables the child to imitate a word for the first time is a powerful reinforcer for parents.

In celebrating successes with the parent, the SLP must ensure that parents attribute this success to their own efforts because a sense of competence and motivation are enhanced when learners attribute success to their own efforts and ability (Wlodkowski, 1993). For this reason, feedback should provide "knowledge of results" (Bruner, 1968), focusing on the specific changes made by parents and on the positive impact these have on their children (e.g., "I noticed that when you waited, Amanda initiated by offering you some of her drink"). This type of feedback is informational in that it allows learners to determine their progress and to appreciate their level of competence. Praise from the SLP, on the other hand, may be counterproductive. For example, saying, "You did a good job of waiting" may appear to be positive, but it fails to convey important information about how a specific behavior affected the child. In addition, praise has the potential to increase the parent's reliance on approval from the SLP, to reduce self-attribution, and to jeopardize the status of the parent as partner in the relationship with the clinician (Wlodkowski, 1993).

ASSESSMENT METHODS TO SUPPORT ONGOING DECISION MAKING

It Takes Two to Talk includes three video feedback consultations that provide opportunities for the SLP to determine the impact of the program on individual parents and children. Observations of parent–child interaction and discussions with the parents concerning the child's progress allow the clinician to initiate joint problem-solving discussions if required. For example, if the child is not motivated to initiate interaction when the parent waits expectantly, other means of enticing children to initiate may be explored, such as environmental manipulations that place desired objects in closed containers or out of the child's reach. Occasionally, additional facets of a child's communication disorder may emerge, adding to the clinician's knowledge of the underlying issues and suggesting alternative routes to treatment. For example, a child with age-appropriate receptive language skills may make no progress in vocabulary acquisition, suggesting a motor speech problem that may require differential diagnosis and a direct treatment model focusing on speech production.

Alternatively, parents may fail to make changes for a variety of reasons that were not apparent at the outset. The motivated parent skips evening sessions without explanation; the talkative parent becomes withdrawn and passive; the enthusiastic parent welcomes the clinician into the home expecting a hands-on therapy session while he or she does the laundry. Home visits permit the clinician to enter the family's environment and learn about some of the realities and stresses each family faces. Unfortunately, some parents will be unable to be their child's primary intervention agent. For these families, 1) expectations may be reduced so that the SLP focuses on helping parents learn just a few of the interactive strategies, or 2) intervention may be intensified so that parents receive more home visits to support their role. Some parents may drop out of the program either because they are unable to cope with its demands or because it may not meet their needs. Because children usually return to the caseload of the referring clinician at the end of It Takes Two to Talk, all children continue to be eligible for alternative service delivery models on an ongoing basis (e.g., consultation, group therapy, individual therapy).

CONSIDERATIONS FOR CHILDREN FROM CULTURALLY AND LINGUISTICALLY DIVERSE BACKGROUNDS

The previous edition of the guidebook *It Takes Two to Talk* (Manolson, 1992) has been translated into many languages (e.g., Chinese, Dutch, French, Hebrew, and Spanish) and is used in many non–English-speaking countries throughout the world. Despite its widespread use, there is a paucity of cross-cultural research on the suitability of specific strategies included in this intervention model for different linguistic and cultural groups. Extant cross-cultural studies of parent–child interactions suggest that the nature of parental language input is strongly influenced by social conventions, cultural values, and norms (van Kleeck, 1994). Consistent with this view, the most widely reported differences attributed to cultural variation involve verbal communicative behavior, such as the amount and type of responsive child-directed language input (Bornstein et al., 1998; Richman et al., 1988). For example, within English-speaking cultures (e.g., Australia, England, North America), contingent responsiveness (i.e., utterances that reflect the content of the child's preceding utterance or share the focus of the child's plan-of-the-moment) is variable and may constitute between 10% and 40% of child-directed speech. In contrast, in other cultural groups (e.g., village cultures in Guatemala and New Guinea), contingent responsiveness is largely nonexistent (Bohannon & Stanowicz, 1989; Nelson, Heimann, Abuelhaija, & Wroblewski, 1989). Thus, cross-cultural expectations may have an important and consistent impact on ways parents respond to their children's communicative attempts. van Kleeck (1994) summarizes additional dimensions of socialization along which parental language input may vary, including aspects of social organization, the value of talk, how status is handled in interactions, beliefs about intentionality, and beliefs about language teaching.

   A second, subtler source of variation reflects the specific linguistic features of the target language and has a significant impact on specific language modeling strategies that parents are taught in It Takes Two to Talk. In Korean, for example, the verb carries a great deal of information about the subject argument, and as a result, Korean child-directed language input teaches object and action labels concurrently (Gopnik, Choi, & Baumberger, 1996; Tardif, Shatz, & Naigles, 1997). In contrast, object categories are unequivocally marked in English; consequently, English language input focuses heavily on object naming. This has direct implications for parent instruction and goal setting for children entering the one-word stage of language development. Korean-speaking parents would use the labeling strategy primarily with action words, whereas English-speaking parents would label objects. This is one subtle example of how direct translation of parent materials and strategies derived for English-speaking families may result in a mismatch with the linguistic features of a different language.

Our understanding of how the interactive model of language intervention applies to different linguistic and cultural groups is still in its infancy. Future research is needed to disentangle the influences of linguistic structure and culture on parental language input before we advocate wholesale adoption of this intervention practice to other cultural groups. Until such research is available, translated versions of It Takes Two to Talk should be used cautiously and only if the clinician and parent both understand and accept that this intervention promotes linguistic and cultural values that may not be consistent with the language and culture of the target child. van Kleeck (1994) recommends that a mainstream program can be altered to fit a family from a different cultural background through frequent and frank discussions of the interaction strategy being recommended and the cultural beliefs from which it is derived. In this way, parents may be freer to select the strategies that work best in their family context.

APPLICATION TO AN INDIVIDUAL CHILD

To illustrate the changes made by parents and children who participated in It Takes Two to Talk, the case of Joshua, a 27-month-old boy, and his family is used.

Preprogram Assessment

During the initial case history interview, Joshua's mother reported that Joshua had a small vocabulary, gestured to communicate his needs, did not imitate words, and had limited pretend play. She also noted that Joshua was often frustrated and lapsed into tantrums when he could not communicate his needs. A family history indicated that Joshua's older brother had been diagnosed with mild learning disabilities and an older sister with attention-deficit/hyperactivity disorder. According to his mother, Joshua's hearing was tested and found to be within normal limits.

Following the parent interview, the SLP videotaped a 5-minute mother–child play interaction. During this interaction, the SLP noted that Joshua's agenda did not include a play partner. Consequently, he did not share joint attention, respond to his mother's questions, or take conversational turns. His mother monitored his play carefully, commented on his ongoing actions, and had a positive manner of interacting with him. However, her strategies to engage Joshua in interaction included 1) asking many test questions that went unanswered and 2) using long and complex utterances to suggest play ideas. Following the videotaped interaction, the clinician asked Joshua's mother to complete the CDIs. Joshua's vocabulary size was 34 words, which was below the 5th percentile for his age group.

Participation in the It Takes Two to Talk Program

Joshua's parents attended all eight evening sessions, although only his mother was present during the assessments and the three video feedback sessions that were conducted in the home. During the first video feedback session, the SLP asked Joshua's mother what she wanted Joshua to learn. She said she wanted him to play with her (as opposed to playing while she watched) and use more words. The SLP suggested that that Joshua would be more likely to learn new words if he was exposed to them during conversational exchanges. Therefore, the objectives of the first video feedback session were to increase Joshua's initiations and the number of turns he took once an interaction began. Joshua's mother was encouraged to 1) pause and wait to encourage Joshua to initiate and 2) respond to Joshua's initiations by imitating, interpreting, or commenting. The SLP helped Joshua's mother accomplish these objectives by stopping the camera and coaching as the activity unfolded. She reminded Joshua's mother to wait expectantly so that Joshua got the message that he was expected to communicate. Joshua did not communicate verbally during this video feedback session, but he initiated far more frequently than in the pretest, using gestures and vocalizations. In evaluating the videotape, Joshua's mother commented that she was surprised to find that pausing and waiting "with anticipation" often resulted in an initiation on Joshua's part (e.g., showing his mother a toy or requesting more) and that she didn't have to work so hard to get him to interact with her. They then discussed in which situations Joshua's mother would make an effort to wait for him to initiate and then imitate, interpret, and comment. They agreed that she would focus on bath time and breakfast and report back at the next evening session.

Because Joshua and his mother were having extended interactions by the second video feedback session, the SLP and Joshua's mother selected 10 target words using the CDIs as a guide. The objective was to help Joshua's mother use focused repetition of these words during a daily routine. With some coaching, Joshua's mother successfully emphasized the words "water," "cup," and "drink" repetitively during a hand-washing routine at the kitchen sink. Later, while observing her videotape, Joshua's mother stated that she felt clearer about the focused stimulation strategy and realized that she could model more than one word in an activity. Joshua did not imitate any words or communicate intentionally during the activity, but he enjoyed the water play and heard many focused repetitions of words that matched his plan-of-the-moment. The SLP suggested that Joshua's mother post signs with the words she was targeting around the house as reminders to use them repetitively.

The third video feedback session focused on strategies to 1) expand on the child's utterances, 2) extend the topic of the child's utterances, and 3) ask questions that maintained longer turn-taking episodes. During a play-dough activity, Joshua interacted frequently with his mother and spontaneously used the words "car," "more," and "spoon." His mother expanded some of these words into short sentences on his topic. She also asked questions that were responsive to his play and were followed by pauses to give Joshua a chance to respond. In reviewing the videotape, the SLP and Joshua's mother focused on increasing the use of expansions. Finally, Joshua's mother and the clinician selected several replacement words for those he used spontaneously.

Postprogram Assessment

A postprogram assessment was conducted 2 weeks after the final program session, when Joshua was 31 months old. In the postintervention videotape, Joshua's mother imitated and interpreted his vocalizations and actions often. She joined in his play and was able to establish long episodes of joint attention by following his lead. She used responsive labeling more frequently and used shorter comments to describe his actions. Because Joshua produced more words during this interaction, his mother was able to expand his utterances frequently. Overall, in comparison with those before taping, the mother–child interaction was more synchronous and Joshua demonstrated greater use of words, more purposeful joint play, and the ability to initiate and respond during conversational turns. A review of Joshua's postprogram CDIs revealed that he acquired 86 new words, showed evidence of word combining, and had begun to use some early morphemes during the 11-week program.

FUTURE DIRECTIONS

Future investigations of the social interactionist model of language intervention are necessary to confirm its usefulness for children with diverse etiologies, for caregivers in different settings (e.g., preschool, child care), and for families from different linguistic and cultural groups. The first thrust of future research projects will be to investigate outcomes for children who have different etiologies. At present, it is unknown whether the focused stimulation version of It Takes Two to Talk is effective for preschool children with receptive and/or expressive language disorders. A replication study to confirm and extend the findings of the focused stimulation version with children who have cognitive and developmental delays would further contribute to our knowledge of this program's effects on language abilities of these children. In addition, studies are needed also determine the efficacy of More Than Words, the adaptation used with families of children with autism spectrum disorders. Future projects will progress from the general question that has motivated past research (i.e., Does "It Takes Two to Talk" work?) to determining the long-term impact of parent training and the relative contributions of various components of the service delivery model (e.g., Is parent-focused intervention more effective when administered individually or in groups?). Increasingly, more children are spending the majority of their day with nonparental caregivers. Therefore, a second research thrust involves training other child care providers to use language facilitation strategies. Currently, the efficacy of Learning Language and Loving It, the adaptation for preschool settings, has been investigated for child care staff and children who are developing normally (Girolametto, Weitzman, & Greenberg, 2003). A follow-up study of this in-service training within integrated preschool settings is required in order to determine the impact on the communication and peer interaction skills of children with language and/or developmental disorders. Finally, a third research thrust concerns the need to identify international partners to complete cross-cultural evaluations of the social interactive model of language intervention. An initial study comparing Italian-speaking with English-speaking mothers has been completed (Girolametto et al., 2002), and successive comparisons for other cultures are required in order to determine the validity of translated versions of It Takes Two to Talk.

RECOMMENDED READINGS

Girolametto, L., Weitzman, E., & Greenberg, J. (2003). Training day care staff to facilitate children's language. *American Journal of Speech-Language Pathology, 12*, 299–311.

Girolametto, L., Weitzman, E., Wiigs, M., & Pearce, P.S. (2000). The relationship between maternal language measures and language development in toddlers with expressive vocabulary delays. *American Journal of Speech-Language Pathology, 8*, 364–374.

Sussman, F. (2000). *More than words: Helping parents promote communication and social skills in children with autism spectrum disorder*. Toronto: The Hanen Centre.

Tannock, R., & Girolametto, L. (1992). Reassessing parent-focused language intervention programs. In S.F. Warren & J. Reichle (Series & Vol. Eds.), *Communication and language intervention series: Vol. 1. Causes and effects in communication and language intervention* (pp. 49–80). Baltimore: Paul H. Brookes Publishing Co.

Weitzman, E., & Greenberg, J. (2002). *Learning language and loving it: A guide to promoting children's social, language, and literacy development in early childhood settings* (2nd ed.). Toronto: The Hanen Centre.

REFERENCES

Achenbach, T., & Edelbrock, C. (1983). *Child Behavior Checklist*. Burlington, VT: University Associates in Psychiatry.

Bohannon, J., & Bonvillian, J. (1997). Theoretical approaches to language acquisition. In J. Berko Gleason (Ed.), *The development of language* (4th ed., pp. 259–316). Boston: Allyn & Bacon.

Bohannon, J., & Stanowicz, L. (1989). Bidirectional effects of imitation and repetition in conversation: A synthesis within a cognitive model. In G. Speidel & K. Nelson (Eds.), *The many faces of imitation in language learning* (pp. 121–150). New York: Springer.

Bornstein, M., Haynes, O., Azuma, H., Galperin, C., Maital, S., Ogino, M., et al. (1998). A cross-national study of self-evaluations and attributions in parenting: Argentina, Belgium, France, Israel, Italy, Japan, and the United States. *Developmental Psychology, 34*, 662–676.

Bronfenbrenner, U. (1974). *Is early intervention effective?* (Publication No. CDH 74–25). Washington, DC: Department of Health, Education, and Welfare, Office of Child Development.

Brown, W., Thurman, S.K., & Pearl, L.F. (1993). *Family-centered early intervention with infants and toddlers: Innovative cross-disciplinary approaches.* Baltimore: Paul H. Brookes Publishing Co.

Bruner, J. (1968). *Toward a theory of instruction.* New York: W.W. Norton.

Bruner, J. (1983). *Child's talk: Learning to use language.* Oxford, England: Oxford University Press.

Conti-Ramsden, G. (1994). Interaction with atypical learners. In C. Gallaway & B.J. Richards (Eds.), *Input and interaction in language acquisition* (pp. 183–196). Cambridge, England: Cambridge University Press.

Crnic, K., & Stormshak, E. (1997). The effectiveness of providing social support for families of children at risk. In M.J. Guralnick (Ed.), *The effectiveness of early intervention* (pp. 209–226). Baltimore: Paul H. Brookes Publishing Co.

Cross, T. (1977). Mother's speech adjustments: The contributions of selected child listener variables. In C. Snow & C. Ferguson (Eds.), *Talking to children: Language input and acquisition* (pp. 157–188). Cambridge, MA: Cambridge University Press.

Cross, T. (1981). Parental speech as primary linguistic data: Some complexities in the study of the effect of the input in language acquisition. In P.S. Dale & D. Ingram (Eds.), *Child language: An interactional perspective* (pp. 215–228). Baltimore: University Park Press.

Dinmore, I. (1997). Interdisciplinarity and integrative learning: An imperative for adult education. *Education, 117*, 452–477.

Donahue-Kilburg, G. (1992). *Family-centered early intervention for communication disorders.* Gaithersburg, MD: Aspen.

Dunst, C., Trivette, C., & Deal, A.G. (1988). *Enabling and empowering families: Principles and guidelines for practice.* Cambridge, MA: Brookline Books.

Dunst, C., Trivette, C., Humphries, T., Raab, M., & Roper, N. (2001). Contrasting approaches to natural learning environment interventions. *Infants and Young Children, 14(2)*, 48–63.

Fenson, L., Dale, P., Reznick, S., Thal, D., Bates, E., Hartung, J., Pethick, S., & Reilly, J. (1993). *The MacArthur-Bates Communicative Development Inventories: User's guide and technical manual.* Baltimore: Paul H. Brookes Publishing Co.

Girolametto, L. (1988). Improving the social-conversational skills of developmentally delayed children: An intervention study. *Journal of Speech and Hearing Disorders, 53*, 156–167.

Girolametto, L., Bonifacio, S., Visini, C., Weitzman, E., Zocconi, E., & Pearce, P.S. (2002). Mother-child interactions in Canada and Italy: Linguistic responsiveness to late-talking toddlers. *International Journal of Communication and Language Disorders, 37*, 153–171.

Girolametto, L., Pearce, P., & Weitzman, E. (1996a). The effects of focused stimulation for promoting vocabulary in children with delays: A pilot study. *Journal of Childhood Communication Development, 17*, 39–49.

Girolametto, L., Pearce, P., & Weitzman, E. (1996b). Interactive focused stimulation for toddlers with expressive vocabulary delays. *Journal of Speech and Hearing Research, 39,* 1274–1283.

Girolametto, L., Pearce, P., & Weitzman, E. (1997). Effects of lexical intervention on the phonology of late talkers. *Journal of Speech, Language, and Hearing Research, 40,* 338–348.

Girolametto, L., Sparks, B., Weitzman, E., & Pearce, P.S. (2003). *The effects of language intervention on the play and behaviour competencies of late talkers.* Unpublished manuscript, University of Toronto, Toronto.

Girolametto, L., Tannock, R., & Siegel, L. (1993). Consumer-oriented evaluation of interactive language intervention. *American Journal of Speech-Language Pathology, 2,* 41–51.

Girolametto, L., Weitzman, E., & Clements-Baartman, J. (1998). Vocabulary intervention for children with Down syndrome: Parent training using focused stimulation. *Infant-Toddler Intervention: A Transdisciplinary Journal, 8,* 109–126.

Girolametto, L., Weitzman, E., & Greenberg, J. (2003). Training day care staff to facilitate children's language. *American Journal of Speech-Language Pathology, 12,* 299–311.

Gopnik, A., Choi, S., & Baumberger, T. (1996). Cross-linguistic differences in early semantic and cognitive development. *Cognitive Development, 11,* 197–227.

Kaiser, A., & Hancock, T. (2003). Teaching parents new skills to support their young children's development. *Infants and Young Children, 16,* 9–21.

Manolson, A. (1992). *It Takes Two to Talk.* Toronto: The Hanen Centre.

Manolson, H.A., Ward, B., & Dodington, N. (1995). *You make the difference in helping your child learn.* Toronto: The Hanen Centre.

McCarthy, B. (1987). *The 4MAT system: Teaching to learning styles with right/left mode techniques.* Barrington, IL: EXCEL.

McLean, L.K., & Woods-Cripe, J.W. (1997). The effectiveness of early intervention for children with communication disorders. In M.J. Guralnick (Ed.), *The effectiveness of early intervention* (pp. 349–428). Baltimore: Paul H. Brookes Publishing Co.

Nelson, K., Heimann, M., Abuelhaija, L., & Wroblewski, R. (1989). Implications for language acquisition models of children's and parents' variations in imitation. In G. Speidel & K. Nelson (Eds.), *The many faces of imitation in language learning* (pp. 305–323). New York: Springer.

Pearce, P., Girolametto, L., & Weitzman, E. (1996). The effects of focused stimulation intervention on mothers of late-talking toddlers. *Infant-Toddler Intervention, 6,* 213–227.

Pepper, J., & Weitzman, E. (2004). *It Takes Two to Talk: A practical guide for parents of children with language delays* (2nd ed.). Toronto: The Hanen Centre.

Pepper, J., Weitzman, E., & McDade, A. (2004). *Making Hanen happen: It Takes Two to Talk—The Hanen Program for Parents. Leader's guide for Hanen certified speech-language pathologists.* Toronto: The Hanen Centre.

Pine, J. (1994). The language of primary caregivers. In C. Gallaway & B.J. Richards (Eds.), *Input and interaction in language acquisition* (pp. 15–37). Cambridge, England: Cambridge University Press.

Richards, B. (1994). Child-directed speech and influences on language acquisition: Methodology and interpretation. In C. Gallaway & B.J. Richards (Eds.), *Input and interaction in language acquisition* (pp. 74–104). Cambridge, England: Cambridge University Press.

Richman, A., LeVine, R., Staples New, R., Howrigan, G., Welles-Nystrom, B., & LeVine, S. (1988). Maternal behavior to infants in five cultures. In W. Damon (Series Ed.) & R. LeVine & M. West (Vol. Eds.), *New directions in child development: Vol. 40. Parental behavior in diverse societies* (pp. 81–97). San Francisco: Jossey-Bass.

Rocissano, L., & Yatchmink, Y. (1983). Joint attention in mother-toddler interaction: A study of individual variation. *Merrill-Palmer Quarterly, 30,* 11–31.

Rogers, C.R. (1961). *On becoming a person: A therapist's view of psychotherapy.* Boston: Houghton Mifflin.

Rossetti, L. (1990). *The Rossetti Infant–Toddler Language Scale: A measure of communication and interaction.* East Moline, IL: LinguiSystems.

Rossetti, L.M. (2001). *Communication intervention: Birth to three.* San Diego: Singular Publishing Group.

Sheldon, M.L., & Rush, D.D. (2001). The ten myths about providing early intervention services in natural environments. *Infants and Young Children, 14(1),* 1–13.

Snow, C. (1994). Beginning from baby talk: Twenty years of research on input in interaction. In C. Gallaway & B.J. Richards (Eds.), *Input and interaction in language acquisition* (pp. 1–12). Cambridge, England: Cambridge University Press.

Snow, C., & Ferguson, C. (Eds.). (1978). *Talking to children.* London: Cambridge University Press.

Tannock, R., & Girolametto, L. (1992). Reassessing parent-focused language intervention programs. In S.F. Warren & J. Reichle (Series & Vol. Eds.), *Communication and language intervention series: Vol. 1. Causes and effects in communication and language intervention* (pp. 49–80). Baltimore: Paul H. Brookes Publishing Co.

Tannock, R., Girolametto, L., & Siegel, L. (1992). Language intervention with children who have developmental delays: Effects of an interactive approach. *American Journal of Mental Retardation, 97,* 145–160.

Tardif, T., Shatz, M., & Naigles, L. (1997). Caregiver speech and children's use of nouns versus verbs: A comparison of English, Italian, and Mandarin. *Journal of Child Language, 24,* 535–565.

van Kleeck, A. (1994). Potential cultural bias in training parents as conversational partners with their children who have delays in language development. *American Journal of Speech-Language Pathology, 3,* 67–78.

Vygotsky, L. (1978). *Mind in society.* Cambridge, MA: Harvard University Press.

Watson, C. (1995, Winter). One language or two? Helping families from other cultures decide how to talk to their language delayed child. *WigWag,* 3–9.

Weistuch, L., & Brown, B. (1987). Motherese as therapy: A program and its dissemination. *Child Language: Teaching and Therapy, 3,* 58–71.

Weistuch, L., & Lewis, M. (1986, April). *Effect of maternal language intervention strategies on the language abilities of delayed two- to four-year-olds.* Paper presented at the Eastern Psychological Association, New York.

Weistuch, L., Lewis, M., & Sullivan, M. (1991). Project profile: Use of a language interaction intervention in the preschools. *Journal of Early Intervention, 15,* 278–287.

Wlodkowski, R.J. (1993). *Enhancing adult motivation to learn: A guide to improving instruction and increasing learner achievement.* San Francisco: Jossey-Bass.

Zimmerman, I.L., Steiner, V.G., & Pond, R.E. (1992). *Preschool Language Scale–3 (PLS-3).* San Antonio, TX: Harcourt Assessment.

4

Appendix

It Takes Two to Talk—The Hanen Program for Parents:
Program Schedule and Content

Week	Session, chapter, and title	Content
1	Group evening session 1: Let your child lead	Stages of communication development are explained and parents learn to describe how (e.g., words, gestures, vocalizations) and why (e.g., to request, label, comment) their child communicates. Parents learn to wait for their child to initiate an interaction and to then respond sensitively.
2	Group evening session 2: Follow your child's lead	Parents learn to follow their child's lead by 1) joining in and playing, 2) imitating what the child says/does, 3) interpreting the child's message, and 4) commenting on the child's focus.
3	Video feedback session 1	Videotaping of parent–child interaction in the home (or center)
4	Group evening session 3: Take turns to keep the interaction going	Parents learn interaction-promoting strategies to support conversational turn taking, such as 1) matching their turns to their child's turn, 2) asking questions to encourage conversation, and 3) using everyday and play routines.
5	Group evening session 4: Add language to the interaction	Parents learn to model language at their child's level by 1) labeling what the child is focused on, and 2) expanding the child's words (i.e., by adding a syntactic or semantic element).
6	Video feedback session 2	Videotaping of parent–child interaction in the home (or center)
7	Group evening session 5: Add language to build understanding	Parents learn to promote their child's receptive language by using more decontextualized language when commenting on the child's activity or topic. Parents also learn how to choose specific communication goals and set up obligatory contexts for their use.
8	Group evening session 6: Let's play!	The stages of play development are described. Parents learn to use play as a context for facilitating general language development and the use of their child's specific communication goals.

Week	Session, chapter, and title	Content
9	Group evening session 7: Sharing books	Parents are taught to use books in an interactive manner to facilitate general language development as well as their child's specific communication goals.
10	Video feedback session 3	Videotaping of parent–child interaction in the home (or center)
11	Group evening session 8: Moving forward with music and program review	Parents learn to use music and songs to facilitate their child's general language development and use of specific communication goals. This final evening session also includes a review of the program strategies.

5

The Picture Exchange Communication System

A Nonverbal Communication Program
for Children with Autism Spectrum Disorders

MARJORIE H. CHARLOP-CHRISTY AND CATHLEEN JONES

ABSTRACT

In the Picture Exchange Communication System (PECS), children are taught functional communication using a picture-based augmentative and alternative communication (AAC) system. Using a system of modeling and decreasing prompts, children move from using pictures to request desired objects to more elaborate communications that may include written language. PECS has primarily been used for children with autism spectrum disorders as well as other severe communication deficits. With few prerequisite requirements, it is seen as particularly promising for children who rarely initiate communication. Its clinical application is broadening to include other populations, and its empirical base has expanded but still consists primarily of case studies and single-subject experimental designs.

INTRODUCTION

The Picture Exchange Communication System (PECS) is an augmentative and alternative communication (AAC) program in which a pictorial system is used for children with autism spectrum disorders and other severe social-communication deficits (Frost & Bondy, 1994). PECS uses basic behavioral principles to teach children functional communication using pictures (black-and-white or color drawings). The first communicative behaviors taught are *mands,* which are words or phrases that specify a reinforcer (e.g., "I want *juice*"). This teaches the child from the outset that communication is functional. Thus, the child learns to communicate because 1) the picture system and the delivery of representational cards for desired items represent a theoretically easier way to communicate than the complex creation of speech, 2) there is a functional and motivational relationship between the communicative act and the retrieval of the desired item, and 3) there is a resulting increased likelihood for spontaneity of communication and continued use (Frost & Bondy 1994; Skinner, 1957).

TARGET POPULATIONS AND ASSESSMENTS
FOR DETERMINING TREATMENT RELEVANCE AND GOALS

There is no formal assessment for deciding who should or should not be taught PECS. The literature on autism has suggested that the children who have acquired speech by the age of 5 years have a better prognosis than children who have not (e.g., Schreibman, 1988). That is, researchers believe that there is a window of opportunity in teaching children with autism, including communication, and that this window occurs before the age of 5 years. The "window" may reflect neuroplasticity of the brain and the ability to learn or make up for what was not learned at developmentally typical ages (e.g., Schreibman, 1988). It has been estimated that 80% of children younger than age 5 years who have a diagnosis of autism do not speak (Bondy & Frost, 1994). This makes the need to teach communication, including communication through speech, imperative. However, the decision to use PECS is controversial.

Bondy and Frost (1994), the creators of PECS, have been fielding criticism that PECS training should be delayed with an individual child until it can be determined that speech is unlikely to emerge or that speech interventions have not been successful. Indeed, a major concern appears to be that the use of PECS will stifle speech development. However, some studies point to subsequent increases in spontaneous speech related to the use of PECS, especially after certain phases (e.g., Bondy & Frost, 1994; Charlop-Christy, Carpenter, Le, LeBlanc, and Kellet, 2002). Charlop-Christy et al. (2002) argued that children should be taught PECS along with traditional speech intervention while more data are being collected to address this question. To determine treatment relevance, then, one should examine the child's progress with traditional speech interventions.

There is a large body of evidence connecting the inability to communicate and the occurrence of behavior problems such as self-injury, aggression, tantrums, and other behaviors that are extremely difficult to treat (e.g., Carr & Durand, 1985). The research on functional communication has shown that when a child has a mechanism to use for communication, whether it is a manual sign, a spoken word, or another method, it can replace the function of the behavior problem and thus decrease or eliminate its occurrence (see also Chapter 19). Children who are nonverbal and display little or no functional communication skills but have severe inappropriate behaviors may be good candidates for PECS (Charlop-Christy, LaBelle, & Jones, 2004).

There are very few prerequisites to PECS training, which makes PECS a highly desirable procedure to teach communication skills. At the beginning of training, a child should simply be able to sit and attend to a two-dimensional stimulus and have the physical ability to hand it to a communicative partner. Whereas many other communication training procedures require eye contact, verbal and/or motor imitation, and match-to-sample skills, PECS does not have these prerequisites (Bondy & Frost, 1994).

THEORETICAL BASIS

The development of PECS was based less on theoretical constructs and more on pragmatics and the observation that children with autism spectrum disorders were not fully benefiting from the existing communication paradigms (Bondy & Frost, 1994). Notwithstanding this fact, there is a coherent set of principles underlying the system. Bondy and Frost (1994) designed PECS to meet these principles. First, the communication system needed to be concrete and representative of the real world. The more concrete or iconic the stimuli (in this case, picture cards), the more easily the task may be learned (Schreibman, 1988). Second, PECS was designed to teach, from the outset, functional communication by teaching mands (requests) before tacts (comments, labels). The child learns from the start of training that communication is meaningful to him or her because the result is the acquisition of a desired item. This makes communication motivating, meaningful, and functional for the child, thus increasing the likelihood that communication will occur again (Skinner, 1957). This is in contrast to the majority of traditional speech paradigms (e.g., Schreibman, 1988). Third, there is a focus on spontaneity in the early phases of PECS by incorporating a time-delay prompt (e.g., Charlop, Schreibman, & Thibodeau, 1985; Charlop & Trasowech, 1991), which increases the likelihood of prompt independence and independent use of PECS. Finally, unlike most other approaches, PECS does not require eye contact (the child does not need to look at the teacher) or imitation (the child does not need to mimic the teacher's behavior).

There are two additional features of PECS that theoretically make it more desirable than other approaches for children with autism spectrum disorders. These are its representation in the visual rather than the auditory modality and its use of communication units that are constant rather than transient in duration.

Communication and the Visual Modality

Since Leo Kanner (1943) first diagnosed a child with autism, it has been well known that these children display great deficits in verbal skills yet may show normal to advanced skills on certain visual tasks such as the Sequin Form Board and other types of puzzle tasks (Peterson, Bondy, Vincent, & Finnegan, 1995; Rimland, 1964; Schreibman, 1988). This discrepancy in visual and verbal skills also has been documented empirically, not just through observation and diagnosis. For example, Peterson and colleagues (1995) assessed

33 individuals with autism (ages 8–29 years) using the Wechsler Intelligence Scale for Children–Revised (WISC-R; Wechsler, 1974) or the Wechsler Adult Intelligence Scale–Revised (WAIS-R; Wechsler, 1981). They found that individuals with autism with a mean IQ score of 76 performed most poorly on the Comprehension subtest, which requires the most verbal reasoning, and best on the Block Design and Object Assembly subtests, which require the most visual skills.

In some cases, samples from individuals with autism did not differ from normal control samples on visual tests, but they did differ on verbal tests. Rumsey and Hamburger (1988) compared men with histories of autism and average verbal and nonverbal intelligence with normal controls on various neuropsychological tests that assess language and visual-perceptual measures. They found that, although the men with autism presented lower scores on the language measures, there were no between-group differences on the visual-perceptual measures.

Ozonoff, Pennington, and Rogers (1991) examined the skills of 23 individuals with autism (ages 8–20 years) with IQs greater than 69. These individuals were matched to controls on IQ, age, sex, and socioeconomic status. Ozonoff et al. (1991) presented the participants with a wide variety of tasks and found that the individuals with autism presented lower scores on verbal memory tests, but there were no between-group differences on the visual tasks. Again, individuals with autism showed deficits in verbal skills but no deficits in visual skills.

Minshew and colleagues (1997) also compared 33 adolescents and young adults with autism with 33 matched controls. All of the participants had IQs greater than 80 and were given a complete neuropsychological test battery. Minshew et al. found that the individuals with autism exhibited impairments in some language domains (i.e., complex language) but not in any visuospatial domains (in which they sometimes presented higher abilities than controls).

Further evidence for the efficacious use of a visually based communication system for children with autism can be derived from observations about very early language development in children who are developing typically. A reliance on visual information is also found in typically developing children, most notably in the first year (e.g., Fagan, 1971). The visual system is an important means for typically developing infants to perceive and understand the world. Visual means are used more extensively than verbal means during the first months of children's lives (Fagan, 1971). For example, a typically developing infant will see a bottle and recognize that it indicates food before they hear and recognize the word "bottle" as an indicator of food. Typically developing children also utilize visual means of communication (gestures) before they utilize verbal means of communication (speech). As children develop typically, verbal means of acquiring and sending information become more important (Rosinski, Pellegrino, & Siegel, 1977). This development does not seem to occur in children with autism (e.g., Charlop & Haymes, 1994; Schreibman, 1988).

It is likely that treatments that incorporate visual representations have been successful due to their reliance on visual information (Schuler & Baldwin, 1981). Bondy and Frost (1994) took advantage of this tendency to learn visually. After years of auditory-based verbal speech paradigms, PECS was designed to focus on the visual modality.

Communication and Duration of the Stimulus

Communication in the visual modality, however, does not ensure that communication stimulus will have a lasting representation. We believe that there are three major modalities of communication training. They are the *auditory-transient, visual-transient,* and *visual-constant* modalities. The auditory-transient modality includes speech as its primary example, because the physical properties of the signal do not persist through time. Words are spoken and then gone. The child with autism needs to attend or "hear" speech, remember it, and then figure out its meaning. It is not a permanent signal. The second type of communication is visual-transient communication in which information is presented visually (it is to be seen) but the representations do not persist through time. Sign language is an example of this visual-transient mode of communication because the body movements used in sign are presented visually but are not long lasting. The child with autism must attend to the sign language, remember it, and figure out what it means. The assumption here is that this modality may reflect the same level of complexity as the auditory-transient modality for children with autism. The third type of communication modality is the visual-constant mode in which communication representations are presented visually and persist through time (constant display). Many forms of AAC—for example, those using the written word—provide examples of a visual-constant mode of communication because the signals are presented visually and are displayed permanently (Quill, 1995). PECS would fall into this category as well. See Table 5.1 for clarification of the modalities and examples.

The visual-constant modality employed by PECS would appear to have definite advantages for children with autism spectrum disorder. When children use the visual-perceptual mechanism, they must still remember what was seen and then ascribe meaning to the previously presented visual stimulus. In visual-constant modalities, the information persists (i.e., the picture cards of PECS are always present, first used in the child's possession, then used in a communicative act, and finally replaced on the PECS notebook). The constant display may serve as a memory aid as well as enhance the acquisition of meaning.

Table 5.1. Different types of presentation formats within communication programs and the manner in which they are perceived

	Presentation format		
	Auditory-transient	Visual-transient	Visual-constant
Stimulus duration	Transient	Transient	Constant (permanent)
Perceptual mechanism	Hearing	Sight	Sight
Examples	Speech, computer-generated vocal-izations	Gestures, sign language	Orthography, picture-point, voice-output communication aids (VOCAs), Picture Exchange Communication System (PECS)

EMPIRICAL BASIS

PECS has grown in popularity prior to its exposure to empirical investigation and experimental validation. Indeed, international popularity may be related to its use of picture cards, which are clear and universally understood. In this section, we summarize and critique the literature on PECS, including several reports and informational articles as well as four experimental investigations. Taken together, these studies constitute the beginnings of a body of scientific evidence to support this intervention. At the end of this section, we demonstrate the varied uses of PECS.

Informational Reports

Several informational reports indicate that children all along the autism spectrum can learn PECS. In the instruction manual for PECS, Bondy and Frost (1994) reported positive outcomes for 85 children who were taught to use PECS. These children were diagnosed with autism spectrum disorder and participated in the Delaware Autistic Program, the public school special education system for children with this diagnosis in the state of Delaware. The children were all between the ages of 2 and 5 years and all displayed severe speech and language deficits and had no means of consistent communication other than gestures. None of the children in this sample was echolalic, although PECS has been effective with children who use echolalia (Bondy & Frost, 1994). For the 66 children who used PECS for more than 1 year, more than 50% acquired speech as their sole communication modality and another 29% combined PECS and speech use. Although these initial children's outcomes provided encouragement for the use of PECS, there are many cautions when incorporating this information as clear evidence supporting PECS. Little descriptive information is provided for the children other than their speech status, age, and diagnosis of autism. Indeed, it was later reported by Frost and Bondy (1994) that successful acquisition and use of PECS may be related to mental age at the time of beginning PECS. It is important to note that these participants were taught PECS based on their individualized education program (IEP) and thus were not part of a formal, controlled study.

Schwartz, Garfinkle, and Bauer (1998) taught PECS to preschool children with autism and other developmental disabilities in an integrated classroom setup. Some of the 18 children produced a very limited amount of speech, whereas the remainder of the children produced no speech at all. The authors reported that the children increased their PECS use, and those who initially had a limited spontaneous vocal repertoire increased spontaneous language following PECS training. However, those children with no initial spontaneous vocalizations did not make gains in vocal behavior. Bondy and Frost (1993) describe the procedures used to train school-based staff in Peru to use the system over a 5-day period. Although no formal data were collected, the school reported that during a 3-month period, approximately 74 children began the PECS training procedures and many children had progressed to the second training phase. That means the children were at least communicating spontaneously by handing over the picture of the desired item.

Anecdotal reports have indicated that the use of PECS may result in a decrease in maladaptive behavior (Peterson et al., 1995). The relationship between lack of communication and inappropriate behaviors is well documented (e.g., Carr & Durand, 1985; Durand & Carr, 1991; Hagopian, Fisher, Thibault-Sullivan, Acquisto, & LeBlanc, 1998; Chapter 19).

Bondy and Frost (1994) examined scores on the Autism Behavior Checklist (Krug, Arik, & Almond, 1980) before and after intervention for three groups of children: speech only, PECS use, and combined speech and PECS. All children demonstrated some reduction in problem behavior, but no specific data or statistical results were provided. Peterson et al. (1995) provided a case report of one child with autism who exhibited decreased levels of self-injurious behavior while using a picture-based communication system compared with using spoken language only. It is important to note that none of these reports has included an experimental research design to eliminate potential confounds such as maturation effects. That is, because measures were taken before and after the academic year, treatment gains could be attributed to a number of factors other than PECS. Specific operational definitions prevent us from gaining a better understanding of the changes reported in the studies. For example, *speech* could mean one or two unclear attempts at uttering a word or it could mean a clear statement of the sentence strip, "I want Cheetos." The term *spontaneous speech* is often defined differently, and in some studies it may actually be "reading" the sentence strip. In addition, we only have general information as to what the children were like.

The majority of this initial information on PECS had been based on its use in the Delaware Autistic Program, the statewide special education program in the public school system. However, these reports have been anecdotal and lack empirical manipulations, such as control groups or the utilization of single-subject experimental methodology.

Experimental Investigations

In the first experimental investigation of PECS, we used a multiple baseline design across subjects to assess the efficacy of PECS with three children with autism (Charlop-Christy et al., 2002). A multiple baseline across subjects design staggers the onset of implementation of treatment across subjects and, therefore, controls for many confounding variables. It is one of the preferred designs for behavioral research with children with autism (e.g., Miltenberger, 1997). Other multiple baseline designs often used include multiple baseline design across settings and multiple baseline design across behaviors. With multiple baseline design across settings, we intervene in one setting at a time for a child, with length of baselines in other settings staggered; with multiple baseline design across behaviors, we intervene for one behavior at a time. In the Charlop-Christy et al. study, one child was presented with the PECS intervention after his baseline, while the other two children remained in baseline. When the second child was presented with the intervention, the third child still remained in baseline. Thus, treatment delivery occurred at three different times, eliminating many threats to internal validity.

In the Charlop-Christy et al. (2002) study, two of the children could imitate merely a few sounds or words and rarely used speech to spontaneously request items prior to the intervention, despite intensive speech treatments. One child was able to imitate a few sounds, but exhibited no spontaneous speech. Baseline was a continuation of traditional procedures of speech-language intervention. The children failed to make gains during baseline. However, when treatment was implemented, the children all learned PECS in a relatively short period of time (less than 200 minutes of direct intervention time). All three children were able to communicate using PECS more frequently and spontaneously than they had using speech. It is important to note that the children also demonstrated concomitant increases in social behaviors, decreases in maladaptive behaviors, and increases in speech following PECS training. These data are promising not only because they were obtained within an experimental design, but also because improvements in communication were accompanied by positive changes outside the communication domain.

Using a multiple baseline design across settings, Kravits, Kamps, Kemmerer, and Potucek (2002) taught a 6-year-old girl with autism to use PECS. For each of four settings, setting-specific icons were taught and later tested for independent use in that setting. The child effectively communicated her setting-specific requests via PECS.

Additional data are being collected in our research program addressing a variety of uses of PECS. We have used PECS as a means to directly decrease problem behaviors (Charlop-Christy et al., 2004). In this study, five children with autism with no speech were taught to communicate via PECS.

Additionally, as their data on PECS acquisition were collected, data on problem behaviors such as tantrums, aggression, and self-stimulation were also kept. We used a multiple baseline design across children, with a reversal within each child, to see if PECS could be used in lieu of the problem behavior to take the function of a problem behavior. That is, when children used aggression to escape work, we taught them to use an appropriate written PECS sentence, such as "I want break," instead of becoming aggressive when they wanted to cease work for a while.

We have also used PECS to teach communication through the use of written words (Charlop-Christy & Daneshvar, 2004; Charlop-Christy & Werner, 2004). In these studies, we first examined whether the children even noticed that a written label of the icon appeared on the PECS card. The children in both studies failed to respond to the separate presentation of the written word after being trained on PECS. Then, a Multiple Cue Training procedure was used (see Schreibman, Charlop, & Koegel, 1982) to teach the children to learn how to respond to both the icon and the written word on the PECS cards. In the Charlop-Christy and Werner (2004) study, the Multiple Cue Training procedure was adapted for PECS and found to be effective. All four children learned to be responders to both icon and written word suggesting that for some children, PECS might be a way to teach communication via words. In the study by Charlop-Christy and Daneshvar (2004), the Multiple Cue Training procedure was incorporated into the original PECS phases to test whether it could be part of traditional PECS training. These results suggested that the four children in this study not only learned to communicate with PECS, but when an additional phase was added after phase 3, the children also communicated with the words instead of the icons used in earlier phases. In both of these studies, a multiple baseline design across subjects was used to provide experimental control.

Finally, we have documented increases in spontaneous speech through the use of PECS (Jones & Charlop-Christy, 2004). Using a multiple baseline design across subjects, five children were taught to use two or three adjectives when speaking. The participants had minimal verbal skills but were taught through PECS to say the words on the sentence strip to request preferred items using two or three attributes (e.g., "I want big, green train"). Although training occurred via PECS, testing was on the target behavior of speech during a free-play format. We counted the number of times the child verbally requested certain items available in the free-play environment using two attributes more than he or she did during baseline. Results suggested that we successfully increased the use of spontaneous requests with the target adjectives to children who did not learn using traditional verbal procedures in baseline.

The empirical studies provide controlled experimental evidence on the efficacy of PECS. However, there are a number of limitations the reader needs to be cautioned about. First, at the date of this writing, there are only two published studies in the peer-reviewed literature. This is a beginning, but not a strong base. In the Charlop-Christy et al. (2002) study, there were three children and in the Kravits et al. study (2002) there was only one child, so clearly we need replication of these results and a broader basis of findings, including reports from group studies. This would provide a stronger basis for generalizing the results of our studies to other children and interventionists. While our lab is producing empirically based research on PECS, as described previously, it is important to point out that this research has not yet been through the peer-review process and at this point remain only promising. Although reliability data collectors, naïve to the purpose of these investigations, participated in each of our studies, it is also important for other researchers to join us in our empirical investigation of PECS. Replication by other authors is necessary to address the well-known challenges of experimenter bias.

PRACTICAL REQUIREMENTS

PECS Materials

A three-ring (6″ × 9″) binder is used as a communication board to teach PECS. The binder contains several strips of Velcro (the sentence strips), an *I want* card, an *I see* card, or *Yes* and *No* cards, and black-and-white pictures (1″ × 1″) of preferred items. These cards are either taken from the *Picture Communication Symbols Combination Book* (Mayer-Johnson, 1994) or constructed from pictures of desired food items as recommended by Frost and Bondy (1994). The sentence strip is a piece of strengthened paper with Velcro on the bottom and top. The strip is attached to the PECS book on the lower right-hand corner, and picture cards could be attached to the top layer of Velcro to create sentences. For initial training trials, the picture cards are 2″ × 2″. Later, the picture cards can be reduced in size to 1″ × 1″. After a preference test for each child, the specific PECS cards used are unique to each individual.

KEY COMPONENTS

Training Sequence

Reinforcer Preference Test   PECS begins by teaching spontaneous requests or mands. In order to do so, the trainer first must learn what the child really wants. Before any of the training phases begin, a preference test is done in which the trainer offers the child various items and then observes which ones the child selects. Once the trainer has identified the child's preferred items, these items are systematically offered a few at a time to determine a hierarchy of preferences.

Phase 1: How to Communicate   In Phase 1 of PECS, the child is taught to communicate without using the spoken word by giving the trainer the picture of the desired item displayed. The child does not yet choose a specific picture but uses the single picture prepared by the trainer. The child is taught to pick up a picture of a desired item, reach over to a communicative partner (the trainer), and give the trainer the picture. The trainer then gives the child the desired item that is displayed in the child's view and that corresponds to the picture on the picture card. If the child needs to be prompted, an assistant sits behind the child and provides manual guidance for the child to pick up the picture card and hand it to the trainer in exchange for the desired item. The assistant sits behind the child to stay out of the communicative interaction. Prompts are faded out as quickly as possible.

Phase 2: Distance and Persistence   During Phase 2, the child using PECS is taught to go farther away to communicate with the trainer. The child must actually travel to the communicative partner by walking increasingly greater distances. This way, the child learns how to be consistent at delivering the pictures, even when the communicative partner is not close at hand. The child also learns to be persistent in the pursuit of the desired item. The child may also need to go get the picture card and then find the communicator in order to acquire the desired item. A communication binder is created, and the one picture that is in use is placed on the front cover of the book while additional pictures of other desired items are stored inside the binder.

Phase 3: Discrimination Between Symbols   Once children have become persistent communicators who reliably approach different people in order to request a variety of desired items, the next step is to teach discrimination between picture cards. Discrimination training begins by presenting the child with a choice of two pictures, and then demonstrating that choosing and exchanging a particular picture results in a specific consequence. At the beginning of Phase 3, the difference between these consequences is exaggerated by using a highly desired item and a non-desired item with corresponding pictures placed on the front of the binder. If the child exchanges the picture of the desired item, the trainer gives the child that item along with some animated social praise. If the child gives the trainer the picture of the non-desired item, he or she is given that item. The child learns that the purpose or function of making the correct discrimination between the cards is to obtain the desired item. Discrimination learning under these circumstances, then, has a very important communicative function for the child.

When this type of discrimination training is learned, the trainer then arranges the two pictures on the front of the binder. More and more pictures are gradually added when the child is taught their meaning through discrimination learning.

Phase 4: Using Phrases   For Phase 4, the child is taught to use a sentence strip. The first sentence that is taught is the request, "I want" plus the desired object's label. The child is taught to construct a two-picture sentence. There is an *I want* picture that is used with the desired item picture (e.g., *cookie*). These are placed on a sentence strip attached to the communication binder. The child then removes the sentence strip and hands it to the communicative partner. The communicative partner then reads back the sentence strip while delivering the requested item (i.e., "You're telling me, 'I want cookie'"). Other sentences such as "I see," "I hear," and "It is" can also be taught.

Phase 5: Answering a Direct Question   The main objective of PECS is to establish a communication method built on the functional use of picture cards. Until Phase 5, the focus has been on the request or mand initiated by the child. By the time the child reaches Phase 5, the child is believed to be ready to engage in response to someone else. Thus, in Phase 4, the child is generally making a request for a tangible reinforcer. Now, the child must focus on a communicative partner's need, not on his or her own need. The first question taught is, "What do you want?" so the tangible reinforcer is not too far away for the child, but the child still must process and respond to the social requirements of the situation with a sentence and delay gratification. Other questions such as "What do you see?" are taught later.

Phase 6: Commenting   By the time children reach this phase, they can communicate via PECS with a variety of people in order to make frequent spontaneous requests using the phrase sentence starter, *I want*. They can answer the question "What do you want?" Their expressive vocabulary consists of a variety of pictures representing preferred items and activities. Children then are taught to use commenting cards such as *I see*. In this phase, only social feedback and praise are provided in order to wean the child off of tangible reinforcers. Another critical step in Phase 6 training is teaching the child to differentially answer "What do you see?" and "What do you want?" by appropriately using the *I see* or the *I want* icon. During this training, multiple opportunities for spontaneous requesting must be created so that the student maintains this skill.

Summary and Table of Phases of PECS

PECS is a pictorial system in which pictures are attached to a child's notebook by Velcro. Children are taught to retrieve pictures from their notebooks and create sentences on a removable sentence strip. Sentences focus on spontaneous requests and responses to questions. The focus is placed on teaching the children to initiate communication by showing their sentences

Table 5.2. Description of each phase of Picture Exchange Communication System (PECS) training according to guidelines set by Frost and Bondy (1994)

Phase	Title	Content
1	Physical exchange	Children are taught to hand a blank picture card to a communicative partner.
2	Expanding spontaneity	Children are taught to go to their PECS board, get a picture card, seek out a communicative partner, and place the card in the partner's hand to receive a reinforcer (mand training). The distance between the child, the board, and the partner (listener) is gradually increased and the response is trained in new settings.
3	Picture discrimination	Children are taught to discriminate among multiple pictures on the PECS board.
4	Sentence structure	Children seek out their PECS board, create a "sentence" on the sentence strip by combining the *I want* card and the card of a desired item, seek out a communicative partner, and give him or her the sentence strip. Listeners read the strip back to the children, inserting a fixed time delay between the words *I want* and the item label. Additional social praise is added if a child independently provides the label during the delay.
5	Answering a direct question	Children are taught to respond to the question, "What do you want?"
6	Commenting	Children are taught to respond to the question, "What do you see?" by selecting a card depicting the same object and combining it with an *I see* card to access an unrelated reinforcer.

to another individual. The communicative partner is then able to pair the children's visual sentence with a verbal sentence by reading the words on the pictures (Bondy & Frost, 1994).

A description of the six phases of PECS is shown in Table 5.2. For a more detailed description of the PECS training procedure, see Frost and Bondy (1994). The criterion for successful completion of each phase is 80% or more trials scored as successful without prompting in a 10-trial block.

APPLICATION TO AN INDIVIDUAL CHILD

Alfonso was a 5-year-old boy who was diagnosed with autism when he was 3 years old. At that time, his autistic characteristics were considered classic for the disorder, and he tended to fall on the lower-functioning end of the spectrum. His strengths were few and his challenges were many. Alfonso had very poor eye contact, and he did not speak or even vocalize, with the exception of the sound [a:] which was not connected to anything in particular. Sometimes, Alfonso would say [a:] while keeping his fingers in his ears, seemingly as a means of changing the sound of it in his head. Alfonso did not respond to commands and produced tantrums much of the time during his therapy sessions. He was not controllable at home so his mother let him roam around and gave him what he wanted. Usually, by bringing her over to the refrigerator and having her guess what it was he wanted, he could communicate with her. He seldom stayed in his seat during therapy but slowly, over time, he began to respond to the behavioral intervention.

During behavioral intervention, we worked with Alfonso on maintaining eye contact, staying in his seat, extinguishing tantrums, complying to simple commands, and increasing attention. We began to teach him a receptive labeling task in which he handed us the requested item out of a two choice discrimination. This was quite difficult for him. We also worked on matching three-dimensional and two-dimensional stimuli. We worked on verbal imitation program and began to get his [a:] under some imitative stimulus control. Occasionally, we began to hear other sounds.

In general, Alfonso's progress was very slow, and his mother said she was very discouraged and depressed. Her real hope was that one day Alfonso would talk. She had a great deal of difficulty appreciating his other improvements because they seemed small in comparison with the skills of other children.

At this time, we initiated the PECS program with Alfonso. When Alfonso's mother thought that we had given up on teaching him speech, we explained that our data indicated that PECS helped encourage speech and that we were hoping that it would do so in this case. At least, Alfonso desperately needed a way to communicate. We began with Phase 1 of PECS in which Alfonso was taught to hand us a PECS card. A prompter sat behind Alfonso and the therapist sat in front of him. The therapist showed Alfonso one of his favorite items (predetermined by a preference test). The PECS card depicting the item was on the table. Alfonso had no difficulty learning to pick up the card and hand it to us in exchange for the item. He easily reached the 80% criterion. He was then presented with Phase 2. We then placed a picture card with the Velcro on the back on his PECS notebook cover. We used picture cards of items that Alfonso liked, such as juice, a particular book, a Barney doll, crackers, and so forth, but one at a time. For example, we placed the picture card of Barney on his notebook and waited for 10 seconds (time delay of 10 seconds) for him to give us the card by taking it off his notebook and putting it in our hand. When Alfonso did this, we provided the Barney doll. Then we changed the picture to the crackers picture and waited until Alfonso handed us the card. Then we gave him a cracker. However, in addition to changing cards on the front of his notebook, we increased the distance of his notebooks so that he would have to seek out the notebook, get the card, and then find someone to give it to. At first, Alfonso needed prompting for this phase. Eventually, he reached the criterion of 80% correct responding without any prompting.

Phase 3 proved very difficult for Alfonso. In this phase, we placed two of his picture cards on his notebook and attempted to teach him to discriminate between cards. That is, he was to choose one of the two cards for one of the two items presented. At first, Alfonso needed prompting for this phase. Prompting consisted of someone sitting behind him and manually taking his hand, placing it on the picture, helping him pick up the picture in his hand, and then moving his hand over to the therapist's hand. Also, it helped to use one highly preferred item and one neutral item. So, when he handed us the card of the highly preferred item, he received that item. But, when he handed us the card of the neutral item, he received the item that he did not necessarily want. We gradually increased the number of cards on his notebook to five, requiring him to pick the card representing an object he wanted from among four other choices.

Phase 4 consisted of using the sentence strip. Through the use of the prompter sitting behind him, Alfonso learned to first get the *I want* card and place it on the Velcro strip. Then he needed to repeat Phase 3 and discriminate between cards to find the card that depicted his desired item. After many trials of this, Alfonso learned to incorporate the *I want* card into his repertoire. At this point, it was unclear as to whether Alfonso understood that the card meant *I want* or he just knew that he now needed to include that card and the desired item card when communicating with his PECS notebook. Phase 6, discrimination between *I want* and *I see,* was not completed before summer vacation.

When Alfonso returned to our program, it was clear that PECS had not been continued at home or in summer school. To make matters worse, Alfonso changed schools and was placed in a classroom where they did not use PECS. We picked up where we left off at Phase 5, the sentence strip. However, Alfonso was not responding and was placing any two pictures and not using the *I want* card. In addition, he started to tantrum when we required him to use his notebook and he started grabbing at the desired items. We wondered if he had been getting the desired items for "free" or by not having to communicate for them. We went back to Phase 3, and he protested using the PECS notebook here also.

We decided that we needed to be very creative with Alfonso. We took photographs of places by our Autism Center that Alfonso indicated a preference for by running to when he first arrived and on breaks. These places included the bike lock-up rack, the outside steps, two different decorative large waterfalls/fountains on campus, and a few other places. We began with Phase 1 and started over. We went to the bike rack, placed the photo of it on a clipboard that we held out in front of Alfonso, with his prompter behind him to motor him through handing the photo to the therapist. We then walked over to the fountain and so on. We easily progressed through the phases up through Phase 5. We also went inside and put back photos of other desired items (e.g., juice, Barney, crackers). At this point, Alfonso was back to using PECS, and we also were able to get his school and family on board. Most important, what had happened during Phase 4, the sentence strip phase, was astonishing: Alfonso started speaking! While using the *I want* and *stairs* cards, Alfonso started to imitate the therapist and provide verbal approximations. He continued to verbalize, using clearer and clearer verbalizations, with most of his cards. Although the emergence of speech had been observed in experimental and nonexperimental contexts (Charlop-Christy, 2002; Frost & Bondy, 1994), we did not expect this to occur with Alfonso.

At present, Alfonso continues to do well with using PECS and his verbalizations continue, although speech outside the context of PECS is still infrequent. We will soon present Phase 5, in which discrimination between *I want* and *I see* will be taught. We predict that this will be difficult for Alfonso, but he has certainly surprised us in the past.

FUTURE DIRECTIONS

We believe that this chapter has suggested some clear future directions for PECS. First, solid empirical data are presently being gathered for a PECS database. Much more evidence is needed, however, to provide a strong foundation, and many questions still remain unanswered. One important question is which children are candidates for PECS. Should all children with disabilities who do not speak by a certain age be taught PECS, or should they be taught other AAC or verbal procedures? A limited amount of data has suggested that PECS has stimulated speech in some children. In what percentage of children is that likely to happen, and can we predict which children are likely to respond in this way?

Comparison studies of PECS and manual sign language would be useful. These studies would help us to determine the extent to which it is the constancy of PECS pictures or their iconicity to which children seem to respond.

Some of our new research has been investigating extensions of the use of PECS, such as written-word communication. Can PECS be extended this way? Can PECS be used as a reading program? We see the potential in a number of uses of PECS, as a communication system with pictures, with words, and other possible training programs such as reading. We call for the continued investigation of this technique.

REFERENCES

Bondy, A.S., & Frost, L.A. (1993). Mands across the water: A report on the application of the picture exchange communication system in Peru. *The Behavior Analyst, 16,* 123–128.

Bondy, A.S., & Frost, L.A. (1994). The Picture Exchange Communication System. *Focus on Autistic Behavior, 9,* 1–19.

Carr, E.G., & Durand, V.M. (1985). Reducing behavior problems through functional communication training. *Journal of Applied Behavior Analysis, 18,* 111–126.

Charlop, M.H., & Haymes, L.K. (1994). Speech and language acquisition and intervention: Behavioral approaches. In J.L. Matson (Ed.), *Autism in children and adults: Etiology, assessment, and intervention* (pp. 213–240). Pacific Grove, CA: Brooks/Cole.

Charlop, M.H., Schreibman, L., & Thibodeau, M.G. (1985). Increasing spontaneous verbal responding in autistic children using a time delay procedure. *Journal of Applied Behavior Analysis, 18,* 155–166.

Charlop, M.H., & Trasowech, J.E. (1991). Increasing autistic children's daily spontaneous speech. *Journal of Applied Behavior Analysis, 24,* 747–761.

Charlop-Christy, M.H. (2002, March). *Assessment of emerging speech and social behaviors and problem behavior reduction as a function of PECS.* Paper presented at the first annual PECS Expo, San Diego.

Charlop-Christy, M.H., Carpenter, M., Le, L., LeBlanc, L.A., & Kellet, K. (2002). Using the Picture Exchange Communication System (PECS) with children with autism: Assessment of PECS use, speech, social behavior, and maladaptive behavior. *Journal of Applied Behavior Analysis, 35,* 213–231.

Charlop-Christy, M.H., & Daneshvar, S. (2004). *Combining multiple cue training during PECS training to teach sight-word recognition to children with autism.* Working paper.

Charlop-Christy, M.H., LaBelle, C.A., & Jones, C. (2004). *Using PECS and FCT to reduce behavior problems of children with autism.* Working paper.

Charlop-Christy, M.H., & Werner, G. (2004). *Using a multiple cue training procedure to teach response to both word and picture during PECS.* Working paper.

Durand, V.M., & Carr, E.G. (1991). Functional communication training to reduce challenging behavior: Maintenance and application in new settings. *Journal of Applied Behavior Analysis, 24,* 251–264.

Fagan, J.F. (1971). Infants' recognition memory for a series of visual stimuli. *Journal of Experimental Child Psychology, 11,* 244–250.

Frost, L.A., & Bondy, A.S. (1994). *The Picture Exchange Communication System training manual.* Cherry Hill, NJ: Pyramid Educational Consultants.

Hagopian, L.P., Fisher, W.W., Thibault-Sullivan, M., Acquisto, J., & LeBlanc, L.A. (1998). Effectiveness of functional communication training with and without extinction and punishment: A summary of 21 inpatient cases. *Journal of Applied Behavior Analysis, 31,* 211–235.

Jones, C., & Charlop-Christy, M.H. (2004). *Using PECS to increase the spontaneous speech of minimally verbal children with autism.* Working paper.

Kanner, L. (1943). Autistic disturbances of affective contact. *Nervous Child, 2,* 217–250.

Kravits, T.R., Kamps, D.M., Kemmerer, K., & Potucek, J. (2002). Brief report: Increasing communication skills for an elementary-aged student with autism using the picture exchange communication system. *Journal of Autism and Developmental Disorders, 32,* 225–230.

Krug, D., Arik, J., & Almond, P. (1980). Autism Behavior Checklist. *Journal of Child Psychology and Psychiatry, 21,* 223–225.

Mayer-Johnson LLC. (1994). *The Picture Communication Symbols Combination Book.* Solana Beach, CA: Author.

Miltenberger, R. (1997). *Behavior modification.* Pacific Grove, CA: Brooks/Cole.

Minshew, N.J., Goldstein, G., & Siegel, D.J. (1997). Neuropsychologic functioning in autism: Profile of a complex information processing disorder. *Journal of International Neuropsychological Society, 3,* 303–316.

Ozonoff, S., Pennington, B.F., & Rogers, S.J. (1991). Executive function deficits in high-functioning autistic individuals: Relationship to theory of mind. *Journal of Child Psychology and Psychiatry, 32*(7), 1107–1122.

Peterson, S.L., Bondy, A.S., Vincent, Y., & Finnegan, C. (1995). Effects of altering communication input for students with autism and no speech: Two case studies. *Augmentative and Alternative Communication, 11,* 93–100.

Quill, K.A. (1995). Visually cued instruction for children with autism and pervasive developmental disorders. *Focus on Autistic Behavior, 10*(3), 10–20.

Rimland, B. (1964). *Infantile autism: The syndrome and its implications for a neural theory of behavior.* New York: Appleton-Century-Crofts.

Rosinski, R.R., Pellegrino, J.W., & Siegel, A.W. (1977). Developmental changes in the semantic processing of pictures and words. *Journal of Experimental Child Psychology, 23,* 282–291.

Rumsey, J.M., & Hamburger, S.D. (1988). Neuropsychological findings in high-functioning men with infantile autism, residual state. *Journal of Clinical and Experimental Neuropsychology, 10*(2), 201–221.

Schreibman, L. (1988). *Autism.* Newbury Park: Sage Publications.

Schreibman, L., Charlop, M.H., & Koegel, R.L. (1982). Teaching autistic children to use extra-stimulus prompts. *Journal of Experimental Child Psychology, 33,* 475–491.

Schuler, A.L., & Baldwin, M. (1981). Nonspeech communication and childhood autism. *Language, Speech, and Hearing Services in the Schools, 12,* 246–257.

Schwartz, I.S., Garfinkle, A.N., & Bauer, J. (1998). The Picture Exchange Communication System: Communicative outcomes for young children with disabilities. *Topics in Early Childhood Special Education, 18,* 144–159.

Skinner, B.F. (1957). *Verbal behavior.* New York: Appleton-Century-Crofts.

Snowling, M., & Frith, U. (1986). Comprehension in 'hyperlexic' readers. *Journal of Experimental Child Psychology, 42,* 392–415.

Wechsler, D. (1974). *Wechsler Intelligence Scale for Children–Revised (WISC-R).* New York: Harcourt Assessment.

Wechsler, D. (1981). *Wechsler Adult Intelligence Scale–Revised (WAIS-R).* New York: Harcourt Assessment.

6

The System for Augmenting Language
AAC and Emerging Language Intervention

MARYANN ROMSKI, ROSE A. SEVCIK, MELISSA CHESLOCK, AND ANDREA BARTON

ABSTRACT

The System for Augmenting Language (SAL) is an augmentative and alternative communication (AAC) intervention approach originally developed as part of a longitudinal research study focused on the language development of school-age children with moderate to severe cognitive disabilities. The SAL consists of five integrated components: 1) a speech-generating device; 2) individually chosen visual-graphic symbols; 3) use in natural everyday environments that encourage, but do not require, the child to produce symbols; 4) models of symbol use by communicative partners; and 5) an ongoing resource and feedback mechanism. The SAL is implemented using a collaborative service delivery model in the home, at school, and in the community. The SAL has been used with school-age children with moderate to severe cognitive disabilities who are at the emerging stage of language development and have at least primitive intentional communication skills. Recently, the use of the SAL has been extended to toddlers and preschoolers with developmental delays.

INTRODUCTION

For more than three decades, the field of AAC has addressed the communication needs of children who cannot consistently rely on speech for functional communication (e.g., Beukelman & Mirenda, 2005; Sevcik & Romski, 2002). Along with many technological advances that support AAC, there have been developments in the empirical knowledge base including new approaches in decision making for clinical assessment and intervention. In particular, research has shown that AAC can be used as part of language inter-

The contributions of the first two authors are equal. Research reported in this manuscript was funded by National Institutes of Health (NIH) Grants HD-06016 and DC-03799. The preparation of manuscript was funded in part by NIH Grant DC-03799.

vention strategies to develop children's speech and language skills. Some
children who use AAC systems may develop vocal and spoken language skills
after experience with AAC. In this chapter, we present information about the
System for Augmenting Language (SAL), a language and AAC intervention
approach that targets the emerging language development by children with
significant disabilities.

TARGET POPULATIONS AND ASSESSMENTS FOR
DETERMINING TREATMENT RELEVANCE AND GOALS

The SAL is a communication intervention approach that was originally developed for use with school-age children and youth whose history included a
number of years of unsuccessful communication experiences and/or interventions, but who had at least primitive intentional communication skills, a
spoken language vocabulary of fewer than 10 intelligible words or word approximations, and gross pointing skills. With respect to clinical/educational
application, individuals who may benefit from this particular approach include a broad range of children and adults with congenital disabilities who
are at the beginning stages of language and communication development, regardless of their chronological age.

These children and adults are actually a heterogenous group including
individuals who have different medical etiologies, can walk or use wheelchairs,
and are usually identified based on communication profiles rather than medical etiologies. Medical etiologies can include, but are not limited to, Down syndrome, autism spectrum disorders, pervasive developmental disorder, deafblindness, cerebral palsy, and seizure disorder; often the etiology is unknown.
Depending on the individual's chronological age and severity of the disability, communication profiles may range from unintelligible speech to a very
limited number of words (e.g., fewer than 10), or no speech at all. A small
number of children or adults with mild or moderate cognitive disabilities who
have specific difficulties with language and/or motor speech output also may
use the SAL. Typically, these are children who have developed speech, but
their speech is often, or almost always, unintelligible to a listener. The majority of children and adults with cognitive disabilities who will use the SAL,
however, are individuals with severe cognitive disabilities. These are children
who never develop any speech, develop only a few words, or are echolalic.
For them, the SAL can provide a means to develop receptive and expressive
language skills. If the school-age children with whom we have worked had
had a conventional way to communicate earlier in their childhood, perhaps
their overall communicative interaction skills and adaptive behavior skills
might not have lagged so significantly behind other children. Recently, the
role that the SAL experience might play in the early language and communication intervention process has been investigated. The SAL intervention is

currently being extended to toddlers and preschoolers who exhibit developmental disabilities and are at significant risk for developing difficulties with spoken language skills.

There are few, if any, standardized measures of language development that assist in determining whether the SAL is an appropriate treatment approach. For the clinical use of the SAL, it is essential that there be a detailed description of the language and communication skill of the child at the onset of intervention so that changes, including the development of speech, attributable to the intervention can be documented. Historically, it was assumed that children with severe disabilities needed to meet certain cognitive and age prerequisites before they could benefit from any type of augmented communication intervention. Research findings have indicated that such cognitive prerequisites are not necessary to begin intervention with the SAL because children without these skills have learned to communicate using augmented means (see Chapter 4; Reichle & Yoder, 1985; Romski & Sevcik, 1996; Romski, Sevcik, & Pate, 1988). Current research and recommended practice documents the effectiveness of communication services and supports for children with a variety of severe disabilities (Brady & McLean, 2000; National Joint Committee on the Communication Needs of Persons with Severe Disabilities [NJC], 2002; Romski, Sevcik, & Forrest, 2001; Rowland & Schweigert, 2000). The types of language and communication skills that must be assessed include speech comprehension skills (see, e.g., Sevcik & Romski, 2002), communication skills and modes (vocalizations, gestures), and speech development. It is also important to assess the environments in which communication will take place so that the SAL can be overlaid on existing routines.

THEORETICAL BASIS

The SAL targets a functional limitation directly to provide supports and compensation for a lack of speech and language skills. The theoretical basis for the SAL approach grows out of two seemingly separate but related theoretical frameworks: how typically developing children learn language and communication skills and how AAC interventions function to compensate for the severe deficits in speech and language development exhibited by children and adults with cognitive disabilities.

Typical Language Acquisition

In order for young children to develop functional language and communication skills, they must be able to comprehend *and* produce language so that they can take on the roles of both listener and speaker in conversational exchanges (Sevcik & Romski, 2002). Young typically developing children learn to speak before the age of 2 years. They do so after spending more than 1 year being exposed to spoken language input from their caregivers. Before actually uttering their first words, children comprehend about 50 words and develop an intentional communication repertoire of vocalizations and gestures that they use to request and to refer to objects and events in their environments (Adamson, 1996; Warren et al., Chapter 3, this volume). The early word learning of typically developing children, then, appears to be couched in their ability to extract relevant information from the linguistic environment and to associate it with their own developing vocal forms in order to express wants and needs (Baldwin & Markman, 1989; Golinkoff, Mervis, & Hirsh-Pasek, 1994; Mervis & Bertrand, 1993). Most children begin talking by gradually building individual vocabularies composed of a range of words (e.g., objects, actions, emotions; Nelson, 1973) until they evidence a vocabulary growth spurt at about 18–20 months of age (Golinkoff et al., 1994). With this spurt, the rate of vocabulary acquisition increases dramatically and the child also begins to combine words to express semantic relations.

The beginning period of communication and language development, then, is rich with opportunities for the young child to develop a firm communication and language foundation even though he or she is not yet talking. This foundation includes opportunities to communicate via vocalizations, gestures, and other means even before he or she uses a conventional output mode such as speech, manual signs, or symbols and to develop language comprehension skills. The literature on typically developing children's communication and language development strongly suggests that these early types of experiences are important for later receptive and expressive language development. It also illustrates the development of communication, language, and speech—three separate but related processes. Language interventions must consider how these communication and receptive and expressive language experiences can be incorporated into intervention strategies during the beginning developmental period through AAC means (Romski & Sevcik, 2005).

Language Intervention, Augmentative Communication, and Severe Cognitive Disabilities

Although the majority of children with cognitive disabilities learn to speak either spontaneously or with the aid of language intervention (Abbeduto, 2003), some children with cognitive disabilities fail to develop speech even after extensive language intervention efforts, or they encounter great difficulty and frustration in attempting to do so. The original rationale for using AAC with children with cognitive disabilities was simply to provide them with an alternative output mode so that they could communicate (Fristoe & Lloyd, 1979). This approach presumed that the child's difficulty in acquiring spoken language was specifically related to deficits in motor speech output. Even after such experience, some children with severe cognitive disabilities continued to experience difficulty learning to communicate. They might have encountered difficulties processing dimensions of the auditory input signal or coordinating fine motor movements, and they might have more generalized receptive and expressive language acquisition impairments (Romski & Sevcik, 1996). More recent teaching efforts for children and youth with significant cognitive disabilities focused on the immediate clinical/educational goal of developing intervention approaches that permit the children to communicate basic functional wants and needs. These interventions have replaced or augmented existing receptive and expressive communication skills with, for example, manual signs or visual-graphic symbols (see Romski, Sevcik, & Fonseca, 2003, for a review).

Current perspectives suggest that the functions AAC can play in language and communication development are broader than just providing an output mode by which individuals can convey information. AAC can augment existing speech and vocalizations, provide an input mode as well as an output mode for communication for individuals with limited speech comprehension skills, and serve as a language teaching tool (Beukelman & Mirenda, 2005). AAC also can replace or mitigate an individual's socially unacceptable behaviors, such as screaming or hitting, with a conventional means of communication (e.g., Mirenda, 1997).

There has been substantial growth in research on the use of AAC with children and adults with cognitive disabilities. This research has eliminated many assumptions about which children and adults can benefit from AAC and how they can be taught. The field's focus has moved away from an assessment of who can use what type of device and a concentration on the technology alone and toward the development of effective language and communication interventions and the broader outcomes of their implementation and use. The AAC device is a tool, a means to an end—functional language and communication skills—but it is not the end. Some studies suggest, for example, that children with severe cognitive disabilities do not require continuous prompting and structured practice in order to learn language and support the use of naturalistic teaching strategies (see Romski, Sevcik, Hyatt, & Cheslock, 2002, for a review). Communication use in natural settings implies that communication instruction can be embedded within the ongoing events of everyday life. Opportunities for joint experiences that occur reliably and result in a routine may facilitate the development of communication (Snyder-McLean, Solomonson, McLean, & Sack, 1984). Using AAC with children with cognitive disabilities requires a focus on language and communication development within the context of a visual-graphic mode. AAC is sometimes thought of as a separate area of practice, and thus practitioners do not always incorporate the information they know about language and communication development as they consider AAC assessment and intervention. It is imperative that these two areas, language intervention and AAC, be linked. The SAL intervention attempts to provide this link.

EMPIRICAL BASIS

Since the early 1980s, our research team has been studying the communication development of children and youth with cognitive disabilities who do not speak. The SAL was developed as part of a study that examined how to inculcate language and communication experiences into classrooms and homes of school-age children with severe cognitive disabilities. Here we present findings from two sets of studies about use of the SAL. First, we review and summarize the findings from a series of studies about use of the SAL by school-age children and youth. Second, we provide a brief overview of findings and a framework for the examination of use of the SAL by younger children with severe disabilities.

Longitudinal Investigation of SAL Use by School-Age Youth

Romski and Sevcik (1996) examined and described changes in the communication skills of 13 school-age participants (mean chronological age = 12 years, 8 months) from baseline through 2 years of intervention at home and at school using the SAL. The children presented with a range of etiologies (including cerebral palsy, Down syndrome, autism spectrum disorders, and unknown) and determination of moderate or severe cognitive disabilities which were based on psychological evaluations that took into account both IQ measures and adaptive behavior and were conducted by certified school psychologists. Each child had an expressive vocabulary of fewer than 10 spoken words and had at least a documented 2-year unsuccessful history learning to communicate via speech and other means prior to participating in this study. The children's communication skills were assessed at the onset of the study, and changes in their vocabulary and communication use were tracked over time. Given their cognitive and communicative profiles as well as their chronological ages at the onset of the study, we were confident that any changes we might observe would not be due to maturational changes. The children were paired (based on chronological age, school placement level, receptive vocabulary skills, and level of cognitive disability) and each member of the pair was randomly assigned to one of two instructional groups (home or school). During the first year of the study, the children assigned to the home group used the SAL only at home and those assigned to the school group used the SAL only at school. In year 2 of the study, all children used the SAL both at home and at school.

We measured two aspects of communicative achievement during the course of the longitudinal study: communication use and vocabulary mastery. To measure communication use, nonparticipant observers coded the children's communications during daily interactions at home and school at regular intervals throughout the 2 years of the study. The *communicative use probes* (CUPs) consisted of live coded observations (using the *commu-*

nication coding scheme [CCS]) with accompanying audiotapes of communicative interactions. The codes and audiotapes were compiled into a language transcript (using the Systematic Analysis of Language Transcripts [SALT]; Miller & Chapman, 1985). The result was a rich transcript of the communicative interaction that permitted us to extract information about the children's and their partners' communications. The four-digit cross-classified event-based CCS reliably coded five types of information: the participant's partner (e.g., adult, peer); the individual participant's role in the communication (e.g., initiation, response); the mode of the communication (e.g., symbol, gesture, vocalization, word, physical manipulation); the function of the communication (e.g., greeting, answering, commenting, requesting); and the success of the communication. After the transcripts were coded using the CCS, we subsequently coded effectiveness defined in terms of how the partner responded to the SAL user's communication (see Romski, Sevcik, Robinson, & Bakeman, 1994, for a complete description of the coding scheme) and vocabulary focus (see Adamson, Romski, Deffebach, & Sevcik, 1992, for a description on the coding scheme). An event contained a referential focus if any of the speaker's acts focused attention on an object or event by, for example, providing a name for or pointing toward a specific food item or toy. An event contained a social-regulative focus if the speaker acted in such a way to call attention to himself, his or her partner, or the communicative link between them. Definitions of referential versus social-regulative vocabulary use may be particularly important when developing language skills beyond single symbol usage.

Vocabulary mastery provided a measure of the participants' comprehension and production of the symbols they were using apart from the contextual framework in which they were used. We developed the *vocabulary assessment measures* (VAMs), a series of 10 structured tasks (four comprehension tasks and six production tasks including one measuring speech production and one measuring printed English word recognition), designed to determine what the participants had learned about the symbols. Each task was administered by an investigator at school in a one-to-one assessment format outside of the communicative use settings (see Romski & Sevcik, 1996, for a full description of the CUPs and VAMs).

The youth integrated the use of their speech-output communication device into their extant vocal and gestural repertoires (Romski, Sevcik, Robinson, et al., 1994). The result was a rich multimodal means of communication that they used to effectively communicate with adults (Romski, Sevcik, Robinson, et al., 1994) and peers (Romski, Sevcik, & Wilkinson, 1994). Individual participant achievements ranged from the communicative use with adults of a modest set of 20–35 symbols to the use of far more than 100 symbols to convey referential and social-regulative symbolic messages in varied daily contexts (Adamson et al., 1992). Seven youth also developed combinatorial symbol skills (Wilkinson, Romski, & Sevcik, 1994) and increased the proportion of words that were rated as intelligible, whereas six youth increased the proportion of printed words that they recognized independent of the symbol (Romski & Sevcik, 1996).

At the completion of the study, two categories of achievement also were identified based on the youth's performance across the study. The first group was described as having an advanced achievement pattern and the second group, a beginning achievement pattern. The nine advanced achievers acquired relatively large symbol vocabularies (50 or more symbols), comprehended and produced most of their symbol vocabularies, and had a swift acquisition of other symbolic skills (e.g., symbol combinations, speech intelligibility, and printed-word recognition). The remaining four youth initially comprehended the symbols better than they used them in production. The overall number of symbols in their vocabulary was also smaller (fewer than 35 symbols) than that of the advanced achievers. They continued to develop vocabulary across the study, although not as quickly as the advanced group.

The descriptive longitudinal approach permitted us to detail the achievements of a relatively small number of participants (a substantial number, however, given the typical number reported in the AAC literature) across a relatively lengthy period of time. Although these findings indicated that the 13 participants developed substantial skills communicating with adults and peers using their vocabulary during this 2-year period (Romski & Sevcik, 1996; Romski, Sevcik, Robinson, et al., 1994; Romski, Sevcik, & Wilkinson, 1994), each child served as his or her own control by comparing performance at the onset of the study with performance across the 2 years of the study. Consequently, we were not able to assert that the use of the SAL was better than no intervention at all, because we did not use an experimental design that permitted us to address this question. The literature, however, had not typically reported gains of this nature for other children with this level of disability using other types of interventions (Light, Beukelman, & Reichle, 2003).

To determine whether broader conclusions about the effects of the SAL could be drawn, two additional studies were conducted (see Sevcik, Romski, & Adamson, 1999, for a discussion). Romski, Sevcik, and Adamson (1999a) employed a repeated measures design and systematically controlled the same 13 SAL users' access to the speech-generating device in a standard interaction with an unfamiliar partner after 5 years of experience with the SAL. These youths were able to convey more conversationally appropriate, clearer (less ambiguous), and more specific information to the unfamiliar adult partner with their devices than without them. Using the same standard partner interaction, Romski, Sevcik, Adamson, and Bakeman (2005) compared the skills of the 13 youths who now had at least 5 years of experience with the SAL (mean chronological age = 19 years, 10 months) to youths who did not speak and who had no SAL experience (Nonspeakers; mean chronological age = 21 years, 3 months) and met the participant selection criteria used in the original study. They also compared the SAL group to youths with cognitive disabilities who used natural speech as their primary means of communication (Speakers; mean chronological age = 18 years, 9 months; MLU = 1.96) on a set of conversational variables (communication mode, rate, engagement, role in the dialogue, conversational content, and communication focus). In general, the SAL users fell in the middle of the range, communicating better than the Nonspeakers (mean effect size d = .45) yet not quite as well as the Speakers (mean effect size d = .84). For example, the SAL users continued to use many more vocalizations and gestures than the Speakers and still lacked the ability to convey information about absent events. These findings highlight the distinct contributions SAL experience made to communication interactions with unfamiliar partners. The comparison group design permitted us to gain support for our initial hypothesis that the use of the SAL intervention was better than no intervention at all.

Studies of SAL Use with Younger Children

The successful communication outcomes from the SAL intervention with school-age children and youth led us to explore adapting the SAL to younger children (toddlers and preschoolers) with similar developmental profiles. After conducting a pilot case study to determine whether this adaptation was feasible (see Sevcik, Romski, & Adamson, 2004, for a description), we undertook a 1-year exploratory study of SAL use by 10 toddlers (mean chronological age = 33 months; range = 26–41 months) with significant developmental delays and severe communication disabilities. At the onset of the study, the children had primitive intentional communication abilities and began the study with fewer than 10 spoken words as observed during initial assessment sessions. On the six items of the Clinical Assessment of Language Comprehension (CALC; Miller & Paul, 1995) Emerging Language Scale, the children's performance ranged from 12–18 months to 24–28 months, suggesting a broad range of speech comprehension skills at the onset of the intervention study. We provided SAL experience as described previously and assessed their comprehension and production symbol and speech skills pre- and postintervention. All 10 toddlers were using symbols to communicate at the end of the year (from 15 to 187 symbols; mean = 62.8 symbols, SD 51.91). Five toddlers had substantial spoken-word vocabularies at the end of 1 year, and five toddlers were still not using any speech at all (Romski, Sevcik, & Adamson, 1999b). These findings suggest that there may be two profiles that emerge in these toddlers. Without further research, however, this exploratory study cannot rule out the role of development or other threats to internal validity in the findings.

The findings from the exploratory study strongly suggested that we had to modify the SAL intervention protocol for younger children to include routines upon which to build communication interactions and to account for a range of speech comprehension skills. We also had to randomly assign children to intervention in order to ensure that we could control for development given the age of the children. Romski, Sevcik, Adamson, and Cheslock (2002) are currently assessing the relative effects of the SAL approach in comparison with two other early communication intervention strategies, one focused only on augmented communication production by the child and the other focused on spoken communication interaction with no augmentation. In this ongoing longitudinal study, 60 toddlers (24–36 months) are being recruited and randomly assigned to one of these three parent-training interventions. Children who participate have severe developmental delay, use fewer than 10 spoken words, and can grossly point at or hit a communication symbol. Each child and his or her parent (primary caregiver) participate in a 12-week parent-implemented intervention protocol and then are followed at 3, 6, and 12 months postintervention. The intervention protocol for all three interventions is focused on teaching the parent to implement specific communication strategies at home during daily routines. Each 30-minute intervention session includes three 10-minute routines around play, book reading, and snack time. Parents first observe the child and an interventionist using the intervention strategies prior to implementing the interaction themselves with coaching from the interventionist. To date, participant recruitment is complete and data collection for all 60 participants is nearing completion. In this context, we expect to be able to articulate the effects of the SAL approach for young children with severe communication disabilities with a range of speech comprehension skills at the onset of the intervention.

In summary, we have reported findings to support the use of the SAL approach with school-age children and the beginnings of our examination of the effectiveness of the SAL for younger children. The successful SAL findings might lead to the question, "Did any children fail to develop communication skills?" We have not had failures per se, but we have had degrees of success. First, all of our participants came to the SAL intervention with at least primitive intentional communication skills and thus were able to engage in communicative exchanges. Second, how success is measured and over what period of time are critical factors to consider in making judgments about success and failure. If in the school study, for example, we had only measured the acquisition of symbol production skills and not included the acquisition of symbol comprehension skills, we would have had to report four failures (Romski & Sevcik, 1996). These potential failures are actually the four beginning achievers. If we had only measured symbol production over a period of 1 month, we again would have had four failures. With this group of children, the length of time an intervention approach is implemented is very important. Often, it takes an extended period of time before a child may demonstrate success, however it is defined. Overall, then, it is important to consider the notion of success along a continuum rather than as an all-or-none phenomenon.

PRACTICAL REQUIREMENTS

The implementation of any AAC intervention approach is time and labor intensive, and the SAL is no different. There are three types of requirements for successful implementation of the SAL: philosophical beliefs about children, setup and instructional planning details, and ongoing support and monitoring of intervention implementation.

First, there are some important philosophical tenets or beliefs that the practitioner must subscribe to in order to implement the SAL. Central to these beliefs is the philosophy that all children can and do communicate (see NJC, 2002, for a full discussion of this viewpoint). It also requires a focus on a collaborative service delivery model and a move away from a traditional pull-out model of speech-language intervention. This model is critical to the belief that children can learn language and communication skills in the natural environment with communication supports to bolster achievement. It also requires a belief that language and communication development focuses on the child's comprehension as well as on production skills.

Second, a number of specific setup and instructional details must occur before the SAL intervention begins. These include purchase of a speech-generating device, selection of the symbol set and the initial lexicon, and instruction of the communication partners. The purchase of the speech-generating device is a particularly important aspect. This process may take some time depending on the individual family's financial circumstances, and it is often wise to have a loaner or a device that can be used so that there is no delay in providing the device to the child. A range of funding sources are available for the purchase of individual speech-generating devices. These include, but are not limited to, local or state educational and/or rehabilitation agencies; private medical insurance; public health assistance; and charitable agencies, foundations, and corporations. (See http://www.aacproducts.org for specific information on individual devices and their potential funding.) The details of device selection are included in the section on Component 1 under the Key Components section.

Instruction is required at two levels. First, to ensure that primary communicative partners (parents, teachers) understand and are comfortable with their roles, they attend a series of three 1-hour instructional meetings that serve several functions prior to the child's introduction to the SAL. During these meetings, the partners receive instruction in the physical operation of the speech-generating device, including charging requirements and maintenance, view videotape samples depicting interactions using the SAL to illustrate examples of communicative use, engage in role playing, and receive coaching about how to utilize communicative opportunities. They also provide input about the choice of specific vocabulary to be placed on the speech-generating device. The child should participate in these decisions at whatever level he or she can. For example, a child's positive or negative response to a specific toy may be used to assist in choosing one toy over another.

Third, there are resource and feedback/coaching strategies (Component 5) that must be incorporated into the intervention on an ongoing basis. The familiar adult (often the parent or the clinician) is probably the person who will be responsible for preparing the device for regular use unless the child can do this for him- or herself. The adult must be comfortable with the mechanical operation of the device (i.e., how to turn it on and off, accessing vocabulary); otherwise, they will not be able to independently operate the device and use it on a daily basis. There also must be some established mechanism for handling maintenance and repair of the device or there may be unnecessary downtime when it is not available for the child's use. With the toddler project, for example, we developed a written intervention protocol manual that leads the clinician and family member through weekly goals and expected outcomes for the 12-week parent instruction protocol.

In summary, the SAL requires a coordinated effort at a number of different levels and by a number of people to succeed. Without this type of planned and targeted support, it is unlikely that the SAL intervention will be successful (Romski & Sevcik, 2003).

KEY COMPONENTS

The SAL is an AAC intervention approach originally developed as part of a longitudinal research study of the language development of school-age children with moderate to severe cognitive disabilities. It was designed to supplement the child's natural, albeit severely limited, language abilities and to facilitate his or her ability to communicate in a conventional manner in everyday environments, most notably at home and at school. The SAL consists of five integrated components: a speech-generating device; individually chosen visual-graphic symbols; use in natural everyday environments that encourage, but do not require, the child to produce symbols; models of symbol use by communicative partners; and an ongoing resource and feedback mechanism. The SAL is implemented using a collaborative service delivery model in natural environments that include home, school, and the community and a variety of communication partners including parents, siblings, peers, classroom teachers, speech-language pathologists, and others with whom the child interacts. This intervention approach was termed a *system* because it consists of five organized components that must work in concert. One component alone, such as the speech-generating device, is not sufficient. We hypothesize that it is the integration of these components that facilitates the language learning process. Practitioners often report that they find speech-generating devices in closets not being used. This lack of use is probably because the device was not integrated within an actual system for ongoing communication and language development.

Component 1: Speech-Generating Devices

The first component of the SAL is a speech-generating device. It was also described as a computer-based speech-output communication device or a VOCA (voice output communication aid). Our initial study actually pre-dated the availability of portable speech-generating devices. During the course of the original research study (Romski & Sevcik, 1996), two different commercially available communication devices were used sequentially: the Words+ Portable Voice II (Words+ Inc.) followed by the SuperWOLF (Adamlab). The Super-WOLF replaced the Words+ device when portable speech-generating devices were able to display symbols at least 1 inch square and produce synthesized speech that was understandable to communicative partners. Rapid changes in software and hardware technology since then have continued until the present. Neither of the above-mentioned devices is still in use. There has been a substantial increase in the quantity and quality of relatively reasonably priced devices now on the market. In our current research efforts with toddlers with significant developmental disabilities who are not speaking, children have used, for example, the Hawk (Adamlab), CheapTalk (Enabling Devices), TechSpeak and TechTalk (AMDI), and the Go Talk (Attainment Company). The SuperWOLF and these more recently developed devices also have the feature of multiple levels so that activity- or routine-specific symbols and vocabulary can be programmed on corresponding display pages. The device can vary depending on the individual needs of the child, and the range of currently available technology can be found at http://www.aacproducts.org. From our perspective, we are not wedded to a specific device. The critical feature with respect to the SAL is the speech output and the child's ability to access it.

Why is speech output a critical component of the SAL? Historically, with the exception of a few early studies (Locke & Mirenda, 1988; Romski et al., 1988; Romski, White, Millen, & Rumbaugh, 1984), manual sign systems and then cardboard communication boards were the choice for able-bodied youth with severe cognitive disabilities. Although a well-established strength of graphic symbols on communication boards is its use of the visual mode (Fristoe & Lloyd, 1979), it requires the communication partner to both monitor the visual channel and attend to the visual communication produced. Romski and Sevcik (1996) have argued that the SAL uses speech-generating devices as the medium for language experiences because the "voice" of a speech-generating device permits the child to compensate for the use of a visual communication system. Use of a synthetic or digitized auditory signal permits partners to hear the "speech" output produced when a symbol is activated and immediately comprehend the message. This feature is particularly important when children are integrated within the general community and interact with unfamiliar communicative partners. The speech-generating device automatically links the child's visual symbol communication with a familiar auditory/spoken modality in social interactional contexts. It permits the child to use a multimodal form of communication including a voice, albeit artificial, while retaining access to the visual modality.

Component 2: Symbols and the Lexicon

The second component of the SAL is a set of visual-graphic symbols and a relevant lexicon. In the original study, lexigrams—arbitrary visual-graphic symbols—were used (Rumbaugh, 1977). Each lexigram was the functional equivalent of one spoken word with the printed English word for each lexigram in reduced size above the symbol to facilitate literate partner interpretation and use. Lexigrams were chosen as the symbol set for this study for two reasons. First, none of the participants had any background with them and thus they all began the study with equivalent symbol set experience. Second, the purpose of this study was to describe the process of learning to communicate symbolically. One critical component of symbolic communication is the use of arbitrary symbols which stand for, and can take the place of, a real object, event, person, action, or relationship (Savage-Rumbaugh, Rumbaugh, & Boysen, 1980). When we began studying the communication development of toddlers, we made a conscious decision to use visual-graphic symbols that were perceived as more age appropriate than arbitrary symbols for younger children. These included symbols that looked like what they represented to adults.

The issues regarding which symbol set to use with an individual are complex and sometimes controversial, and they deserve further study (for detailed discussions of this issue, see Mineo Mollica, 2003; Sevcik, Romski, & Wilkinson, 1991). The main issue of concern is the symbol set's level of arbitrariness. Symbols that are arbitrary do not resemble the vocabulary item they represent, whereas nonarbitrary symbols do resemble, in varying degrees, the meanings they represent. For example, the arbitrary printed English word *hat* does not resemble the piece of clothing that you wear on your head, whereas the Mayer-Johnson symbol for *hat* looks like a line drawing of the object it represents.

Different symbol set choices are often made in research as compared with practice. In research, the purpose of the study will often dictate the symbol set used. We chose a symbol set that was arbitrary because we wanted to learn about language development. In clinical or educational practice, our experience is that the decision is often a subjective one determined by what the practitioner "thinks" the individual can use and what symbol set might be the easiest for the practitioner to use. For example, many practitioners choose to use Picture Communication Symbols from the Mayer-Johnson Company because they come in an organized format and can generate displays of symbols via a computer software program. Recently, Mineo Mollica (2003) suggested that practitioners should consider the skills the child brings to the task as well as considering the type of representation, the number of representations presented simultaneously, and the arrangement of representations when determining what symbol set(s) to use.

The lexicon that is available for understanding and expression plays a very important role in language learning through augmented means. It provides a foundation upon which communicative interaction is built. Although individuals with little or no functional speech are often exposed to a spoken input vocabulary comparable to that of a speaking child, their output is likely to be externally constrained by the number of visual-graphic symbol vocabulary items available on the symbol display. Ironically, one of the features that has been proposed to facilitate learning via augmented means, the use of recognition rather than recall memory (Fristoe & Lloyd, 1979), may also limit symbol use capabilities because of the limited number and type of vocabulary items that are available at any one time. For this project, we used comprehension of symbols as the criterion for expanding a child's vocabulary. We used this criterion because we wanted to ensure that the children had some understanding of the symbols on the display panel before more symbols were added to the display. Often, easily depictable lexical items have been chosen for children with cognitive disabilities. The rationale is that these words are concrete and more easily learned than less depictable and more abstract words. Initially, we were hesitant to place nonreferential symbols on the participants' displays. However, when we did place social-regulative symbols (e.g., *more, please, thank you, I'm finished*) on the display, we found that the children readily used them (Adamson et al., 1992).

Component 3: Teaching Through Natural Communicative Exchanges

Component 3, along with component 4, illustrates the teaching dimensions of the SAL. This teaching method includes the location and type of communicative experiences the child has with the speech-generating devices. Loosely structured naturalistic communicative experiences are provided to encourage, but not require, the children's use of the symbols during daily activities. These natural communicative experiences are embedded into routines that the children engage in during the course of their daily activities. Such an approach is consistent with contemporary research and theory which recommends the implementation of AAC interventions in natural environments in order to emphasize the functional nature of language, facilitate the generalization of communicative routines to diverse contexts, and increase the spontaneity of communicative exchange (see Romski et al., 2003, for a review).

Teaching through natural communicative exchanges may be the most difficult component of the system for some to implement because it is a fairly radical departure from more traditional treatment approaches. One basic decision to be made is where the instruction will take place. While traditional interventions have occurred in isolated settings where the practitioner and child interact independently, the literature strongly advocated for the use of natural, integrated settings as the preferred environments for communicative instruction (Beukelman & Mirenda, 2005; Romski, Sevcik, Hyatt, et al., 2002). Settings such as home, school, and community provide familiar locations for the typical occurrence of such shared communicative experiences. Depending on the child's skills, introduction during one or more than one routine can be determined.

Component 4: Partner's Use of the Device

The partner's active role in communicative interactions is the fourth component of the SAL. Partners play two rather obvious roles in the communication exchange: they are speakers providing communicative input to the children who are their partners and they also are listeners who then respond to the child's communications. By virtue of the visual component, the ways in which the partner communicates with the child are modified. An instructional focus that encompasses partners must then include considerations of both their speaker and listener roles. Additionally, some emphasis needs to be placed on instruction directed toward the partner's operation of the device itself (see Practical Requirements of the SAL).

With the SAL, communicative partners were encouraged to integrate the use of the devices into their own spoken language communications by using augmented input. Augmented language input is characterized as the incoming communication/language from a child's communicative partner that includes speech and is supplemented by AAC symbols, the speech output produced by the AAC device when the symbol is activated, and the environmental context (Romski & Sevcik, 2003). In the example, "Tommy, let's go OUTSIDE and ride your BIKE," *OUTSIDE* and *BIKE* are symbols touched on the board, produced by the speech-generating device, and simultaneously spoken by the partner. This communicative model permits each family member or teacher to incorporate the device's use more simply into his or her individually specific communicative interactions.

Partner augmented input, in turn, serves several functions for the participant. First, it provides a model for how the SAL can be used, in what contexts, and for what purposes. When the child's communicative partners uses SAL as input, the pairing of the visual symbol with the synthetic speech output may permit the child to extract previously unobtainable spoken words from the language-learning environment. The specific way in which the symbols are produced and paired with synthetic speech segment the critical word/symbol from the natural stream of speech (e.g., "Let's see your DRESS") and may facilitate the matching of the symbol/word with its physical referent. Second, it has the potential to reinforce the effectiveness of using the system; when a partner incorporates the SAL in successful communicative exchanges, it provides the child with real-world experiences that illustrate the meaning of symbols and the varied functions they serve. The child then experiences the potential utility and power of the SAL. Finally, and perhaps most importantly, partner augmented input makes an implicit statement to the participant that the SAL provides an acceptable vehicle for communicating, a vehicle which the partner is willing to use with the youth (Romski & Sevcik, 2003; Sevcik & Romski, 2002; Sevcik, Romski, Watkins, & Deffebach, 1995).

Component 5: Monitoring Ongoing Use

The fifth and final component of the SAL is a resource and feedback mechanism that monitors ongoing use by child and partner. This resource and feedback mechanism consists of gaining regular information from the child and the primary partners. The practitioner can then use this information, coupled with the assessment tools to be described later, to gain insights into patterns of communicative use, SAL accomplishments and/or difficulties that might be experienced, as well as operational challenges in the settings of use. To gather this type of information, we developed the Parent/Teacher Questionnaire (QUEST; Romski & Sevcik, 1996) to provide a standard format by which to gain a systematic index of the communicative partners' perception of the participant's performance during a given interval. Regular meetings can also be held with the partners to provide an opportunity for face-to-face interactions to discuss progress and problems.

Why is it important to have a plan to monitor ongoing use? A monitoring plan is important because the successful implementation of the SAL depends on having a systematic way to monitor the partners' perceptions of the child's SAL use so that changes can be made as needed. This process serves to keep everyone on track and address issues regarding SAL use in a timely fashion.

ASSESSMENT METHODS TO SUPPORT ONGOING DECISION MAKING

The SAL often is a long-term language intervention approach that requires ongoing learning and use, and then maintenance and expansion of the child's language skills. Thus, assessment of progress is an ongoing process assessed via multiple measures including monthly measures of vocabulary development in comprehension and production, biweekly measures of communicative use across settings and contexts, and biweekly ratings of child and partner perceptions of success (as described in component 5). Romski and Sevcik (1996) described a multifaceted approach to capture changes in SAL communicative patterns in different settings and symbol knowledge outside of contextual constraints. First, communicative use probes (CUPs) are a series of live observations, with accompanying audiotapes, during communicative interactions with both adults and peers. Using communication coding schemes (CCSs) to code communicative events within the CUPs, data can be gathered about people with whom the youth communicated (i.e., communication partner), the role of the communication participant (i.e., initiation, response), how they communicated (i.e., mode of communication), what communication functions were used, and the success and effectiveness of the communication interactions. Language transcripts, using both natural speech and symbol communications on a communication device with synthesized or digitized speech, can be compiled and analyzed using the SALT software program (Miller & Chapman, 1985). Second, Romski and Sevcik (1996) designed VAMs to determine what the 13 youth had learned about the meanings of the symbols that they were using apart from the supporting contextual framework in which the symbols were used. The VAMs are composed of 10 tasks, four comprehension measures and six production measures. They also include measures of the child's word production and printed English word recognition skills. CUPs and VAMs can first be administered to gain a baseline measure of the child's communicative performance prior to the onset of SAL experience. To measure progress, they can be administered at regular intervals, as they were throughout the intervention study. As a child's symbol comprehension and production and communicative success expand, new symbol vocabulary can be introduced to expand the child's communication.

The SAL assessment model provides a comprehensive approach for monitoring ongoing changes in communicative symbol knowledge and use in natural environments. While the SAL was originally developed for research, it can be adapted easily for practical use in educational, home, and clinical settings by incorporating measures of communication use, symbol knowledge, and partner perception as an approach to measuring a variety of dimensions of symbol development. For the toddler study, we added a specific measure that asks the parent to rate their perception of the child's language and communication development as well as the intervention the child is receiving (Romski, Sevcik, Adamson, Cheslock, & Smith, 2004). This systematic assessment information can then be used to make decisions regarding initial and continued intervention goals such as vocabulary development, increased utterance length, development of communicative function use, and communication partner instruction.

Although the SAL primarily is focused on symbol comprehension and symbol production and use, it also is important to monitor the emergence of intelligible speech and recognition of printed English. Thus, assessing changes in the quality and quantity of children's vocalizations as well as printed English recognition is an essential component of the continual assessment process.

CONSIDERATIONS FOR CHILDREN FROM CULTURALLY AND LINGUISTICALLY DIVERSE BACKGROUNDS

Children who have used the SAL represent diverse cultural and linguistic backgrounds. Culture permeates the development of an individual's identity (Soto, Huer, & Taylor, 1997), and it is important for researchers and practitioners to take into account cultural differences if intervention is to be successful. The

SAL key components have been modified easily to accommodate children from culturally and linguistically diverse backgrounds. The speech-generating device is an integral component of the SAL for reasons discussed previously and should be selected individually for any child, respecting the family's cultural values. Some features of the device to keep in mind include its appearance, the intelligibility of the speech output on the device (e.g., digitized versus synthetic speech output), and the adaptability of the device. Some cultures may find that an speech-generating device draws attention to the child and the disability. In this case, it is important to work with the family to ensure that the family can integrate the device in a culturally appropriate way.

Vocabulary also plays a very important role in learning through augmented means. Because it is always chosen with the family's input, vocabulary should be culturally appropriate to the child's primary language. Light et al. (2003) noted that all too often, AAC systems for children reflect the language of the school system and fail to address the cultural values and language of the family, isolating the child from his or her family and cultural community. Soto and colleagues (1997) have also indicated that communication is less effective if vocabulary is selected by an individual from a different cultural background than that of the AAC user. Culturally appropriate vocabulary must also be represented in a culturally appropriate manner. Many symbol sets are currently commercially available to meet the diverse needs of the growing number of children who may use the SAL. For example, the Boardmaker software program (Mayer-Johnson Co.) offers a variety of symbols that represent people and objects from various racial and ethnic backgrounds. Because the SAL is used during communicative exchanges in natural settings such as home, school, and community, it is essential that all communication partners take an active role by providing augmented communicative input and responding to the child's communications. Clinicians and teachers can easily integrate augmented input strategies into the intervention programs of AAC users from many different backgrounds by respecting cultural norms of child participation and customary ways of interacting during daily activities. It is critical for clinicians and teachers to honor parent perceptions of their child's development, respect the family's time constraints, and highlight the importance of becoming active partners in parent–child communication exchanges during culturally appropriate activities. By monitoring ongoing SAL use, the fifth component of SAL, researchers and practitioners are able to gain insights into a family's culturally appropriate pattern of communicative use, their symbol acquisition accomplishments, and difficulties they experience.

APPLICATION TO AN INDIVIDUAL CHILD

Romski and Sevcik (1996) have described the application of the SAL with J.A., who was a 13-year, 3-month-old youth with a diagnosis of moderate cognitive disabilities and "autistic-like" tendencies when we first met him. He had resided in foster home placements since early childhood and he attended a local public school. He was an almost completely silent young man whose only differentiated vocalizations appeared to serve a self-stimulatory function. He primarily communicated through the use of pointing gestures and some manual signs that were not easily understood by others in his school environment though his foster mother indicated she could communicate with him at home. Even though he could not express himself easily, he received an age-equivalent score of 7 years, 0 months on the Arthur Adaptation of the Leiter International Performance Scale (Arthur, 1952). He also had an age-equivalent receptive vocabulary score of 2 years, 3 months on the Peabody Picture Vocabulary Test–Revised (Dunn & Dunn, 1981). His performance on the Assessment of Children's Language Comprehension (ACLC; Foster, Gidden, & Stark, 1983) revealed that he correctly identified 94% of one-word utterances that were assessed, 100% of two- and three-word utterances that were assessed, and 50% of the four-word utterances. He also recognized some printed English words. J.A. was a participant in the study described earlier (Romski & Sevcik, 1996). His use of the SAL was monitored over 2 years as part of the research study. Then, the school district continued to provide communication services and supports so that his communication skills continued to grow until he transitioned to adulthood.

J.A. was immediately successful with his device. He liked it so much that he became distressed when it needed repair or was otherwise unavailable. He learned and used new symbols the first time he had access to them so that his vocabulary potential was almost limitless. He was one of 4 (out of 13) participants who achieved skills in every domain we assessed. He communicated with adults and peers, produced symbol combinations, improved his speech intelligibility ratings, and expanded his vocabulary to more than 100 symbols that he readily used. He also was able to rapidly map, retain, and generalize the names of four novel nonsense words-plus-symbols even though he had little exposure and no intervening naturalistic communicative experience with the novel words-plus-symbols. In fact, more than 3 months after the study was completed, J.A. demonstrated that he still retained his knowledge of one novel word-plus-symbol. At that time, J.A. was being assessed to determine if he was an appropriate candidate for another study that included a new speech-generating device with an alphanumeric keyboard and an LED screen. While he was exploring the new device, he was observed to type out *witzor* (incorrect spelling of *wiztor*), one of the nonsense words from the study. The investigator, amazed at what J.A. had typed, retrieved the stimuli from the study and asked him what the item was. J.A. correctly identified it as *wiztor*.

J.A.'s outgoing, friendly personality emerged as he initiated appropriate conversations with unfamiliar as well as familiar partners. He truly became an independent communicator. After 5 years of SAL experience, he had a vocabulary of more than 100 symbols that he readily combined with gestures and vocalizations for communication.

Although his foster mother initially was not particularly supportive of J.A. using the speech-generating device, his enthusiasm and insistence that he use the device at home resulted in an increased level of acceptance on her part. J.A.'s communication skills advanced beyond the capacity of his speech-generating device, the WOLF, and he faced the transition from high school to work. The school team recommended that he obtain a new, more sophisticated speech-generating communication device to meet his needs. J.A.'s mother took the recommendation and independently spearheaded the funding of a new speech-generating device for him (i.e., a laptop computer with Words+ software) by petitioning the local Kiwanis and Knights of Columbus organizations to provide funds for its purchase. She then worked with the school team to obtain the most appropriate device for J.A. J.A. has worked at a local grocery store since he completed his school experience and continues to use his new speech-generating device that guarantees his ability to communicate independently into the future. J.A. is one example of the communication successes we have had when the SAL is used by school-age children (see Romski & Sevcik, 1996, Chapter 8, for additional examples).

FUTURE DIRECTIONS

The SAL has continued to undergo additional refinement with the development of a structured parent-training protocol for the ongoing randomized control study with toddlers. The outcomes of this study will permit us to systematically examine the use of the SAL with younger children, refining it for use with children across different levels of comprehension.

In addition to the current children who can benefit from the use of the SAL, there are two other populations of children for whom it will be important to specifically examine how well the SAL may facilitate their early communication development. Children with autism spectrum disorders or pervasive developmental disorder who are not speaking may also benefit from the approach employed. In the Romski and Sevcik (1996) study, two of the children had a diagnosis of autism and severe cognitive disabilities; both children communicated via the SAL and were characterized as advanced achievers. As well, to date the SAL has been used with children who have at least the physical motor skills to access symbols via a gross point. It is also important to consider how well the SAL can be adapted to the needs of children with more severe physical disabilities who must access speech-generating devices through other means such as scanning. Although there is no reason to believe that children with more severe physical disabilities would be any less successful than children who access the speech-generating device through direct selection, it is important to examine how they would use this intervention approach.

One particularly important, yet challenging, area of research need is the development of language and communication measurement tools (Romski &

Sevcik, 2005; Sevcik et al., 1999). Attention must be focused on the development of assessment tools that provide a fine-grained analysis of the child's language and communication skills across modes including speech and written language and that measure a range of SAL intervention outcomes over time. Some outcomes of using the SAL, and other AAC techniques, go beyond the development of specific comprehension and production vocabulary and grammatical skills and have been somewhat elusive to quantitative measurement. These include how the use of the SAL can change the quality of a child's life in inclusive settings and across transitions from school to work, in family interactions, and in the perceptions and attitudes of others toward a child who does not speak (Romski & Sevcik, 1996). Such communication access also may prevent the emergence of secondary disabilities such as challenging behaviors and this relationship should be investigated. The development of tools that permit measurement of these secondary outcomes is important and should form the basis for future research.

Finally, the translation of the SAL research findings to practice is essential. Since the completion of the study, we have worked closely with the school district in which the study was originally conducted to implement the components of SAL and develop Project FACTT (Sevcik, Romski, Collier, et al., 1995). Our efforts have expanded from the SAL intervention into a broad model for the implementation of AAC service delivery in school districts (Sevcik & Romski, in press).

RECOMMENDED READINGS

Beukelman, D.R., & Mirenda, P. (2005). *Augmentative and alternative communication: Supporting children and adults with complex communication needs* (3rd ed.). Baltimore: Paul H. Brookes Publishing Co.

National Joint Committee (NJC) for the Communication Needs of Persons with Severe Disabilities (2002). Access to communication services and supports: Concerns regarding the application of restrictive eligibility criteria. *Communication Disorders Quarterly, 23,* 145–153.

Reichle, J., Beukelman, D.R., & Light, J.C. (2002). *Exemplary practices for beginning communicators: Implications for AAC.* Baltimore: Paul H. Brookes Publishing Co.

Romski, M.A., & Sevcik, R.A. (1996). *Breaking the speech barrier: Language development through augmented means.* Baltimore: Paul H. Brookes Publishing Co.

REFERENCES

Abbeduto, L. (Ed.) (2003). *International review of research in mental retardation: Language and communication.* New York: Academic Press.

Adamson, L.B. (1996). *Communication development during infancy.* Boulder, CO: Westview.

Adamson, L.B., Romski, M.A., Deffebach, K., & Sevcik, R.A. (1992). Symbol vocabulary and the focus of conversations: Augmenting language development for youth with mental retardation. *Journal of Speech and Hearing Research, 35,* 1333–1343.

Arthur, G. (1952). *The Arthur Adaptation of the Leiter International Performance Scale.* Washington, DC: Psychological Service Center Press.

Baldwin, D., & Markman, E. (1989). Establishing word-object relations: A first step. *Child Development, 60,* 381–399.

Beukelman, D.R., & Mirenda, P. (2005). *Augmentative and alternative communication: Supporting children and adults with complex communication needs* (3rd ed.). Baltimore: Paul H. Brookes Publishing Co.

Brady, N.C., & McLean, L.K. (2000). Emergent symbolic relations in speakers and non-speakers. *Research in Developmental Disabilities, 21,* 197–214.

Dunn, L.M., & Dunn, L.M. (1981). *Peabody Picture Vocabulary Test–Revised.* Circle Pines, MN: American Guidance Service.

Foster, R., Gidden, J., & Stark, J. (1983). *Assessment of Children's Language Comprehension (ACLC).* Palo Alto, CA: Consulting Psychologists Press.

Fristoe, M., & Lloyd, L. (1979). Nonspeech communication. In N.R. Ellis (Ed.), *Handbook of mental deficiency: Psychological theory and research* (pp. 401–430). Hillsdale, NJ: Lawrence Erlbaum Associates.

Golinkoff, R., Mervis, C., & Hirsh-Pasek, K. (1994). Early object labels: The case for lexical principles. *Journal of Child Language, 21,* 125–155.

Light, J.C., Beukelman, D.R., & Reichle, J. (Eds.). (2003). *Communicative competence for individuals who use AAC: From research to effective practice.* Baltimore: Paul H. Brookes Publishing Co.

Locke, P., & Mirenda, P. (1988). A computer-supported communication approach for a nonspeaking child with severe visual and cognitive impairments. *Augmentative and Alternative Communication, 4,* 15–22.

Mervis, C., & Bertrand, J. (1993). Acquisition of early object labels: The role of operating principles. In S.F. Warren & J. Reichle (Series Eds.) & A.P. Kaiser & D. Gray (Vol. Eds.), *Communication and language intervention series: Vol. 2. Enhancing children's communication: Research foundations for intervention* (pp. 287–316). Baltimore: Paul H. Brookes Publishing Co.

Miller, J., & Chapman, R. (1985). *Systematic analysis of language transcripts (SALT).* Madison, WI: Waisman Center on Mental Retardation and Human Development.

Miller, J.F., & Paul, R. (1995). *The clinical assessment of language comprehension.* Baltimore: Paul H. Brookes Publishing Co.

Mineo Mollica, B. (2003). Representational competence. In J.C. Light, D.R. Beukelman, & J. Reichle (Eds.), *Communicative competence for individuals who use AAC: From research to effective practice* (pp. 107–145). Baltimore: Paul H. Brookes Publishing Co.

Mirenda, P. (1997). Supporting individuals with challenging behavior through functional communication training and AAC: Research review. *Augmentative and Alternative Communication, 13,* 207–225.

National Joint Committee for the Communication Needs of Persons with Severe Disabilities. (2002). Access to communication services and supports: Concerns regarding the application of restrictive "eligibility" policies. *Communication Disorders Quarterly, 23*(3), 145–153.

Nelson, K. (1973). Structure and strategy in learning to talk. *Monographs of the Society for Research in Child Development, 38*(1–2), Serial No. 139.

Reichle, J., & Yoder, D. (1985). Communication board use in severely handicapped learners. *Language, Speech, Hearing Services in Schools, 16,* 146–157.

Romski, M.A., & Sevcik, R.A. (1996). *Breaking the speech barrier: Language development through augmented means.* Baltimore: Paul H. Brookes Publishing Co.

Romski, M.A., & Sevcik, R.A. (2003). Augmented input: Enhancing communication development. In J.C. Light, D.R. Beukelman, & J. Reichle (Eds.), *Communicative competence for individuals who use AAC: From research to effective practice* (pp. 147–162). Baltimore: Paul H. Brookes Publishing Co.

Romski, M.A., & Sevcik, R.A. (2005). Early intervention and augmentative communication: Myths and realities. *Infants and Young Children, 18,* 174–185

Romski, M.A., Sevcik, R.A., & Adamson, L.B. (1999a). Communication patterns of youth with mental retardation with and without their speech-output communication devices. *American Journal on Mental Retardation, 104*, 249–259.

Romski, M.A., Sevcik, R.A., & Adamson, L.B. (1999b, March). Toddlers with developmental disabilities who are not speaking: Vocabulary growth and augmented language intervention. In A.P. Kaiser (Chair), *Early language intervention: Vocabulary growth and development.* Symposium conducted at the annual Gatlinburg Conference on Research and Theory in Mental Retardation and Developmental Disabilities, Charleston, SC.

Romski, M.A., Sevcik, R.A., Adamson, L.B., & Bakeman, R. (2005). Communication patterns of individuals with moderate or severe cognitive disabilities: Interactions with unfamiliar partners. *American Journal on Mental Retardation, 110,* 226–239.

Romski, M.A., Sevcik, R.A., Adamson, L.B., & Cheslock, M. (2002, August). *Exploring communication development in toddlers who are not speaking.* Paper presented at the biennial meeting of the International Society for Augmentative and Alternative Communication, Odense, Denmark.

Romski, M.A., Sevcik, R.A., Adamson, L.B., Cheslock, M., & Smith, A. (2004, November). *Measuring parent perception of early communication development and intervention.* Poster presented at the annual meeting of the American Speech-Language-Hearing Association, Philadelphia.

Romski, M.A., Sevcik, R.A., & Fonseca, A. (2003). Augmentative and alternative communication for persons with mental retardation. In L. Abbeduto (Ed.), *International review of research in mental retardation.* New York: Academic Press.

Romski, M.A., Sevcik, R.A., & Forrest, S. (2001). Assistive technology and augmentative communication in inclusive early childhood programs. In M.J. Guralnick (Ed.), *Early childhood inclusion: Focus on change* (pp. 465–479). Baltimore: Paul H. Brookes Publishing Co.

Romski, M.A., Sevcik, R.A., Hyatt, A., & Cheslock, M.B. (2002). Enhancing communication competence in beginning communicators: Identifying a continuum of AAC language intervention strategies. In J. Reichle, D.R. Beukelman, & J.C. Light (Eds.), *Exemplary practices for beginning communicators: Implications for AAC* (pp. 1–23). Baltimore: Paul H. Brookes Publishing Co.

Romski, M.A., Sevcik, R.A., & Pate, J.L. (1988). The establishment of symbolic communication in persons with mental retardation. *Journal of Speech and Hearing Disorders, 53,* 94–107.

Romski, M.A., Sevcik, R.A., Robinson, B.F., & Bakeman, R. (1994). Adult-directed communications of youth with mental retardation using the system for augmenting language. *Journal of Speech and Hearing Research, 37*, 617–628.

Romski, M.A., Sevcik, R.A., & Wilkinson, K.M. (1994). Peer-directed communicative interactions of augmented language learners with mental retardation. *American Journal on Mental Retardation, 98*, 527–538.

Romski, M.A., White, R., Millen, C.E., & Rumbaugh, D.M. (1984). Effects of computer-keyboard teaching on the symbolic communication of severely retarded persons: Five case studies. *The Psychological Record, 34,* 39–54.

Rowland, C., & Schweigert, P. (2000). Tangible symbols, tangible outcomes. *Augmentative and Alternative Communication, 16,* 61–78.

Rumbaugh, D.M. (1977). *Language learning by a chimpanzee: The LANA project.* New York: Academic Press.

Savage-Rumbaugh, E.S., Rumbaugh, D.M., & Boysen, S. (1980). Do apes have language? *American Scientist, 40,* 40–51.

Sevcik, R.A., & Romski, M.A. (1997). Comprehension and language acquisition: Evidence from youth with severe cognitive disabilities. In L.B. Adamson & M.A. Romski (Eds.), *Communication and language acquisition: Discoveries from atypical development* (pp. 187–202). Baltimore: Paul H. Brookes Publishing Co.

Sevcik, R.A., & Romski, M.A. (2002). The role of language comprehension in establishing early augmented conversations. In J. Reichle, D.R. Beukelman, & J.C. Light (Eds.), *Exemplary practices for beginning communicators: Implications for AAC* (pp. 453–474). Baltimore: Paul H. Brookes Publishing Co.

Sevcik, R.A., & Romski, M.A. (in press). *A school district's guide to augmentative communication service delivery.* Baltimore: Paul H. Brookes Publishing Co.

Sevcik, R.A., Romski, M.A., & Adamson, L.B. (1999). Measuring AAC interventions for individuals with severe developmental disabilities. *Augmentative and Alternative Communication, 15*, 38–44.

Sevcik, R.A., Romski, M.A, & Adamson, L.B. (2004). Augmentative communication and preschool children: Case example and research directions. *Disability and Rehabilitation, 26*, 1323–1329.

Sevcik, R.A., Romski, M.A., Collier, V., Rayfield, C., Nelson, B., Walton-Bowe, A., Jordan, D., & Howell, M. (1995). Project FACTT: Meeting the communication needs of children with severe developmental disabilities. *Technology & Disability, 4*, 233–241.

Sevcik, R.A., Romski, M.A., Watkins, R., & Deffebach, K. (1995). Adult partner-augmented communication input to youth with mental retardation using the system for augmenting language (SAL). *Journal of Speech and Hearing Research, 38*, 902–912.

Sevcik, R.A., Romski, M.A., & Wilkinson, K. (1991). Roles of graphic symbols in the language acquisition process for persons with severe cognitive disabilities. *Augmentative and Alternative Communication, 7*, 161–170.

Snyder-McLean, L., Solomonson, B., McLean, J., & Sack, S. (1984). Structuring joint action routines: A strategy for facilitating communication and language development in the classroom. *Seminars in Speech and Language, 5*, 213–228.

Soto, G., Huer, M.B., & Taylor, O. (1997). Multicultural issues. In L.L. Lloyd, D.R. Fuller, & H.H. Arvidson (Eds.), *Augmentative and alternative communication: A handbook of principles and practices* (pp. 406–413). Boston: Allyn & Bacon.

Wilkinson, K.M., Romski, M.A., & Sevcik, R.A. (1994). Emergence of visual-graphic symbol combinations by youth with moderate or severe mental retardation. *Journal of Speech and Hearing Research, 37*, 883–895.

7

Language is the Key

Constructive Interactions Around Books and Play

KEVIN N. COLE, MARY MADDOX, AND YOUNG SOOK LIM

ABSTRACT

The Language is the Key: Constructive Interactions Around Books and Play (LIK) model is designed to optimize language development of young children with unmet communication needs, as well as children who are limited in English proficiency. Its most innovative features involve the use of common language facilitation techniques (e.g., use of open-ended questions, expansion of child utterances) during shared book-reading tasks (i.e., dialogic or interactive book reading). The model is designed to be delivered by a wide range of individuals, including professionals, paraprofessionals, and family members. In addition, we advocate that parents speak to their children using the language the parents know best in order to enhance early language acquisition, while professionals facilitate English in the school environment. The efficacy of the model has been supported by research with children with disabilities and with children whose parents speak a language other than English at home.

INTRODUCTION

The LIK model consists of training materials and procedures to encourage parents and other caregivers to use language facilitation techniques with children when looking at books together and during play. The target behaviors include 1) making comments about the child's interests, 2) asking questions related to the child's interests, and 3) responding to child utterances by adding a little more information. In addition, the training content includes providing wait time for the child to respond after an adult speaks.

TARGET POPULATIONS AND ASSESSMENTS FOR DETERMINING TREATMENT RELEVANCE AND GOALS

The primary target group for the LIK model is young children with delayed language who are functioning developmentally below approximately the 4-year-old level. Materials we have developed also make the approach appropriate for young children whose parents are most proficient in a language other than English. It is important to note that the model is also useful for young children who are developing typically or who may even be advanced in development (Whitehurst et al., 1988). Because of this, the speech-language pathologist (SLP) can implement this model through parent groups without the need to separate out parents who have children who are struggling with language development. Thus, an SLP could use this model to provide support to organizations such as Head Start, to child care, and to other inclusive environments that are appropriate for the general population as well as for families of children with special needs.

Children with specific language impairment (i.e., children with typical cognitive development and delayed language development) and children with developmental lag language impairment (i.e., exhibiting equivalent delays in cognitive development and language development) appear to benefit equally from services by SLPs (e.g., Cole & Fey, 1996). Children who have unmet communication needs benefit from SLP involvement, regardless of the relationship between their IQ scores and language assessment scores. Because of this, we make no distinction between these two broad groups in recommending language facilitation services, including use of the LIK model.

Appropriate assessments can include a wide range of receptive and expressive language measures in the early childhood age range. Measures derived from language samples, including rate or number of utterances, mean length of utterance (MLU), and vocabulary diversity, have been used in past research to indicate change. Indications that a child is ready to participate in the intervention are 1) the ability to remain in proximity to the adult, and 2) interest (or, at a minimum, lack of aversion) toward the book or play activity. Thus, very young children and infants may be talked to in the context of books and play, although assessments may need to include developmentally appropriate measures including body orientation, gaze, mood state assessment, and joint attention. Contraindications for the intervention may include reluctance to interact, or the child's self-redirection to other objects or activities.

Although young children with unmet communication needs are the final target population, the model encourages SLPs to provide training to other stakeholders who can, in turn, use the language facilitation methods with children. In this sense, a secondary target population is parents and early childhood service providers, including Head Start staff, child care providers, librarians, paraprofessionals, and others who may interact with young children in book interactions and play activities.

THEORETICAL BASIS

Although this intervention is relatively simple and straightforward, it is based on several diverse theoretical foundations. In this section, we outline the theoretical elements supporting 1) the value of picture book and play interactions in facilitating language and early literacy development, 2) the use of the intervention with minority language populations, 3) the benefit of facilitating the child's heritage language in the home as an avenue to English acquisition, and 4) the importance of encouraging sustainable routines in the home when providing language intervention support to parents.

Using Picture Book and Play Interactions to Facilitate Language and Literacy Development

Children with delayed language are clearly at risk for school failure. Follow-up studies have documented that children with language delays are much more likely to have academic, social, and linguistic deficits later in life than are children with adequate language development (e.g., Catts, Fey, Tomblin, & Zhang, 2002; Stothard, Snowling, Bishop, Chipchase, & Kaplan, 1998). Early intervention can, however, significantly improve language and academic functioning by the time children enter the primary grades (Cole, Mills, & Dale, 1989; Whitehurst et al., 1994).

At the broadest theoretical level, this intervention is consistent with a connectionist model of development (Elman et al., 1996), grounded in the notion that the child's interactions with his or her environment are critical to neurobehavioral development. Maturation alone, without specific types of environmental stimulation, is thought not to be sufficient for language development to occur. The LIK approach also adheres to a constructivist developmental model of child growth (e.g., Leong & Bodrova, 1995). Although we recognize the essential role of key adult interaction in language development, we also acknowledge the role of the child in guiding his or her own development. Thus, we incorporate the developmentally appropriate practices of following the child's lead in activities and making available materials and activities that are in the appropriate range of development for the child. The role of books and play within this broader theoretical framework is more practical.

Interactions between adults and children around picture books provide a very rich opportunity for young children to learn language and preliteracy skills (Ninio & Bruner, 1978; Wells, 1985). It is important to note that picture book interactions may not involve reading at all. In terms of promoting language development in very young children, it may be more beneficial for adults *not* to read, but rather to use books as a point of departure for talking and listening. Thus, appropriate books for this model might include picture books with no text at all, as well as books that include both text and pictures, with a larger focus on the pictures.

In a seminal study involving preschoolers with typical language, Whitehurst et al. (1988) demonstrated empirically that specific techniques used during picture book time can have very positive effects on language development. Significant differences in grammatical complexity and verbal description of objects between experimental and control groups were found after only two 30-minute training sessions provided to parents. Although these effects were somewhat diminished later, they were still observed at a 9-

month follow-up. Perhaps the most convincing argument for the use of picture book interaction techniques described above is the cost–benefit ratio of the intervention. A brief period of parent training leads to meaningful gains in the children's language performance.

The rationale for the success of picture book interactions is more practical than theoretical. Books provide a specific shared context for interactions, and they are often associated with undivided adult attention and comfort. In addition, a well-chosen picture book will be developmentally appropriate and of interest to the child. Book interactions may be reinforcing to the adult in their use as mood regulators for the child (e.g., a calming activity before bedtime) and as positive social routines with the child that are inherently enjoyable.

Using Communication Around Play to Facilitate Language and Literacy Development

Conversations with adults in everyday activities are as important as picture book interactions in providing critical language experience (Wells, 1981). Studies have found strong relationships between play and language development (e.g., Bates, Benigni, Bretherton, Camaioni, & Volterra, 1979; McCune-Nicolich & Bruskin, 1982; Shore, 1986), especially for children with disabilities (e.g., Cunningham, Glenn, Wilkinson, & Sloper, 1985; Dansky, 1980; Kennedy, Sheridan, Radlinski, & Beeghly, 1991; Ogura, Notari, & Fewell, 1991). Furthermore, language use by parents with children during play and other daily activities has proven to be a strong predictor of later language development (Hart & Risley, 1995).

Using Picture Book Interactions and Communication Around Play with Language Minority Children with Disabilities

Training provided by the LIK model prepares staff and parents to use picture book interactions and play to facilitate language. The U.S. Department of Education has estimated that approximately 175,000 teachers are still needed to serve the nation's English language learner (ELL) students (i.e., children whose home language is other than English; Schmidt, 1992). Finding specialty personnel (e.g., early childhood special educators, speech pathologists) who are trained to teach ELLs is even more difficult. Schools often supplement their programs for language minority students with bilingual paraprofessionals who help students who are limited in English proficiency negotiate the instructional environment. However, for many low-incidence languages even bilingual aides are unavailable to provide support and the only instructional option, by default, is an English-only approach. In these circumstances, the picture book and play contexts in English can be enhanced through the use of the LIK model, and parent training can provide a concurrent language enhancement in the parents' most proficient language at home.

The picture book and play contexts are natural ways to add a heritage language component to preschool programs by involving parents who have limited English proficiency in the education of their children. Picture book and play strategies do not place parents in the unnatural and frequently unwanted role of "teaching" their children (Winton & Turnbull, 1982) and do not require the high costs associated with time-intensive parent training. It is important to note that the picture book and play techniques do not require literacy in either English or the family's first language. Instead, the strategies are easy to learn and give parents tools they can use in typical family contexts. Because literacy is not a prerequisite for use of these techniques, more parents can benefit from the methods.

The LIK model is designed to facilitate language, preliteracy, and play activities that are appropriate for a variety of cultures and ethnic groups. Books and play are rich environments for communication development for young children across cultures (Lim & Cole, 2002; Nagasaki, Katayama, & Morimoto, 1993; Teale, 1986). Valdez-Menchaca & Whitehurst (1992), for example, successfully used picture book language facilitation techniques to improve typically developing children's language through training provided to child care providers in Mexico. Chao (1995) suggested that, even though mothers' specific tactics may vary across Western and Chinese cultures, they share the desire to teach skills necessary for a successful future and developing relationships. Furthermore, functional similarities can be identified in typical parent–child interactions across Western and Chinese cultures. For example, due to the complexity of Chinese orthography, Chinese parents may reserve reading or working with the printed word for older children (Johnston & Wong, 2002). Even so, a functional equivalent to storybooks can be found in family photo albums or other material that does not focus primarily on text.

The LIK model also addresses effective use of interpreters in working with parents. Many programs use interpreters to communicate with parents. As American society becomes increasingly heterogeneous, cross-cultural communication skills are essential for early interventionists (Barrera, 1992; Lynch & Hanson, 1992). Yet staff are frequently unprepared to work with interpreters and translators and risk miscommunicating with parents. The LIK model provides information about this topic, including how to select interpreters and translators, when it is appropriate or not appropriate to use family members as interpreters, and the best formats for using interpreters, as well as other issues related to speaking style and privacy concerns.

Benefits of Facilitating the Child's Heritage Language at Home in Addition to English at School

The LIK model generally encourages use of the child's heritage language (L1) as well as English (L2) in the picture book and play contexts to help the child develop language and succeed in school. Research since the early

1980s has suggested that strengthening a child's heritage language will also support the development of English and help ensure that the child's acquisition of academic content and skills does not suffer (Cummins, 1981; Gutierrez, 1993; Wong-Fillmore & Valadez, 1986). Research has also substantiated that learners whose L1 proficiency is better developed acquire cognitively demanding aspects of L2 proficiency more rapidly than learners with less well-developed L1 skills (Cummins, 1980; Ekstrand, 1977; Genesee, 1978). Thus, children who get their parents' best language at home, even if it is not English, probably learn English faster when they are exposed to it in school. As a side benefit to this approach, the children may be more likely to maintain their heritage language in addition to English. There may also be cognitive and linguistic benefits of being bilingual. For example, several studies have reported that bilingual children are more cognitively flexible in certain respects and are better able to analyze linguistic meaning than monolingual children (e.g., Albert & Obler, 1978; Cummins, 1979).

Maintaining Sustainable Routines

For a language intervention method to work, it must not only be effective, it must actually get used. This rather fundamental notion may be especially relevant when we work with parents and child care staff. Odom (1988) used the term *impact* to describe the relationship between an intervention's effectiveness and its likelihood of being implemented. Thus, *Impact = Effectiveness × Likelihood of Implementation* (Odom, McConnell, & McEvoy, 1992). If we ask parents to attend 6-week evening workshops to learn how to work with their children, and then ask them to rearrange their schedules to build new activities into their daily routines, the likelihood of implementation may be reduced. Even if the intervention is remarkably powerful, it cannot be effective if it is not used. Consequently, the LIK model is designed to be learned quickly and to dovetail into existing family, school, and child care facility routines.

In summary, the LIK model is based on connectionist theory and constructivist theory, as well as basic behaviorist principles (i.e., if the activity is enjoyable it will be conducted more frequently, and the impact of a model is related to its use).

EMPIRICAL BASIS

The effectiveness of language facilitation in the context of picture book interactions has been examined with children who are developing typically, children with delayed language development, children from middle and lower socioeconomic environments, and children whose first language is other than English. Studies are described in the following sections.

One of the seminal studies (Whitehurst et al., 1988) included parents and typically developing 2-year-old children from middle to high socioeconomic status families. Following random assignment, parents in the intervention group received a home-based intervention of two half-hour sessions. The control group received no training but read to their children as often as the intervention group.

Audiotapes of parent–child interactions at home were analyzed, and the mothers in the intervention group performed significantly better at using the target language facilitation techniques. The target behaviors included asking "what" questions and open-ended questions, following answers by the child with a question, repeating what the child says, praising the child, helping the child as needed, following the child's interests, expanding what the child says, and having fun. Whitehurst et al. referred to this model as *dialogic reading* to differentiate between this language facilitation focus and simply reading a body of text to the child.

Posttests after approximately 6 weeks, consisting of grammatical complexity and expressive language measures, revealed significant gains for the children in the intervention group relative to the control group with changes from pretest to posttest of at least 6 months in skill development. These effects were maintained at a 9-month follow-up. The results were especially striking because the children were already functioning at an advanced level in language ability, and parents were already reading to their children frequently. Researchers found these results promising and began examining the use of the methods with other target groups, including children from low socioeconomic backgrounds, children with disabilities, and children who spoke languages other than English.

Whitehurst and colleagues (1994) and Lonigan and Whitehurst (1998) examined the use of these picture book interaction methods with typical preschoolers from low socioeconomic status families. Whitehurst et al. (1994) randomly assigned 3-year-old children to one of three conditions: Exposure to dialogic reading from child care staff and parents, exposure from child care staff only, and exposure to play activities rather than book interaction. Significant differences were found favoring the intervention groups over the play condition, and effects were again maintained at a 6-month follow-up. The combined child care and home condition produced greater gains than the child care only condition. A replication of this study was conducted by Lonigan and Whitehurst (1998) and included one additional condition: picture book interactions with parents only. Again they found significant gains for the school–home combined intervention groups, and no significant difference was seen between the school-only and control groups. Thus, the greatest gains in both studies were found in groups that involved parents.

The work of Whitehurst and colleagues with typically developing children indicated that the specific picture book interactions, such as asking questions, expanding on child responses, and providing descriptions, resulted in improvements in children's language performance regardless of who implements the procedures and the context within which they are used. Building on the work of Whitehurst and colleagues, other researchers explored whether this same type of approach would also be effective with children with language delays and their parents (Dale, Crain-Thoreson, Notari-Syverson, & Cole, 1996). This study also examined the relative efficacy of the picture book interaction training in comparison with the more traditional training around conversational use of language facilitation techniques during play.

Dale et al. (1996) randomly assigned parent–child dyads to either the dialogic reading training or a conversational training. Children in the study ranged in age from 3 to 7 years. They exhibited language delays in the mild to moderate range. The dialogic reading training consisted of mothers viewing a videotape developed by Whitehurst, followed by a brief group discussion. The conversational training consisted of viewing a videotape describing and modeling the use of informational talk (describing what the child is doing or seeing), using expansions of child utterances, encouraging open-ended questions, and showing interest in the child's activities. Thus, the two conditions involved the same procedures but varied the context—either book reading or conversation.

Pretest and posttest language samples were gathered and analyzed for both parent and child behaviors. Parent behaviors included asking yes/no questions and open-ended questions, expansions, information talk, and imitations. Child behaviors included making statements, asking questions, imitating adult utterances, and nonverbal attending. Parents in the picture book intervention produced significantly more what/who questions, open-ended questions, and imitations than did the conversational intervention. Children in the picture book intervention also produced significantly more different words than did the children in the conversational intervention. Dale et al. (1996) found that there was a correlation between parent use of the techniques and child gains, supporting the interpretation that the intervention resulted in child change.

The efficacy of picture book interactions with children who have language delays was also examined by Hargrave and Senechal (2000). They compared two types of book interactions—dialogic reading and traditional book reading—with preschool children delayed in expressive vocabulary only. The traditional book-reading situation involved parents reading to their children with no emphasis on interacting with the child about the contents of the book. This was compared with dialogic reading. Both the traditional book reading condition and the interactive book use resulted in vocabulary gains from pretest to posttest, but the interactive method resulted in significantly more gains than the traditional reading method. Similar results were found by Crain-Thoreson and Dale (1999). They trained parents and early childhood special education staff in interactive reading methods under three conditions: parent instruction with one-to-one practice, staff instruction with one-to-one practice, and staff instruction without one-to-one practice.

They then examined language development over an 8-week period for children with mild to moderate language delays across a range of developmental levels. Delays included both isolated language delays and delays occurring as one aspect of overall developmental delay. They found that all three conditions resulted in longer utterances by children, more diverse vocabulary use, and more frequent utterances during book interactions. Again, the magnitude of change in children's language performance was correlated with the use of the techniques presented in the training.

These findings indicated that children with disabilities benefit from parent training in specific picture book interaction methods. In fact, comparisons of book interaction and play as contexts for the use of language intervention have indicated that where differences exist, they favor book reading. Available studies also suggest that information presented to parents in videotape format can be an effective component of intervention. The efficacy of a videotape format, an important element of the LIK model, was supported in a study by Arnold, Lonigan, Whitehurst, and Epstein (1994) with children developing typically. Parent–child dyads were assigned randomly to three conditions: A direct training group received instruction by a trainer in dialogic reading during two sessions and was given written descriptions of the intervention components. The video training group received training via videotape, as well as the written instructions. The group in the control condition received no training. All groups looked at approximately the same number of books per week during the 4 weeks of intervention.

Posttests were administered to children, including the Expressive One-Word Picture Vocabulary Test (EOWPVT; Brownell, 2000), the Peabody Picture Vocabulary Test–Revised (PPVT-R; Dunn & Dunn, 1981), and the Illinois Test of Psycholinguistic Abilities-Verbal Expression subtest (ITPA-VE; Kirk, McCarthy, & Kirk, 1968). The video group performed significantly higher than the control group on each of these measures. The direct training group outperformed the control group on the ITPA-VE, but not on the other measures. The video condition was also compared with the training condition. The video group scored significantly higher on the EOWPVT and the PPVT-R. The authors suggested that the video training may have been more effective because it consisted of a more standardized presentation. They also postulated that the videotape's inclusion of mothers modeling behaviors may have been more effective than modeling by professionals, and it may have allowed the mothers to see more clearly the effect of the methods on children.

In addition to evidence of general efficacy with typically developing children and those with language delays, several studies have indicated that specific language facilitation methods used in the context of picture book reading are effective with adult–child dyads who speak a language other than English. Valdez-Menchaca and Whitehurst (1992) trained staff in a Mexican child care program to use picture books to facilitate language with 2-year-old children from lower socioeconomic backgrounds who were thought to be typically developing. A control group of children received arts and crafts training from the same teacher. The intervention group scored significantly higher on both standardized language measures and on measure of language production.

To examine whether the picture book interaction methods might also be appropriate and useful for Asian families, Lim and Cole (2002) conducted a study with Korean families. Twenty-one children, ages 2–4 years, and their mothers participated. The children were considered by their parents to be developing typically. The mean MLU in words (MLU-W) for the children was 2.28. Korean was the parents' first language, and it was spoken in the home. Dyads were assigned randomly to a treatment or control condition. The treatment group received approximately 1 hour of instruction in specific language facilitation techniques around picture book interactions. The control group received approximately 1 hour of instruction in general emergent literacy development and the importance of first language acquisition. The parent intervention then lasted approximately 6 weeks. Results from pretest-posttest language samples indicated significant between-group differences in parents' use of methods and in children's language production, both favoring the treatment group. Specifically, the treatment group parents made significantly more gains in asking questions to children, responding to children's talking, and providing time for children to respond. The children in the treatment group had significantly longer MLU-W, produced more utterances, and used a greater variety of vocabulary than did the children in the control group. The mean effect size for children in this study was 1.8 for the treatment group, indicating that changes were large enough to be educationally meaningful.

Lim and Cole (2003) then conducted a follow-up of the treatment and control groups 1 year after the initial study. They found that the children in the treatment group still produced significantly more utterances (effect size = 1.82) and significantly more diverse vocabulary during picture book interactions with their parents (effect size = 1.53) than did the children in the control group. Parents were still asking questions (effect size = 1.82) and making comments (effect size = 1.50) more often than parents in the control condition. When they were contacted to participate in the follow-up study, many of the parents in the treatment group apologized because they felt they were no longer using the methods (when, in fact, they were still using them). They apparently had internalized the use of the techniques to the degree that it had become transparent to them.

In addition to research in school and clinical settings, the efficacy of picture book interactions has been examined in a broad dissemination through a city library system (Huebner, 2000). Librarians were trained as trainers in picture book interaction methods and then taught the methods to parents during two 1-hour sessions. Parents were assigned randomly to the intervention group or to a group that received only information in general library services. After 6 weeks, pretest-posttest comparisons indicated a significant advantage for the interactive picture book group on expressive vocabulary development.

In summary, research regarding specific methods of interaction around picture books by parents and teachers indicates both short- and long-term gains in language production and development for children with delayed language and children who are developing typically. In addition, the methods appear to be culturally appropriate for families who speak a language other than English at home. We have not yet evaluated the LIK model for play activities specifically, although play has traditionally been a medium for language facilitation.

PRACTICAL REQUIREMENTS

The LIK model is implemented through a training program that can be used in different settings (e.g., clinic, home, center-based early childhood program, child care facility) and with a wide variety of different people (e.g., professionals, paraprofessionals, volunteers, parents, family members, older school children). The videotapes and written materials provide resources that facilitate both basic and in-depth training aimed at preparing adults to apply basic language facilitation techniques.

Basic Training for All Staff and Parents

A very basic training scenario for staff or parents in a center-based early childhood program might be conducted as follows:

Session I   Parents view and then discuss the *Talking and Books* videotape. This takes approximately 1 hour. The materials include answers to frequently asked questions, and "refrigerator" handouts (in several languages) are given to remind parents and service providers of the techniques to be used. The basic techniques (e.g., commenting, asking questions, responding by adding a little more, and giving time to respond) are modeled and practiced. A more detailed description of these techniques is included in the Key Components section.

Session II   Parents view and then discuss the *Talking and Play* videotape. This 1-hour session includes a review of the language facilitation techniques presented at the first session but demonstrates their use in a different setting: play activities. Handouts and discussion guidelines are provided in the training manual.

In-Depth Training for Staff

In addition to training in the use of the basic techniques, the LIK model also offers guidelines for providing training to parents and other staff. Handouts and other written material are provided with the LIK video materials to support this in-depth training. Training suggestions include structured peer support among teachers/paraprofessionals or parents. Guidelines for peer coaching are provided in the training manual. The LIK manual also includes information to address frequently asked questions about the methods, suggestions for books to select, and extended examples of the basic methods. We allow (and encourage) SLPs to make copies of the videotapes and materials to distribute to parents and other professionals. This practice, paired with the training-of-trainers materials included in the manual, facilitates wider dissemination of the model.

Using the Program in a Clinical Setting

In a clinical setting, the SLP may choose to work with parents individually to prepare them to use the language facilitation techniques during book and play time at home. Parents of target children can take the videotapes home and view them independently or view them in the treatment setting followed by a debriefing by the clinician. Streaming video opportunities are also available at http://www.UWTV.org for parents who have high-speed access to the Internet. Group meetings during which parents view the videotapes and have an opportunity to ask questions and discuss the procedures also can be used. This setting allows for interaction among parents and gives the trainees an opportunity to discuss the concepts and strategies with the SLP as a participant.

A basic, one-page handout for each language version of the Language is the Key program is provided for parents who are ELLs. Each handout provides a 2- to 6-word summary of each language facilitation technique that is presented in acronym form for easy recall. The handout is intended to be taken home by the trainees as a reminder of the techniques presented in the videos. Parents are encouraged to look at books and play with their children daily. We suggest 15 minutes a day as a general rule but encourage parents to follow the child's lead in determining the actual length of interactions.

Materials Used in This Intervention

We encourage trainers to bring a variety of books and toys to training sessions so they can model offering children a selection of several books or toys from which to choose. The most important factor in selecting books and toys that will stimulate language is the individual child's interests, which can only be determined by observing and working with the child.

Choosing Books   We have observed that children may be less likely to converse when presented with counting books, name-the-color or object-type books, and alphabet books. We have also found that children are more stimulated to talk when books have lively pictures that vary significantly in content from page to page and are colorful. Parents are encouraged to allow children to choose the same book over and over, view the book from front to back, or flip pages until they come to one they like. We encourage trainees, especially with younger children, to focus on facilitating language rather than stressing the teaching of book conventions (e.g., starting at the front, turning one page at a time).

Choosing Toys   When toys are used to facilitate language, observing the child's interests and following his or her lead will help trainees choose specific toys. Adults may want to observe their children carefully during a free play time to identify the toys that encourage talking for a given child. An individual child's interests may vary between manipulative toys and representational toys, or the child may prefer one over the other. For many children, the play setting may not be as stimulating as the book setting for language production. Children tend to talk about what they are doing with objects during play (Bloom & Tinker, 2001); however, language production has been shown to decrease during play activities that involve construction activities, such as blocks or sand table (Kahneman, 1973; van Geert, 1991). For children who have difficulty interacting during play, SLPs can encourage parents to focus on language facilitation during book time.

We generally present book interactions first to parents. Book reading often is already in their repertoire, while floor play may be a newer activity for some parents. In addition, books provide a concrete, shared context, so practice in the LIK methods may be somewhat easier to master in that context. Play, in contrast, can be much more fluid, and the referent for conversations may be less clear to the adult, especially in more open-ended, imaginary play interactions. Because of this, we suggest conducting a session for use of the LIK methods in the context of play after training in use of the methods around books. An exception to this practice is when parents do not come from a culture that has a history of literacy. In this case, looking at books may be a less familiar activity than play and it may be appropriate to conduct training around play first.

KEY COMPONENTS

LIK provides an intervention for children with language disorders and promotes language skills in children who are developing typically. The basic goals of the intervention are general targets in form, content, and use of language.

For example, the research noted earlier has reported gains in MLU, improvements on receptive and expressive language tests, and increase in frequency of utterance production.

Content

The basic skills promoted in the materials are commenting, asking questions, responding by adding a little more, and giving time to respond. In addition, we encourage following a child's interests in selecting materials and choosing topics. Examples of each of the techniques are provided in Table 7.1.

Setting

The goals typically are addressed one on one wherein the child and adult engage in the prescribed language-stimulating activities (looking at books or engaging in play), with the adult coaching and offering encouragement in the form of comments, questions and expansions, recasts, and expatiations. In a center-based program setting, small groups of two to three children also can benefit from this intervention, although individual interaction may have some advantages, depending on the child's abilities and characteristics (Lonigan & Whitehurst, 1998). The one-on-one format, however, may be more effective in allowing the adult to follow the child's interests and in providing wait time for the child to respond. Our frequent observation of group interaction around books is that children who are more verbal produce the greatest number of responses, and children who need more time to process responses miss opportunities to practice language use. In addition, children who have difficulty shifting their attention to new topics may have less interest in group interactions.

Clinical Role of the Speech-Language Pathologist

In a clinical setting in which parents are taught to use language facilitation techniques, as incorporated in the LIK model, the SLP's role is to refine the parents' use of the techniques through discussion and demonstration and by providing feedback on parent performance. To monitor implementation at

Table 7.1. Basic skills promoted in Language is the Key

Skill	Example
Commenting: The adult notices what the child is interested in with the book or toy and makes a comment (and waits).	(Child points to a ball). Adult says, "I like to play ball."
Asking questions: The adult, guided by what the child seems to be interested in, asks a question appropriate to the child's developmental level (and waits).	(Child knocks a stack of blocks over). Adult says, "What happened?" or (Child looks at a picture and says, "House"). The adult says "What color is the house?"
Responding by adding a little more: After the child talks, the adult expands, recasts, or expatiates the utterance (and waits).	(Child says, "Ball"). Adult says, "Big blue ball" or (Child says, "Get on bus." The adult says "You are ready to go to school."

home, the SLP can encourage parents to keep a log of the times they look at picture books or play with their child and to audiotape samples of book and play time.

We conducted parent interviews to gather qualitative information about parents' perceptions of the LIK methods. Observations from these parent reports may be of use to SLPs in following up on parent training. Parents reported that they had the greatest difficulty making comments and giving the child time to respond after the adult talked. In addition to these parent reports, we also noted observationally that following the child's lead was a relatively difficult skill to learn for some parents, although modeling and coaching were effective in getting parents to let the child turn the pages of the book or, during play, to talk about what the child was doing.

In developing the videotapes, we took into account the relative difficulty of the tasks and included more examples and more instructional redundancy for the difficult tasks. We recommend that discussion and modeling by the SLP for parents also reflect the relative difficulty of the tasks and that more time be spent on *commenting* and *waiting* to be sure these skills are adequately understood and implemented.

SLPs will also find that some children may resist the transition from having a parent simply read the book to having the parent talk about the book. This appeared to be the case for some children above the developmental age of 3 years. In this situation, parents were most successful if they responded to the child's request to read the text for a period of time, then gradually added comments or questions. Switching to a less familiar book or a wordless book can also help with this transition.

For videotape materials in languages other than English, we taught a strategy to be used when the parent spoke in the heritage language, and the child responded in English. We encouraged parents to repeat the child's English language utterance in the heritage language. For example, if a child said, "Vamos a la store," the adult might respond with a model, "Vamos a la botega." Our goal was to facilitate the heritage language. With parents who are most comfortable speaking their heritage language, this strategy is very easy to learn and employ. However, we observed that, among bilingual parents who are very comfortable with English and their heritage language, this strategy was frequently converted to direct teaching in which the parent says a word and asks the child to repeat it. Clinicians may want to look for this behavior and redirect parents to the strategy, *Repeat again in Spanish (or the appropriate heritage language),* which is a response to the child's code switching rather than direct teaching of the heritage language.

Obviously, parents who are less successful at engaging their children in language facilitation will require more intensive intervention. In instances in which child language production is particularly limited, the SLP may want to provide additional tools for parents to increase social engagement and motivation to communicate. For example, SLPs might encourage increased use of facial expressions and other aspects of affect in interacting with the child. The SLP may also want to demonstrate other methods for encouraging engagement, such as "playful obstruction" (Greenspan & Weider, 1997), in which the adult interaction partner joins in and gently impedes the child's play (e.g., "accidentally" sitting in front of a desired toy) to encourage communication. This type of "sabotage" is common in many forms of language intervention (cf. Fey, 1986; Chapter 3, this volume). The LIK model helps provide a foundation for successful language facilitation between children and caregivers, but it is not meant to be a substitute for finely targeted language intervention that considers the specific needs of the parents and child.

Goals

As noted earlier in this chapter, the goals addressed by the LIK model are very broad: General language stimulation and increased opportunities for responding are the key outcomes of the model. Targeting more specific goals at home (e.g., asking parents to try to elicit specific vocabulary items or classes of syntactic forms) could interrupt the comfort of picture book time and playtime. We attempted this in early stages of development of our model by putting sticky notes in books that cued parents to ask particular questions or make specific comments. Parents reported (and our observations confirmed) that this was not particularly effective. We postulated that these cues conflicted with the parents' attempts to follow the child's lead, which may be a key aspect of successful interaction at the target age range.

Although specific skill targeting may not be appropriate for many parents to implement, SLPs and early childhood special education staff can, of course, use picture book interactions and play as very effective methods of facilitating specific language targets. When very specific language targets are practiced to mastery with the SLP or teacher in the context of a particular book or toy, the same materials may then be used at home to encourage carryover to the different setting and different communication partners.

Training-of-Trainers Role for the Speech-Language Pathologist

In addition to the role of direct service provider and support to parents in specific language facilitation services, the LIK materials allow the SLP to provide general language facilitation support to the community. To encourage this "training-of-trainers" dissemination, we encourage SLPs to make copies of the videotapes and written materials to give away to people they train. We require only that they not be sold.

ASSESSMENT METHODS TO SUPPORT ONGOING DECISION MAKING

To monitor and assess child progress with the broad language facilitation goals around which the LIK model is built, we recommend the use of relatively broad language measures. These may include standardized measures of receptive and expressive vocabulary and morphosyntactic form. We would also suggest measures derived from language samples, including frequency of utterances (or rate per minute), MLU, and semantic diversity such as number of different words. Changes in pragmatic language skill in response to the LIK model have not yet been examined; however, the kinds of interactions that often occur around books and play (e.g., requesting information, responding on topic, turn taking) may affect this language domain as well.

It may be as important to assess the behavior of the parents and caregivers around books and play as it is to monitor child change. We suggest asking parents to audiotape samples of their book and play interactions. It may also be helpful to use a notebook that passes back and forth between the SLP and the parent that cues the parent to identify books read and to note any concerns the parent might have. Although most parents appear to be able to learn the methods in a short period of time, we recommend periodic informal monitoring to support parents in aspects of the model that may be more difficult. For example, parents reported in interviews that waiting after they talked was quite difficult, and our direct observation of parents indicated that making comments was an interaction skill that was somewhat difficult to acquire relative to the other techniques (Lim & Cole, 2002). Thus, SLPs might also anticipate that more difficult skills, such as commenting and providing wait time, could be encouraged and monitored more regularly. An anecdote from our initial study with young children with disabilities (Dale et al., 1996) reinforces the need for parent monitoring. As part of the research protocol, we advised parents to have fun and try to interact with their child "about 15 minutes a day." In a follow-up interview we asked how the activity went. One parent replied, "Well, there were lots of tears sometimes, but we did it 15 minutes a day." Contact between the clinician and parents and other caregivers should be maintained following initial training. Gathering audiotapes or videotapes of adult–child interactions may also allow more refined follow-up suggestions to be provided by the clinician.

CONSIDERATIONS FOR CHILDREN FROM CULTURALLY AND LINGUISTICALLY DIVERSE BACKGROUNDS

Approximately 20% of students enrolled in U.S. schools live in families for which English is not the primary language (U.S. Bureau of the Census, 2000). According to the Head Start Bureau (2000), 26% of children enrolled in Head Start programs are from families that speak languages other than English. The development of heritage language literacy skills by bilingual children entails no negative consequences for their overall academic or cognitive growth or for their linguistic and social development (Hakuta, 1986; McCardle, Kim, Grube, & Randall, 1995), and there may be significant educational benefits. This appears also to be true for children with language delays (Bruck, 1982). There is considerable evidence of interdependence of literacy-related or academic skills across languages (Cummins, 1991), such that the better developed a child's first language is, the more likely the child will be to develop similarly high levels of conceptual abilities in a second language. Cummins (1986) also advances the theory that there is a common underlying proficiency between languages. Skills, ideas, and concepts a child learned in the first language readily transfer to the second language. Simultaneous language learners learn many words that are exclusive to one language and naturally use code switching. We found that this happened even though mothers spoke only in Korean when they interact with their children during book interaction. For example, one child counted, "*Hana* (one), *dul* (two), three, *net* (four), and this" (pointing as she counted objects in a book). In another example, the child said, "And then, hold on to *korae*'s *kori*" in which she used *korae* (a whale) in Korean but used -*s* for possessive, the English rule, and she used *kori* (a tail) in Korean, mixing two languages in the same context (Lim & Cole, 2002).

Picture book reading has long been recognized as a useful language facilitation activity. It creates a context in which language is repetitive and predictable and provides extra linguistic cues to meaning. In addition, parents are available to scaffold the use of new language forms (Dale et al., 1996). As noted earlier, picture book interactions are common across a variety of cultures, although differences exist in specific styles of interacting. Ochs (1982), for example, found that one of the most striking characteristics of Samoan child–adult interactions is the absence of expansions. Children who are highly referential are reinforced in middle class American culture. Mothers tend to view naming as a sensible and intelligent way to use language. To a Samoan mother, however, naming is more likely to be seen as "talking to no purpose." We found a similar view with some Spanish-speaking cultures when we conducted focus groups to help guide our development of materials. Two informants from different Spanish-speaking countries advised us against teaching what they both termed, "that Anglo thing." They were both referring to the practice of describing to the child what was in the environment even though it did not appear to be of particular interest to the child or have any clear communicative function (e.g., saying to a child in a shopping cart who is looking at something else: "Look here at the big stack of tomatoes. Aren't they a pretty red color?"). To avoid teaching "that Anglo thing," we stressed in our materials that the adult should follow the child's interests in books and play. This is inherent in the general principle of following the child's lead.

Another difference among cultures may be found in the importance of play. Western cultures tend to value parent–child interactions in play as a means of developing language and social skills (Kaderavek & Sulzby, 1999). However, Chinese parents may not view the use of play activities as a context for language teaching because they see less potential for learning in them. On the other hand, they might be willing to create explicit language lessons rather than embedding their teaching in play (Johnston & Wong, 2002).

A study regarding Japanese children's language development through mother–child conversation during picture book reading shows that Japanese mothers are more oriented toward development of affect, and they are less information-oriented than American mothers. They value affective communication more and linguistic ability less than do American mothers (Fernald & Morikawa, 1993). Similarly, Korean mothers reported that book reading could provide an emotional bond between mothers and children while sharing their time together during a picture book reading intervention (Lim & Cole, 2002).

Mothers can successfully acquire specific language facilitation techniques, such as following the child's lead, commenting, questioning, responding by adding a little more, and repeating in the heritage language when a child uses code switching following one session of training (Lim & Cole, 2002). This indicates that these types of interactive behaviors can be taught to parents within different cultural contexts. Parents can be encouraged to practice them during storybook reading with their children.

Texts or storybooks can also be very useful in providing representations of cultural values. Illustrations play an important part in the literacy development of children because illustrations are identified as being extremely significant in the processes children undergo as they construct meaning about cultural and personal identity (Makin & Diaz, 2002). Simply translating original stories into a second language without considering values and beliefs may not produce texts viewed as authentic across cultures. For example, the use of culturally appropriate pictures improved the language performance of African American children (Cazden, 1970).

Parents may use well-practiced narratives, supported by pictures, family photo albums or oral story telling without books to create the context of language learning if their cultures typically do not read to young children. If parents do not have literacy skills in their own language, it may be more useful for the SLP to focus on interactions around play first then introduce picture books at a later time. It may also be helpful to introduce picture books that have no text at all to alleviate the fear of embarrassment that may be associated with illiteracy by the parents.

APPLICATION TO AN INDIVIDUAL CHILD

When the LIK model was first implemented for him, Manuelito was a 3-year-old boy whose parents were first generation immigrants from Mexico. Manuelito scored 2 standard deviations (*SD*) below the mean on the Spanish version of the PPVT and 1.5 *SD* below the mean on the English PPVT-3. He qualified for early childhood special education services based on test scores and observation of functional performance, and he was referred to the SLP. Manuelito's early childhood special education teacher had 15 children in her class. She had one educational assistant. She also had parent volunteers 2 days a week as well as upper-grade student volunteers at times.

As one aspect of intervention, the SLP increased general language stimulation in both English at school and Spanish at home through training of parents, siblings, and staff in the LIK model. When Manuelito's parents were contacted, the SLP learned that they had been using English at home with Manuelito because they wanted to be sure he learned to speak the language and had a better chance of succeeding. It was evident from the conversation, however, that the model of English that they were providing was incomplete and sometimes incorrect. Manuelito's older sister, who was in sixth grade, also attended the meeting. She appeared to have well-developed basic interpersonal communication skills in English, and the English as a Second Language teacher reported that the sister's cognitive and academic language proficiency were roughly typical.

The SLP provided training to the parents using the Spanish-language videotapes and handouts. She advised the parents to use their most well-developed language (Spanish) when communicating with Manuelito. Manuelito's sister also was encouraged to read and talk about books to Manuelito in either English or Spanish. The SLP worked with the classroom staff to enhance their skills in using picture books and play to facilitate language. A parent volunteer and a sixth-grade volunteer viewed the training videotapes (in English) and worked with Manuelito one-on-one using English, with monitoring by the classroom teacher and the SLP. After family and staff were comfortable and consistent with using books to facilitate language, the SLP presented the videotape showing the same techniques used in the context of play.

FUTURE DIRECTIONS

We anticipate several new directions in model development and research in the future. We are still working to determine the best service delivery practices for the existing materials and plan to implement a variety of exploratory, efficacy, and effectiveness studies to validate their use. For example, we do not currently know the relative effects of presenting parents with the videotape only, compared with providing them with the videotape training paired with staff modeling. We are currently implementing a study to compare these two variables with the play videotape. We hope to replicate that study using the picture book videotape as well. We would also benefit from knowing more about best practices for follow-up after training. For example, would a weekly phone follow-up with parents in the first few weeks after training help them in implementing the techniques? Would it be useful, or too intrusive, to request that parents keep a brief log of reading time? Are group trainings of parents more or less effective than individual training sessions? More information about these and other refinements may add value to the intervention.

Finally, one of our most central interests is to determine whether the language intervention presented with literacy materials very early in children's lives limits their risks for later reading problems (Catts et al., 2002). Finding answers to this question, however, poses a very significant challenge to researchers.

In addition to refining the service delivery model, we also anticipate an expansion of similar materials to other age groups and other populations. It may be helpful to develop language facilitation procedures around book interactions for children in the developmental or chronological age range of 4–7 years. This might include facilitation of more advanced linguistic, cognitive, and social skills such as predicting what might happen next in a story, promoting theory of mind (e.g., questions such as, "Why do you think he did that?" or "How did she know?"), reviewing what has already happened in a story, developing alternative endings, and so forth.

Finally, SLP and early childhood special education staff who have used the existing materials have suggested that additional materials be developed for specific populations they serve. These have included children who are deaf or hearing impaired, children who exhibit characteristics of autism or pervasive developmental disability, and children who have very limited cognitive and communication development.

The LIK model does not provide new intervention techniques. The use of appropriate questions with children, modeling language in a communicative context, following the child's interests, scaffolding language input to the level of the child's development, providing enough time for the child to respond, and providing recasts, expansions, and expatiations for child utterances are all part of standard practice. Instead, the LIK model provides an effective, cost-efficient, and easy-to-disseminate set of materials to get these methods used in the home and in the classroom.

RECOMMENDED READINGS

Many of the references in this chapter provide specific details related to the Language is the Key model. The three recommended readings expand into the adjacent areas of early emergent literacy and cultural issues.

Notari-Syverson, A., O'Connor, R.E., & Vadasy, P.F. (1999). *Ladders to literacy: A preschool activity book*. Baltimore: Paul H. Brookes Publishing Co.

Tabors, P.O. (1997). *One child, two languages: A guide for preschool educators of children learning English as a Second Language*. Baltimore: Paul H. Brookes Publishing Co.

Whitehurst, G.J., & Fischel, J.E. (2000). Reading and language impairments in conditions of poverty. In D.V.M. Bishop & L.B. Leonard (Eds.), *Speech and language impairments in children: Causes, characteristics, intervention, and outcome* (pp. 53–71). Philadelphia: Psychology Press.

REFERENCES

Albert, M.L., & Obler, L.K. (1978). *The bilingual brain.* New York: Academic Press.

Arnold, D., Lonigan, C.J., Whitehurst, G.J., & Epstein, J.N. (1994). Accelerating language development through picture book reading: Replication and extension to a videotape training format. *Journal of Educational Psychology, 86,* 235–243.

Barrera, R.B. (1992). The cultural gap in literature-based literacy instruction. *Education and Urban Society, 24,* 227–243.

Bates, E., Benigni, L., Bretherton, I., Camaioni, L., & Volterra, V. (1979). *The emergence of symbols.* New York: Academic Press.

Bloom, L., & Tinker, E. (2001) The intentionality model and language acquisition: Engagement, effort and the essential tension in development. *Monographs of the Society for Research in Child Development, 66*(4, Serial No. 267).

Brownell, R. (2000). *Expressive One-Word Picture Vocabulary Test–2000 Edition (EOWPVT).* Minneapolis, MN: Pearson Assessments.

Bruck, M. (1982). Language impaired children's performance in an additive bilingual education program. *Applied Psycholinguistics, 3,* 45–60.

Catts, H., Fey, M., Tomblin, J., & Zhang, X. (2002). A longitudinal investigation of reading outcomes in children with language impairments. *Journal of Speech, Language, and Hearing Research, 45,* 1142–1157.

Cazden, C.B. (1970). The neglected situation in child language research and education. In F. Williams (Ed.), *Language and poverty: Perspectives on a theme* (pp. 81–101). Chicago: Markham.

Chao, R. (1995). Chinese and European American cultural models of the self reflected in mothers' childrearing beliefs. *Ethos, 23,* 328–354.

Cole, K.N., & Fey, M.E. (1996). Cognitive referencing in language assessment. In S.F. Warren & J. Reichle (Series Eds.) & K.N. Cole, P.S. Dale, & D.J. Thal (Vol. Eds.), *Communication and language intervention series: Vol. 6. Assessment of communication and language* (pp. 143–160). Baltimore: Paul H. Brookes Publishing Co.

Cole, K., Mills, P., & Dale, P. (1989). Comparison of effects of academic and cognitive curricula for young handicapped children one and two years post-program. *Topics in Early Childhood Special Education, 9(3),* 110–127.

Crain-Thoreson, C., & Dale, P. (1999). Enhancing linguistic performance: Parents and teachers as book reading partners for children with language delays. *Topics in Early Childhood Special Education, 19,* 28–39.

Cummins, J. (1979). Linguistic interdependence and the educational development of bilingual children. *Review of Educational Research, 49*(2), 222–251.

Cummins, J. (1980). The cross-lingual dimensions of language proficiency: Implications for bilingual education and the optimal age issue. *TESOL Quarterly, 14,* 174–187.

Cummins, J. (1981). The role of primary language development in promoting educational success for language minority students. In *Schooling and language minority students: A theoretical framework* (pp. 3–49). Los Angeles: California State University, Evaluation, Dissemination, and Assessment Center.

Cummins, J. (1986). Empowering minority students: A framework for intervention. *Harvard Educational Review, 56*(1), 18–36.

Cummins, J. (1991). Interdependence of first- and second-language proficiency in bilingual children. In E. Bialystok (Ed.), *Language processing in bilingual children* (pp. 70–89). New York: Cambridge University Press.

Cunningham, C., Glenn, S., Wilkinson, P., & Sloper, P. (1985). Mental ability, symbolic play, and receptive and expressive language of young children with Down syndrome. *Journal of Child Psychology and Psychiatry, 26,* 255–265.

Dale, P., Crain-Thoreson, C., Notari-Syverson, A., & Cole, K. (1996). Parent-child storybook reading as an intervention technique for young children with language delays. *Topics in Early Childhood Special Education, 16,* 213–235.

Dansky, J.F. (1980). Cognitive consequences of sociodramatic play and exploration training for economically disadvantaged preschoolers. *Journal of Child Psychology and Psychiatry, 20*, 47–58.

Dunn, L.M., & Dunn, L.M. (1981). *Peabody Picture Vocabulary Test–Revised.* Circle Pines, MN: American Guidance Service.

Ekstrand, L.H. (1977). Social and individual frame factors in second language learning: Comparative aspects. In T. Skutnabb-Kangas (Ed.), *Papers from the first Nordic conference on bilingualism.* Helsinki, Finland: Helsingfors Universitet.

Elman, J.L., Bates, E.A., Johnson, M.H., Karmiloff-Smith, A., Parisi, D., & Plunkett, K. (1996). *Rethinking innateness: A connectionist perspective on development.* Cambridge, MA: The MIT Press.

Fernald, A., & Morikawa, H. (1993). Common themes and cultural variations in Japanese and American mothers' speech to infants. *Child Development, 64*, 637–656.

Fey, M. (1986). *Language intervention with young children.* San Diego: College-Hill Press.

Genesee, F. (1978). Is there an optimal age for starting second language instruction? *McGill Journal of Education, 13*, 145–154.

Greenspan, S.I., & Weider, S. (1997). *The child with special needs: Encouraging intellectual and emotional growth.* Reading, MA: Perseus Books.

Gutierrez, K.D. (1993). Biliteracy and the language minority child. In B. Spodek & O. Saracho (Eds.), *Language and literacy in early childhood education* (pp. 82–101). New York: Teachers College Press.

Hakuta, K. (1986). *Mirror of language: The debate in bilingualism.* New York: Basic Books.

Hargrave, A., & Senechal, M. (2000). Book reading intervention with preschool children who have limited vocabularies: The benefits of regular reading and dialogic reading. *Early Childhood Research Quarterly, 15*, 75–90.

Hart, B., & Risley, T. (1995). *Meaningful differences in the everyday experience of young American children.* Baltimore: Paul H. Brookes Publishing Co.

Head Start Bureau. (2000). *Celebrating cultural diversity in Head Start.* Washington, DC: Commissioner's Office of Research and Evaluation and Head Start Bureau.

Huebner, C.E. (2000). Promoting toddlers' language development through community-based intervention. *Journal of Applied Developmental Psychology, 21*, 513–535.

Johnston, J.R., & Wong, M.Y.A. (2002). Cultural differences in beliefs and practices concerning talk to children. *Journal of Speech, Language, and Hearing Research, 45*, 916–926.

Kaderavek, J., & Sulzby, E. (1999). Issues in emergent literacy for children with language impairments. *CIERA* (Center for the Improvement of Early Reading Achievement) Report #2–002.

Kahneman, D. (1973). *Attention and effort.* Upper Saddle River, NJ: Prentice Hall.

Kennedy, M., Sheridan, M., Radlinski, S., & Beeghly, M. (1991). Play-language relationships in young children with developmental delays: Implications for assessment. *Journal of Speech and Hearing Research, 34*, 112–122.

Kirk, S.A., McCarthy, J.J., & Kirk, W.D. (1968). *Illinois Test of Psycholinguistic Abilities-Verbal Expression Subtest (ITPA-VE).* Chicago: University of Illinois Press.

Leong, D.J., & Bodrova, E. (1995). *Tools of the mind: A Vygotskian approach to early childhood education.* Upper Saddle River, NJ: Prentice Hall.

Lim, Y.S., & Cole, K.N. (2002). Facilitating first language development in young Korean children through parent training in picture book interactions. *Bilingual Research Journal, 26*, 367–381.

Lim, Y.S., & Cole, K.N. (2003). *One-year follow-up of Korean parent training in picture book interactions.* Manuscript submitted for publication.

Lonigan, C.J., & Whitehurst, G.J. (1998). Relative efficacy of parent and teacher involvement in a shared-reading intervention for preschool children from low-income backgrounds. *Early Childhood Research Quarterly, 13*, 263–290.

Lynch, E., & Hanson, M. (1992). *Developing cross cultural competence: A guide for working with young children and their families*. Baltimore: Paul H. Brookes Publishing Co.

Makin, L., & Diaz, J. (2002). *Literacies in early childhood: Challenging practice*. Sydney: MacLennan & Petty.

McCardle, P., Kim, J., Grube, C., & Randall V. (1995). An approach to bilingualism in early intervention. *Infants and Young Children, 7*, 63–73.

McCune-Nicolich, L., & Bruskin, C. (1982). Combinatorial competency in symbolic play and language. In D. Pepler & K. Rubin (Eds.), *The play of children: Current theory and research* (pp. 30–45). Basel, Switzerland: Karger.

Nagasaki, T., Katayama, H., & Morimoto, T. (1993). Early language interaction using a joint attention routine. *Japanese Journal of Special Education, 31*, 23–33.

Ninio, A., & Bruner, J.S. (1978). The achievement and antecedents of labeling. *Journal of Child Language, 5*, 1–15.

Ochs, E. (1982). Talking to children in Western Samoa. *Language in Society, 1*, 77–104.

Odom, S. (1988). Research in early childhood special education. In S. Odom & M. Karnes (Eds.), *Early intervention for infants and children with handicaps: An empirical base* (pp. 1–21). Baltimore: Paul H. Brookes Publishing Co.

Odom, S., McConnell, S., & McEvoy, M. (1992). Implementation of social competence interventions in early childhood special education classes: Current practices and future directions. In S. Odom, S. McConnell, & M. McEvoy (Eds.), *Social competence of young children with disabilities* (pp. 277–306). Baltimore: Paul H. Brookes Publishing Co.

Ogura, T., Notari, A., & Fewell, R. (1991). The relationship between play and language in young children with Down syndrome. *Japanese Journal of Developmental Psychology, 2*, 18–24.

Schmidt, P. (1992, February 12). Shortage of trained bilingual teachers is focus of both concern and attention. *Education Week*, p. 10.

Shore, C. (1986). Combinatorial play, conceptual development, and early multiword speech. *Developmental Psychology, 20*, 872–880.

Stothard, S., Snowling, M., Bishop, D., Chipchase, B., & Kaplan, C. (1998). Language impaired preschoolers: A follow-up into adolescence. *American Journal of Speech, Language, and Hearing Research, 41*, 407–418.

Teale, W.H. (1986). Home background and young children's literacy development. In W.H. Teale & E. Sulzby (Eds.), *Emergent literacy* (pp. 173–206). Norwood, NJ: Ablex.

U.S. Bureau of the Census. (2000). *U.S. Census Bureau: The official statistics*. Washington, DC: Author.

Valdez-Menchaca, M.C., & Whitehurst, G.J. (1992). Accelerating language development through picture book reading: A systematic extension to Mexican daycare. *Developmental Psychology, 28*, 1106–1114.

Van Geert, P. (1991). A dynamic systems model of cognitive and language growth. *Psychological Review, 98*, 3–53.

Wells, G. (1981). *Learning through interaction*. Cambridge, England: Cambridge University Press.

Wells, G. (1985). Preschool literacy-related activities and success in school. In D.R. Olson, N. Torrance, & A. Hildyard (Eds.), *Literacy, language and learning* (pp. 229–255). Cambridge, England: Cambridge University Press.

Whitehurst, G.J., Arnold, D., Epstein, J.N., Angell, A.L., Smith, M., & Fischel, J.E. (1994). A picture book reading intervention in day care and home for children from low-income families. *Developmental Psychology, 30*, 679–689.

Whitehurst, G.J., Falco, F.L., Lonigan, C.J., Fischel, J.E., DeFarshe, B.D., Valdez-Menchaca, M.C., & Caulfield, M. (1988). Accelerating language development through picture book reading. *Developmental Psychology, 24*, 552–558.

Winton, P., & Turnbull, A. (1982). Dissemination of research to parents. *Exceptional Parent, 12*, 32–36.

Wong-Fillmore, L., & Valadez, C. (1986). Teaching bilingual learners. In M.S. Wittrock (Ed.), *Handbook on research on teaching* (pp. 648–685). New York: Macmillan.

8

Focused Stimulation Approach to Language Intervention

SUSAN ELLIS WEISMER AND SHARI ROBERTSON

ABSTRACT

In focused stimulation, a child is exposed to multiple exemplars of a specific linguistic target (e.g., a specific vocabulary item or grammatical morpheme) within meaningful communicative contexts. Following exposure to such models, the child may be given opportunities to produce the linguistic construction, although this is not an obligatory feature of the approach. Imitation procedures are not used; instead, an attempt is made to elicit spontaneous productions of the target by taking advantage of naturalistic conversational contexts promoting the use of that target. Focused stimulation can be used to promote the form, content, and/or use of language and typically involves a contextually based service delivery model implemented by clinicians and/or parents. This approach is used with toddlers with early language delay (late talkers), as well as with preschool and early school-age children with specific language impairment and developmental disabilities.

INTRODUCTION

Focused stimulation is a long-standing treatment approach that has been used widely with various populations. In an article summarizing methods for facilitating language abilities in children with specific language impairment (SLI), Leonard (1981) described an approach that he referred to as *focused stimulation,* distinguishing this from a *general stimulation* approach. The distinction between the two approaches, which both entail types of modeling, rests on whether particular linguistic constructions are targeted. In focused stimulation, the child is provided with concentrated exposures of specific linguistic forms/functions/uses within naturalistic communicative contexts. In the original specification of this approach, Leonard described variations of this approach in which there is no attempt to evoke productions of the targets following exposure and those in which opportunities for target produc-

Focuses on input rather than output

tion are included. Two sample excerpts of clinical interactions are provided in Table 8.1 to illustrate the use of the focused stimulation approach. In the first case, specific vocabulary items (action and object labels) are modeled repeatedly, with no attempt to elicit productions of these words by the child. In the second case, focused models of locative forms (prepositions) are provided along with opportunities for the child to use the target forms. Some focused stimulation approaches have also incorporated recasts of children's spontaneous productions of linguistic targets to encourage the development of more complex language. Several investigators have recently provided definitions and descriptions of focused stimulation approaches that are similar to the original characterization of this approach (Ellis Weismer, 2000b; Lederer, 2001), although some researchers have placed relatively heavier emphasis on interactive components, linking this approach to the interactive model of language intervention used in parent training (e.g., Girolametto, Weitzman, & Clements-Baartman, 1998).

TARGET POPULATIONS AND ASSESSMENTS FOR DETERMINING TREATMENT RELEVANCE AND GOALS

Focused stimulation is primarily designed for and has been most thoroughly studied with late-talking toddlers, children with specific language impairment, and children with mental retardation. Secondary populations for whom this approach may prove useful include bilingual children with language delay and children who have phonological disorders with concomitant language delay; this approach may be particularly useful for the latter group when opportunities to produce phonological targets are incorporated within the treatment program (Camarata, 1995).

The developmental range for this approach includes toddlers through early elementary school-age children, with a focus on promoting vocabulary skills and early grammatical development. Prerequisite skills include joint attentional abilities and some degree of sustained attention to process multiple exemplars of selected linguistic input within ongoing communicative exchanges. Furthermore, the child needs to display at least a minimal level of social engagement for this type of interactive, naturalistic treatment approach to be appropriate. Although published reports of the efficacy of focused stimulation for children with autism spectrum disorders (ASD) are not available, this approach might be useful for higher functioning children who have the requisite social skills. The emphasis within focused stimulation is on input rather than output, so this approach can be used with children who have limited productive capabilities as well as with those who are more verbal.

As a first step, some combination of standardized tests, parent-report instruments, and language sample analysis would be used to determine the linguistic capabilities of a child and identify the need for treatment (see Paul, 2001). Once the need for treatment is established, dynamic assessment might

Table 8.1. Sample excerpts of focused stimulation

Sample 1. Use of focused stimulation to model target vocabulary (*dig* and *sand*) during sandbox play. Focused models are provided with no attempts to elicit production:

Clinician: Let's make something in the *sand*. Look at all this *sand*. Do you like to play with *sand*?

Child: Uh-huh.

Clinician: I do too. I like to *dig* in the *sand*. I can *dig* with my shovel. Do you want to *dig*? (Clinician hands the child the shovel.)

Clinician: Yes, *dig* the *sand*. Wow, look at you *dig*. Now we have a pile of *sand*. Look at all this *sand*. Uh, oh. Look at the floor! We got *sand* on the floor.

Sample 2. Use of focused stimulation to model locative forms *beside, in front*, and *behind* during a searching game. Focused models are provided along with opportunities for nonimitative productions of the target form:

Clinician: Let's play a game with Nemo (toy fish). Nemo swims all around the ocean. He looks for his dad beside the cave. Look, he's *beside* the cave. Now he looks *in front of* the rock. He's swimming *in front of* it.
   His dad isn't there. He swims *behind* the rock. Look on the other side. I don't see him *behind* the rock. Kisha, you tell Todd where Nemo should look. Where should Nemo swim now? (Clinician gives the toy fish to Todd.)

Kisha: The ship.

Clinician: Where?

Kisha: *Beside* the ship.

Clinician: Great, Nemo is looking *beside* the ship. He's *beside* it now. But I don't see his dad anywhere. Now it's Kisha's turn to make Nemo swim. Where should we look now, Todd?

Todd: By the fish.

Clinician: I don't know where you mean. Should he look beside the big fish?

Todd: *Behind*.

Clinician: *Behind* the fish—I see. Kisha, make Nemo swim *behind* that big fish. Great, now Nemo's *behind* the big blue fish.

---

be used to decide whether a focused stimulation approach appeared to be appropriate for the specific goals selected for that individual child (Bain & Olswang, 1995; Olswang, Bain, & Johnson, 1992). That is, the clinician would undertake an evaluation of the child's potential for change relative to the selected targets, using a focused stimulation treatment approach. For example, if the child demonstrates variable use of copula *be* forms, the clinician might first establish the baseline level of the child's correct use of this construction in a short spontaneous language sample. Then the clinician could provide a number of focused examples of utterances containing the target construction within a meaningful communicative context, in order to prime the child's use of this form. Finally, another spontaneous sample would be obtained to determine whether this supportive context facilitated more consistent use of the copula form. If intervention goals focus on early vocabulary usage, an assessment of the child's phonemic inventory should be completed along with other areas of language assessment, because it has been shown that young children are more likely to produce new words containing sounds within their current repertoire than words that contain sounds they have not yet acquired (Leonard et al., 1982; Schwartz & Leonard, 1982). It is common for "in-phonology" words to be selected as target vocabulary in treatment studies that have investigated the efficacy/effectiveness of focused stimulation (Ellis Weismer, Murray-Branch, & Miller 1993; Girolametto, Pearce, & Weitzman, 1996; Girolametto et al., 1998; Lederer, 2001).

THEORETICAL BASIS

Support for the use of focused stimulation to address language delays may be drawn from a variety of theoretical viewpoints. Although discussed separately below, the likelihood of a single theory accounting for the deficits of all children for whom the approach is appropriate is clearly limited. Whereas much support for focused stimulation can be drawn from theories that posit deficits in organizing and storing information, extracting patterns, and abstracting rules within the social context, it is highly probable that the actual explanation lies in a combination of tenets from these, and other, theoretical foundations. Furthermore, the theoretical perspectives discussed in this section are not mutually exclusive but rather work together to provide insight to guide clinical decision making. Regardless of why children are seen as having difficulty in extracting information about the ambient language, the rationale for using focused stimulation to improve language skills, and hence the common strand linking each of these theoretical models, is that the quality of the linguistic input, as nested within the social context, is of critical importance to language learning.

Social Theories as a Rationale/Foundation for Focused Stimulation

Social theories of learning propose bidirectional interactions between the unique cognitive characteristics of the learner, the environment, and the people within that environment. In contrast to behavioristic theories, in which all learning is viewed as the result of a conditioned response to a given stimulus, these models view individuals as cognitively active in the learning process and emphasize the importance of the social context to the speed and durability of the learning. Children with language delays are believed to be unable to extract and process information from the natural social context as effectively as children with more typical language learning capabilities. From this perspective, a more structured, focused, and enriched version of the language input than would occur naturally in typical parent–child interactions is believed to facilitate the language learning for children who manifest linguistic deficits.

Social Learning Theory   Bandura's (1977) classic theory of social learning suggests that human behaviors are learned through the observation of events, concepts, or activities modeled by others. In this way, with seemingly little effort, children who are typically developing are able to learn complex linguistic forms such as extracting the rules of syntax from models that occur naturally in their surrounding linguistic environment.

Approaches to language intervention that stem from this theory have in common the belief that attention is a critical component of learning (Fey, 1986). Furthermore, interactions between social factors and the individual characteristics of the learner heavily influence the level of attending which, in return, affect the individual's ability to perceive and retain information. For example, a toddler may be interested enough in a group of toy farm animals to attend to the verbal stimuli long enough to learn the labels when his or her mother is in the room; however, the same child may not attend to the stimuli at all if the mother leaves unexpectedly or another child starts to grab the referents.

Social Constructionist Theory   Theories stemming from this perspective (Bruner, 1983; Vygotsky, 1978) emphasize the role of the adult in fostering the child's learning across a variety of developmental domains. In effect, the adult and child work together within the dyad to construct meaning. Generally, the adult's role is to provide input that is of appropriate complexity and frequency for the child's developmental level. As the child's skills increase, the adult provides more complex input and less support, allowing the child to take more control in the learning process.

Transactional Model of Language Development   A more recent interpretation of social theory is the transactional model of language development as described by Yoder and Warren (1993). This model suggests that early disruptions in the development of a child's language system can have a negative impact on the child's ability to learn effectively within the natural social context. Reciprocal interactions between caregiver and child are envisioned during participation in social discourse that provides natural and positive rewards for each member of the dyad. Typically, a parent provides a language model (e.g., "See the monkey?") and the child imitates the model (e.g., "Monkey"). The success of the exchange encourages both members of the dyad to engage in future interactions with one another.

Alternatively, parents of children who are unable to participate effectively in communicative exchanges may find interacting with their children to be less enjoyable. They may respond to a child's lack of verbal responses by reducing the number of linguistic models they provide. Consequently, the child is exposed to fewer and less idealized models than might be provided to a more verbally responsive child when, in fact, what the child needs is a significant increase in exposure to appropriate verbal models. This phenomenon has been termed by Rice (1993) and others as a *negative social spiral.*

Theories stemming from social theories of language emphasize the critical role of the interactive context in which language learning occurs. From this perspective, focused stimulation addresses both the linguistic and social deficits associated with language delay as described by each of the variations of the theory discussed. Specifically, the concentrated models that are the hallmark of this intervention technique provide the child with multiple opportunities to observe language models—the critical requirement for learning according to social learning theory—which is presumed to lead to a more advanced level of language development. Because the language targets are preselected and modeled by the adult based on the child's current level of linguistic functioning, the child is provided with a scaffold within the dyad from which to begin to construct a functioning language system.

At the same time, high-frequency exposure to linguistic stimuli provides a child with language delays with input that has the potential to reverse the negative social spiral within the parent–child dyad. When more linguistic stimuli are provided, the child is given more opportunities to participate in social discourse. This may, in turn, lead to more attempts by the child to produce language. Furthermore, because the intervention method is fairly straightforward, parents can be taught to implement focused stimulation after appropriate training. This has the potential to yield increases in both the linguistic and social domains by extending the intervention into the child's home environment.

Information Processing Models as a Rationale/Foundation for Focused Stimulation

Some researchers believe that deficits in language learning are the result of a deficit in the child's cognitive processing abilities (e.g., Just & Carpenter, 1992; Montgomery, 1995); specifically, in the ways in which the brain attends to, organizes, and stores information. Originally arising from computer modeling, various information processing models have been used to describe human learning, but most models include components related to attention, discrimination, organization, memory, recall, and transfer of old information to new settings.

Information processing frameworks argue that all processing begins with input and ends with output. In human learning, a variety of mental operations may occur between input and output. Information may be attended to, transformed into some type of mental representation, compared with information already stored in the system, or used to formulate a response. Each component must work in concert with the others in order for information to move smoothly and efficiently through the human learning system. When this does not occur, learning is compromised. As an example, when a child is unable to effectively attend to an auditory stimulus, such as a word, the information is not moved into the central systems for processing and storage. Hence, the word does not become part of the long-term storage system and is not learned. Similarly, even if a child is able to attend to the input, if the capacity of the processing mechanism is unable to internally refresh the information while it is being processed (that is, keep it active in the working memory component), the signal will degrade and eventually be lost rather than be integrated into the cognitive system.

Parallel Distributed Processing   Traditionally, human information processing was believed to occur in a sequential or serial fashion. Information was posited to be processed singly, one piece at a time. However, alternative models describe human learning through parallel distributed processing (PDP) which posits a series of interconnected networks of processors (activation nodes) through which information is processed simultaneously (Rumelhart & McClelland, 1986). In this model, a unit of information (such as a word) is not believed to be stored in a single node. Rather, the information is represented in the specific pattern of activation across multiple nodes—some related to the sounds included in the word, some to its meaning, and so forth. Often referred to as *connectionism* due to the way in which the nodes are linked or connected, PDP describes learning as a modification of the strengths of the links between the activation nodes. As the links between nodes strengthen, the individual is able to access the information stored in the nodes more quickly and more efficiently. In other words, the stronger the links between nodes, the better the information is learned.

Learning in a connectionist sense involves three possible mechanisms: modifying the strength of the connections between units, creating new connections, or reducing the strength of old connections. Consequently, the amount and timing of input are crucial to establishing the desired links between nodes. Simply put, the more often the link between nodes is activated, the stronger the connection becomes. Given enough time, the system learns to detect certain patterns between nodes so that similar links are more easily established. In this way, even higher level linguistic input, such as complex grammatical rules, can be learned more quickly when related rules have already been processed through the system (see Vigil & van Kleeck, 1996, for a more in-depth discussion of PDP and language).

Limited Capacity Models   Various investigators have suggested that the human information-processing system is of limited capacity in terms of the cognitive resources that can be allocated to the tasks performed by the individual components of the system (Baddeley, 1986; Just & Carpenter, 1992; Lahey & Bloom, 1994). From this perspective, when task demands exceed the available resources, the learning system breaks down and both processing and storage of information is compromised.

The notion of limited capacity is most often applied to the component of the information processing system in which input is initially received and processed. In contrast to the virtually infinite amount of information that can be stored in long-term memory components, Baddeley and Hitch (1974) termed the information processing system that allows individuals to process and store information simultaneously as *working memory*. Because of its limited capacity, the traces of information within this space do not last long without constant reactivation, either through an internal method (such as verbal rehearsal) or through repeated input of the original external stimuli (i.e., repetition of the input).

From this viewpoint, success in comprehending and producing language is dependent on the resources available to maintain and integrate linguistic information in working memory. For example, to accomplish successful discourse the listener must hold the speaker's entire set of utterances in working memory while processing the meaning of each word within the context of the individual utterances. If the capacity of the working memory is not adequate to meet the demands of the linguistic task, the communicative interaction breaks down.

Recent research related to working memory suggests that capacity limitations constrain language performance in some individuals more than others (Just & Carpenter, 1992). From this perspective, children's linguistic deficits may be related more to deficits in their ability to hold and retain information in working memory than in their ability to learn language per se (Gathercole & Baddeley, 1990; Montgomery, 1995). Linguistic breakdowns occur, therefore, when the demands of a particular interaction exceed the resources available in working memory. This is believed to set up a series of trade-offs among selected language domains. For example, as the syntactic complexity of the input increases, the child's comprehension of the semantic and/or phonological information embedded within the utterance decreases. In his "surface account," Leonard (1998) argues that linguistic forms that are weakly represented in the speech stream (e.g., inflectional suffixes, auxiliary verbs, nominative pronouns, articles) are especially vulnerable when children with slow processing abilities attempt to extract meaning from complex input. Consequently, these forms are processed incompletely by children with SLIs and take them much longer than normal to learn. In general, then, children with more limited-capacity systems may require input that is less complex, more salient, or more frequent for them to be able to process it effectively (see Ellis Weismer, 1996, 2000a, 2004, for a more complete exploration of the impact of limited-capacity models on language processing by children with language impairment).

From an information-processing view, the language system of children with linguistic deficits is believed to be fundamentally intact. That is, there is no specific assumption of a broken grammar or vocabulary "module." Rather, the deficits in linguistic skills are seen as the result of underlying limitations in the processing components of the human learning system. Consequently, manipulation of the input to make it more salient, as provided through focused stimulation techniques such as high-density repetitions or exaggerated stress, is believed to assist children in processing, organizing, and ultimately integrating the targeted information into their cognitive system.

Because it is preselected to match the child's current linguistic levels, the input provided through focused repetition is generally less complex than language used in normal conversational interactions. If, as suggested by some researchers, the deficit in processing is a result of a limited capacity in working memory, less complex input should enhance the child's ability to process and store the linguistic information while more repetitions will help strengthen the connections between and among activation nodes.

EMPIRICAL BASIS

There has been increasing discussion within our field concerning the need to consider different levels of evidence with respect to the evaluation of treatment approaches (Dollaghan, 2002; Fey, 2002; Olswang, 1998; Robey & Schultz, 1998). In this chapter, we will distinguish between *exploratory* evidence (which includes observational and feasibility studies according to the continuum proposed by Fey [2002]), as well as *efficacy* versus *effectiveness* evidence. Most of the published treatment studies investigating the use of focused stimulation consist of efficacy studies. Efficacy studies investigate the effects of a treatment under ideal, controlled conditions and typically focus on specific, short-term language outcomes. A few studies also have examined the effectiveness of focused stimulation approaches. Effectiveness research identifies the usefulness of a treatment under the conditions of everyday practice and usually includes broader measures of language gains and functional outcome measures in related areas such as social skills, school readiness, or perceptions of quality of life. With respect to the levels of classification identified by the World Health Organization (1980, 2001), efficacy research tends to focus on *impairment* issues, whereas effectiveness research emphasizes *activity* (formerly, *disability*) and *participation* (formerly, *handicap*) outcomes.

Studies that have examined the use of a focused stimulation approach have varied with respect to specific intervention targets and the ancillary areas that have been assessed following treatment. As discussed in the following review, these have included various aspects of child language abilities (vocabulary repertoire, category use, early word combinations, use of grammatical morphemes, phonology), as well as social skills and sociocommunicative interactions. Certain measures of parental interactive behavior (talkativeness, directiveness, topic contingency) and parental perceptions have also been examined following the use of treatments involving focused stimulation. There is evidence to support the use of focused stimulation across different types of service delivery models and intervention agents (direct clinician-implemented treatment or indirect parent training programs) and treatment contexts (individual or group; laboratory, preschool/child care center, classroom, or home).

Clinician-Implemented Approaches

There is evidence to support the use of clinician-administered focused stimulation from studies that have employed group designs and single-case design methodology. This evidence consists of experimental studies of lexical learning (Leonard et al., 1982; Rice, Buhr, & Nemeth, 1990; Schwartz, 1988), as well as treatment studies focused on vocabulary and grammatical goals (Culatta & Horn, 1982; Ellis Weismer et al., 1993; Olswang, Bain, Rosendahl, Oblak, & Smith, 1986; Robertson & Ellis Weismer, 1999; Wilcox, Kouri, & Caswell, 1991). The results of an exploratory study conducted by Thordardottir, Ellis Weismer, and Smith (1997) suggest that focused stimulation techniques are useful in facilitating vocabulary skills when incorporated within a bilingual (Icelandic–English) treatment program, as well as a monolingual approach.

Variations occur in the implementation of focused stimulation procedures within clinician-administered programs. One variation pertains to whether or not active attempts are made to elicit (nonimitative) productions of the target form by the child. Both variations have been shown to be successful. For instance, children were never asked to produce the experimental words in the study by Leonard et al. (1982), although spontaneous uses were noted. On the other hand, Culatta and Horn (1982) specifically arranged the situational and interactional contexts to provide opportunities for children to use the grammatical forms being targeted as part of their treatment program. Another variation in the use of focused stimulation relates to modifications of the linguistic input, such as use of emphatic stress on the targets to increase the saliency of the modeled forms. Ellis Weismer (1997) summarized experimental evidence regarding the impact of emphatic stress on language learning and discussed clinical applications of these findings for intervention. This evidence indicates that use of emphatic stress during the training on novel words results in significant increases in production of these words by children who are typically developing and children with language impairment. Several studies have included emphatic stress on target forms in treatment programs incorporating focused stimulation (e.g., Culatta & Horn, 1982; Robertson & Ellis Weismer, 1999).

As noted previously, various investigations of lexical learning provide supportive evidence for the use of focused stimulation, although their main purpose was to study the nature of language acquisition rather than the efficacy of the language facilitation techniques. These studies have involved examiner-implemented use of focused stimulation in one-on-one interactions (such as play with toys or listening and responding to questions about a story) that were designed to provide a naturalistic communication context. For example, Leonard et al. (1982) examined early lexical learning in preschoolers (ranging in age from 2 years, 8 months to 4 years, 2 months) with specific language impairment. Children were exposed to 16 unfamiliar object and action labels, along with their referents. The examiner provided focused models (five repetitions per session) of the experimental words in sentence-final position (e.g., "Here's the shell," "Watch the baby kneel") during ten 45-minute play sessions that were conducted over a period of about 1 month. A control group of children participated in 10 play sessions that were identical to those of the experimental group, except that the sessions did not include the focused stimulation component (i.e., no models of the unfamiliar object and action labels were provided). The mean number of target words comprehended at posttest by the children in the experimental group was 7.14, compared to a mean of 0.02 words comprehended by the control group. Similarly, the mean number of words produced was much higher for the experimental group than for the control group, 3.50 versus 0.01. Thus, the children in the experimental group clearly outperformed those in the control group in their comprehension and production of the unfamiliar words, demonstrating the effects of this concentrated linguistic stimulation.

A classic example of a treatment study that used a variation of focused stimulation was conducted by Culatta and Horn (1982). This four-step intervention program was designed to promote generalization of grammatical rules to spontaneous discourse in four children with language impairment who ranged in age from 4 to 6 years. In each step of the program, naturalistic situations were enacted through dramatic play (such as setting up a grocery store or getting ready for school) that were used to expose children to focused models of the target forms and to provide opportunities for children to use the targets through the clever arrangement of the situational context. Across the different steps of the treatment program, the complexity of the communicative situation was increased and the frequency of focused models of the grammatical targets was decreased. Through the use of a multiple baseline design, Culatta and Horn demonstrated that target grammatical forms were used more frequently in conversational discourse than were untreated (control) forms. Similar gains were observed when this treatment program was later initiated for the untreated forms. Furthermore, the original treatment goals were maintained at mastery levels in spontaneous discourse following intervention.

Robertson and Ellis Weismer (1999) investigated the effects of an interactive, child-centered intervention on linguistic and social skills of late-talking toddlers. Twenty-one toddlers were randomly assigned to a treatment group ($n = 11$) or delayed-treatment (control) group ($n = 10$). The treatment group received a 12-week clinician-implemented language intervention program focused on promoting vocabulary skills and use of two- or three-word combinations. This intervention was an eclectic language stimulation approach that combined a number of standard techniques that were commonly used in the center-based birth-to-3 program where the study was conducted. These techniques included parallel talk, expansion, and recasts, as well as focused repetition of specific language targets, presented within structured routines and theme-based activities. Focused repetition of vocabulary was used relatively more frequently than expansion or recasts. The effects of treatment were measured via the use of a parent report measure (MacArthur-Bates Communicative Development Inventories [CDIs]; Fenson et al., 1993), spontaneous language sample analysis during play, a standardized test of social skills (Socialization Domain of the Vineland Adaptive Behavior Scales; Sparrow, Balla, & Ciccetti, 1984), and a self-report parental stress measure (Parenting Stress Index–Child Domain; Abidin, 1995).

Following treatment, Robertson and Ellis Weismer (1999) found significant gains in lexical repertoire (based on the CDIs), total number of words produced, number of different words, and mean length of utterance (MLU) (as measured by language sampling). More notably, significant changes were observed in areas that had not been specifically targeted by the treatment program; the percentage of children's intelligible utterances increased, their social skills improved (independent of language and communication gains), and parental stress was reduced.

This investigation represents a hybrid of efficacy and effectiveness research. Several features of the study are consistent with efficacy research, including the tightly controlled participant criteria, careful monitoring of treatment fidelity, and the collection of specific linguistic measures related to the intervention targets shortly after treatment. Yet, this investigation used a combined treatment package reflective of actual clinical practice and examined the impact of treatment beyond the language targets (social skills, parental perceptions); these features provide evidence regarding the broader construct of effectiveness of the approach.

Parent-Based Approaches

Lederer (2001) conducted an exploratory study to investigate the use of a parent–child intervention group, referred to as TOTtalk, that was designed to promote vocabulary development in late-talking toddlers. Ten late-talking toddlers (23–29 months old) and their mothers participated in 11 weekly 90-minute sessions (in groups of no more than six toddler–parent pairs). This treatment program involved the use of a focused stimulation approach, which Lederer described as a "naturalistic, interactive approach to language stimulation, which requires the pretreatment selection of target vocabulary" (p. 227). Although production of the targets was not required, attempts were made to elicit either imitative or spontaneous use of the target words by the toddlers through verbal prompts or through the play context in which the child was engaged. Target words were carefully selected for each child based on criteria established from prior research, including the following: 1) all words began with a sound in the child's phonemic inventory (Leonard et al., 1982); 2) target words had been reported to be acquired by at least 50% of 24-month-olds (Fenson et al., 1994); and 3) pretreatment comprehension of target words was not required because this has not been shown to be a necessary prerequisite for successful treatment focused on production (Leonard et al., 1982; Wilcox et al., 1991). Additional guidelines for target vocabulary in this study included selecting words that could be gestured easily and attempting to choose targets that were appropriate for all of the toddlers participating in these group sessions.

The Lederer (2001) study provides quantitative and qualitative data related to the use of this particular program, using a single-group, pre- to post-treatment, quasi-experimental design (Schiavetti & Metz, 2002). Quantitative data regarding total words produced and number of context categories expressed were derived from an adaptation of a parent report measure, the Language Development Survey (LDS; Rescorla, 1989); parents were instructed only to report words that the child produced spontaneously three times in at least three different contexts. Functional outcomes of the treatment program were explored through assessment of parental perceptions. Following treatment, data were obtained from a parent perception survey regarding the child's vocabulary and socialization skills, as well as parental anxiety, language facilitation abilities, parent–peer support, and preference for type of program. Lederer (2001) reported gains in target and overall vocabulary and very positive perceptions by parents in areas extending beyond linguistic improvements for all areas except peer support.

Girolametto and colleagues have conducted a series of controlled group-design studies investigating the efficacy of using interactive focused stimulation within a parent-based treatment program (Girolametto, Pearce, & Weitzman, 1996, 1997; Pearce, Girolametto, & Weitzman, 1996). They have employed the Hanen Program (Manolson, 1992) in research utilizing an interactive model of language intervention. Within the general stimulation version of the interactive model, parents are taught to stimulate their child's language by providing models at a developmentally appropriate level within ongoing activities, but specific targets are not identified. This version of the interactive model has not been shown to have substantial effects on the language abilities of children with developmental delay (Tannock & Girolametto, 1992). Therefore, researchers have explored the viability of a focused stimulation version of the interactive model in which parents are trained to follow the child's lead and to use various techniques to promote interaction, while also providing frequent presentations of specific language targets. This approach, which is described in detail in Girolametto and Weitzman (see Chapter 4), has been demonstrated to foster vocabulary and phonological development among late-talking toddlers.

Some evidence indicates that parent-based treatments using focused stimulation can be useful with young children who have cognitive impairments as well as language delays. Two early exploratory studies reported that parents' use of focused stimulation led to increases in vocabulary and use of early word combinations in children with cognitive delays (primarily Down syndrome) (Cheseldine & McConkey, 1979; McConkey, Jeffree, & Hewson, 1979). Focused stimulation involving clear modeling of target words/ constructions was reported to result in more improvement than other approaches such as imitation, direct questioning, or expansion (Cheseldine & McConkey, 1979). However, these studies did not include a control group, so it is difficult to determine whether the effects observed over the course of the 10–14 weeks of intervention were actually related to the treatment program or to other confounding variables such as maturation. Girolametto and colleagues (1998) observed positive, if somewhat limited, results of this approach on the vocabularies of children with Down syndrome. These findings suggest that parent-implemented interactive focused stimulation has positive short-term effects on target word learning for children with concomitant cognitive and language impairments. See Girolametto and Weitzman (Chapter 4) for further discussion of these points.

Comparison of Clinician and Parent Approaches

A focused stimulation approach has been shown to be useful in facilitating grammatical abilities in children with language impairment when administered by a clinician or by parents. Fey, Cleave, Long, and Hughes (1993) compared the effectiveness of a 4½-month treatment program that emphasized grammatical targets; the program employed focused stimulation procedures and used a cyclical goal-attack strategy. Thirty preschool children (ranging in age from 3 years to 5 years) were randomly assigned to a clinician treatment group, parent treatment group, and a delayed-treatment (control) group. This is a particularly strong experimental design that allows for direct comparisons of these two methods of presenting focused stimulation, and it also controls for the effects of maturation through the inclusion of the delayed-treatment group. The children participating in this study had marked grammatical delays and displayed discrepancies between their language and cognitive abilities; however, they did not meet the standard criteria for SLI (nonverbal IQ ranged from 73 to 130). Instead of being narrowly defined within standard research specifications, this sample was more typical of clinical populations of preschoolers receiving treatment for language impairment.

Primary and secondary treatment outcomes were calculated on the basis of language samples obtained from child–caregiver interactions. The primary measure used to determine effectiveness of the treatments was Developmental Sentence Score (DSS) (Lee, 1974; using the DSS Module of Computerized Profiling by Long & Fey, 1989). Secondary measures included mean main verb score per sentence, mean personal pronoun score per sentence, and percentage of sentences that received a sentence point (i.e., sentences that were semantically and grammatically acceptable). On average, the control group displayed no gain on these variables during the no-treatment interval. Conversely, large treatment effects were found for the clinical treatment and parent treatment groups for three of the four measures examined (DSS, main verbs, sentence point). Although the two treatment groups were not significantly different with respect to their performance on these measures, additional analyses indicated that the effects were more consistent across trials for the clinician treatment than for the parent treatment. Overall, these findings provide strong evidence that focused stimulation, whether provided by a clinician or a parent, is an effective treatment approach for improving grammatical delays. It is interesting to note that a follow-up study by Fey and colleagues (1994) indicated that this grammar facilitation program did not have an indirect effect on the phonological skills of preschoolers with language impairment as measured by the percent of consonants correctly produced; it is unclear whether other measures of phonological abilities might have reflected indirect treatment effects, as in the case of the Girolametto et al. (1997) study. In contrast to the findings of Fey et al., Girolametto and colleagues observed significant gains in phonological complexity of late talkers who had received the parent-administered focused stimulation vocabulary intervention.

PRACTICAL REQUIREMENTS

Implementation of the focused stimulation approach requires little expenditure of either financial or physical resources. Consequently, it has been used successfully in a variety of clinical contexts including the home environment (Girolametto et al., 1996), small playgroups (Lederer, 2001), group center-based intervention (Robertson & Ellis Weismer, 1999), and individual therapy (Ellis Weismer et al., 1993). A key characteristic of these applications is the careful selection of the linguistic targets, using normal development as a guide. Although focused stimulation can be used with children across a variety of developmental levels, children should minimally demonstrate communicative intent and the ability to participate in joint attending (see Warren et al., Chapter 3, this volume).

The basic requirements of the focused stimulation approach include the facilitator (e.g., clinician, trained parent), the child (or children), and a social context. Manipulation of the environment to provide opportunities for joint attending to selected stimuli that support the use of the linguistic targets is crucial. For example, when targeting specific vocabulary, the clinician must be able to provide a visual representation (picture of a cat), the actual object (the cat), or an opportunity to experience the meaning of the targeted word (e.g., *pet, soft, purr*). Obviously, multiple opportunities to provide the linguistic model must be provided and a method of tracking the input, particularly in terms of a frequency count, is also necessary. These data may be collected via a clinician-designed protocol such as that found in the Appendix, which was designed for use with a toddler who demonstrated delayed onset of expressive language. A tick or slash mark was placed next to the targeted vocabulary word each time it was modeled during a treatment session. Spontaneous productions of the target by the child were noted by an *X*. Although the specific number of models required for optimal learning has not been established clearly in the empirical research base, most studies of vocabulary treatment involving focused stimulation have used 10 as the minimum provided per target per session (e.g., Girolametto et al., 1996; Lederer, 2001). There is some evidence that number of target models needed may be much higher for grammatical constructions than for words (M.E. Fey, personal communication, July, 2003).

From a practical standpoint, focused stimulation is an exceptionally cost-effective therapeutic strategy. It requires no specialized equipment, no computer software or hardware, and, once targets have been selected, relatively limited pretraining even for nonprofessionals. Therapeutic materials gleaned from the child's natural environment are at least as effective as those obtained from commercial sources. Data collection protocols can be quickly developed and require little time or effort to use (see the Appendix). In addition, as mentioned previously, parents can be trained to provide focused stimulation of selected targets—as either a supplement to traditional clinician-administered intervention or as an alternative to more traditional service delivery models—with positive results (see Girolametto et al., 1996).

KEY COMPONENTS

As discussed in previous sections, a key component of focused stimulation is the deliberate manipulation of preselected linguistic targets to increase the saliency of the input. Given this, there are many therapeutic variations of focused stimulation in use by practicing clinicians. Generally, the manipulation of the input provided to the child is in the form of multiple repetitions of preselected language targets presented in an unambiguous context. However, when the language model is more complex than a single word, the input can be manipulated further by placing additional emphasis (stress) on the target form or by placing it at the beginning or end of the carrier phrase to draw the listener's attention to the target. It is important to ensure that the use of stress is pragmatically felicitous. One way to accomplish this is to establish a contrast and then use emphatic stress to highlight the contrast (see the example that follows for addressing auxiliary *be*).

In one version of the focused stimulation approach, no response from the child is expected. However, spontaneous repetitions/attempts to use the form by the child are acknowledged with a positive response from the clinician such as "Yes! That is a funny dog." In other applications, the child is prompted, usually by a direct request to name an object or event, to produce the target after a substantial amount of modeled input has been provided. To further encourage spontaneous use of the target, the environment in which the intervention is implemented can be manipulated to increase the likelihood that the targeted form will be produced in context by both the adult and the child. For example, if vocabulary targets happen to be animals, small plastic representatives of the targets can be hidden in a tub of rice so that they can be "discovered" by the child during play. This provides the adult with a natural context in which to provide the label and may eventually evoke a spontaneous production of the appropriate label from the child. Because elements of both clinician-directed (e.g., preselected targets, manipulation of input) and child-centered (e.g., natural context, following the immediate interest of the child) therapy exist, focused stimulation has traditionally been considered a hybrid intervention technique (Fey, 1986).

Focused stimulation is appropriate for remediation of a wide variety of linguistic deficits. Due to methodological constraints, the research literature has generally only reported the use of this technique in studies related to vocabulary and syntax development. However, focused stimulation can be used clinically to address deficits in language use (pragmatics) as well as in content (semantics) and form (phonology, morphology, and syntax). Although important for any intervention strategy, accurate assessment of the child's language abilities is especially critical so that the input that is provided to the learner is at the appropriate level. Obviously, input that is too advanced will not be processed effectively while input that is not challenging enough will not assist the child in moving forward linguistically. In the subsections that follow, key components are described as they apply to goals involving language form (e.g., grammatical morphemes, sounds), language content (e.g., lexical items), and language use (e.g., requesting, greeting).

Using Focused Stimulation to Address Language Form

The use of focused stimulation to address deficits in a child's morphosyntactic system has received considerable attention in the literature. Once a child's current level of expressive language has been assessed, the clinician chooses appropriate syntactic or morphological forms to target, generally based on typical patterns of language development. As an example, one of the grammatical morphemes that children typically acquire relatively early is the present progressive ending (-*ing*) (Balason & Dollaghan, 2002; Lahey, Liebergott, Chesnick, Menyuk, & Adams, 1992). Consequently, this would be a reasonable target for a child who has begun to combine words and is starting to demonstrate use of certain grammatical morphemes, but is not yet demonstrating use of this morpheme. To address this target, the clinician would manipulate the environment so that the child would have access to props and materials that would lend themselves to parallel talk (i.e., adult talks aloud about what the child is doing while he or she is doing it) that included the present progressive form. While the child and adult are playing together with a dollhouse, for example, the clinician could provide input such as "The baby is sleeping," "The mother is cooking," or "The boy is eating." In the block area, clinical models might include "You are stacking," "I am pushing," or "The block is falling," depending on what the child or clinician is doing at the time. Generally, the clinician will increase the saliency of the input by using linguistic constructions that place the targeted form at the end of the phrase (as above). In other cases in which it is linguistically appropriate, the clinician may also attempt to increase saliency by stressing and lengthening the production target. For example, when targeting free morphemes, such as auxiliary *be,* the clinician can manipulate discourse so that it is appropriate to place secondary or even primary stress on the otherwise phonetically weak morpheme (e.g., "*Is* he knocking? I don't hear him. Oh, yes he *is*. He *is* knocking on the door"). Multiple repetitions of the same phrase are common and even desirable in order to help the child process the information more effectively. In this paradigm, the child is not required to attend to a specific prop or activity any longer than seems natural. Rather, the clinician provides parallel talk that includes the targeted form referring to the objects and events to which the child has chosen to attend.

The same form could be targeted in a more clinician-directed intervention by directing the child's attention to a clinician-chosen picture or prop, asking for the child's attention, and then producing the targeted form. The clinician might produce a picture of a child on a playground, prompt for attention with a phrase such as "Look at this picture," followed by the model, "The boy is sliding." The model is produced multiple times within varying sentence contexts before moving on to the next picture (e.g., "He is sliding fast. The girl is sliding, too. They are sliding").

Specific phonological targets can be addressed in a similar manner. As illustrated previously, once the appropriate targets are identified, the clinician provides high-density input of the selected words and/or sound(s) without requiring the child to attempt to produce a correct model (Camarata, 1995). Again, the sound is generally stressed within the word and usually words are chosen in which the targeted sound occurs at the beginning. If the child spontaneously produces the word or sound, a positive response is provided for the attempt, but errors are ignored. This is especially important when a child produces a correct label but uses an incorrect phonological form. For example, the child says "tup" in response to a picture of a cup. Feedback such as "No, that's a cup" has the potential to confuse children who, because they are unaware of the phonological features of the target, may assume they have provided the incorrect label. Instead, the clinician might respond, "Yes, that's a cup" so that the child has an immediate correct model of their attempted sound and word.

Using Focused Stimulation to Address Language Content

Focused stimulation may also be used to facilitate oral vocabulary of preschool-age children with significantly delayed language. Once the words that are in the child's current expressive (and/or receptive) repertoire are established, the clinician chooses a set of words to target during intervention. Generally, words are selected with consideration of the ease in which they can be represented in the intervention setting (such as a playroom or home) and to reflect the state of the child's current level of phonological sophistication. The targets are then modeled by the clinician in the presence of an unambiguous referent. As before, the child is not required to try to name the object. Rather, the child's job is to interact with the clinician and the referent while the clinician provides high-density repetitions of the target word.

There is flexibility in the number of words targeted and the scheduling of the presentations. Given a list of target words, the clinician may choose to model all of the words during each session and repeat this procedure until the child begins to use these words in spontaneous productions, or concentrate on presenting only a few of the words more times each session, adding new words only when the child begins to produce the initial targets. Clinicians could also choose to use a cyclical approach, targeting a certain number of words for a specific number of sessions and then moving on to a new set of words before coming back to the original targets. Some clinicians may also choose to pair the verbal stimulation with a formal sign or gesture, providing the child with a visual cue to match the verbal input.

Using Focused Stimulation to Address Language Use

Sometimes, what we want children to pay attention to is not the particular words or grammatical form of an utterance, but rather the function of the utterance within a communicative interaction. Although less common than addressing form or content, language functions, such as greetings, inquiries, conversational initiations, and requests, may also be modeled using a focused stimulation paradigm. Emphasis is placed on what is occurring during the interaction to help the child focus on the use of language. For example, to encourage requests for an object, the clinician orchestrates the environment so that the child is tempted by an object that is not accessible (e.g., placing favorite toys or food out or reach but within the child's range of vision). When the child indicates a desire to attain the object (e.g., pointing, leading clinician near the object, gazing at the object), the clinician provides a number of repetitions of appropriate verbal requests (e.g., "I want the cookie,"

"Cookie, please," "May I have the cookie?") and then gives the desired object to the child.

Similarly, to address the pragmatic function of a greeting, the clinician might place a number of toys that could be "greeted" within the environment (such as teddy bears, dolls, and puppets). Each time a child looks at or reaches for the object, the clinician models an appropriate greeting such as "Hello, teddy" or "Hi, dolly." The clinician might also use the toys or puppets to role play greetings with the clinician using parallel talk while one toy "greets" another. Specifically, the clinician holds a dog puppet and a bird puppet facing one another. The clinician bends the dog puppet and says, "Hello, bird." The clinician then bends the bird puppet and says, "Hello, dog." In each situation, the noun could be eliminated so that the puppet only provides the greeting (i.e., "Hello") depending on the linguistic capabilities of the child. Finally, multiple models of greetings when the child, or anyone else, enters the room or play space would further support the development of this important pragmatic function.

ASSESSMENT METHODS TO SUPPORT ONGOING DECISION MAKING

When using a focused stimulation approach, the clinician may use various methods to assist in decision making regarding evidence of progress, need for changes in the treatment plan, or termination of treatment. With respect to charting progress or making adjustments in the treatment plan, a combination of direct assessment measures and parent- or teacher-report measures could be used. These might include the following:

1. Periodic informal probes of the target constructions following treatment sessions

2. Comparison of target form usage to that of untreated control forms

3. Language sample analysis to evaluate use of treatment targets as well as to assess cascading effects of intervention and development on other aspects of language development

4. Parental report measures such as the MacArthur-Bates CDIs (Fenson et al., 1993) or the LDS (Rescorla, 1989) to assess early lexical and grammatical abilities

5. Use of parent logs to document the child's production of target words or grammatical structures at home

6. Completion of parent or teacher surveys to compile perceptions of the child's linguistic skills, as well as perceptions of broader domains relating to social skills and academic readiness or performance.

This range of options proceeds from direct evidence of short-term changes on the treatment targets to ecological indices of the overall effects of the treatment program.

The assessment methods described above might be used in combination with standardized tests to determine when it is appropriate to terminate treatment. In that case, the clinician would not only assess a child's progress relative to his or her own baseline performance but would be interested in determining the child's language level relative to peers. That is, both standardized and criterion-referenced measures may be used in the decision-making process (assuming that standardized tests are available that were developed and normed on children from the same background as the child being evaluated). Most of the informal assessment measures discussed previously represent the types of assessment methods that have been suggested as more appropriate for culturally and linguistically diverse groups than standardized tests, although even language sample analysis has been shown to be sensitive to differences in SES (Dollaghan et al., 1999).

CONSIDERATIONS FOR CHILDREN FROM CULTURALLY AND LINGUISTICALLY DIVERSE BACKGROUNDS

The flexibility of the focused stimulation approach makes it applicable for children from culturally and linguistically diverse backgrounds. In cases where the child is not from the mainstream culture or a native speaker of English, a clinician who speaks both dialects/languages would provide concentrated models of targets appropriate to the linguistic patterns of the child's particular dialect or language. As noted previously, there is some preliminary evidence supporting the use of focused stimulation techniques with children who are second language learners, as well as in bilingual treatment programs for children with language impairment (Thordardottir et al., 1997). This suggests that focused stimulation approaches could be useful, for example, in supporting language facilitation for the increasing number of children in this country who are Spanish–English bilingual speakers (Brice, 2002), some of whom exhibit delays in both languages.

The nature of focused stimulation makes it adaptable to various cultural interaction styles. Focused stimulation can be contrasted with direct instruction methods or certain Milieu Teaching procedures (mand-model) in which "test questions" or prompts are used that require the child to name objects or make comments in situations where the information is known to both speakers ("What's this?"). This type of test questioning violates sociolinguistic expectations of certain cultural groups, such as African American speakers (Wyatt, 2002). Because the focused stimulation approach does not entail these types of questions/prompts, it avoids potential incompatibilities in this regard. Another possible area of cultural incompatibility with certain treatment methods pertains to the reinforcement of correct responses. As noted by Harris (1998), any type of attempt to manipulate the behavior of another person, such as through the use of contingent reinforcement, would be viewed as a violation of Navajo cultural values. Given the emphasis on input within the focused stimulation approach, there is no requirement for child responses or reinforcement that is dependent on the child's performance. In most cases, the flexible nature of the focused stimulation approach means that it is possible to match the teaching procedures/learning opportunities of the home culture and the clinical treatment (see Ellis Weismer, 2000a, for further discussion of culturally compatible teaching approaches).

For any intervention approach, it is important to take into account differing sociocultural perspectives with respect to disabilities, the need for intervention, the role that the family is comfortable assuming in the treatment process, and their expectations with regard to the child's language and communication skills (Brice, 2002; Harris, 1998; Kayser, 2002). In the book, *The Spirit Catches You and You Fall Down,* Fadiman (1998) provides a dramatic portrayal of these issues surrounding the clash between the health care system in the United States and the family of a young child with a seizure disorder who is a member of the Hmong community. When considering the use of a parent-based treatment approach, it is also necessary to remember that typical parent–child interactions differ across various cultural groups; therefore, care must be taken regarding the use of parent training that emphasizes mainstream cultural interaction patterns (see van Kleeck, 1994).

APPLICATION TO AN INDIVIDUAL CHILD

Drew, at 23 months of age, was using few words to communicate. He had not yet begun to combine words or use pseudophrases such as "All gone" or "So big." Drew's primary method of communication was through gestures, grunts, or temper tantrums. His parents reported that his birth and general developmental history were unremarkable. Drew's cognitive, physical, and receptive language skills all fell within age expectations.

Completion of the MacArthur-Bates CDIs (Fenson et al., 1993) by Drew's mother indicated that the extent of his expressive vocabulary was 18 words, placing him below the 5th percentile compared with other boys his age. Of these, three words represented food items, four were labels for animals, two were family names, one was a pet name, two were clothing items, and five were toys. In addition to these words, Drew used the word *no.* Thus, Drew's expressive repertoire did not include verbs or adjectives. His phonetic inventory consisted primarily of vowels, bilabials, liquids, and stops. He generally produced one-syllable words (or reduced multisyllable words to one syllable) and deleted the final consonant of most words.

Given this information, the clinician selected 10 words as targets for Drew based on criteria suggested in recent studies employing focused stimulation with toddlers (e.g., Girolametto et al., 1996; Lederer, 2001). Specifically, the target words consisted of VC, CV, or CVC syllable shapes, began with sounds that were currently a part of Drew's phonetic repertoire, were based on his current knowledge and interests, and were easily represented with a physical prop. Seven of the targets were nouns (*cow, hat, bug, cup, ball, egg, pot*) and two were verbs (*eat, hug*); the relational word *more* was also targeted. Drew was provided with at least 10 presentations of each of the targeted words during biweekly play-based intervention sessions. Treatment data were collected via the protocol in the Appendix. Each clinician-provided model was noted as a slash or tick mark. If at any time during the session Drew spontaneously produced one of the target words, an *X* was marked next to the word.

Drew's parents were provided with training that included observing the play session and direct training of the focused stimulation technique. In addition, they were given the list of target words and appropriate props and/or suggestions for providing exposure to these words in Drew's home environment. Two home visits were undertaken during the intervention interval to provide parental support and guidance in the use of focused stimulation. At the end of 10 weeks, Drew had produced all of the targeted words and his overall vocabulary had grown by 30 words as measured with the CDIs. Use of many of the words reported by the parents was confirmed through language sample analysis. With respect to phonological and grammatical gains, Drew had begun to close final syllables and demonstrated two multiword utterances ("Moon ball" and "Go car").

FUTURE DIRECTIONS

The focused stimulation approach to language intervention has well-established theoretical and empirical bases. Future investigations should strive to continue to refine the approach in line with the most current theories addressing the interplay of social, cognitive, and language development. Additional empirical work is particularly needed regarding the viability and efficacy of implementing this approach with children who have developmental disabilities, such as Down syndrome, as well as with children with other types of language and cognitive impairments. More broadly, further research is warranted to examine the interactions between various child characteristics (e.g., age level, cognitive abilities, linguistic/cultural background, learning style) and the degree of responsiveness to focused stimulation treatment. Additional areas of exploration should include direct comparisons between clinician and parent-implemented treatments and comparisons between different types of conventional and experimental treatments, such as those described in this text. Finally, because we have only begun to investigate functional outcomes of focused stimulation treatment, we need effectiveness studies to firmly establish the impact of this language treatment approach on social and academic areas (see Fey, Catts, & Larrivee, 1995; Robertson & Ellis Weismer, 1999) and on family functioning (Robertson & Ellis Weismer, 1999).

RECOMMENDED READINGS

Ellis Weismer, S. (2000). Language intervention for young children with language impairments. In L. Watson, E. Crais, & T. Layton (Eds.), *Handbook of early language impairment in children: Assessment and treatment* (pp. 173–198). Albany, NY: Delmar/ Thomson Learning.

Fey, M., Cleave, P., Long, S., & Hughes, D. (1993). Two approaches to the facilitation of grammar in children with language impairment. *Journal of Speech and Hearing Research, 36*, 141–157.

Girolametto, L., Pearce, P., & Weitzman, E. (1996). Interactive focused stimulation for toddlers with expressive vocabulary delays. *Journal of Speech and Hearing Research, 39*, 1274–1283.

Leonard, L. (1998). *Children with specific language impairment.* Cambridge, MA: The MIT Press.

REFERENCES

Abidin, R. (1995). *The Parenting Stress Index.* Charlottesville, VA: Pediatric Psychological Press.

Baddeley, A. (1986). *Working memory.* New York: Clarendon Press/Oxford University Press.

Baddeley, A.D., & Hitch, G.J. (1974). Working memory. In G.H. Bower (Ed.), *Recent advances in learning and motivation, Vol. 8.* San Diego: Academic Press.

Bain, B., & Olswang, L. (1995). Examining readiness for learning two-word utterances by children with specific expressive language impairment: Dynamic assessment. *American Journal of Speech-Language Pathology, 4*, 81–91.

Balason, D.V., & Dollaghan, C.A. (2002). Grammatical morpheme production in 4-year-old children. *Journal of Speech, Language, and Hearing Research, 45*, 961–969.

Bandura, A. (1977). *Social language theory.* Englewood Cliffs, NJ: Prentice Hall.

Brice, A.E. (2002). *The Hispanic child: Speech, language, culture, and education.* Boston: Allyn & Bacon.

Bruner, J. (1983). *Child talk: Learning how to use language.* Cambridge, England: Cambridge University Press.

Camarata, S. (1995). A rationale for naturalistic speech intelligibility intervention. In S.F. Warren & J. Reichle (Series Eds.) & M.E. Fey, J. Windsor, & S.F. Warren (Vol. Eds.), *Communication and language intervention series: Vol. 5. Language intervention: Preschool through the elementary years* (pp. 63–84). Baltimore: Paul H. Brookes Publishing Co.

Cheseldine, S., & McConkey, R. (1979). Parental speech to young Down's syndrome children: An intervention study. *American Journal of Mental Deficiency, 83*, 612–620.

Culatta, B., & Horn, D. (1982). A program for achieving generalization of grammatical rules to spontaneous discourse. *Journal of Speech and Hearing Disorders, 47*, 174–180.

Dollaghan, C.A. (2002, November). *An evidence-based approach to clinical practice in communication disorders.* Seminar presented at the American Speech-Language-Hearing Association annual convention, Atlanta.

Dollaghan, C., Campbell, T., Paradise, J., Feldman, H., Janosky, J., Pitcairn, D., & Curs-Lasky, M. (1999). Maternal education and measures of early speech and language. *Journal of Speech, Language, and Hearing Research, 42*, 1432–1443.

Ellis Weismer, S. (1996). Capacity limitations in working memory: The impact on lexical and morphological learning by children with language impairment. *Topics in Language Disorders, 16*, 33–44.

Ellis Weismer, S. (1997). The role of stress in language processing and intervention. *Topics in Language Disorders, 17*, 41–52.

Ellis Weismer, S. (2000a). Language intervention for children with developmental language delay. In D. Bishop & L. Leonard (Eds.), *Speech and language impairments: From theory to practice* (pp. 157–176). Philadelphia: Psychology Press.

Ellis Weismer, S. (2000b). Language intervention for young children with language impairments. In L. Watson, E. Crais, & T. Layton (Eds.), *Handbook of early language impairment in children: Assessment and treatment* (pp. 173–198). Clifton Park, NY: Thomson Delmar Learning.

Ellis Weismer, S. (2004). Memory and processing capacity. In R.D. Kent (Ed.), *MIT encyclopedia of communication disorders* (pp. 349–351). Cambridge, MA: The MIT Press.

Ellis Weismer, S., Murray-Branch, J., & Miller, J. (1993). Comparison of two methods for promoting productive vocabulary in late talkers. *Journal of Speech and Hearing Research, 36*, 1037–1050.

Fadiman, A. (1998). *The spirit catches you and you fall down: A Hmong child, her American doctors, and the collision of two cultures.* New York: Farrar, Straus, & Giroux.

Fenson, L., Dale, P., Reznick, S., Thal, D., Bates, E., Hartung, J., Pethick, S., & Reilly, J. (1993). *The MacArthur-Bates Communicative Development Inventories: User's guide and technical manual.* Baltimore: Paul H. Brookes Publishing Co.

Fenson, L., Dale, P.S., Reznick, J.S., Bates, E., Thal, D.J., & Pethick, S.J. (1994). Variability in early communication development. *Monographs of the Society for Research in Child Language Development, 59*(5).

Fey, M. (1986). *Language intervention with young children.* San Diego: College-Hill Press.

Fey, M. (2002, February). *Intervention research in child language disorders: Some problems and solutions.* Paper presented at the 32nd annual Mid-South Conference on Communicative Disorders, Memphis.

Fey, M., Catts, H., & Larrivee, L. (1995). Preparing preschoolers for the academic and social challenges of school. In S.F. Warren & J. Reichle (Series Eds.) & M.E. Fey, J. Windsor, & S.F. Warren (Vol. Eds.), *Communication and language intervention series: Vol. 5. Language intervention: Preschool through the elementary years* (pp. 3–17). Baltimore: Paul H. Brookes Publishing Co.

Fey, M., Cleave, P., Long, S., & Hughes, D. (1993). Two approaches to the facilitation of grammar in children with language impairment. *Journal of Speech and Hearing Research, 36*, 141–157.

Fey, M., Cleave, P., Ravida, A., Long, S., Dejmal, A., & Easton, D. (1994). Effects of grammar facilitation on the phonological performance of children with speech and language impairments. *Journal of Speech and Hearing Research, 37*, 594–607.

Gathercole, S., & Baddeley, A. (1990). Phonological memory deficits in language disordered children: Is there a causal connection? *Journal of Memory and Language, 29*, 336–360.

Girolametto, L., Pearce, P., & Weitzman, E. (1996). Interactive focused stimulation for toddlers with expressive vocabulary delays. *Journal of Speech and Hearing Research, 39*, 1274–1283.

Girolametto, L., Pearce, P., & Weitzman, E. (1997). Effects of lexical intervention on the phonology of late talkers. *Journal of Speech, Language, and Hearing Research, 40*, 338–348.

Girolametto, L., Weitzman, E., & Clements-Baartman, J. (1998). Vocabulary intervention for children with Down syndrome: Parent training using focused stimulation. *Infant-Toddler Intervention, 8*, 109–125.

Harris, G.A. (1998). American Indian cultures: A lesson in diversity. In D.E. Battle (Ed.), *Communication disorders in multicultural populations* (2nd ed., pp. 117–156). Boston: Butterworth-Heinemann.

Just, M., & Carpenter, P. (1992). A capacity theory of comprehension: Individual differences in working memory. *Psychological Review, 99*, 122–149.

Kayser, H.R. (2002). Bilingual language development and language disorders. In D.E. Battle (Ed.), *Communication disorders in multicultural populations* (3rd ed., pp. 205–232). Boston: Butterworth-Heinemann.

Lahey, M., & Bloom, L. (1994). Variability and language learning disabilities. In G. Wallach & K. Butler (Eds.), *Language learning disabilities in school-age children and adolescents* (pp. 354–372). New York: Macmillan.

Lahey, M., Liebergott, J., Chesnick, M., Menyuk, P., & Adams, J. (1992). Variability in children's use of grammatical morphemes. *Applied Psycholinguistics, 13,* 373–398.

Lederer, S.H. (2001). Efficacy of parent–child language group intervention for late-talking toddlers. *Infant-Toddler Intervention, 11,* 223–235.

Lee, L. (1974). *Developmental sentence analysis.* Evanston, IL: Northwestern University Press.

Leonard, L.B. (1981). Facilitating linguistic skills in children with specific language impairment. *Applied Psycholinguistics, 2,* 89–118.

Leonard, L.B. (1998). *Children with specific language impairment.* Cambridge, MA: The MIT Press.

Leonard, L.B., Schwartz R.G., Chapman, K., Rowan, L.E., Prelock, P.A., Terrell, B., et al. (1982). Early lexical acquisition in children with specific language impairment. *Journal of Speech and Hearing Research, 25,* 554–564.

Long, S.H., & Fey, M.E. (1989). *Computerized profiling* (Version 6.2). Ithaca, NY: Computerized Profiling.

Manolson, A. (1992). *It takes two to talk: A parent's guide to helping children communicate.* Toronto: The Hanen Centre.

McConkey, R., Jeffree, D., & Hewson, S. (1979). Involving parents in extending the language development of their young mentally handicapped children. *British Journal of Disorders of Communication, 14,* 203–218.

Montgomery, J. (1995). Sentence comprehension in children with specific language impairment: The role of phonological working memory. *Journal of Speech and Hearing Research, 38,* 177–189.

Olswang, L. (1998). Treatment efficacy research. In C. Frattali (Ed.), *Measuring outcomes in speech-language pathology* (pp. 134–150). New York: Thieme.

Olswang, L., Bain, B., & Johnson, G. (1992). The zone of proximal development: Dynamic assessment of language disordered children. In S. Warren & J. Reichle (Eds.), *Perspectives on communication and language intervention: Development, assessment, and remediation* (pp. 187–216). Baltimore: Paul H. Brookes Publishing Co.

Olswang, L., Bain, B., Rosendahl, P., Oblak, S., & Smith, A. (1986). Language learning: Moving performance from a context dependent to independent state. *Child Language Teaching and Therapy, 2,* 180–210.

Paul, R. (2001). *Language disorders from infancy through adolescence: Assessment and intervention* (2nd ed.). St Louis: Mosby.

Pearce, P.S., Girolametto, L., & Weitzman, E. (1996). The effects of focused stimulation intervention on mothers of late-talking toddlers. *Infant-Toddler Intervention, 6,* 213–227.

Rescorla, L. (1989). The language development survey: A screening tool for delayed language in toddlers. *Journal of Speech and Hearing Disorders, 54,* 587–599.

Rice, M.L. (1993). "Don't talk to him, he's weird": A social consequences account of language and social interactions. In S.F. Warren & J. Reichle (Series Eds.) & A.P. Kaiser & D. Gray (Vol. Eds.), *Communication and language intervention series: Vol. 2. Enhancing children's communication: Research foundations for early language intervention* (pp. 139–158). Baltimore: Paul H. Brookes Publishing Co.

Rice, M., Buhr, J., & Nemeth, M. (1990). Fast mapping word-learning abilities of language-delayed preschoolers. *Journal of Speech and Hearing Disorders, 55,* 33–42.

Robertson, S.B., & Ellis Weismer, S. (1999). Effects of treatment on linguistic and social skills in toddlers with delayed language development. *Journal of Speech, Language, and Hearing Research, 42,* 1234–1248.

Robey, R.R., & Schultz, M.C. (1998). A model for conducting clinical outcome research: An adaptation of the standard protocol for use in aphasiology. *Aphasiology, 12*, 787–810.

Rumelhart, D.E., & McClelland, J.L. (1986). *Parallel distributed processing*. Cambridge, MA: The MIT Press.

Schiavetti, N., & Metz, D.E. (2002). *Evaluating research in communicative disorders* (4th ed.). Boston: Allyn & Bacon.

Schwartz, R.G. (1988). Early action word acquisition in normal and language impaired children. *Applied Psycholinguists, 9*, 111–122.

Schwartz, R.G., & Leonard, L.B. (1982). Do children pick and choose? An examination of phonological selection and avoidance in early lexical acquisition. *Journal of Child Language, 9*, 319–336.

Sparrow, S.S., Balla, D.A., & Ciccetti, D.V. (1984). *Vineland Adaptive Behavior Scales*. Circle Pines, MN: American Guidance Service.

Tannock, R., & Girolametto, L. (1992). Reassessing parent-focused language intervention programs. In S.F. Warren & J. Reichle (Series & Vol. Eds.), *Communication and language intervention series: Vol. 1. Causes and effects in communication and language intervention* (pp. 49–80). Baltimore: Paul H. Brookes Publishing Co.

Thordardottir, E.T., Ellis Weismer, S., & Smith, M.E. (1997). Vocabulary learning in bilingual and monolingual clinical intervention. *Child Language Teaching and Therapy, 13*, 215–227.

van Kleeck, A. (1994). Potential cultural bias in training parents as conversational partners with their children who have delays in language development. *American Journal of Speech-Language Pathology, 3*, 67–78.

Vigil, A., & van Kleeck, A. (1996). Clinical language teaching: Theories and principles to guide our responses when children miss our language targets. In J. Smith & J. Damico (Eds.), *Childhood language disorders* (pp. 64–96). New York: Thieme.

Vygotsky, L. (1978). *Mind in society*. Cambridge, MA: The MIT Press.

Wilcox, M., Kouri, T., & Caswell, S. (1991). Early language intervention: A comparison of classroom and individual treatment. *American Journal of Speech-Language Pathology, 1*, 49–62.

World Health Organization. (1980). *ICIDH: International classification of impairments, disabilities, and handicaps*. Geneva: Author.

World Health Organization. (2001). *ICF: International classification of functioning, disability, and health*. Geneva: Author.

Wyatt, T.A. (2002). Assessing the communicative abilities of clients from diverse cultural and language backgrounds. In D.E. Battle (Ed.), *Communication disorders in multicultural populations* (3rd ed., pp. 415–450). Boston: Butterworth-Heinemann.

Yoder, P.J., & Warren, S.F. (1993). Can developmentally delayed children's language development be enhanced through prelinguistic intervention? In S.F. Warren & J. Reichle (Series Eds.) & A.P. Kaiser & D. Gray (Vol. Eds.), *Communication and language intervention series: Vol. 2. Enhancing children's communication: Research foundations for early language intervention* (pp. 35–62). Baltimore: Paul H. Brookes Publishing Co.

8

Appendix

*Sample Data Collection
Protocol for Focused Stimulation*

Client: _____

Date of session: _____

Target	**Frequency count**
Cow	_____
Bug	_____
Cup	_____
Ball	_____
Egg	_____
Pot	_____
Eat	_____
Hug	_____
More	_____

Directions: Record each instance of input of the model with a slash or tick mark. Record spontaneous productions by the client with an X.

9

Enhanced Milieu Teaching

TERRY B. HANCOCK AND ANN P. KAISER

ABSTRACT

Enhanced milieu teaching (EMT) is a naturalistic, conversation-based strategy for teaching language and communication skills to children in the early stages of language development (mean length of utterance [MLU] 1.0–3.5). More than 50 empirical studies have provided evidence for the efficacy and effectiveness of EMT for preschool children with significant cognitive and language delays; children with autism spectrum disorders; and children from high-risk, low-income families. EMT is a hybrid intervention based on three components: environmental arrangement, responsive interaction (RI), and milieu teaching (MT). Effective use of EMT requires high fidelity in the implementation of these three components and precise teaching of specific child targets. This chapter describes EMT procedures and their theoretical and empirical bases with a specific emphasis on parent-implemented applications.

INTRODUCTION

EMT is a naturalistic language teaching procedure that combines RI strategies (contingent semantic feedback, modeling language targets in descriptive talk, expansions, balanced turn taking) and MT procedures to prompt language production (elicitive models, mands, time delays, and incidental teaching). EMT focuses on promoting children's functional use of productive language skills in naturalistic interactions.

TARGET POPULATIONS AND ASSESSMENTS FOR DETERMINING TREATMENT RELEVANCE AND GOALS

EMT derives from a set of naturalistic teaching procedures that have been used since the middle 1970s (Hart & Risley, 1975; Hart & Rogers-Warren [Kaiser], 1978). EMT and its precursors have been used with a wide range of children in the early stages of communication development including children with mental retardation (Hamilton & Snell, 1993; Hemmeter & Kaiser, 1994; Warren & Bambara, 1989), children with autism (Hemmeter & Kaiser,

1994; Kaiser, Hancock, & Nietfeld, 2000), children with specific language impairments (Warren, McQuarter, & Rogers-Warren, 1984), and children with severe disabilities (Halle, Marshall, & Spradlin, 1979; Kaiser, 1993).

Although EMT can be used effectively for many children, children with the following characteristics are most likely to show rapid changes in their communication skills (Kaiser, Yoder, & Keetz, 1992):

- Children who are verbally imitative

- Children who have at least 10 productive words

- Children with MLUs between 1.0 and 3.5

Verbal imitation is a prerequisite because the core MT techniques (modeling, mand modeling, time delay, and incidental teaching) rely on adult modeling and child imitation to practice the response in a functional context. Children who already show some spontaneous production of single words present the adult using EMT with opportunities to both provide expanded models in response to the child and to practice the functional use of existing language within the scaffolded context of the EMT session. EMT appears to be ideally suited to teaching children who are in the early stages of language learning, particularly children who do not verbalize frequently and who are learning vocabulary or early semantic relationships.

In general, EMT is suitable for any parent who is willing to commit time and energy to learning and practicing the EMT intervention. Typically, the parents take 24–36 sessions to learn the intervention. This translates to approximately 3–5 months of the parent attending sessions twice per week. Parents must be willing to engage as learners and be coached by another adult. Some parents may feel uncomfortable with our direct teaching approach that includes feedback and coaching in every session. We feel that an important component of the intervention is working with parents and children in their home environment so they can apply the principles they learn to interactions with their child at home. Occasionally we have encountered parents who were not comfortable having a professional come to their home. In these cases, professionals need to decide how important a home component is for their intervention goals. Parents who participate in our EMT intervention have been willing to spend time, energy, and resources coming to our center. Self-selected parents may be different from parents in the general population. Among our middle income sample of parents, parents' age, education, or gender has not been predictive of their success in learning the EMT intervention. With low-income parents, the amount of life stress they are experiencing is predictive of their success in completing the EMT program. Because our training is conducted one-on-one with parents, we individualize for a parent's needs and learning styles. Professionals who conduct EMT in a group format may have to consider the skills and backgrounds of parents who can benefit from less individualized instruction.

THEORETICAL BASIS

EMT procedures derive from three distinct theoretical perspectives on early language learning. The MT procedures, which are used to prompt functional use of target language, reflect a behavioral perspective on language learning and instruction (Hart & Rogers-Warren, 1978). In this view, stimuli set the occasion for language, children's responses are related to those stimuli, and the consequences that follow child communicative responses are important to the subsequent use of those forms. In everyday terms, the use of communication forms will occur in specific contexts when use results in desired positive consequences. The antecedent-behavior-consequence paradigm creates instructional opportunities from which children can learn new language skills. In a behavioral approach to language, modeling, imitation, and prompted practice of productive language skills are key processes. Basically, the adults who are teaching prompt children to use language by presenting antecedent stimuli (e.g., models, mands, time delays) that tell the child when to talk and what to say. Children responding to these prompts are reinforced by the consequences adults provide contingent on their communication. Reinforcement plays an important role in the behavioral modeling of language learning because it serves both to increase the frequency with which children make communicative responses and to provide differential feedback for relatively more effective and appropriate target language forms. Hart and Risley's (1968, 1975) early adaptations of the behavioral paradigm to teach language in natural environments linked typical behavioral teaching/learning procedures to instruction in functional contexts for children. At its core, EMT remains grounded in behavioral principles for prompting, reinforcing, modeling, and shaping new language. Imitation and production practice with feedback are essential child behaviors for learning in this framework. Embedded in the four milieu teaching procedures (model, mand-model, time delay, and incidental teaching) are strategies for shifting control of the child responses from imitation (model), to responses to questions and mands (mand-model), to the child initiating requests and comments (time delay and incidental teaching). The behavioral paradigm dictates what will be taught in EMT: specific targets that are functional in the child's immediate environment.

Selection of targets in EMT is, however, driven by both functional and developmental considerations. A general developmental sequence for semantic and syntactic forms is followed in selecting targets for the early stages of learning (e.g., Brown's stages I–IV), and specific lexical items (e.g., nouns, verbs, modifiers) are typical words for early language learners. Targets are vocabulary, semantic, and early syntactic classes, but the specific examples taught are those that are immediately functional in the child's environment. Thus, the behavioral emphasis on functional communication is maintained while the general content being taught is consistent with developmental sequences derived from observations of typical language learners.

The behavioral perspective dictates a strong interest in critical phases of learning: acquisition, generalization, and maintenance. Many children with significant language delays, particularly children with mental retardation, will have difficulty with generalizing newly learned forms to other contexts, people, and settings (Goldstein, 1993; Kaiser & Warren, 1987; Yoder & Warren, 1998). EMT embodies the core principles for promoting generalization that were first outlined by Stokes and Baer (1977), including teaching multiple exemplars, teaching with multiple trainers, teaching in multiple settings, loose training (allowing natural variations in stimuli and reinforcers to occur), and training specifically to promote generalization to functional contexts.

A second theoretical strand in EMT is a social interactionist perspective on the learning of language through meaningful communicative interactions (Bruner, 1975). From this perspective, language is learned in the context of social interaction, particularly interactions between children and their caregivers. The responsiveness of the caregiver to the child's communicative attempts provides a framework in which models of new language (without prompts to imitate) occurring contiguously with the child's focus of attention and actions support the child's learning new forms and meanings. The learning of language in this model is driven by the social purpose of communication, but the adult plays a critical role in reading the child's intentions and providing language that maps the child's interests and focus. The child's ability to learn from adult models in social context is presumed to be based in the child's emergent cognitive skills. Ideal targets would include those for which the child already has the underlying concept or some features of the concept. Modeling language in the context of the child's attentional focus would be sufficient to assist the child in mapping his underlying knowledge and/or social intention with spoken language.

EMT emphasizes reciprocity, turn taking, following the child's lead in play and conversation, semantically contingent (meaningful) feedback, and expansions of child utterances to model more complete forms. Language learning results from responsive modeling of increasingly complex forms in social, dyadic interactions. Developmental studies have shown these interactional strategies to be associated with optimal language learning in typical mother–child dyads (Moerk, 1992). It is relatively easy to blend procedures derived from behavioral and social interactionist perspectives because both perspectives maintain the importance of modeling language in context to promote acquisition of meaning and forms. Both teach new communication forms during ongoing social interaction and promote responding to children's communication attempts while introducing more complex forms for communication contingent on children's expressed intentions. The difference between the two perspectives lies in the explicit use of prompting strategies to promote production in a behavioral model versus relying on children's spontaneous imitation of forms in the social interactionist model. In a behavioral perspective, child practice in producing new target forms is presumed to be necessary for mastering those forms. In addition, while a behavioral perspective makes reinforcement an explicit process in learning, a social interactionist approach relies on social relationships between children and their caregivers to maintain children's interest in learning and using language. In the latter case, the child is presumed to be the active constructor of new language knowledge; cognition drives the child's analysis, acquisition, and integration of new language forms in his or her emergent communication repertoire. In sum, when these differences are seen as points on a common continuum representing learning forms and functions of language in social contexts, it is possible to anchor EMT in both theoretical perspectives, as we have done.

A third perspective that informs EMT, as described in this chapter, is the emphasis on parents as language teachers. Both behavioral and developmental social interactionist theories support the involvement of primary caregivers in child language intervention. The behavioral perspective emphasizes that language is learned when it is functional for communication; such learning occurs in environments that provide both stimuli (e.g., contexts, setting events, specific social communicative events) and contingencies for a child's attempts to communicate. Generalization is promoted when the stimuli and consequences of language occur in the natural environment; thus, parents in everyday settings are likely to use both naturally occurring stimuli (events, objects, interaction) to teach language and the child is likely to be reinforced by the functional consequences of his communication. In the social interactionist perspective, the ongoing interactions between child and parent provide social meaning, physical proximity, and an affective relationship that will be supportive of language learning. Parents are ideal teachers because of their likely responsiveness to child communicative attempts, ability to closely monitor child communicative attempts based on proximity to the child, and their ability to provide language that elaborates those attempts. In typical learners, parent linguistic modeling and responsiveness to communication shapes early language development; thus, a social interaction perspective on early intervention places parents in the key role as teachers of new language in the context of ongoing parent–child interactions.

EMPIRICAL BASIS

Since 1978, the authors have been engaged in a series of research studies investigating the effects of naturalistic language interventions implemented by parents, teachers, and therapists. In the course of this research, four approaches to naturalistic teaching have been developed and tested 1) MT, 2) RI, 3) EMT, and 4) blended EMT and behavior intervention (see Table 9.1). EMT is a hybrid of the MT and RI approaches. The synthesis of these approaches is ideal for parent implementation because it builds responsiveness

Table 9.1. Naturalistic teaching approaches

Approach	Description	Key components
Milieu teaching (Alpert & Kaiser, 1992)	Parent teaches functional language in context of natural conversations. Prompts are used in conjunction with functional consequences	Environmental arrangement Modeling Mand modeling Time delay Incidental teaching
Responsive interaction (Kaiser et al., 1996)	Parent models developmentally appropriate language in conversational interactions. Models, meaningful recasts, and expansions are contingent on child communication.	Following child's lead Semantically responsive feedback Model talk at target level Expansions Balanced turn taking
Enhanced milieu teaching (EMT) (Hemmeter & Kaiser, 1994)	Parent's use of milieu teaching prompt strategies are embedded in responsive conversational interactions with child.	Environmental arrangement Responsive interaction Milieu teaching
Blended EMT and behavior intervention (Hancock, Kaiser, & Delaney, 2002)	Parent uses the EMT approach and also positively supports the child's behavior.	Environmental arrangement Responsive interaction Milieu teaching Behavior support techniques

within the parent–child relationship while providing the child with specific support for language production. We developed the blended EMT and behavior intervention approach for children who present with both language delays and specific behavioral problems that make it difficult for the parent and child to play together. In this variation of EMT, we teach parents strategies for giving instructions effectively and ways to manage their child's behavior consistent with a naturalistic teaching paradigm (increased responsiveness to child's communication attempts, descriptive feedback about behavior, environmental arrangement to promote engagement).

Milieu Teaching

MT is a conversation-based model of early language intervention that uses child interest and initiations as opportunities to model and prompt language use in everyday contexts (Hart & Rogers-Warren, 1978). Experimental applications of MT typically have included four sequential steps: 1) arranging the environment to increase the likelihood that the child will initiate to the adult; 2) selecting specific language targets appropriate to the child's skill level; 3) responding to the child's initiations with prompts for elaborated language consistent with the child's targeted skills; and 4) functionally reinforcing the child's communicative attempts by providing access to requested objects, continued adult interaction, and feedback in the form of expansions and confirmations of the child's utterances.

More than 50 studies incorporating variants of MT have been conducted (see Kaiser et al., 1992, for a partial review). Our model of MT extended and specified the incidental teaching model of Hart and Risley (1968, 1975) to include four related procedures: 1) elicitive model, 2) mand-model, 3) time delay, and 4) incidental teaching.

In an early efficacy study, Alpert and Kaiser (1992) investigated the effects of teaching six mothers of preschoolers with language impairments to use these four milieu language training procedures: model, mand-model, time delay, and incidental teaching. The children participating in the study were all boys between the ages of 35 and 51 months who had at least a 10-month expressive delay (range = 11–27 months) at the beginning of the study. Additionally, four of the six boys had a severe articulation disorder. A multiple baseline design across pairs of mother–child dyads and within each dyad across milieu techniques was used to evaluate the effects of training. All mothers learned the milieu procedures; all children in the study increased their use of total and spontaneous targets during their mothers' implementation of the MT procedures. All mothers used MT during home observation sessions. Mothers also generalized use of these techniques to two nontraining situations (domestic chore and television on) and showed acceptable levels of maintenance 3 months after training was completed. Comparison of child language behaviors at baseline and maintenance showed improvements in three areas for four of the six children: 1) average monthly gains in MLU exceeded or were approximately equal to the increase predicted for normally developing children; 2) number of total words produced and number of novel words produced more than doubled; and 3) increases occurred in the number of children's communicative requests. Two of six children did not show clinically significant gains on these developmental measures. Note that developmental measures were collected by an adult not involved in training. Transcription was completed by trained coders who were not otherwise associated with the study. The findings of this study suggested that mothers could be taught to correctly apply milieu language teaching procedures and that use of these procedures may have a positive effect on children's acquisition of new vocabulary, early syntactic/semantic forms, and appropriate use of requests.

Responsive Interaction

RI includes a set of behaviors (e.g., following the child's lead, responding to the child's verbal and nonverbal initiations, providing meaningful semantic feedback, expanding the child's utterances) that maintain the child's interest in the conversation and provide linguistic models slightly in advance of the child's current language (Kaiser & Delaney, 2001). We began by comparing MT with RI in a series of studies with parents and teachers. In one of the early efficacy studies, Kaiser and colleagues (1990) compared the effects of parent-implemented RI with parent-implemented MT on children's language outcomes. Thirty-six preschool-age children with developmental disabilities and their parents were randomly assigned to either the RI condition ($N = 18$) or MT ($N = 18$). Parents in both groups completed 24 individualized sessions and similar child language targets were taught in the RI and MT interventions. The majority of parents reached preset criterion levels for the strategies taught in their assigned intervention group. No main effects for treatment type were observed; children in both groups showed improvements in language skills from pre- to posttesting. Children at the lower end of the language continuum of children enrolled in the study (MLU < 1.8) appeared to respond better to the MT intervention while children at the upper end of the language continuum of children enrolled in the study (MLU > 3.0) responded somewhat better to the RI intervention.

In one of the later efficacy studies, Kaiser and colleagues (1996) evaluated the effectiveness of parent-implemented RI on the language and communication skills of preschool children with disabilities. Twelve parents participated in individual training sessions. A multiple baseline design across groups of families was used to evaluate the parents' use of the intervention strategies and the effects of the intervention on the children's language skills. Results indicated that all parents learned to use the procedures after 20 sessions in the clinic and generalized their use of the procedures to interaction sessions conducted in the home. Although there was variability in child outcomes, positive effects were observed for all children. Maintenance sessions conducted with nine of the 12 parents 6 months after the end of training indicated that all of these parents maintained their use of the procedures. In addition, seven of the nine children who participated in the maintenance sessions were observed to use their targeted language spontaneously at levels comparable to or higher than the levels achieved during intervention. All parents indicated that they were highly satisfied with their participation in the intervention and the effects of the intervention on the language and communication skills of their children.

Enhanced Milieu Teaching

Although these comparison studies did suggest differential treatment effects for some children, they also suggested that the majority of children could benefit from either RI or MT. Based on these findings, EMT emerged. EMT is the third generation of naturalistic teaching strategies, building on the principles of incidental teaching (Hart & Risley, 1968) and MT (Hart & Rogers-Warren, 1978) and adding systematic principles for responsive conversational style. EMT blends three components: 1) environmental arrangement to support language learning and language teaching (i.e., choosing activities of interest to the child, arranging for natural opportunities to prompt language, and natural positive consequences of using language); 2) RI; and 3) limited MT episodes.

In an early efficacy study, Hemmeter and Kaiser (1994) examined the effects of training four parents to use EMT with their preschool-age children with developmental delays. A multiple baseline design across three intervention strategies was used to assess the parents' acquisition of the strategies. A multiple-probe design across two families, replicated across two additional families, was used to assess the effects of parents' implementation of the strategies on their children's communication skills. The parents learned to use the strategies in the clinic and generalized them to the home. Positive effects were observed on children's spontaneous communication and target use and on parent and child affect. Evidence of positive effects on language development measures was observed for three of the four children. Three of four children showed gains of 12 months or more (> 2 standard deviations [SD]) on their receptive skills as measured by the Sequenced Inventory of Communication Development–Revised (SICD-R; Hedrick, Prather, & Tobin, 1975); two children showed gains on their expressive skills as measured by the SICD-E (> 1.5 SD). All children had more spontaneous words at the posttest; three children more than doubled their spontaneous words in the language sample. MLU increases were not significant for any of the children.

In a later efficacy study, Kaiser and Hancock (2000) compared parent-implemented RI with EMT implemented by parents and EMT implemented by therapists. Seventy-three preschool-age children in the early stages of language learning (performance on standardized tests indicating approximately 24 months language age; 10 productive words) with significant cognitive and language delays and their parents were recruited to the study. Children were then randomly assigned to one of the three intervention conditions: 1) RI-Parent ($N = 18$), 2) EMT-Parent ($N = 19$); 3) EMT-Trainer ($N = 18$), or 4) a nontreatment control group ($N = 18$). Child participants were an average of 45 months of age (range = 30–77 months), had an IQ of 66 (range = 40–119), and had an MLU of 1.58 (range = 1.00–2.43) at the beginning of the study. A typical parent was a Euro-American mother who was married and had a high school education. The mean age of parents was 34 years. Parents in the four groups did not differ significantly in age, education, or family resources. For the intervention groups, child and parent measures were collected during baseline (5–7 sessions), treatment (24 sessions), follow-up (once per month for 6 months), and home generalizations were conducted pre- and posttreatment.

RI and EMT implemented by both therapists and parents were effective in teaching language targets during the intervention. All three intervention approaches produced positive effects on language development (e.g., MLU, productive syntax measured by the SICD-E, Peabody Picture Vocabulary Test–Revised [PPVT-R]; Dunn & Dunn, 1981) assessed 6 months after the intervention. Children whose parents were trained to use RI or EMT performed better on measures of productive language (SICD-E, MLU) at the 6-month follow-up than did the EMT-Trainer group who got the intervention directly from a clinician (the effect size, or $d = .3$ for parent versus trainer-implemented interventions). Differences between the two parent-implemented interventions on measures of children's productive syntax were small, with children in the EMT-Parent group gaining an average of 1.2 months for every month of intervention versus children in the Parent-RI group gaining an average of 0.73 months for every month of intervention.

Kaiser et al. (1990) observed that children with lower language skills benefited more from the MT intervention whereas children with higher language skills learned more from the RI intervention. Kaiser and Hancock (2000) did not replicate this aptitude by treatment interaction, however. There are two possible explanations for the failure to replicate. First, the sample of children enrolled in the Kaiser and Hancock (2000) study were relatively homogenous in terms of language skills at the beginning of the study (ranging between 24 and 28 months for receptive and productive language age). Second, the addition of RI strategies to the MT procedures to form the EMT hybrid model used in this study may have reduced critical differences between the two procedures such that the procedures no longer affected children with varied aptitudes differentially.

Presently, we are investigating how EMT can affect communication development not only in preschool children with significant disabilities, but also in children who are at risk because of poverty and early emergent language delays and behavior problems. These are two very different populations of children; children with significant cognitive delays in the early stages of learning (MLU < 2.5) and children with no specific cognitive delays but general language delays and clinical or subclinical levels of behavior problems (MLUs ranging from 2.0 to > 3.5).

Blended EMT and Behavior Intervention

Our recent work specifically examines how children with early emergent behavior problems and delayed language are affected by naturalistic teaching of both language and positive social behavior. Into the EMT model we have embedded strategies for giving children instructions and following through on compliance and noncompliance that are consistent with naturally occurring communication in everyday settings. We teach parents to give instructions that match the child's communication skills, to map child compliance with descriptions of child behavior as well as praise, and to reframe their child's noncompliance, at least in part, as a breakdown in communication.

In a later efficacy study, Hancock and colleagues (2002) used an AB single-subject design replicated across five participants to assess the effects of an EMT and behavior intervention that taught parents to support their preschool children's communication skills and manage their behavior. Children with language delays and emergent behavior problems and their parents from low-socioeconomic status backgrounds participated. Parents attended 30 individual sessions and were taught to be responsive to their children's communication and to provide contingent consequences for their children's behavior. Generalization to interactions at home and maintenance of intervention efforts were assessed. Parents learned the strategies, generalized these strategies to interactions at home, and maintained positive changes 6 months after the intervention. Children showed positive changes in language and behavior during the intervention, but maintenance and generalization of these effects were more variable. For example, children's average MLU during the baseline sessions was 2.25. At the end of intervention, their average MLU had increased to 3.00, and during the follow-up sessions their average MLU was 3.04, approximately the same MLU observed at the end of intervention. All children decreased their frequency of noncompliant/negative behavior from baseline (average = 3.7) to the end of intervention (average = 1.8) to the follow-up sessions (average < 1). Three of the five children generalized their gains from the training setting to interactions with parents at home. The other two children showed limited evidence of positive changes in communication with their parents at home. The average frequency of noncompliant/negative behavior observed at home before the intervention began was 5.5 per session and after the intervention 1.6 per session.

Throughout these studies, and in the evolution of our model of EMT, we have been almost equally concerned with two issues: 1) improving children's language development and communication use, and 2) changing the support for language learning provided by significant partners. Thus, our concern has been with the child, the parent, and the transactions that support teaching and learning.

PRACTICAL REQUIREMENTS

Learning EMT procedures generally takes parents from 20 to 36 individual sessions, depending on the parent's entry skills and the child's communication level. Typically, parents require about 20 sessions to reach the criterion on all components of the procedures. Thus, the 36 sessions allow a substantive period of time in which the parent implements EMT at criterion levels to teach child targets. Child-specific language targets are usually introduced within the first five sessions. Parent and child data during clinic interaction sessions are monitored continuously throughout the training as a basis for feedback to parents. We have conducted training sessions in our clinic, in parents' homes, in an extra room at child care centers, or in schools. We have conducted training sessions with parents in a group context and individually, but for the last 10 years we have primarily conducted EMT interventions with parents in individual, criterion-based training sessions.

A typical EMT parent session lasts approximately 45 minutes to 1 hour. The first 15 minutes is devoted to reviewing child and parent progress and introducing new information. Role playing or viewing videotapes may by used to provide concrete examples of EMT procedures. The parent is invited to ask questions, report progress or concerns at home, or modify the proposed agenda to fit his or her concerns. Typically, the child is not present during this parent-teaching period. The child joins the parent for a period of practicing the new EMT procedure for approximately 15–20 minutes. The professional coaches and gives brief feedback while the parent and child interact in a play-based context. Parent–child interactions are videotaped for review by the professional after the session. During the last 10–15 minutes of the session, the parent is invited to reflect and evaluate the practice session. The clinician provides information in response to parent comments and concerns and supplies additional feedback about the parent's implementation of the procedures. A few minutes are spent helping the parent plan for interactions at home, and brief homework assignments are given. Instruction on how to use EMT at home, handouts on home activities, and discussion of parent use of EMT at home are included in each session. Sessions always end with summary-level positive feedback to the parents about their progress in implementing EMT procedures and their children's language progress.

We have examined applications of EMT by therapists, parents, and classroom teachers, but our research has focused primarily on examining changes in child communication skills resulting from parent-implemented EMT and related naturalistic communication approaches. We have also conducted studies addressing strategies for training professionals to work with parents (Hester, Kaiser, Alpert, & Whiteman, 1996; Kaiser, Hester, Alpert, & Whiteman, 1995). In the course of conducting these studies, we have trained more than 40 early childhood professionals, special educators, psychologists, social workers, and speech pathologists who have taught more than 200 parents in our research programs. From both a research perspective and our clinical experience, we have learned that there is a minimal set of skills needed for professionals to be effective in teaching EMT strategies to parents. These skills can be grouped into two general areas: 1) skills in applying EMT strategies directly with children and 2) skills in teaching parents the intervention.

EMT Skills

Professionals need knowledge of and experience in applying the EMT procedures they will teach parents. We have found that professionals need to have intervened with a minimum of three children individually before they have the experience necessary to teach parents. Simply put, professionals cannot teach what they do not know. The professional's skills and experience in the EMT intervention allow him or her to model the procedures with the child, provide the practical knowledge about the types of adaptations that may be required for this child to learn, and establish with the parent the credibility of both the EMT procedures and the professional's skill.

Skills with Parents

Teaching parents requires skills that are different from those required to teach children, but most training programs do not address professional skills that are important when working with adults. We have specifically investigated strategies for training professionals to work with parents and found that parent learning and performance were directly linked to the use of 1) positive examples and 2) coaching and feedback (Hester et al., 1996). Verbal instructions and explanations were found to be less effective than examples provided through in vivo modeling by the professional, videotaped examples of other parents demonstrating EMT techniques, or role playing EMT procedures with the parent. When the professional is able to model new skills and join in the ongoing parent–child interaction without overwhelming the parent, in vivo modeling can be an excellent way of providing positive examples. Role playing, in which the parent assumes the roles of both interventionist and child across several practice opportunities, can assist the parent in gaining insight into the child's need for models, prompts, and feedback to support new communication skills and the time to practice the specific steps of each strategy without the demands presented by the child.

Professionals must have skills in coaching and giving parents feedback in their use of EMT skills. Coaching supports the parents in being immediately successful in implementing newly learned EMT strategies. Professionals must provide assistance to parents while staying in the background of the parent–child interactions. In order to coach effectively and give differential feedback about the parent's use of procedures, the professional must know each step of the intervention procedures and be able to offer specific suggestions during the course of the parent–child interaction. Coaching is most effective when professionals offer support while parents are practicing; however, this requires mastery and fluency in EMT and skill in tactfully providing precise information to parents. Effective feedback and coaching require that the professional has good adult interaction skills, a conceptual understanding of the purpose of each component of EMT, the ability to problem solve as issues arise in the parent–child interaction, and the ability to give precise feedback about parent behavior. The degree to which the professional is able to be precise, supportive, and clear about critical behavior changes greatly influences how quickly a parent learns EMT strategies.

KEY COMPONENTS

The components of EMT are taught sequentially, with environmental arrangement taught first, followed by RI strategies, and lastly MT procedures. Parents do not move to the next skill in the sequence until they master the skill they are being taught. Criterion performance for each skill is set in advance and the parent demonstrates the criterion for the current strategy for two consecutive sessions before moving to the next skill. See Table 9.2 for the specific sequence of strategies as they are generally introduced to parents in an EMT intervention. Table 9.3 describes the criteria the parent needs to meet for each strategy before being taught the next strategy in the sequence.

The component of environmental arrangement is designed to increase the child's engagement with the physical setting which then can provide more frequent opportunities for the parent to communicate with the child, to elicit communicative responses, to model appropriate language forms, and to respond contingently to the child's verbal and nonverbal communication attempts. Parents are taught to *select* toys and materials that are of interest to the child and will provide the child a reason to talk, to *arrange* the materials in a way that will elicit initiated communication by their child, and to *manage* the toys so their child maintains play engagement and there are functional reasons for their child to communicate. Table 9.4 summarizes the environmental arrangement principles and gives examples for selecting, arranging, and managing toys and materials.

In the RI component of EMT, emphasis is placed on developing a conversational style of interaction that promotes balanced communication between parent and child as well as models of appropriate language. Parents

Table 9.2. Sequence for enhanced milieu teaching (EMT) intervention

Session*	Content
Session 1	General principles of interacting with your child, play and routines as a context for child learning, following your child's lead
Session 2	Choosing materials that interest your child and arranging the environment to promote your child's engagement and requesting
Sessions 3 and 4	Turn-taking strategies: nonverbal turn taking (mirroring) and verbal turn taking (pausing)
Sessions 5 and 6	Respond to what your child communicates
Sessions 7 and 8	Talk at your child's target level
Session 9	Expansions
Sessions 10 and 11	Expansions at the child's target level
Sessions 12 and 13	Principles of environmental arrangement to build child initiations and requests
Session 14	Identifying your child's verbal and nonverbal requests
Sessions 15–18	Incidental teaching I: using models after child requests
Sessions 19–22	Incidental teaching II: using mand/models after child requests
Sessions 23 and 24	Choice-making mands/questions versus open-ended mands/questions
Sessions 25 and 26	Time-delay procedure
Sessions 27–30	Putting it all together: balancing responsiveness and milieu teaching

*This is an approximate timeline for teaching the EMT intervention to parents. In our program, decisions about moving to the next strategy are data driven. Total number of sessions needed depends on the entry skill level of the parent and can vary from 20 to 30 total sessions.

Table 9.3.   Criteria for parent strategy use before introducing a new strategy

Strategy	Measure	Criterion
Balanced parent/ child turns	Discrepancy of turns (based on number of parent verbal turns minus number of child verbal and nonverbal turns). This is not a matched-turns criterion (adult takes a turn then child takes a turn) but is total number of turns taken by the adult or the child.	0
Parent pausing for child initiations	Number of parent pause errors (i.e., two or more consecutive parent utterances without a 5-second pause for child to respond)	<5
Parent responsiveness to child verbal behavior	Percentage of child verbalizations followed by responsive feedback	> 80%
Parent talk at the child's target level	Percentage of all parent utterances that are at the child's targeted level (i.e., no more than two or three words longer than the child's target construction) (total frequency of parent target utterances/total frequency of parent utterances)	> 50%
	Number of different child targets used (usually three to four different targeted forms)	All
Parents expansions of child utterances	Percentage of child utterances that parent expanded	≥40%
Milieu teaching procedures	Number of episodes attempted	> 5 and <10
	Percentage of episodes that included correctly executed steps and at the child's target level	≥80%

learn basic principles of interaction (responsiveness, following the child's lead, facilitating turn taking, matching, and extending the child's topic) and basic language modeling strategies (matching the child's linguistic level, imitating or mirroring the child, expansions of child utterances, descriptive talk). To some extent, these strategies extend the basic principles learned in the environmental arrangement component and apply them in ways that enrich the child's language learning environment and provide a basis for conversational interaction.

The RI component of EMT greatly enhances the naturalistic qualities of MT. RI sets a social context for language in the same way that environmental arrangement sets a physical context. Together, responsive conversational style and environmental arrangement create a supportive interactional context for conversation-based teaching. MT, the third component of EMT, is a prompting procedure in which the child's interest in the environment is used as a basis for eliciting elaborated child communicative responses. MT in EMT is embedded in the arranged environment and the conversational style taught in the first and second components of the model. The MT episodes should be relatively few and carefully matched to the child's interest and intended lan-

Table 9.4.   Environmental arrangement principles for parents

Selecting materials

1.   Select toys/materials that are high preference and interesting to your child.

2.   Select toys with multiple parts (such as Legos, Mr. Potato Head) or add-ons (for example, add the barnyard animals to your child's bathtub).

3.   Select toys that require assistance opening (such as playdough) or putting together (like a train track).

4.   Select toys/tasks that require you to be a partner with your child (like throwing and catching a ball, hiding and finding an object). Nonverbal turn taking provides a foundation for verbal turn taking (balanced conversation).

Arranging materials

1.   Limit the number of materials/toys you make available to your child at any one time. Limiting materials helps your child attend to the toys you are playing with rather than being overwhelmed by too many toys. It also may provide an opportunity for your child to request additional materials.

2.   Have some toys in your child's view but out of reach (like on a high shelf or in plastic containers up on a counter).

3.   Keep toys in containers that your child will need assistance opening.

Managing materials

1.   Be a gatekeeper. Place yourself between your child and the materials or keep some portion of the materials in your control.

2.   When your child seems to start losing interest, add in materials to keep the play going. Have fun and be creative as you mix toys and materials that may not generally go together. For example, add food coloring to water play or have the barnyard animals go through the car wash made for the Matchbox cars.

3.   When you do not give your child all of the toys or materials at once, there is an opportunity for your child to request more. For example, give him or her two Lego blocks instead of the whole container of Legos.

4.   You can also provide an opportunity for your child to communicate with you by not providing all the materials he or she might need for an activity. For example, you could give your child paint but no paintbrush, or a paintbrush but no water so he or she will need to ask for the material.

5.   Your child may communicate with you when something happens that he or she does not expect. For example, if you put Mr. Potato Head's arm where his eye goes, your child may use language to tell you that it is wrong or to move it to the right location.

guage functions. Generally, we limit MT to 8–10 episodes per 20-minute EMT interaction. This is based on our clinical experience in maintaining a naturalistic, responsive interaction. We focus on using prompts in response to child requests so that the episode is functional for the child and there is a natural limit to the number of episodes. Using a high number of prompts in a short amount of time can feel like "drill and practice," and the responsive nature of the interaction may be lost.

There are four core MT procedures: 1) modeling, 2) the mand-model procedure, 3) the time-delay procedure, and 4) the incidental teaching procedure. *Modeling* may be considered the most fundamental MT strategy. The parent first establishes joint attention by focusing attention on the child and on the child's specific interest. Next, the parent presents a verbal model that is related to the child's interest. If the child imitates the model correctly, immediate positive feedback (which includes an expansion of the child's response) and the material of interest are given to the child. If the child does not respond to the initial model or responds with an unintelligible, partial, incorrect, or unrelated response, the parent establishes joint attention again and presents the model a second time (a corrective model). A correct child response again results in immediate positive feedback and expansion of the child's response and access to the material. If an incorrect response follows the corrective model, the parent provides corrective feedback by stating the desired response and then gives the material to the child. All milieu procedures have a modeling component that includes the steps described here (see Table 9.5 for an example of the model procedure).

The mand-model procedure differs from modeling by including a verbal prompt in the form of a question (e.g., "What do you need?") or a choice (e.g., "We have milk or juice; which one would you like?") or a mand (e.g., "Tell Mommy what you want."). The presentation of corrective models of appropriate responses when a child responds incorrectly or fails to respond to the mand (i.e., question, choice, or request) is identical to the sequence in the model procedure. When the parent and child are playing together, for example, the parent can use a mand to give the child a choice of play materials ("Do you want to play with the cars or the balls next?"). If the child gives an appropriate response, the parent can respond positively and descriptively (e.g., "You want to play with the race cars") and provide the requested material. If the child does not respond or gives an incorrect response, the parent provides a model for the child to imitate. By presenting choices among interesting materials, toys, or activities, the parent allows the child to make

Table 9.5. An example of the strategy of modeling

Steps	Example
Establish joint attention by attending to the child's focus of interest	Hunter and his mom, Celia, are playing with cars that go down a track. Hunter is looking at the box of cars his mom is opening.
Present a verbal model	Celia prompts, "Say 'want car.'"
If the child responds correctly, acknowledge response with expansion and material	When Hunter responds with "Want car," Celia expands with "You want the blue car" and gives him the car.
If the child doesn't respond or doesn't repeat the model exactly, give another model	When Hunter answers with only a partial response such as "Car," Celia again prompts, "Say 'want car'" and really emphasizes *want* since Hunter missed that part the first time.
If the child responds correctly, acknowledge response with expansion and material	If Hunter then responds with "Want car," Celia expands with "You want the race car" and gives him the car.
If the child doesn't respond or doesn't repeat the model exactly, state the correct response and give the child the material.	If Hunter doesn't respond or responds with only a partial response such as "Car," Celia says, "Want car" and gives Hunter the car.

language immediately functional in indicating his or her choice (see Table 9.6 for an example of the mand-model procedure).

Conversation should involve not only responding to another person's models and mands for verbalization but also initiating communication about various aspects of the environment. The time-delay procedure was developed to establish environmental stimuli for child initiation instead of simply presenting models and mands as cues for verbalization. The effects of the time-delay procedure alone were experimentally demonstrated in studies by Halle and his colleagues (Halle, Baer, & Spradlin, 1981; Halle et al., 1979). Adults in these studies (e.g., caregiving staff members and teachers) were instructed to attend to individual students by introducing a time delay in situations where the students were likely to need assistance or materials (see Table 9.7 for an example of the time-delay procedure).

Time delay may be especially useful with children who are echolalic (e.g., frequently imitate or repeat the exact words spoken to them). Often children with autistic characteristics repeat the last words of a prompt. These echoic repetitions can be functional; that is, the child may be communicating a specific intention such as greeting the parent or indicating agreement with a parent statement or signaling that he or she does not understand the parent's request. By observing the context in which the child uses an echoic utterance, it may be possible to use the occasion to prompt for a more standard, spontaneous utterance that serves the same function. The use of this nonverbal prompting helps avoid the automatic echoing of a response and teaches the child to respond to nonverbal cues for initiating language.

Table 9.6. An example of the mand-model strategy

Steps	Example
Establish joint attention by attending to the child's focus of interest	Hunter and his mom, Celia, are playing with Mr. Potato Head. Hunter watches as she picks up the hat and the glasses.
Present a verbal mand/question	Celia can use a mand, "Tell me what you want, Hunter" or a choice question, "Do you want the hat or the glasses?"
If the child responds correctly, acknowledge response with expansion and material	When Hunter says, "Want hat," which is a target, Celia says, "You want the baseball hat" and gives him the hat.
If child doesn't respond or doesn't respond to the mand at the targeted level, give another mand or a model depending on level of support the child needs	When Hunter points to the hat without responding verbally, Celia prompts him: "Say 'want hat.'"
If child responds correctly, acknowledge response with expansion and material	When Hunter repeats her model exactly, Celia expands with "You want the funny hat" and gives him the hat to put on Mr. Potato Head.
If child doesn't respond to the mand at the targeted level, or doesn't repeat the model exactly, state the correct response and give child the material	When Hunter responds to the model or mand with "Hat," which is not complete and at the target level, Celia corrects with "Want hat" and gives him the hat.

Table 9.7.   An example of the time-delay strategy

Steps	Example
Establish joint attention by attending to the child's focus of interest	Hunter is carefully watching his mom, Celia, as she blows bubbles through a wand.
Wait for the child to initiate a request or comment	After Celia has blown bubbles several times, she puts her mouth up to the wand but does not blow and looks expectantly at Hunter.
If the child initiates a request/comment at the target level, acknowledge with expansion and material	When Hunter says, "Blow bubbles" Celia blows bubbles, laughs, and says, "I blow big bubbles!"
If the child doesn't initiate at the target level, give a mand or a model depending on level of support the child needs	When Hunter does not respond, Celia can either give a mand, "Tell me what you want" or a model, "Say 'blow bubbles.'"
If the child responds correctly, acknowledge response with expansion and material	When Hunter repeats the model accurately, Celia says, "I blow bubbles for you" and blows lots of bubbles.
If the child doesn't respond to mand or doesn't repeat the model exactly, state the correct response and give the child the material	If Hunter doesn't respond or says, "Bubbles" Celia says, "Blow bubbles" and then blows the bubbles.

The fourth MT strategy, incidental teaching, was developed for teaching more elaborate language and for improving conversational skills about particular topics. Incidental teaching is used when a child makes a request. The first step in the incidental teaching procedure is for the parent to arrange the environment in ways that encourage the child to request materials and assistance. The child who verbally or nonverbally requests materials or assistance is identifying the reinforcer at that moment. The parent responds by modeling, manding, or delaying for a more elaborated response or for a targeted language response. When the child responds appropriately, the parent gives the item of interest while affirming and repeating the answer in an expanded fashion, thereby presenting a model of more complex language for future child responses (see Table 9.8 for an example of the incidental teaching procedure).

If the child does not respond appropriately to the time-delay prompts, the parent can either provide a model for the child to imitate or give a mand, cuing the child about possible responses. The parent then confirms the accuracy of the child's response, expands what the child said, and gives the child whatever he or she requested. Because teaching to a reinforcer is possible only as long as the item or event is really of interest to the child, episodes are brief and positive in nature. Ability to request verbally or nonverbally and ability to imitate target forms are the only prerequisite child skills for incidental teaching (see Figure 9.1 for the core milieu pattern).

Two general guidelines apply when parents are selecting which one of the four milieu procedures is most appropriate. First, parents should select the procedure that is the most natural to the ongoing interaction with their child.

Table 9.8. An example of the incidental teaching strategy

Steps	Example
Arrange the environment to encourage the child to request assistance or materials.	Hunter and his mom, Celia, enjoy painting together. Celia gives him a paintbrush and paper but no paint.
Wait for the child to initiate a request or comment.	Hunter looks at Celia and says, "Want paint."
If the child initiates a verbal or nonverbal request, respond by using model, mand-model, or time-delay procedures, depending on the level of support needed by the child.	Celia smiles at Hunter, gives him the paint, and says, "You want the paint box." If Hunter points to the paint without speaking or says, "Paint," which is not a target, Celia can respond with the procedure she thinks is the most appropriate support for Hunter.

For instance, asking a question (using the mand-model procedure) is natural when a child's intentions or desires are not clear or when asking for specification would be usual (e.g., "Would you like milk or juice?"). The model procedure is used whenever the child does not know the appropriate response. If the child does not know the name of an object, however, it is appropriate for the parent to begin by modeling the label for the child to imitate (e.g., "These are Lego blocks").

Second, parents should use the procedure that provides the level of support their child needs to make an appropriate communicative response. Modeling provides maximum support for a child's response. The mand-model procedure provides a middle level of support and can be tailored to fit a child's skills by either asking a question only or providing two named choices followed by a question (e.g., "I have a cheese sandwich and a peanut butter sandwich. What do you want?"). Time delay provides no initial verbal support.

Incidental teaching differs from the other three procedures because it always follows a child request. Thus, incidental teaching should be used by parents only when their child has made a request. Requests can be verbal, vocal, or gestural. How the parent responds to the child's request in order to prompt elaborated language depends on the level of support the child requires to respond appropriately. In all uses of the milieu procedures, incomplete or incorrect child responses are followed by support for a correct response (i.e., if a child cannot respond to a mand, a model of the correct response is offered). Every episode includes a positive consequence, continuing communication, and modeling of an expanded form of the prompted response. The goals in all applications of the procedures are to ensure that the interaction is as communicative, natural, and positive as possible and that interactions end with the child gaining the specified reinforcers.

EMT is more complex and more naturalistic than earlier versions of MT (Alpert & Kaiser, 1992). The emphasis on responsiveness shifts the focus from proactive teaching to responsive teaching and embeds prompts into con-

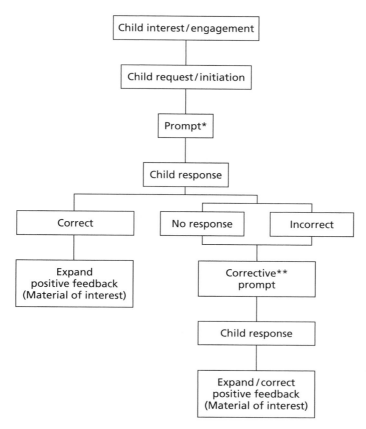

Figure 9.1. Core milieu pattern. *Prompt, mand, model, time delay. **Corrective, mand, model, time delay; repeated.

versations and engaging play interactions. These changes, although subtle, require teaching parents a different approach to communicating with their child and require a high level of skill and extensive experience with EMT procedures by the professional who is working with parents.

ASSESSMENT METHODS TO SUPPORT ONGOING DECISION MAKING

In our research studies, child outcomes of EMT are assessed from both pre- and poststandardized measures as well as session-by-session observational measures. Standardized measures have included general receptive and expressive skills, receptive and expressive vocabulary, and MLU and vocabulary diversity derived from language samples. Observational data from individual sessions generally include frequency measures of total child utterances, spontaneous utterances, total target language, elicited target language, spontaneous target language, dyadic turn taking, MLU, and diversity. Typically, language targets are vocabulary, early syntactic/semantic forms (e.g., agent–

action–object constructions, and requests at the child's target level). Multiple exemplars of these classes of targets are taught in the intervention. The activity and the child's focus of interest always determine specific exemplars.

We have found it useful to generate lists of examples for targets (e.g., examples of modifier + noun; agent–action–object; preposition–object) and to provide parents with specific examples that can be taught with a particular toy. For a toy race track with cars, for example, the list of examples for an agent–action target might include: *I/you/we race; Car roll; Car stop; Car go; I/you push; Car crashes; We crash.* Table 9.9 shows some measures of child language outcomes that can be obtained from language samples. We have frequently taught students and classroom teachers to collect language samples and analyze them using Systematic Analysis of Language Transcripts (SALT; Miller & Chapman, 1998).

Parent training in EMT is criterion based so assessment of parent use of the strategies drives the timing of when the next skill in the sequence is introduced. Parent behaviors that are assessed include frequency of pause errors, frequency and percentage of responsive feedback, frequency and percentage of expansions, frequency and percentage of language at the child's targeted level, and frequency and correctness of MT episodes.

Our research has emphasized generalization to home interactions and maintenance of parent and child gains over time. Parents and children are observed before, during, and after training at home during typical household activities and play. Follow-up observations at home and in the clinic extend over 6–18 months. The same observational measures used in the training setting are used to estimate generalization and maintenance. We further examine child generalization and maintenance through probes across other

Table 9.9. Example of language sample data sheet

Measure[a]	Data	
Mean length of utterance	1.83	
Total number of utterances	145	
Number of different words	62	
Number of one-word utterances	51	
Number of two-word utterances	27	
Number of three-word utterances	12	
Number of four- and four+-word utterances	10	
Target frequency[b]	Spontaneous	Prompted
1. Two-word request	4	2
2. Action–object	5	1
3. Modifier + noun	2	1
Target examples	Spontaneous	Prompted
1. Two-word request	Want milk	Want bubbles
2. Action–object	Play ball	Blow bubbles
3. Modifier + noun	Red ball	Little bubble

[a]Automatically calculated by Systematic Analysis of Language Transcripts (SALT).
[b]Counted from transcript.

adults. We are just beginning to measure children's generalized use of target forms systematically in peer and sibling interactions.

Additionally, informal assessment of parent and child progress takes place at the beginning and end of each intervention session. At the beginning of the session, the therapist asks the parent about the use of EMT at home since the last training session, what worked, and what may have been problematic. The therapist is able to assess the parent's understanding of EMT principles and use this information to help the parent build on his or her working knowledge, to troubleshoot any problems, and possibly as a frame for where the parent might need support in the upcoming session with the child. At the end of the session, the therapist conducts an informal assessment of how the parent felt about implementing the strategies with the child. This gives the therapist the opportunity to again troubleshoot and help the parent integrate the strategies in a way that makes sense for his or her child and context. The therapist also asks about how the parent is going to implement the newly learned strategy at home before the next session, and this is an opportunity for the therapist to troubleshoot and help the parent apply the strategies to the home environment.

Without systematic data collection and review of the implementation of EMT procedures, even the most experienced professional is likely to be inconsistent or imprecise in training parents. Ideally, implementation data are collected in each session by the professional (and occasionally by a second person), plans are written for every meeting with the parent, and accomplishments are evaluated after each session. The EMT implementation checklist (see Table 9.10) is one tool the professional can use to evaluate the parent's use of procedures. Data on child behavior are the anchor for each training session. Data on parent performance are used to support specific targeted feedback and planning for future sessions. Data can be collected in a variety of ways, but data collection and use directly affect how quickly children will learn new language and how well parents will learn EMT procedures.

CONSIDERATIONS FOR CHILDREN FROM CULTURALLY AND LINGUISTICALLY DIVERSE BACKGROUNDS

When using EMT with different cultural and linguistic groups we must consider the intersect between the cultural or linguistic group and 1) specific EMT strategies, 2) specific EMT behavioral outcomes, and 3) the venue for EMT intervention, including toys and materials used in the play-based interaction.

EMT Strategies

EMT is an intervention that is anchored in a responsive, contingent adult–child interaction. When considering the appropriateness of applying an EMT intervention within any culture, it would be important to consider the

Table 9.10.   Enhanced milieu teaching implementation checklist

Strategy	Not observed	Needs more practice	Satisfactory
1. Environmental arrangement			
Play area is well organized			
Appropriate selection of materials			
Arrangement encourages engagement			
Arrangement encourages initiations			
2. Parent style and affect			
Parent responds quickly to child			
Parent is warm and positive			
Parent listens to child			
Parent often at child's eye level			
3. Parental responsiveness			
Parent engages in child's activity			
Parent allows child to lead play activity			
Parent engages in conversation with child			
Parent balances turns with child			
Parent pauses for child to initiate			
Parent talks about what child is doing			
Parent responds to content of child's talk			
Parent asks for clarification when child not understood			
Parent talks at child's target level			
Parent expands child's utterances			
Parent expands at child's target level			
4. Milieu teaching			
Parent teaches in response to child requests			
Parent prompts language at child target level			
Parent follows through on prompts for language			
Parent stops prompting when child loses interest			
Parent prompts no more than once per minute			
Parent prompts all of child's target forms			
Accuracy of model procedure			
Accuracy of mand-model procedure			
Accuracy of time delay procedure			
Accuracy of incidental teaching procedure			
5. Overall quality of session			

norms for responsiveness within that culture, especially as they relate to adult–child interactions. It would be particularly important to consider the culture's norms around behaviors that are foundational to responsiveness, such as eye contact, touch, and physical closeness. If the professional is unfamiliar with a culture, some of this information may be determined by observing naturally occurring parent–child interactions within that culture. The families with whom we are working have some baseline rate of the strategies we are trying to teach, but we are often asking them to implement the strategies more frequently or more systematically than they are using them in their natural interactions. A cultural informant independent from the parent may also provide some helpful information that will allow the professional to determine the appropriateness of EMT strategies within that culture and if what is being observed with the parent may be individual variation within that culture.

EMT Outcomes

A second consideration when determining the appropriateness of EMT for members of a specific cultural/linguistic group involves the language forms targeted for the EMT intervention. Successful language outcomes of EMT are often driven by the extent to which the adult can model and elicit developmentally appropriate targets for individual children. One implicit requirement in implementing EMT successfully is that adults must be relatively competent in the language in which they will teach children. Competence includes sufficient vocabulary and grammatical knowledge to make the adjustments needed when talking at the child's targeted language level. The teaching adult's language skills can be an issue when the parent's first language is other than English, but issues can also arise when parents themselves have learning or language-related difficulties. We have had parents who were English speakers who were not metalinguistically sophisticated enough to be able to teach their child's specific targets. These parents had difficulty when children's targets were longer than 3 words (e.g., agent–action–preposition–object). Although these parents did learn to increase their responsiveness and to globally expand their children's utterances, they had difficulty modeling specific linguistic structures and sometimes giving systematic corrective feedback during MT episodes. It is important, regardless of cultural background or first language, to determine if a parent's language competence will support teaching specific linguistic targets beyond a three-word level.

EMT Venue

Because the EMT intervention generally occurs within a play context, it is important for an interventionist to select culturally appropriate toys and materials. Often this may mean supplementing existing toys so there are more culturally appropriate choices. For example, when we are working with African American families, we use African American dolls and add culturally appropriate hair products to our hairdressing play scheme. Open communication with parents from all backgrounds and gathering information from cultural informants can be helpful in determining creative and appropriate ways to supplement toys and materials or to choose activities that are familiar to the child and parent. In addition, in some cultures, sustained play with a child does not occur in the home. Although the goal of EMT is use across everyday environments, initially teaching and practicing EMT skills is easiest using play as a context. We discuss our rationale for this approach with parents. We ask them to participate in play during training and encourage them to create a comfortable context for engaging with their child at home to practice the EMT strategies.

We have systematically asked every parent in our project to give us written and informal verbal feedback about our teaching procedures, the materials and toys, and expectations for practice at home. Although these assessments have been uniformly positive, we believe there is much to be learned about adapting EMT for families from varied cultures.

APPLICATION TO AN INDIVIDUAL CHILD

Our current research has two foci. First, we are studying the effects of combining therapist and parent-implemented EMT to maximize child communication development across settings and time with preschool children with developmental disabilities. Second, we are examining the preventive effects of teaching low-income parents of preschoolers with language delays and behavior problems to support their children's communication and social skills. The following two case studies are composites of children we have worked with who represent the typical course and outcome of EMT with each of these two distinct populations.

Child with Developmental Disabilities

Hunter was 42 months old when he participated in our intervention and had been diagnosed with autism. He had some spoken language but much of what he said was rote; for instance, when he met someone new he said, "Hi Hunter." He often made his needs known by taking his mother's hand and leading her to what he wanted. He enjoyed playing with cause-and-effect toys such as the cars that go down the race track and the balls that go down a series of chutes. Hunter's mom, Celia, agreed to participate in the EMT intervention research study, which meant she came with Hunter to our center twice each week for individual sessions which lasted for approximately 6 months. During this intervention phase, we visited Celia and Hunter at home at least six times and helped her apply EMT principles to her everyday activities at home. At the end of the intervention, she agreed for us to complete booster sessions, once per month for an additional 6 months, which we have learned is important support for parents in their continued use of EMT. Before the intervention began, Hunter was assessed with the Preschool Language Scale–3 (Zimmerman, Steiner, & Pond, 1992), the PPVT-R, and the Expressive Vocabulary Test (Williams, 1997), and a language sample was also completed. Hunter's standardized test scores were all more than 2 SD below the expected mean. His MLU during the language sample was 1.45 and his diversity of word roots was 65. Five parent–child play interaction sessions were videotaped before beginning the intervention phase, in order to obtain a baseline on Celia and Hunter's communication and interaction behaviors before we taught Celia any of the EMT strategies. Celia and Hunter appeared to have a good time playing during these sessions. Celia sat close to Hunter and tried to engage him in the play and conversation. She asked lots of questions and directed his attention to the toys: "Look, Hunter. This race car can go really fast down this track. Vroom. Vroom. The race car is loud! Why don't you take the red race car and mommy will take the green race car? How does that sound?" Hunter usually looked at Celia when she tried to engage him in this way but did not respond verbally.

At the beginning of intervention, we talked to Celia about environmental arrangement and balancing her turns with Hunter. We showed her videotapes of other parents, role played with her, and gave her handouts that she took home and read at her convenience. Instead of allowing Hunter full access to all toys and materials, we instructed Celia to put the race cars within his sight, but out of reach in plastic containers that required adult assistance, since this set up a functional reason for him to communicate with her. We also instructed her to wait until Hunter initiated communication either verbally or nonverbally (e.g., when he reached for the toys) and then respond to his initiation with one brief, related comment. By about the fifth intervention session, Celia was consistently following Hunter's lead and responded contingently to his communicative initiations. The next step was for her to talk frequently at Hunter's target level. From the pretesting and transcriptions of Hunter's communicative utterances in the language sample and the play sessions with his mom, we determined that Hunter's target level was generally two-word utterances that specifically included: 1) agent–action verb, 2) action verb–object, 3) adjective–noun, and 4) requests, specifically want + object. (See Table 9.11 for a target handout given to Celia.) Celia quickly incorporated Hunter's target-level utterances in all the responsive strategies she learned, including expanding what Hunter said. By session 12, we began to teach milieu prompts, starting with models, then mand-models, time delays, and lastly the incidental teaching procedure. Generally, Celia used milieu prompts no more than 10 times during a session so it felt playful

Table 9.11. Language targets for Hunter

Toy	Target form	Target example
Ball	Agent – action	"Mommy throws"
	Action – object	"Throw ball"
	Adjective – noun	"Big ball"
	Want + object	"Want ball"
Cars	Agent – action	"Mommy drives"
	Action – object	"Drive car"
	Adjective – noun	"Fast car"
	Want + object	"Want track"
Babies	Agent – action	"Baby cries"
	Action – object	"Feed baby"
	Adjective – noun	"Sleepy baby"
	Want + object	"Want bottle"
Playdough	Agent – action	"I open"
	Action – object	"Make snake"
	Adjective – noun	"Red playdough"
	Want + object	"Want roller"

and responsive to Hunter. Before we began the MT phase, Hunter initiated twice as much to his mother as he had before the intervention began, but he was only using target language at a slightly higher rate. After the third session in which Celia used milieu prompts, Hunter's use of targets doubled in the session and continued to increase at a steady rate.

By the end of intervention, Celia was using all of the EMT procedures at a high rate of accuracy, and the interaction between her and Hunter looked very natural. At posttesting, Hunter made substantial gains on the standardized language assessments (e.g., his pre-PPVT-R standard score was 68 and his post-PPVT-R standard score was 78 (a gain of > 2 *SEM*). Additionally, his MLU on the language sample was 2.20 (versus 1.45 preintervention) and diversity of word roots almost doubled from his preintervention rate (65 preintervention to 125 postintervention). More importantly, Celia reported that Hunter now initiated communication with other adults (something he had not done before intervention) and had stopped taking her hand to get what he wanted because he could verbalize many of his immediate needs.

Child Who Is at Risk

Destiny was 39 months old when she first participated in our intervention and was attending a daily child care program that primarily served families who were low income. Her mother, Gina, worked hard to provide for her family and better her circumstances. She took adult classes to help her pass her General Educational Development (GED) exam and was employed at a local retail center earning the minimum hourly wage. Destiny had no contact with her father but did spend time with her maternal grandmother and several cousins. When our program offered a free language and behavior screening for all preschool children enrolled in Destiny's child care program, Gina promptly returned her permission form allowing us to assess Destiny. She had some concerns about Destiny's frequent temper tantrums and aggression toward other classmates, and she had questions about whether Destiny's language skills were at the level expected for her age. Destiny's tested language skills were about 1.5 *SD* below the expected mean. Both her teacher and her mother rated her problem behavior in the clinical range; aggression and noncompliance were the two most problematic areas. We met with Gina and explained the EMT program and what would be involved if she decided to participate. We proposed to meet with Gina and Destiny at the child care center before Gina's GED classes. We told her if she and Destiny came twice each week, it would take about 12 weeks to complete the program. Gina was concerned about trying to fit these sessions into her very full schedule. Destiny's teacher told her about other families who had participated in the program. After talking to her mother, who offered to pick Destiny up from child care two afternoons per week to give Gina more time to study or work at her job, Gina decided to participate in the program.

Although Gina was shy at first, over time she built a relationship with Barbara, her EMT therapist. Gina later told us that after a few weeks she really looked forward to the sessions. She could tell a difference in how Destiny was talking after about 10 sessions. Destiny was also minding her better, which made Gina's life easier. Barbara worked with Gina to adapt the environmental arrangement strategies to Gina and Destiny's needs. Barbara taught Gina several things she could do to get Destiny talking more so she could practice her language skills. Barbara also showed Gina some ways she could arrange the environment at home so she would not have to worry about Destiny's safety all the time. Making her home safer then decreased the number of instructions Gina was giving Destiny. By the middle of training, the few instructions Gina did give were almost always followed by a consequence, so Destiny seemed to obey her more often. Barbara talked to Gina about RI and how important it was for her to respond when Destiny talked to her. Nobody had ever told Gina that she was Destiny's most important language teacher. After hearing about her important role in her daughter's learning, Gina took the responsibility very seriously. Now when she talked to Destiny, she tried to use language that was as descriptive as possible, with lots of labels and adjectives. Talking at Destiny's target level also included giving instructions at her target level to ensure that Destiny would understand what Gina was asking her to do. During the play session, Barbara purposefully changed toys several times so Gina could practice giving Destiny short, direct instructions for putting away each toy during the transitions. When it was time for Gina to learn the milieu prompting strategies, Barbara focused mainly on choice questions. This not only served to support Destiny in using language to communicate her wants and needs but also gave her some control over her environment. Gina's use of the EMT procedures both supported Destiny's developing language skills and helped set boundaries for appropriate behavior. Gina was extremely proud of the EMT certificate she was given at the end of 28 intervention sessions. Six months after the intervention ended, Destiny's language skills were assessed and her results showed a gain of 0.66 *SD*. Her behavior as rated by her parent and teacher decreased by 1 *SD,* which was now close to or within normal limits. More importantly, Gina felt less stressed by parenting Destiny, more competent in her role as a parent, and now enjoyed playing with her child.

FUTURE DIRECTIONS

A relatively unexplored aspect of parent-implemented EMT is the effect of this intervention on the parent–child relationship and subsequent effects on the child's social interactions with peers. In the first generation of parent-training studies, concerns were raised about the potential of parent-implemented interventions disrupting or inhibiting the naturally occurring relationship between children and caregivers (Hanson & Hanline, 1990; Vincent & Beckett, 1993). Although there has been little empirical evidence of negative effects of parent-implemented interventions, controversy about the effects of these interventions on parent–child relationships remains (Kaiser et al., 1999; Kelly & Barnard, 1999; Mahoney et al., 1999; Winston, Sloop, & Rodriquez, 1999). There are indications that parent-implemented EMT may have positive effects on parent–child relationships (Kaiser, 1993; Kaiser, Hancock, & Hester, 1998). First, parents' evaluations of parent-implemented interventions consistently refer to positive changes in their relationship with their child (Hemmeter & Kaiser, 1994; Kaiser et al., 1998; Kaiser & Delaney, 2001; Kaiser & Hancock, 2003; Kaiser et al., 2000). Second, generalized changes in parental responsiveness, especially when those changes are sustained over time, may be an indicator of potentially positive changes in the parent–child relationship (Delaney & Kaiser, 2001; Hancock et al., 2002; Kaiser et al., 2000). Parental responsivity has been a key variable assessed as an indicator of quality of parent–child interactions with young children who have developmental disabilities (Dunst & Trivette, 1986; Mahoney & Powell, 1988) as well as in facilitation of language development (Yoder, McCathren, Warren, & Watson, 2001; Yoder & Warren, 2001). Third, whereas parent-implemented EMT has focused on improving children's use of language in naturalistic communication contexts, there are a number of similarities between this approach to supporting communication and more general strategies for improving parent–child relationships (Barnard & Martell, 1995; McCollum & Hemmeter, 1997). Fourth, there is some evidence that parents who participate in EMT training report less stress related to parenting and more positive social behavior by their children (Hancock et al., 2002).

Interactions with peers are a second important type of social relationship in the lives of young children (Hartup, 1992). Children with developmental disabilities typically have difficulty in peer interactions and many of these difficulties are related to their deficits in communication development (Guralnick, 1999). Although there is a literature on peer-mediated strategies for increasing verbal interactions between children with developmental disabilities and their typical peers (Brown & Conroy, 2001; Odom et al., 1999), there is little known about the effects of EMT by parents on children's interactions with their peers.

RECOMMENDED READINGS

Hancock, T.B., Kaiser, A.P., & Delaney, E.M. (2002). Teaching parents of preschoolers at high risk: Strategies to support language and positive behavior. *Topics in Early Childhood Special Education, 22(4),* 191–212.

Kaiser, A.P., & Hancock, T.B. (2003). Teaching parents new skills to support their young children's development. *Infants and Young Children, 16,* 9–21.

Kaiser, A.P., Hancock, T.B., & Nietfeld, J.P. (2000). The effects of parent-implemented enhanced milieu teaching on the social communication of children who have autism. *Journal of Early Education and Development [Special Issue], 4,* 423–446.

REFERENCES

Alpert, C.L., & Kaiser, A. (1992). Training parents as milieu language teachers. *Journal of Early Intervention, 16*(1), 31–52.

Barnard, K.E., & Martell, L.K. (1995). Mothering. In M.H. Bornstein (Ed.), *Handbook of parenting: Vol. 3. Status and social conditions of parenting* (pp. 3–26). Mahwah, NJ: Lawrence Erlbaum Associates.

Brown, W.H., & Conroy, M.A. (2001). Promoting peer-related social-communicative competence in preschool children. In H. Goldstein, L.A. Kaczmarek, & K.M. English (Eds.), *Promoting social communication: Children with developmental disabilities from birth to adolescence* (pp. 173–200). Baltimore: Paul H. Brookes Publishing Co.

Bruner, J.S. (1975). From communication to language: A psychological perspective. *Cognition, 3*(3), 255–287.

Delaney, E.M., & Kaiser, A.P. (2001). The effects of teaching parents blended communication and behavior support strategies. *Behavioral Disorders, 26*(2), 93–116.

Dunn, L.M., & Dunn, L.M. (1981). *Peabody Picture Vocabulary Test–Revised.* Circle Pines, MN: American Guidance Service.

Dunst, C., & Trivette, C. (1986). Looking beyond the parent-child dyad for the determinants of maternal styles of interaction. *Infant Mental Health Journal, 7,* 69–80.

Goldstein, H. (1993). Structuring environmental input to facilitate generalized language learning by children with mental retardation. In S.F. Warren & J. Reichle (Series Eds.) & A.P. Kaiser & D. Gray (Vol. Eds.), *Communication and language intervention se-*

ries: Vol. 2. Enhancing children's communication: Research foundations for early language intervention '(pp. 317–334). Baltimore: Paul H. Brookes Publishing Co.

Guralnick, M.J. (1999). Family and child influences on the peer-related social competence of young children with developmental delays. *Mental Retardation and Developmental Disabilities, 5*(1), 21–29.

Halle, J.W., Baer, D.M., & Spradlin, J.E. (1981). Teachers' generalized use of delay as a stimulus control procedure to increase language use in handicapped children. *Journal of Applied Behavior Analysis, 14*, 387–400.

Halle, J.W., Marshall, A.M., & Spradlin, J.E. (1979). Time delay: A technique to increase language use and facilitate generalization in retarded children. *Journal of Applied Behavior Analysis, 12*, 431–440.

Hamilton, B., & Snell, M.E. (1993). Using the milieu approach to increase spontaneous communication book use across environments by an adolescent with autism. *Augmentative and Alternative Communication, 9*, 259–272.

Hancock, T.B., Kaiser, A.P., & Delaney, E.M. (2002). Teaching parents of preschoolers at high risk: Strategies to support language and positive behavior. *Topics in Early Childhood Special Education, 22*(4), 191–212.

Hanson, M.J., & Hanline, M.F. (1990). Parenting a child with a disability: A longitudinal study of parental stress and adaptation. *Journal of Early Intervention, 14*(3), 234–248.

Hart, B.M., & Risley, T.R. (1968). Establishing the use of descriptive adjectives in the spontaneous speech of disadvantaged preschool children. *Journal of Applied Behavior Analysis, 1,* 109–120.

Hart, B.M., & Risley, T.R. (1975). Incidental teaching of language in the preschool. *Journal of Applied Behavior Analysis, 8,* 411–420.

Hart, B.M., & Rogers-Warren, A.K. (1978). Milieu teaching approaches. In R.L. Schiefelbusch (Ed.), *Bases of language intervention* (Vol. 2, pp. 193–235). Baltimore: University Park Press.

Hartup, W.W. (1992). Peer relations in early and middle childhood. In V. Van Hasselt & M. Hersen (Eds.), *Handbook of social development* (pp. 257–281). New York: Kluwer Academic/Plenum.

Hedrick, D.L., Prather, E.M., & Tobin, A.R. (1975). *Sequenced Inventory of Communication Development.* Seattle: University of Washington Press.

Hemmeter, M.L., & Kaiser, A.P. (1994). Enhanced milieu teaching: Effects of parent-implemented language intervention. *Journal of Early Intervention, 18,* 269–289.

Hester, P.P., Kaiser, A.P., Alpert, C.L., & Whiteman, B. (1996). The generalized effects of training trainers to teach parents to implement milieu teaching. *Journal of Early Intervention, 20*(1), 30–51.

Kaiser, A.P. (1993). Functional language. In M.E. Snell (Ed.), *Instruction of students with severe disabilities* (4th ed., pp. 347–379). New York: Macmillan.

Kaiser, A.P., Alpert, C.L., Fischer, R., Hemmeter, M.L., Tiernan, M., & Ostrosky, M. (1990, October). *Analysis of the primary and generalized effects of milieu and responsive-interaction teaching by parents.* Paper presented at the annual meeting of the Division of Early Childhood, Albuquerque.

Kaiser, A.P., & Delaney, E.M. (2001). Responsive conversations: Creating opportunities for naturalistic language teaching. *Young Exceptional Children Monograph Series No. 3,* 13–23.

Kaiser, A.P., & Hancock, T.B. (2000, April). *Supporting children's communication development through parent-implemented naturalistic interventions.* Presented at the 2nd annual conference on Research Innovations in Early Intervention (CRIEI), San Diego.

Kaiser, A.P., & Hancock, T.B. (2003). Teaching parents new skills to support their young children's development. *Infants and Young Children, 16,* 9–21.

Kaiser, A.P., Hancock, T.B., & Hester, P.P. (1998). Parents as co-interventionists: Research on applications of naturalistic language teaching procedures. *Infants and Young Children, 10*(4), 46–55.

Kaiser, A.P., Hancock, T.B., & Nietfeld, J.P. (2000). The effects of parent-implemented enhanced milieu teaching on the social communication of children who have autism.
Journal of Early Education and Development [Special Issue], 4, 423–446.

Kaiser, A.P., Hemmeter, M.L., Ostrosky, M., Fischer, R., Yoder, P.J., & Keefer, M. (1996).
The effects of teaching parents to use responsive interaction strategies. *Topics in
Early Childhood Special Education, 16*(3), 375–406.

Kaiser, A.P., Hester, P.P., Alpert, C.L., & Whiteman, B.C. (1995). Preparing parent trainers: An experimental analysis of effects on trainers, parents, and children. *Topics in
Early Childhood Special Education, 14*(4), 385–414.

Kaiser, A., Mahoney, G., Girolametto, L., MacDonald, J., Robinson, C., Safford, P., & Spiker,
D. (1999). [Rejoinder] Toward a contemporary vision of parent education. *Topics in
Early Childhood Special Education, 19,* 173–176.

Kaiser, A.P., & Warren, S.F. (1987). Pragmatics and generalization. In R.L. Schiefelbusch
& L.L. Lloyd (Eds.), *Language perspectives: Acquisition, retardation, and intervention* (2nd ed.). Austin, TX: PRO-ED.

Kaiser, A.P., Yoder, P.J., & Keetz, A. (1992). Evaluating milieu teaching. In S.F. Warren &
J. Reichle (Series & Vol. Eds.), *Communication and language intervention series:
Vol. 1. Causes and effects in communication and language intervention* (pp. 9–47).
Baltimore: Paul H. Brookes Publishing Co.

Kelly, J.F., & Barnard, K.E. (1999). Parent education within a relationship-focused model.
Topics in Early Childhood Special Education, 19, 151–157.

Mahoney, G., Kaiser, A., Girolametto, L., MacDonald, J., Robinson, C., Safford, P., & Spiker,
D. (1999). Parent education in early intervention: A call for a renewed focus. *Topics in
Early Childhood Special Education, 19,* 131–140.

Mahoney, G., & Powell, A. (1988). Modifying parent-child interaction: Enhancing the development of handicapped children. *The Journal of Special Education, 22,* 82–96.

McCollum, J.A., & Hemmeter, M.L. (1997). Parent-child interaction when children have disabilities. In M.J. Guralnick (Ed.), *The effectiveness of early intervention* (pp. 549–576).
Baltimore: Paul H. Brookes Publishing Co.

Miller, J., & Chapman, R. (1998). *SALT: Systematic analysis of language transcripts.*
Baltimore: University Park Press.

Moerk, E.L. (1992). *A first language taught and learned.* Baltimore: Paul H. Brookes
Publishing Co.

Odom, S.L., McConnell, S.R., McEvoy, M.A., Peterson, C., Ostrosky, M., Chandler, L.K.,
Spicuzza, R.J., Skellenger, A., Creighton, M., & Favazza, P.C. (1999). Relative effects of
interventions supporting the social competence of young children with disabilities.
Topics in Early Childhood Special Education, 19, 75–91.

Stokes, T.F., & Baer, D.M. (1977). An implicit technology of generalization. *Journal of
Applied Behavior Analysis, 10*(2), 349–367.

Vincent, L.J., & Beckett, J.A. (1993). Family participation. In S. L. Odom & M. E. McLean
(Eds.), *DEC recommended practices: Indicators of quality in programs for infant
and young children with special needs and their families* (pp. 19–29). Reston, VA:
Council for Exceptional Children, Division for Early Childhood, Task Force on Recommended Practices.

Warren, S.F., & Bambara, L.M. (1989). An experimental analysis of milieu language intervention: Teaching and action-object form. *Journal of Speech and Hearing Disorders,
54,* 448–461.

Warren, S.F., McQuarter, R.J., & Rogers-Warren, A.K. (1984). The effects of teacher mands
and models on the speech of unresponsive language-delayed children. *Journal of
Speech and Hearing Research, 51,* 43–52.

Williams, K.T. (1997). *Expressive Vocabulary Test.* Circle Pines, MN: American Guidance Service.

Winton, P.J., Sloop, S., & Rodriquez, P. (1999). Parent education: A term whose time is past.
Topics in Early Childhood Special Education, 19, 157–171.

Yoder, P.J., McCathren, R.B., Warren, S.F., & Watson, A.L. (2001). Important distinctions in measuring maternal responses to communication in prelinguistic children with disabilities. *Communication Disorders Quarterly, 22,* 135–147.

Yoder, P.J., & Warren, S.F. (1998). Maternal responsivity predicts the prelinguistic communication intervention that facilitates generalized intentional communication. *Journal of Speech, Language, and Hearing Research, 41*(5), 1207–1219.

Yoder, P.J., & Warren, S.F. (2001). Relative treatment effects of two prelinguistic communication interventions on language development in toddlers with developmental delays vary by maternal characteristics. *Journal of Speech, Language, and Hearing Research, 44,* 224–237.

Zimmerman, I.L., Steiner, V.G., & Pond, R.E. (1992). *Preschool Language Scale–3.* San Antonio, TX: Harcourt Assessment.

10

Conversational Recast Intervention with Preschool and Older Children

STEPHEN M. CAMARATA AND KEITH E. NELSON

ABSTRACT

The purpose of conversational recast intervention is to parallel natural language acquisition by responding to children's initiations with recasts, language models that both reflect and go beyond the forms and functions they currently are using. An example of a recast would be, "*The* cow *is* jump*ing*" in response to a child's production, "Cow jump." The recast in this example includes auxiliary (*is*), progressive (*ing*), and article (*the*) forms that were absent in the child's initiation. This is a procedure that can be applied broadly in many different approaches rather than a specific "package" of its own. It has been applied to a wide variety of disabilities, including specific language impairment, mental retardation (including Down syndrome), hearing impairment, and autism spectrum disorders and to a variety of targets, including vocabulary, grammar, and phonology. It has most often been applied with toddler and preschool children, although the procedure has been used with older children who are functioning at the preschool developmental level. Although untested experimentally, it could also apply to school-age language learning. This chapter includes a detailed description of conversational recast procedures and theoretical and empirical support for the model.

INTRODUCTION

The purpose of this chapter is to describe basic procedures used in many speech and language interventions falling under the broad rubric of *conversational recast* approaches. A recast is defined as a response to an imma-

---

Preparation of this manuscript was supported by Grants P50 DC03282 from the National Institute on Deafness and Other Communication Disorders and P30 HD15052 from the National Institute of Child Health and Human Development. The Scottish Rite Foundation of Nashville also supported this work.

Background research and reflection underpinning the ideas and data presented in this paper were provided by grants to the authors from the National Science Foundation (BNS-8013767) and the National Institutes of Health (MH 19826h, HD 06254, R01-NS26437, R01DC00508, and 1P50 DC0382–01898).

ture or incorrect child production that includes additional semantic, grammatical, and/or phonological information and generally corrects the child's error. An example of a grammatical recast could be, "She eats the cookie" in response to the child's production, "She eat cookie." A crucial aspect of conversational recast intervention is that it is focused on specific, developmentally appropriate speech and language skills. This chapter will describe the application of recast intervention and discuss the theoretical underpinnings and evidence to support this approach.

TARGET POPULATIONS AND ASSESSMENTS FOR DETERMINING TREATMENT RELEVANCE AND GOALS

Target Populations and Developmental Levels

The target populations for conversational recast intervention include any preschool group requiring language and/or speech intervention. This approach also extends to 6- to 9-year-old children who are functioning at prelinguistic or preschool language levels. In theory, it could also extend to language learning in older children and even to reading disorders, but there are no studies available to determine whether these theoretical applications are, in fact, effective. Empirical support is available for application to specific language impairment (SLI; Camarata, Nelson, & Camarata, 1994; Nelson, Camarata, Welch, Butkovski, & Camarata, 1996), phonological disorder (Camarata, 1993, 2001), autism (Heiman, Nelson, Tjus, & Gillberg, 1995; Koegel & Koegel, 2001; Koegel, O'Dell, & Koegel, 1987; Nelson, Heiman, & Tjus, 1997), hearing impairment (Prinz & Nelson, 1985, and see the review in Nelson & Camarata, 1998), and mental retardation (Yoder et al., 1995). In terms of developmental language level, the approach has been studied as a component of an approach for prelinguistic attainments (Yoder & Warren, 1998, 2001a, 2001b; see Warren et al., Chapter 3) through complex sentence acquisition (Camarata et al., 1994; see Ellis Weismer & Robertson, Chapter 8). Research has been primarily focused on lexical acquisition and grammatical acquisition. In addition, it has been applied to sign language acquisition in deaf children (Prinz & Masin, 1985) and to phonemes in phonological disorders and reading disability (Nelson et al., 1997). Although most of the research cited in this section has served to demonstrate the use of recasts to promote the acquisition of specific language forms (i.e., speech sounds, words, and grammatical forms), evidence also exists that the approach can be used as part of much more comprehensive intervention programs (e.g., Fey, Cleave, & Long, 1997; Fey, Cleave, Long, & Hughes, 1993; Leonard, Camarata, Brown, & Camarata, 2004).

Assessment for Determining Treatment Relevance

In general, assessment should focus on what aspects of the child's disabilities provide impediments to the conversational process. In conversational recast intervention, for example, the adult follows the child's initiations with responses specifically tailored to the child's own production and to the child's needs. An important pretreatment assessment issue, then, is the frequency of the child's spontaneous initiations, either nonverbally in the case of prelinguistic children (e.g., using joint attention) or verbally. If the frequency of child conversational contributions is low, the method will need to be modified to include adult presentation of self-recast patterns. For example, the adult can follow a simple adult utterance with a more complex recast of his or her own utterance (as in Baker & Nelson, 1984). The adult may also work to increase the child's participation by using some form of extrinsic motivation. Natural reinforcers might be added, for example, as in the natural language paradigm for autism (Koegel & Koegel, 1995; see also the models described by Halle et al. [Chapter 19], Hancock & Kaiser [Chapter 9], and Warren et al. [Chapter 3]).

A crucial aspect of conversational recast intervention is that it is focused on specific, developmentally appropriate speech and language skills. Consequently, determining which speech and/or language forms are to be targeted is a crucial aspect of the evaluation process (see Chapter 8). Conversational recast intervention is designed to teach/support the child's acquisition of the forms that are used in speech and language (and the social contexts associated with these forms), and the assessment should be focused on the child's preintervention developmental speech and language abilities. Thus, the actual goals of conversational recast intervention are words, suffixes, phonological forms, and syntax rather than "special skills" (e.g., sound discrimination, auditory processing, sensory defensiveness; Fuchs, 1979) hypothesized to impede speech and language acquisition. It should be noted that much of the research on recast intervention has included specific goals. Therefore, preintervention assessment for conversational recast intervention (and we would argue any other speech and/or language intervention) should include a detailed analysis of the child's actual speech and language abilities.

The literature on parent–child interaction suggests that parents and other caregivers automatically deliver recasts without explicit knowledge of speech and language structure. Therefore, one could wonder why targeting explicit, specific speech and language goals is an emphasis for conversational recast intervention. Specific goals are targeted because children with disabilities are more likely than typically developing children to require greater frequency and salience for sounds, words, word endings, and syntactic structures. Thus, the approach includes assessment to highlight those linguistic structures that are appropriate for the child's developmental level and within the constraints of the disabling condition(s).

Actual goals for intervention, for example, could include acquisition of a set of words a child needs in the preschool context, use of grammatical morphemes, such as progressive aspect (*be* + verb + *-ing*), auxiliaries (e.g., forms of *be, do,* and *have* preceding a lexical verb), copula (forms of *be* used as the main verb), tense (e.g., *-s, -ed* attached to the lexical verb), and an increase in the proportion of complex sentences (e.g., infinitives, relative clause, conjoined forms, other embedded forms). Goals could also include individual phonemes (e.g., [s], [z], [k]). The data on conversational recast interventions also indicate that secondary effects can be seen on broader intermediate goals, or basic goals, such as increases in mean length of utterance (MLU) and overall intelligibility (e.g., Yoder, Camarata, & Gardner, in press). In summary, the goals for recast intervention, at least in theory, could be any linguistic form, including phonemes, words, grammatical morphemes, grammar, and/or complex sentences that the child is ready to produce but is consistently omitting or otherwise producing incorrectly.

Assessment should also be completed to determine whether there are any sensory or perceptual deficits that may reduce or impede processing of the adult recast model. For example, a hearing impairment could reduce or preclude a child's ability to process the adult's verbal model so that the recast could be delivered via visual models such as sign language. Note that this assessment is not focused on a determination of the presence or absence of *sensory integration deficit* (SID) or *central auditory processing deficits* (CAPD). These diagnostic categories do not as yet have methods widely regarded as psychometrically valid (e.g., see the review in Cacace & McFarland, 1998, on CAPD). Rather, this assessment consideration should be focused on well-established procedures such as audiometry and traditional vision testing using standardized, psychometrically valid testing and well-established measures of speech and language. Stated directly, a diagnosis of SID or CAPD should *not* be used to exclude children from conversational recast intervention on the assumption that these conditions preclude a child's ability to process the adult recast. Many children labeled as having SID and/or CAPD have been included in our studies of conversational recasts, and, although none were given sensory integration or auditory treatment, most have displayed significant language and/or speech growth (Camarata et al., 1994; Leonard et al., 2004; Nelson et al., 1996).

THEORETICAL BASIS

Origins in Normal Language: Transactional Model of Language Development

Although the debate on how children acquire language continues unabated, including nativist accounts that minimize the importance of language input (Chomsky, 1965, 1975; Pinker, 1994, 1999), detailed observation of mother–

child interaction has provided a number of interactional characteristics that are likely to facilitate language learning (cf. Conti-Ramsden, 1990; Moerk, 1992; Shatz, 1983; Yoder & Warren, 1993). These characteristics include the generous provision of indirect repetitive feedback to the child, extensive contextual support (i.e., routines), contingent responses (i.e., attention, verbal interaction), and reductions in the complexity of speech and language models directed to the child. In a transactional model of mother–child interaction (Sameroff & Fiese, 1989), these learning opportunities are most powerful when they are coordinated in the language-learning environment (see also Nelson, 1989). More important from an intervention perspective, speech and language learning is viewed as an ongoing interaction (transaction) between child behaviors and parent behaviors that are mutually supporting and lead to advances in the child's language (Camarata & Yoder, 2002). Simply stated, aspects of the child's productions prompt specific classes of responses from the parent. These parent responses are associated with speech and language advances in the child, which then prompt more advanced responses from the parent and so on, across the course of normal speech and language development (Camarata, 1996; Camarata & Yoder, 2002; Nelson, 1989; Sameroff & Fiese, 1989; Yoder & Warren, 1993).

When the infant produces relatively frequent and stable speech-like vocalizations, for example, parents will often respond with linguistic input (often lexical mapping, wherein the parent says an actual word in response to the infant's nonverbal forms; see Snow, Perlmann, & Nathan, 1987; Yoder & Warren, 1993; see also Chapter 3). For example, if a toddler uses the canonical vocalization, [nanana], the child's mother may respond using the lexical form *mama* saying, "Mama, yes, mama." Even those who hypothesize that parental input has little direct impact on language development hypothesize that these transactions may be important for lexical acquisition (Pinker, 1999). After the child learns early words, the parent often responds with two- and three-word utterances. Similarly, when the child strings two- and three-word utterances together, the parent responses will often include grammatical morphemes that the child omitted (see Moerk, 1992; Nelson, 1989; Nelson et al., 1996), sounds that were mispronounced, or words that were omitted or used incorrectly. Although it is difficult to determine causality in these kinds of bidirectional naturalistic associations without experimental tests (but see sections below), it is clear that a number of these factors often coalesce during language learning.

Because parent responses are a critical element in the transaction, the child's linguistic initiations are extremely important; these serve as antecedent events that trigger the parent response (Moerk, 1992). Similarly, in order for the transaction to occur and be sustained, the linguistic level of the parent's response should add complexity to the child's form but also be sufficiently simple for the child to process the added information. It is important to note that many of these speech and language advances are observed in typically developing children while they have relatively immature neurological systems (Molfese & Molfese, 2000) and relative poor perception of static and dynamic acoustic cues in speech (Ohde & Haley, 1997). Indeed, one could argue that speech and language transactions are crucial for the neural organization of speech and language in the developing brain (see Camarata & Yoder, 2002; Neville & Mills, 1997) and also facilitate more accurate processing of key static and dynamic acoustic cues (Ohde & Haley, 1997; Yoder & Molfese, 2002).

Most children with language disorders, including those with SLI, Down syndrome, and global intellectual disabilities, display at least some degree of motivation for social communication. If provided with a supportive setting, these children will usually use verbal (or nonverbal) initiations that can then be recast by the clinician. Children with autism (Koegel & Koegel, 1995) display a reduced or even absent motivation for social communication and often require external reinforcers to engage in social communication. In children with autism, planning must be more extensive in order to provide opportunities for recasts. It should be noted that rate of initiations is a predictor of level of verbal communication in autism (Koegel, Koegel, & Brookman, 2003), and recast elements are included in treatment for autism (e.g., natural language paradigm; Koegel et al., 1987). It should also be noted that a diagnosis of autism spectrum disorder does *not* preclude using conversational recasts. Rather, as a practical consideration, any child with reduced levels of initiations may require adaptation of the technique to increase initiations and/or to ensure that recasts are delivered to a higher proportion of existing initiations and to enhance attention to recasts when presented.

Finally, in order for an accurate, child-appropriate grammatical or phonological recast to be delivered, the initiation must be intelligible. That is, the adult must be able to map at least a minimal degree of meaning to the child's verbal (or nonverbal) initiation in order to provide a relevant recast. A clue into this practical consideration can be seen in the following example, drawn from a clinical case in our Down Syndrome Clinic. The child, a male, age 8;3 was playing Birthday Party with the clinician and said "[ka]." An obvious interpretation of this production would be *cake* as the child's form and the context (which included a birthday cake), and the clinician responded with a recast using "cake" as part of the platform utterance. At this point, the interaction shifted because the child corrected the clinician by shaking his head and saying, "No [kak], [ka]!" which was then followed by four turns of child–clinician interaction attempting to establish intelligibility for the child form. Eventually, the clinician was able to determine that [ka] in this case was *cat* (it turned out that there was a cat depicted on the paper plates used in the birthday party). The point here is that intelligibility for the child's intended message is needed for the clinician to deliver a developmentally appropriate recast.

Development of Speech and Language Interventions from an Interactive Perspective

Because a transactional model of speech and language development includes simultaneous integration of a number of elements in the adult–child interaction, a full experimental evaluation of this model with speech and language-impaired populations has not yet been completed. However, a number of interventions have included elements of the model and generally provide support for the model. We refer to approaches that include one or more transactional elements as *interactive*. The more widely studied of these approaches are discussed in this section.

Incidental Teaching   Incidental teaching was perhaps the first attempt to move from strictly analog imitation and drill procedures toward more naturalistic learning contexts (Hart & Risley, 1968, 1974, 1995; Hart & Rogers-Warren, 1978; see also Chapters 3, 9, and 19). Incidental teaching retains many elements of the traditional imitation and drill (discrete trials) but integrates these teaching episodes into play activities while delivering secondary reinforcers that are consistent with those occurring in the natural environment. Thus, rather than providing edibles or other tangible items to reinforce prompted imitative productions, as was characteristic of early didactic language teaching models, incidental teaching may be conducted in a playroom that requires adult mediation for access to toys. When the children imitate the prompted toy names (or their colors or other targeted attributes), the adult provides access to the toy (Hart & Risley, 1968).

Although incidental teaching is very effective for establishing production of a variety of language goals in the training context, and it often results in improvements in more general language abilities, these productions also sometimes fail to generalize to contexts less directly under adult control (Warren & Kaiser, 1986). From a transactional perspective, although incidental teaching includes appropriate nonverbal responses to the child's productions (e.g., providing a toy the child has named), the earliest versions did not systematically include adult verbal response modeling of more advanced language forms that were directly contingent on child initiations; that is, the earlier versions did not include the use of recasts (Hart & Risley, 1968). Specifically, incidental teaching focuses on teaching the child a verbal repertoire using operant conditioning methods and does not include responses to child initiations. Thus, based on the transactional model described here, one might predict that incidental teaching would be highly effective for training specific language forms in relatively structured contexts, but would be less likely to result in more generalized improvements in language because the reinforcers and clinician prompts used to elicit the child forms are not generally present in the ambient environment. Despite these potential limitations, incidental teaching laid the conceptual groundwork for transferring operant methodology to language learning contexts that more closely parallel typical normal language acquisition and served as the basis for the milieu intervention that followed.

Milieu Teaching   Milieu teaching combines prompting and requests for imitation with naturalistic support (cf. Warren & Kaiser, 1986; Chapters 9 and 19, this volume). The key components of incidental teaching are retained and augmented by shifts to more interactive adult responses. That is, the adult not only controls delivery of the stimulus materials but models language targets in the form of developmentally appropriate responses. The imitative prompts are then provided within this context. This approach has been researched extensively and has been evaluated in a number of training contexts and with a variety of language goals among many different groups of children (see the review in Kaiser, 1993). A number of studies have indicated that milieu procedures are associated with acquisition of specific language targets and are also associated with more general gains in language (see the review in Kaiser, Yoder, & Keetz, 1992). However, Kaiser et al. concluded: "In general, the studies [reviewed] have not provided a sufficiently rigorous set of conditions for determining the effects of milieu teaching on performance outside the intervention context, on generalized knowledge, or on global language development" (1992, p. 40). Despite this, elements consistent with a transactional model are an integral part of milieu teaching.

Rare Event Learning Applied to Conversational Recasts   Unlike the models reviewed above, conversational recast intervention was developed originally from primarily cognitive models of language acquisition, such as the rare event learning mechanism (RELM; Nelson, 1977, 1980, 1981, 1987, 1989). Nelson argued that learning will occur when a number of factors occur simultaneously in the language environment. Specifically, children will learn new language structures when 1) the child production lacks advanced language structure (i.e., certain grammatical and/or syntactic elements are missing), 2) the parent responds with an utterance that maintains the basic elements of the child's previous production and includes some of the forms missing in the child's production (i.e., presents a structural challenge relative to the child's form), 3) this adult–child exchange directly follows the child's utterance so that the child can more easily process the differences in his or her production and the adult response, and 4) the child maintains working memory focus and actually encodes new structural information. Nelson stated that these elements occur relatively rarely in the stream of adult–child interaction (hence the designation *rare event learning mechanism*) but produce rapid acquisition of language forms when they do occur simultaneously, at least in children who are developing typically. Nelson and his colleagues have demonstrated these effects in a number of studies of normal language (e.g., Baker & Nelson, 1984; Nelson, Baker, Denninger, Bonvillian, & Kaplan, 1985). More recently, Camarata and Nelson adapted the model for use in children with language impairments. The results of these studies (Camarata & Nelson, 1992; Camarata et al., 1994; Gillum, Camarata, Nelson, & Camarata, 2003; Nelson et al., 1996) indicate that the conversational recast intervention is more effective in producing generalized spontaneous target use than imitation and drill used in discrete therapy activities for language-impaired children at Brown's stages IV and V (Brown, 1973).

Transactional Model and the Development of Speech Intelligibility

It is perhaps easy to overlook the importance of speech intelligibility as a factor in development. In the transactional model (see Figure 10.1), a child's initiation that is partially intelligible is paired with a contingent adult response that provides additional phonological information to the child's platform utterance. In the lexical domain, a child's joint attention, object-oriented point, and CV production could be followed by an adult presentation of a word, and that word would be modeled using more advanced phonology than the child's initiation. For example, a child's "ba" while playing with and pointing to a ball may yield a number of contingent adult models for the word *ball* which add the adult model of the CVC form and the correct final consonant that was

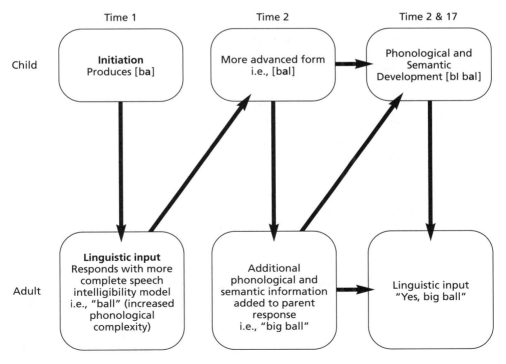

Figure 10.1. Underlying assumptions regarding conversational recast intervention.

deleted in the child's initiation. As the child's speech (and speech intelligibility) develops, more sophisticated exchanges occur wherein the adult models provide more and more complex information (cf. Nelson et al., 2002).

The transactional process hinges directly on the intelligibility of the child's initiation. For example, assume that a child is playing with several objects and says, "a." Was the child's initiation *ball, block, water, bottle, car, fall,* or any one of a large number of possible lexemes? An unintelligible child production reduces the probability that the adult's response will facilitate later child lexical development. For example, consider the recent finding that children with Down syndrome who use early sign language may demonstrate superior oral word use later in development as compared with children who did not receive sign language training (Sedey, Rosin, & Miller, 1991). One speculative explanation of this finding is that children with Down syndrome often develop speech intelligibility much more slowly than other children so that many of their productions do not elicit teaching responses from parents, teachers, or peers. Sign language teaching may provide parents, teachers, and peers with more intelligible initiations for which they can provide an appropriate verbal or sign response; meaningful conversational exchanges may thus be more frequent and also more positive socially-emotionally, and vocabulary challenges may be more easily processed and in turn support the child's subsequent increase in oral vocabulary. The point here is that unintelligible communication can have a devastating impact on child lexical development (see also Camarata, 1996; Smith & Camarata, 1999), and improving intelligibility could shift interactional communication in many respects and have broader impacts on language and social development.

Underlying Assumptions Regarding Conversational Recast Intervention

The primary assumption underlying the conversational recast approach is that children with disabilities can learn in the same manner as typically developing children if the transactions are adjusted to accommodate the parameters of the disability that impede access to transactions or to learning from them. For example, a child with autism displays reduced or even absent motivation for social communication (Koegel & Koegel, 1995). Because of this, the child displays reduced initiations and is less likely to attend to adult models in response to those initiations that do occur. It is revealing that Koegel et al. (2003) reported that level of spontaneous initiation is a strong predictor of language growth in autism. In order for conversational recast interventions to be effective in this population, it may be necessary to provide extrinsic motivation for social interaction and for attending to adult responses. Indeed, Koegel and his colleagues have provided evidence that elements of conversational recast intervention can be effective in autism.

Similarly, an assumption in conversational recast intervention is that children with speech and language disorders often will learn in a manner similar to typically developing children, but that they may be helped by a narrower focus for adult conversational responses with an increased frequency of speech/language structures within that focus (see Proctor-Williams, Fey, & Frome-Loeb, 2001). This is where the special expertise of speech-language pathologists (SLPs) is crucial because assessment of developmental level and focus on specific speech and language skills provide the targets for conversational recast intervention.

A further assumption is that typically developing children have immature and inaccurate speech processing ability (Ohde & Camarata, 2004; Ohde & Haley, 1997) and that, consistent with their language delays, children with speech and language disorders display delayed development in some aspects of speech processing. Because typical development does not include special training in speech processing, slowed speech, or drill designed to teach speech discrimination or establish phoneme boundaries, the usual developmental advances in speech processing may also be a by-product of parent–child transactions (Camarata & Yoder, 2002). That is, it is unlikely that adult levels of speech perception are required for speech and language learning and that children with disabilities require training on speech perception in order to make gains in speech and language abilities.

The relative contribution of training in speech processing by itself to overall speech and language acquisition in populations with disabilities remains an open question because these programs (e.g., Fast ForWord; Tallal, Miller, Jenkins & Merzenich, 1997; see Chapter 18) often include a combination of speech processing training and training on lexical and grammatical forms. A method then used to improve the language disorder focuses on "remediating" this special deficit by using numerous presentations of speech stimuli that are "slowed" and teach the child to discriminate these altered forms. However, because such programs often also include presentations of words and phrases, simply increasing the exposure to these forms may be just as likely to account for any gains as is the slowed speech. That is, when a speech processing treatment package includes training on vocabulary words, prepositions, and grammatical forms in addition to slowed speech, it is difficult to determine the relative contribution of any individual factor, including slowed speech or speech processing, to observed growth. Thus, an assumption within conversational recast treatment is that children with speech and language disorders can learn new sounds, words, morphemes, and syntax without requiring specialized speech processing training. It is perhaps noteworthy that many speech processing approaches to treatment include training on "real" words and phrases in addition to the speech processing procedures and are not usually completed exclusively on the elements hypothesized to underlie the speech and language disorders (e.g., see Chapter 18). This is noteworthy because there is a relatively large number of studies indicating that children can acquire words, grammatical morphemes, and syntax without teaching speech processing. In addition, a randomized clinical trial (Cohen et al., in press) indicates no significant advantage for this kind of training as compared with other procedures that do not include speech processing training. The assumption, therefore, is that multiple exposures to speech and language targets in predictable contexts using conversational recasts do not require a preliminary course of speech processing training.

EMPIRICAL BASIS

Conversational recast intervention is a procedure that can be applied broadly across many interventions and can include a parent, clinician, and/or teacher model of semantic, syntactic, and/or phonological information in response to a child's initiation. Elements of recasting are often included in multifactor parent-implemented (e.g., Fey et al., 1993; Gibbard, 1994) and clinician-implemented treatment (e.g., Leonard et al., 2004). In addition, one could argue that because recasts are a naturally occurring part of adult–child interaction, it is a latent part of treatments that ostensibly focus on other procedures. In Camarata et al. (1994), for example, treatment fidelity checks indicated that clinicians sometimes delivered a recast in response to a child's incorrect production within the discrete trials condition. Although this occurred at a much lower rate than in the conversational recast condition, recasts are a normal response to an error, and we hypothesize that some recasts are delivered in nearly all interventions. It is perhaps noteworthy that the reverse was not true in Camarata et al. (1994); there were virtually no imitative prompts or overt reinforcers delivered during the conversational recast condition. This should be borne in mind when examining the empirical basis for any intervention. In most cases, unless tight experimental control is maintained, conversational recasts could be delivered. For example, a sensory integration session (see Chapter 17) for a child with a language impairment was recently observed wherein the child was undergoing brushing of his arm and "joint compression." During this treatment, the clinician was talking to the child quite frequently and this interaction included frequent recasts. If language gains were observed during this procedure, this confound would have to be accounted for in the analysis because the source of the language growth, at least in part, could be attributable to the language interaction and recasting rather than to the brushing. This kind of potential confound is often a challenge in determining treatment effects (Snow, Swisher, McNamara, & Kiernan, 1996).

   In general, there are two forms of evidence in support of a conversational recast approach to speech and language intervention. First, there are a few studies that focus on the effects of recasting as compared with control and/or alternative treatments (e.g., Yoder et al., 1994). These studies can be used to estimate the overall effect size of the treatment for language targets or more general measures of language growth (e.g., MLU, standardized testing). A second level of evidence comes from studies that include recasts as a component of a broader treatment package (e.g., Fey et al., 1993, 1997). These studies include one or more additional treatments and cannot be used to determine the specific effects of conversational recasts on the outcome measures. However, if growth is observed under such treatments, it seems reasonable to assume that recasts were an important factor in development, because of the already existing support for their effects in studies with tighter controls on the application of recasts. Examples of both types of empirical evidence for conversational recast treatment are provided in the next section.

In a direct comparison of intervention methods, Camarata and colleagues (1994) compared discrete trial intervention on grammatical forms to conversational recasting in 21 children with SLI. They reported that grammatical targets were acquired following a mean of 63.6 recasts as compared with a mean of 150.7 presentations in the imitation condition. The dependent measure in this study was generalized use of the targets within spontaneous language samples. The size of this effect, in standard deviation units, was 1.10. This method of estimating relative effect size is generated by dividing the mean difference by the pooled standard deviation, and the value obtained indicates a substantial advantage for the children who received recasts. Thus, the results of Camarata et al. (1994) can be viewed as supporting the application of conversational recast to teach grammatical targets in children with SLI as compared with discrete trial procedures.

Similarly, Gillum and colleagues (2003) reported that children with SLI who scored significantly below the normative standard score on the sentence imitation subtest of the Test of Language Development–Primary (TOLD-2:P; Newcomer & Hammill, 1988) performed much poorer with regard to grammatical target acquisition in imitation-based intervention as compared with conversational recast intervention. In this case, there was a mean difference of 57.9 presentations and an estimated effect size of .83. This interaction between imitation ability and treatment type is intuitively appealing; children with SLI who at pretreatment were relatively poor imitators performed significantly more poorly when grammatical targets were taught using imitation treatment. It should be noted that relatively strong imitation skills were not associated with higher gains in imitation treatment. To summarize, there was an overall main effect favoring the use of recasts, and there was a significant interaction effect wherein low imitators performed particularly poorly in imitation treatment.

Finally, Proctor-Williams and colleagues (2001) directly examined the relationship between parents' use of recasts and later target use in children with SLI and compared this with children who were typically developing. They examined copula and article recast use by 10 parents of children with SLI and 10 parents of younger language-matched children in a nonintervention context. They then followed up with these same children and examined productions of these same forms at three points across an 8-month period. A strong positive relation was observed between the copula recasts used by parents of children with SLI at Time 1 and their children's use of copulas 8 months later. In contrast, however, the correlations between recasts of articles by parents and later production of articles by their children were not statistically significant. Most important, there were no apparent relationships between early parental recast rates and later child use of articles or copulas among the group of children with SLI. This finding seems to conflict with other reports that children with SLI respond well to recast interventions. Proctor-Williams et al. (2001) argued that children with SLI can benefit substantially from the grammar-facilitating properties of recasts, but only when the recasts are presented at rates that are much greater than those available in typical conversations with young children. This suggests that recasts available from parents in the ambient environment may not be sufficient for children with SLI to learn key grammatical structures so that a goal of intervention could be to increase these recasts by parents and/or teachers as well as by SLPs.

In addition, even in studies indicating a main effect for recast, there have been individual differences in outcomes. Camarata and Nelson (1992), for example, reported that specific grammatical targets may be better suited to recasts than others. For instance, passive structures, which are used in spontaneous language samples when the subject of the conversation is the object of an action in the sentence (e.g., "I was driving my truck yesterday. It was hit by another car"), may be illustrated in the conversational interaction used in recast interventions. In contrast, attributes, such as relative clauses, may be specifically illustrated and modeled within more structured interactions. In this vein, Fey and Loeb (2002) reported that recasts in the form of inverted yes/no questions did not facilitate acquisition of auxiliary forms in 16 children with SLI. In this latter case, the use of auxiliaries by these children was not different in the recast treatment as compared with a control group that participated in play sessions with an adult who did not recast the child's utterances.

Another factor that may influence the effects of recast intervention is the developmental language level of the children. Yoder and colleagues (1991) reported that the effects of a responsive interaction treatment in that study, which included systematic use of recasts, was significantly greater in children at higher MLU levels as compared with children at the one- and two-word level. At this lower developmental level, Yoder et al. reported that a treatment that included imitation was significantly greater than responsive interaction. Again, there is an intuitive appeal to this finding; early vocabulary (particularly nouns) and early two-word semantic relations can be quickly and efficiently trained using discrete trial methods. In contrast, generalized use of more sophisticated grammar may be better facilitated using recast procedures, which model complex grammar within an interactive, conversational context.

In the studies mentioned above, the outcome measures included tracking of specific language targets, including grammatical forms, lexical items, and early semantic relations. However, another method of testing treatment effects focuses on the results of standardized testing and/or broad language markers (e.g., MLU), which reflect goals Fey (1986) has described as intermediate or basic, rather than specific in scope (see Chapter 1). Yoder et al. (1995), for example, compared responsive interaction with milieu teaching in a total of 38 children who were included in classroom-based treatment. Rather than tracking individual targets, Yoder et al. included broad measures of language growth including MLU, scores on standardized tests, and measures of lexical density. No significant effects were reported for number of utterances per minute or for percentage of different words. They reported that both treatments were associated with significant growth in MLU, and in performance on the Sequenced Inventory of Communication Development (receptive and expressive; Hedrick, Prather, & Tobin, 1975), the Peabody Picture Vocabulary Test (Dunn & Dunn, 1981), and the Expressive One-Word Vocabulary Test (Gardner, 1990). After establishing significant growth in these parameters, Yoder et al. tested the interaction effect between treatment group and pretreatment language level predicting expressive and receptive language at the posttreatment period reported that milieu teaching facilitated expressive language and receptive vocabulary level better than responsive interaction for children who entered intervention with relatively poorer receptive and expressive language levels. In contrast, children with initially higher pretreatment expressive and receptive language levels made significantly larger gains in responsive interaction than in milieu language teaching. The effect sizes were in the low-to-moderate range (R^2 change for interaction effects of .06 to .18). Because both milieu teaching and responsive interaction include recasts as a part of the intervention procedure and, in the case of RI in this study, very extensive use of recasts, this can be viewed as evidence in support of the effects of recasting on broad measures of language.

Additional evidence parallels what could be occurring in the Yoder et al. (1995) study of milieu treatment. For example, Leonard and colleagues (2004) studied grammatical morpheme acquisition in the context of a treatment that included conversational recasts during semistructured interactions, but this treatment also included scripted stories that focused on the targeted grammatical morphemes. The results of this study indicated that the targeted grammatical morphemes increased significantly as compared with control forms, but this growth cannot be attributed exclusively to conversational recasts. Indeed, there is no way of knowing the specific contribution (if any) to the overall growth for this particular element in the intervention (see the arguments in Snow et al., 1996). There are a number of studies that include conversational recasts as a part of a broader intervention package. These include natural language paradigm for autism (Koegel et al., 1987, and see Koegel, Carter, & Koegel, 2003, for a review), parent-delivered and clinician-delivered enhanced milieu teaching (see Delaney & Kaiser, 2001; Chapter 9), and focused stimulation approaches that may even be delivered by parents (Fey et al., 1993; Chapter 8). Indeed, it appears that conversational recasts are a rather ubiquitous component of many intervention programs that have reported gains in speech (e.g., Yoder et al., 2005) and in language (e.g., Leonard et al., 2004).

In summary, there is extensive evidence that conversational recasts can facilitate language acquisition, and there are several studies (e.g., Camarata et al., 1994) indicating a relatively large effect. However, there are also studies that indicate that recasts may not be effective for certain language structures (e.g., relative clause; Camarata & Nelson, 1992) or for auxiliary verbs when taught using inverted yes/no recasts to children not yet using auxiliaries (Fey & Loeb, 2002). Furthermore, the relative effect can vary across developmental language levels (e.g., Yoder et al., 1991). Finally, many treatments include recasts as part of a broader intervention package. Although these studies can be viewed as providing indirect support for this approach (e.g., Leonard et al., 2004), the relative contribution of recasts to the overall gain is unknown in these studies.

PRACTICAL REQUIREMENTS

Because conversational recasts require a specific type of contingent response to the child's initiations, one-on-one or small-group settings are helpful, especially if recasts are designed to provide focus on specific forms. To date, most work on conversational recasts has included direct interactions between parents or clinicians and children. This treatment can be delivered in group settings and in classrooms. Of course, parent implementation is often completed in a home environment, and teachers, clinicians, and caregivers providing home visits (e.g., in early intervention programs) could also use recasts in home settings. If general responses to initiations are the focus of treatment (i.e., the recast approach is not target specific), then any social partner could be included in the intervention program. This could include parents, teachers, peers, and social workers. Training to these partners should be provided to ensure that they learn to apply developmentally appropriate recasts that are contingent on the child's utterances.

If target-specific recasts are used, as has been principally advocated in this chapter, additional expertise (and training) are needed. Goal selection requires careful consideration of the child's developmental language level, which requires expert knowledge of speech and language acquisition. Fey et al. (1993) and Gibbard (1994) trained parents to use approaches that included recasts of specific forms. Although this was done successfully, it required more than 10 parent education sessions as well as consistent monitoring and updating the list of goals. It is likely that an SLP will be needed to provide the requisite expertise in assessing speech and language.

KEY COMPONENTS

The key components of this intervention include 1) child initiation; 2) a parent, teacher, or clinician teaching response; and 3) a speech and/or language goal that is developmentally appropriate. These components are applied within an interactive context that is interesting and motivating for the child. This context could include playing with a favorite toy, taking part in a preferred activity, or reading an engaging storybook. The key here is *not* a specific package of materials (although any set of materials including prepackaged materials could be used); rather, the focus is on the recast process, which is a specific form of interaction between adult and child.

When these key components are delivered effectively, several additional key components are directly or indirectly also incorporated. The adult, in the case of specific linguistic targets (e.g., grammatical, phonological, lexical), provides a teaching response that can be processed by the child (Nelson, 1989, 2000). The simple term *process* takes in substantial cognitive territory. In Nelson's formulation (Nelson, 2001), this includes ensuring that the child's attention, motivation, and auditory system are sufficiently activated to compare the incorrect forms stored in long-term memory with the accurate forms the adult provides within recasts.

It should be noted, however, that these latter key components are typically brought into play in procedures of recast treatment. That is, when the clinician responds positively to a child initiation, the child's attention and motivation and emotional regulation are likely to be high as the clinician is engaging and the topic of interaction is presumably of interest to the child. If one adopts a limited set of targets for recasting, then multiple and redundant presentation of these forms in treatment could support auditory processing and facilitate short- and long-term storage of the forms. Thus, the focus of the intervention is squarely on transactional components. Although our current working hypothesis indicates that delivering recasts properly and frequently is sufficient so that special skills training is not required, it is an interesting and as yet unanswered question whether auditory processing or memory training could enhance recast effectiveness for certain children.

A final key component is the nature of the targets (goals) included in recasts. Much of our own work has argued for and provided data to support the notion of delivering a high frequency of target-specific recasts. Other researchers (e.g., Fey et al., 1993, 1997; Fey & Loeb, 2002) have also stressed the need for focus on specific targets. Alternatively, there is some evidence to suggest that broader recasting intervention procedures that provide structural recast variation but without the adult narrowing his or her focus to a small set of specific structures can also be effective for grammar (Nelson et al., 1996; and for language-typical children, Nelson, Carskaddon, & Bonvillian, 1973), for phonology (Smith & Camarata, 1999), and for speech intelligibility (Yoder et al., 2005).

ASSESSMENT METHODS TO SUPPORT ONGOING DECISION MAKING

Our own research (e.g., Camarata et al., 1994) and that of others (Fey & Loeb, 2002; Yoder et al., 2005) indicates that recast treatments will be effective for a majority of children and a majority of targets, but will not be effective for all targets in all children. This then raises the question of how one can determine whether the intervention is in fact effective. Camarata (1995) argues that no one clinical approach should be applied to all children or all targets. Rather, the clinical process is used to establish which levels of support are needed for the child to learn. Although it would be a tremendous boon to speech and language intervention if one magic bullet were available to treat all children with disabilities, the reality is that no such universal intervention is likely to be forthcoming. This applies to recast treatment as described herein. An assessment process must be included to determine who is learning and what is learned within this process. Therefore, an assessment process must be incorporated into the treatment.

Additionally, a clinician must decide whether to implement target-specific or broader, less target-specific recasts. If a clinician uses either target-specific or broadly targeted recasts, a representative language sample is needed, as is a careful analysis of that sample. For grammatical objectives, one could perform an Assigning Structural Stage type of analysis (Miller, 1981) or a Developmental Sentence Scoring analysis (Lee, 1974). Ongoing assessments also need to involve language sampling of some type. If a clinician opts instead for a broad, non–target-specific approach, a lack of growth in language sample or broad measures of language would warrant a switch to target-specific recast procedures.

At the first level, this assessment process should focus on the child outcomes. From a global level, this includes whether speech and language skills are advancing. This requires testing that is sensitive to the goals of intervention but must also be ecologically valid in terms of having an impact on the child's disorder. This question is further complicated by the fact that children with disabilities can make gains without specific intervention (e.g., see Nelson et al., 1996; Paul, 2000). Therefore, the assessment should first ensure that the targets are in fact being learned and if so, that this is diminishing the level of disability and handicap. Second, it is not sufficient to establish that growth is occurring, as this may be associated with simple maturation or with factors that are not related to the treatment. Although often challenging in clinical contexts, to address this issue some form of control could be introduced in the assessment process as well. For example, this could include monitoring untreated targets (as in Nelson et al., 1996), using single-case designs such as reversal designs or multiple baseline designs, or gathering accurate information on preintervention growth levels for comparison to growth rates within treatment. This latter step can be utilized when there is a time lag in the initial assessment and enrollment in treatment. A broad measure such as

MLU could be applied during the initial assessment and at the onset of treatment to estimate untreated growth. This rate of growth could then be compared over a similar time span following enrollment in treatment.

The information given in the previous paragraphs should be applied to any intervention, including those involving recasts. Assessment that is specific to recasting would include measuring the primary key components. This includes periodic sampling of child initiation rates and rate of clinician (or parent) recast of the child's forms (as in Nelson, 2000). In goal-specific recasting, this should also include assessment of whether the recasts actually deliver the intended target. Additionally, one could argue that because the fundamental purpose of goal-specific recast intervention to preschoolers is to increase use of the targeted forms, the evaluation process should include examining regular spontaneous speech and language samples to determine whether forms appearing in the treatment context are appearing elsewhere and are being used appropriately (see Nelson, 1989; Spradlin & Siegel, 1982). As mentioned previously, recasting is unlikely to be effective for all speech and language targets in all children. An assessment process *must* be included that allows the clinician to detect when the procedure is and *is not* working. If the procedure is not working, other levels of support should be applied and these, in turn, should be evaluated. If an alternative treatment is applied, it should be 1) monitored for effect and 2) selected from alternatives that offer a priori objective evidence to support use (e.g., discrete trials for some cases).

CONSIDERATIONS FOR CHILDREN FROM CULTURALLY AND LINGUISTICALLY DIVERSE BACKGROUNDS

Because the transactional model (Sameroff & Fiese, 1989), the RELM (rare event learning mechanism; Nelson, 1989), and rationales underlying recast intervention appear to have broad applicability across targets and across disability typologies (Nelson, 2001; Yoder & Warren, 1993), there do not appear to be any a priori limitations on the applicability of this method to culturally and linguistically diverse populations. Clearly, one should be cautious in goal specific recasting to ensure that the intervention targets are appropriate for the target population. This requires foreknowledge of the dialectal variations of a particular group (e.g., Washington, 1996; Washington & Craig, 2004).

As this chapter was written, the focus on cultural and linguistic diversity appears to have been primarily in the area of assessment and only recently has a standardized measure of dialectal variation become widely available (Seymour et al., 2003). Less is known regarding treatment of speech and language disorders in children from diverse backgrounds. Unkefer-Craig and Camarata (2004) have completed a preliminary study of recast intervention in four children with SLI from AAE dialectal backgrounds and a subset of the children in our previous intervention studies have been from culturally diverse backgrounds but were not studied specifically. Unkefer-Craig and Camarata found that recast intervention was associated with growth in targeted linguistic forms that were absent in baseline language samples but obligatory in AAE dialect; however, there is a clear need for additional study on this topic.

The current paucity of data should not prevent a clinician from employing the procedure with culturally and linguistically diverse groups and the assessment methods described above should be applied to evaluate whether the treatment is useful. Bear in mind that any intervention is child specific and should be applied and evaluated within this context. There is ample theoretical justification for applying conversational recast treatment to culturally and linguistically diverse populations, although the clinician must be educated with regard to appropriate goal selection for the target group.

APPLICATION TO AN INDIVIDUAL CHILD

One of the strengths of a conversational recast treatment is that the procedure is ultimately an individualized procedure, tailored to the child's interests and language level. As noted earlier, this is a procedure rather than a highly regimented program, and so it can have broad applicability in many different intervention approaches. Several case descriptions from our own clinic may be useful to illustrate this.

The first case is a fairly typical application and is selected to illustrate short-term goals and monitoring. This preschool boy (age 4;7) was identified as having mixed expressive-receptive language disorder (American Psychiatric Association, 1994) and met our criteria for SLI, including standard scores on the Test for Auditory Comprehension of Language–Third Edition (Carrow-Woolfolk, 1999) and on the PLS-3 below the 2nd percentile. Like many children with SLI, he used few grammatical morphemes and his MLU was significantly less than age-level expectations. A goal-specific recast procedure was employed. The targets were copula *is* (she *is* nice, he *is* little) and third person singular *–s* (she walk*s*). Untreated targets that were monitored included auxiliary *is* (she *is* running, he *is* walking) and possessive *'s* (mommy*'s* book).

Notice that the phonological form of the treated and untreated targets was similar so that any growth observed under treatment could not be attributable to ease of production. Also, notice that the goals emerge and are mastered at relatively similar points in development so that differences could not be attributed to developmental order (i.e., treating an "easy" target and monitoring a "hard" target). Treatment was provided twice per week for 4 months (0.5-hour sessions), and language samples were gathered prior to treatment in the clinic and at home. Monthly language samples were gathered during treatment and at home. We realize that many clinicians may not have the resources for home language sample collection, but the in-clinic sampling may be practical. In our clinic, we often have parents provide a video of home interaction, which can be used for language sample analysis. For this child, all targets were at 0% use before treatment. After 4 months, the targets increased strongly to 67% for copula and to 92% for third person singular. Note that for copula, we counted disagreement in tense and/or number as correct use (e.g., "We is nice" was counted as correct use for copula). The untreated forms occurred with substantially lower frequencies. Although the child did sometimes use *his* and *mine,* he did not use the bound possessive morpheme in any of the samples. The auxiliary *be,* like the copula, was counted correct if present, even if an error in tense and/or number was evident. Auxiliary usage increased weakly from 0% in the baseline home sample to 11% in the final home sample. This example illustrates progress on the specific goals being taught, but it does not address progress in broader language. In this case, the child's expressive scores increased on the PLS-3 (baseline expressive quotient of 68 to posttest quotient of 81). One must be cautious in assigning the global gain on the PLS to learning directly and indirectly associated with these particular goals, but there is evidence that the intervention was effective for this child.

The second case illustrates the application of speech-intelligibility recasts to a girl, age 5;3, with autism and phonological disorder. She presented with a diagnosis of pervasive developmental disorder-autism, which was associated with reduced frequency of spontaneous initiations. To further complicate the situation, when she did speak the words were difficult to understand. Although clinicians who were not part of our clinic had attempted picture use and sign language previously, this child did not use these latter forms outside of the treatment sessions. In addition to the pictures and the sign language, the previous treatment had also included traditional, imitation-based, sound-by-sound phonological treatment (discrete trials of articulation therapy). As with many children with autism, this child resisted imitative prompting, and her level of disruptive behavior during articulation training was very high so that this was discontinued. Recast intervention for phonology was then employed in our clinic.

In autism, a key component of the intervention is to determine when the child initiates, as this is much rarer than is the case for typically developing children. In our case, the child vocalized with some regularity when favorite toys were placed in a basket on a shelf behind the clinician. Therefore, a set of three toys was placed in the basket and changed across sessions. The toys were preselected to include reasonably diverse phonemic structure that the child could produce, even with her limited phonetic inventory. Because these were favored toys, the child would initiate using a vocalization that was distinguishable within the controlled therapy context. For example, one set of toys included a doll, a key, and a puppy, which were initially produced as [ba], [bi], and [baba], respectively. The treatment targets were [d], [k], and [p]. When the child attempted one of these words, the clinician provided a toy from the basket regardless of the accuracy of the child's attempt. In response to the child's vocalization, the clinician recast the word using the appropriate phonemes. The sessions were transcribed by a person unfamiliar with the child, and the order of the tapes was randomized prior to transcription to ensure that simply becoming more familiar with the child did not result in higher posttreatment production accuracy ratings. Treatment was provided twice per week for 30 minutes over 6 months, and a follow-up sample was obtained 2 months after treatment. The child's percentage accuracy for the targeted phonemes increased from 0% in baseline to more than 40% at posttest 8 months later. Control targets, including [t] and [g], increased much less, from 0% in baseline to 11% at the 8-month follow-up. This child would not cooperate well enough to permit standardized testing, but it appears that gains were associated, at least in part, with the recast intervention.

FUTURE DIRECTIONS

There are many future directions to be explored with recasts. An overarching direction would be to further refine the intervention so that the issues of goal selection (broad versus specific), goal domains (lexical, grammatical, phonological), and populations (cultural and linguistically diverse, disability typologies) would be better understood. At this time, the results are promising and the theoretical underpinnings are relatively broad. However, the limits of the intervention are not yet known, both in terms of specific child characteristics and in terms of effective clinical factors (dose, effective developmental level, settings).

In addition, the interface between cognitive factors such as cognitive level, processing speed, memory, auditory processing, and recast delivery have not been examined in detail—although recasting has generally proven effective without any specific accompanying procedures to improve children's skills in such domains. At an even more basic level, it is unclear whether recast interventions, which have been applied nearly exclusively to expressive goals, will be effective for receptive language goals as well. Similarly, there are few studies of whether intervention that is associated with growth in a reasonably diverse set of specific goals relates to growth in broader measures (but for exceptions, see Nelson, Craven, Xuan, Arkenberg, & Lauck, 2002, and Yoder et al., 2005). Given the theoretical underpinnings of these latter studies, it is not surprising that Camarata and Nelson have focused primarily on individual language target use in their analyses. An interesting question is whether broader, less target-specific forms of recasting will also prove effective. There has been some preliminary evidence to suggest that broader, less focused responses can lead to associated growth (e.g., Yoder et al., in press).

Another intriguing direction is the relationship between neural organization and speech and language growth. Camarata and Yoder (2002) argued that speech and language intervention provides a useful paradigm for studying several issues in this area, including neural plasticity and the relative contribution of receptive language ability to treatment response. Specifying individual traits that predict response to treatment is a related area of future study. For example, if a child has relatively strong receptive language, would this factor predict response to conversational recast intervention? Of all possible directions, it may be most important that strengths and the limitations of recast treatment are studied systematically relative to other high-profile interventions. This type of information is crucial to clinicians' application of evidence to the intervention process.

RECOMMENDED READINGS

Camarata, S. (1995). A rationale for naturalistic speech intelligibility intervention. In S.F. Warren & J. Reichle (Series Eds.) & M.E. Fey, J. Windsor, & S.F. Warren (Vol. Eds.), *Communication and language intervention series: Vol. 5. Language intervention: Preschool through the elementary years* (pp. 63–84). Baltimore: Paul H. Brookes Publishing Co.

Camarata, S., Nelson, K.E., & Camarata, M. (1994). A comparison of conversation based to imitation based procedures for training grammatical structures in specifically language impaired children. *Journal of Speech and Hearing Research, 37,* 1414–1423.

Nelson, K.E. (1989). Strategies for first language teaching. In M.L. Rice & R.L. Schiefelbusch (Eds.), *The teachability of language* (pp. 263–310). Baltimore: Paul H. Brookes Publishing Co.

Proctor-Williams, K., Fey, M., & Frome-Loeb, D. (2001). Parental recasts and production in copulas and articles by children with specific language impairment and typical language. *American Journal of Speech-Language Pathology, 10,* 155–168.

Yoder, P.J., & Warren, S.F. (1993). Can the prelinguistic intervention enhance the language development of children with developmental delays. In S.F. Warren & J. Reichle (Series Eds.) & A.P. Kaiser & D. Gray (Vol. Eds.), *Communication and language intervention series: Vol. 2. Enhancing children's communication: Research foundations for early language intervention* (pp. 35–62). Baltimore: Paul H. Brookes Publishing Co.

REFERENCES

American Psychiatric Association. (1994). *Diagnostic and statistical manual of mental disorders* (4th ed.). Washington, DC: Author.

Baker, N.D., & Nelson, K.E. (1984). Recasting and related conversational techniques for triggering syntactic advances by young children. *First Language, 5,* 3–22.

Brown, R. (1973). *A first language: The early stages.* Cambridge, MA: Harvard University Press.

Cacace, A., & McFarland, D. (1998). Central auditory processing disorder in school-aged children: A critical review. *Journal of Speech, Language, and Hearing Research, 41,* 355–373.

Camarata, S. (1993). The application of naturalistic conversation training to speech production in children with speech disabilities. *Journal of Applied Behavior Analysis, 26,* 173–182.

Camarata, S. (1995). A rationale for naturalistic speech intelligibility intervention. In S.F. Warren & J. Reichle (Series Eds.) & M.E. Fey, J. Windsor, & S.F. Warren (Vol. Eds.), *Communication and language intervention series: Vol. 5. Language intervention: Preschool through the elementary years* (pp. 63–84). Baltimore: Paul H. Brookes Publishing Co.

Camarata, S. (1996). On the importance of integrating naturalistic language, social intervention, and speech-intelligibility training. In L. Koegel, R. Koegel, & G. Dunlap (Eds.), *Positive behavior support* (pp. 333–351). Baltimore: Paul H. Brookes Publishing Co.

Camarata, S. (2001). *Clinical update: Phonological disorders in children.* Paper presented at the annual developmental disabilities clinical update series, Johns Hopkins University, Baltimore.

Camarata, S., & Nelson, K. (1992). Treatment efficiency as a function of target selection in the remediation of child language. *Clinical Linguistics and Phonetics, 6,* 167–178.

Camarata, S., Nelson, K.E., & Camarata, M. (1994). A comparison of conversation based to imitation based procedures for training grammatical structures in specifically language impaired children. *Journal of Speech and Hearing Research, 37,* 1414–1423.

Camarata, S., & Yoder, P. (2002). Language transactions during development and intervention: Theoretical implications for developmental neuroscience. *International Journal of Developmental Neuroscience, 20*(3–5), 459–465.

Carrow-Woolfolk, E. (1999). *Test for Auditory Comprehension of Language–Third Edition (TACL-3).* Austin, TX: PRO-ED.

Chomsky, N. (1965). *Aspects of a theory of syntax.* Cambridge, MA: The MIT Press.

Chomsky, N. (1975). *Reflections on language.* New York: Pantheon.

Cohen, C., Hodson, A., O'Hare, A., Boyle, J., Durrani, T., McCartney, E., Mattey, M., Naftalin, L., & Watson, J. (in press). Effects of computer-based intervention using acoustically modified speech (Fast ForWord-Language®) in severe mixed receptive-expressive language impairment: Outcomes from a randomized controlled trial. *Journal of Speech, Language, and Hearing Research.*

Conti-Ramsden, G. (1990). Maternal recasts and other contingent replies to language-impaired children. *Journal of Speech and Hearing Disorders, 55,* 262–274.

Delaney, E., & Kaiser, A. (2001). The effects of teaching parents blended communication and behavior support strategies. *Behavioral Disorders, 26,* 93–116.

Dunn, L.M., & Dunn, L.M. (1981). *Peabody Picture Vocabulary Test–Revised.* Circle Pines, MN: American Guidance Service.

Fey, M.E. (1986). *Language intervention with young children.* Austin, TX: PRO-ED.

Fey, M.E., Cleave, P., & Long, S. (1997). Two models of grammar facilitation in children with language impairments: Phase 2. *Journal of Speech and Hearing Research, 40,* 5–19.

Fey, M.E., Cleave, P., Long, S., & Hughes, D. (1993). Two approaches to the facilitation of grammar in children with language impairment: An experimental evaluation. *Journal of Speech and Hearing Research, 36,* 141–157.

Fey, M.E., & Loeb, D. (2002). An evaluation of the facilitative effects of inverted yes-no questions on the acquisition of auxiliary verbs. *Journal of Speech, Language, and Hearing Research, 45,* 160–174.

Fuchs, D. (1979). Reading and perceptual-motor performance: Can we strengthen them simultaneously? *Journal of Special Education, 13,* 265–273.

Gardner, M. (1990). *Expressive One-Word Vocabulary Test.* Novato, CA: Academic Therapy Publications.

Gibbard, D. (1994). Parental-based intervention with pre-school language-delayed children. *European Journal of Disorders of Communication, 29,* 131–150.

Gillum, H., Camarata, S., Nelson, K.E., & Camarata, M. (2003). Pre-intervention imitation skills as a predictor of treatment effects in children with specific language impairment. *Journal of Positive Behavior Intervention, 5*(3), 171–178.

Hart, B., & Risley, T. (1968). Establishing use of descriptive adjectives in the spontaneous speech of disadvantaged preschool children. *Journal of Applied Behavior Analysis, 1,* 109–120.

Hart, B., & Risley, T. (1974). Using preschool materials to modify the language of disadvantaged children. *Journal of Applied Behavior Analysis, 7,* 243–256.

Hart, B., & Risley, T. (1995). *Meaningful differences in the everyday experience of young American children.* Baltimore: Paul H. Brookes Publishing Co.

Hart, B., & Rogers-Warren, A. (1978). A milieu approach to teaching language. In R.L. Schiefelbusch (Ed.), *Language intervention strategies* (pp. 193–235). Baltimore: University Park Press.

Hedrick, D.L., Prather, E.M., & Tobin, A.R. (1975). *Sequenced Inventory of Communication Development.* Seattle: University of Washington Press.

Heimann, M., Nelson, K.E., Tjus, T., & Gillberg C. (1995). Increasing reading and communication skills in children with autism through an interactive multimedia computer program. *Journal of Autism and Developmental Disorders, 25,* 459–480.

Kaiser, A. (1993). Enhancing children's social communication. In S.F. Warren & J. Reichle (Series Eds.) & A.P. Kaiser & D. Gray (Vol. Eds.), *Communication and language intervention series: Vol. 2. Enhancing children's communication: Research foundations for early language intervention* (pp. 3–10). Baltimore: Paul H. Brookes Publishing Co.

Kaiser, A.P., Yoder, P.J., & Keetz, A.L. (1992). Evaluating milieu teaching. In S.F. Warren & J. Reichle (Series & Vol. Eds.), *Communication and language intervention series: Vol. 1. Causes and effects in communication and language intervention* (pp. 9–47). Baltimore: Paul H. Brookes Publishing Co.

Koegel, L., Carter, C., & Koegel, R. (2003). Teaching children with autism self-initiations as a pivotal response. *Topics in Language Disorders, 23,* 134–145.

Koegel, R., & Koegel, L. (1995). *Teaching children with autism.* Baltimore: Paul H. Brookes Publishing Co.

Koegel, R., Koegel, L., & Brookman, L. (2003). Empirically supported pivotal response interventions for children with autism. In A. Kazdin (Ed.), *Evidence-based psychotherapies for children and adolescents* (pp. 341–357). New York: Guilford Press.

Koegel, R.L., O'Dell, M.C., & Koegel, L.K. (1987). A natural language paradigm for teaching non-verbal autistic children. *Journal of Autism and Developmental Disorders, 17,* 187–199.

Lee, L. (1974). *Developmental sentence analysis.* Evanston, IL: Northwestern University Press.

Leonard, L., Camarata, S., Brown, B., & Camarata, M. (2004). Tense and agreement in the speech of children with specific language impairment. *Journal of Speech, Language, and Hearing Research, 47,* 1363–1379.

Miller, J. (1981). *Assessing language production in children.* Austin, TX: PRO-ED.

Moerk, E. (1992). *A first language taught and learned.* Baltimore: Paul H. Brookes Publishing Co.

Molfese, D.L., & Molfese, V.J. (2000). The continuum of language development during infancy and early childhood: Electrophysiological correlates. In C. Rovee-Collier, L.P. Lipsitt, & H. Hayne (Eds.), *Progress in infancy research, Vol. 1* (pp. 251–287). Mahwah, NJ: Lawrence Erlbaum Associates.

Nelson, K.E. (1977). Facilitating children's syntax acquisition. *Developmental Psychology, 13,* 101–107.

Nelson, K.E. (1980). Theories of the child's acquisition of syntax: A look at rare events and at necessary, catalytic, and irrelevant components of mother-child conversation. *Annals of the New York Academy of Sciences, 345,* 45–67.

Nelson, K.E. (1981). Toward a rare-event cognitive comparison theory of syntax acquisition. In P.S. Dale & D. Ingram (Eds.), *Child language: An international perspective* (pp. 229–240). Baltimore: University Park Press.

Nelson, K.E. (1987). Some observations from the perspective of the rare event cognitive comparison theory of language acquisition. In K.E. Nelson & A. van Kleeck (Eds.), *Children's language: Vol. 6* (pp. 289–331). Hillsdale, NJ: Lawrence Erlbaum Associates.

Nelson, K.E. (1989). Strategies for first language teaching. In M.L. Rice & R.L. Schiefelbusch (Eds.), *The teachability of language* (pp. 263–310). Baltimore: Paul H. Brookes Publishing Co.

Nelson, K.E. (2000). Methods for stimulating and measuring lexical and syntactic advances: Why Fiffins and lobsters can tag along with other recast friends. In L. Menn & N.B. Ratner (Eds.), *Methods for studying language production* (pp. 115–148). Hillsdale, NJ: Lawrence Erlbaum Associates.

Nelson, K.E. (2001). Dynamic tricky mix theory suggests multiple analyzed pathways (MAPS) as an intervention approach for children with autism and other language delays. In S. von Tetzchner & J. Clibbens (Eds.), *Understanding the theoretical and methodological bases of augmentative and alternative communication* (pp. 141–159). Toronto: ISAAC Press.

Nelson, K.E., Baker, N.A., Denninger, M., Bonvillian, J., & Kaplan, B. (1985). Cookie versus do-it-again: Imitative-referential and personal-social-syntactic-initiating language styles in young children. *Linguistics, 23,* 433–454.

Nelson, K., & Camarata, S. (1998). Improving English literacy and speech acquisition learning conditions for children with severe to profound hearing impairments. *Volta Review, 98,* 17–41.

Nelson, K.E., Camarata, S.M., Welsh, J., Butkovsky, L., & Camarata, M. (1996). Effects of imitative and conversational recasting treatment on the acquisition of grammar in children with specific language impairment and younger language-normal children. *Journal of Speech and Hearing Research, 39,* 850–859.

Nelson, K.E., Carskaddon, G., & Bonvillian, J. (1973). Syntax acquisition: Impact of experimental variation in adult verbal interaction with the child. *Child Development, 44,* 497–504.

Nelson, K.E., Craven, P.L., Xuan, Y., Arkenberg, M.E., & Lauck, G. (2002, July). *Acquisition of passive sentence structures by children during intervention and under naturalistic conditions.* Paper presented at the joint conference of the International Association for the Study of Child Language and the Symposium on Child Language Disorders. Madison, WI.

Nelson, K.E., Heimann, M., & Tjus, T. (1997). Theoretical and applied insights from multimedia facilitation of communication skills in children with autism, deaf children, and children with motor or learning disabilities. In L.B. Adamson & M.A. Romski (Eds.), *Research on communication and language disorders: Contributions to theories of language development* (pp. 296–325). Baltimore: Paul H. Brookes Publishing Co.

Neville, H., & Mills, D. (1997). Epigenesis of language. *Mental Retardation and Developmental Disabilities Research Reviews, 3,* 282–292.

Newcomer, P., & Hammill, D. (1988). *Test of Language Development-2: Primary.* Austin, TX: PRO-ED.

Ohde, R.N., & Camarata, S.M. (2004, June). *Cue weighting of static and dynamic vowel properties by adults and children with normal language and specific language impairment.* Paper presented at the conference "From Sound to Sense: Fifty + Years of Discoveries in Speech Communication." MIT, Cambridge, MA.

Ohde, R.N., & Haley, K.L. (1997). Stop consonant and vowel perception in 3- and 4-year-old children. *Journal of the Acoustical Society of America, 102,* 3711–3722.

Paul, R. (2000). Predicting outcomes of early expressive language delay: Ethical implications. In L.B. Leonard & D.V.M. Bishop (Eds.), *Speech and language impairments in children: Causes, characteristics, intervention and outcome* (pp. 195–209). Philadelphia: Psychology Press.

Pinker, S. (1994). *The language instinct.* New York: William Morrow & Co.

Pinker, S. (1999). *Words and rules: The ingredients of language.* New York: Basic Books.

Prinz, P.M., & Masin, L. (1985). Lending a helping hand: Linguistic input and sign language acquisition. *Applied Psycholinguistics, 6,* 357–370.

Prinz, P., & Nelson, K.E. (1985). Alligator eats cookie: Acquisition of writing and reading skills by deaf children using the microcomputer. *Applied Psycholinguistics, 6,* 283–306.

Proctor-Williams, K., Fey, M., & Loeb, D. (2001). Parental recasts and production in copulas and articles by children with specific language impairment and typical language. *American Journal of Speech-Language Pathology, 10,* 155–168.

Sameroff, A., & Fiese, B. (1989). Transactional regulation and early intervention. In S.J. Meisels & J. Shonkoff (Eds.), *Early intervention: A handbook of theory, practice, and analysis* (pp. 119–149). Cambridge, MA: Cambridge University Press.

Sedey, A., Rosin, M., & Miller, J. (1991, November). *A survey of sign use among children with Down syndrome.* Paper presented at the annual conference of the American Speech-Language-Hearing Association, Atlanta.

Shatz, M. (1983). On transition, continuity, and coupling: An alternative approach to communicative development. In R. Golinkoff (Ed.), *The transition from prelinguistic to linguistic communication* (pp. 43–55). Hillsdale, NJ: Lawrence Erlbaum Associates.

Smith, A., & Camarata, S. (1999). Increasing language intelligibility of children with autism within regular classroom settings using teacher implemented instruction. *Journal of Positive Behavior Intervention, 1,* 141–151.

Snow, C., Perlmann, R., & Nathan, D. (1987). Why routines are different. In K.E. Nelson & A. van Kleeck (Eds.), *Children's language: Vol. 6* (pp. 65–97). Hillsdale, NJ: Lawrence Erlbaum Associates.

Snow, D., Swisher, L., McNamara, M., & Kiernan, B. (1996). A potential limitation of treatment efficacy research: A comment on Camarata, Nelson, and Camarata (1994). *Journal of Speech and Hearing Research, 39,* 221–222.

Spradlin, J., & Siegel, G. (1982). Language training in natural and clinical environments. *Journal of Speech and Hearing Disorders, 47,* 2–6.

Tallal, P., Miller, S., Jenkins, W., & Merzenich, M. (1997). The role of temporal processing in developmental language-based learning disorders: Research and clinical implications. In B. Blachman (Ed.), *Foundations of reading acquisition and dyslexia: Implications for early intervention* (pp. 49–66). Mahwah, NJ: Lawrence Erlbaum Associates.

Washington, J. (1996). Issues in assessing the language abilities of African American children. In K.E. Pollock & A.G. Kamhi (Eds.), *Communication development and disorders in African American children: Research, assessment, and intervention* (pp. 35–54). Baltimore: Paul H. Brookes Publishing Co.

Washington, J., & Craig, H. (2004). A language screening protocol for use with young African American children in urban settings. *American Journal of Speech-Language Pathology, 13,* 329–340.

Warren, S., & Kaiser, A. (1986). Generalization of treatment effects by young language-delayed children: A longitudinal analysis. *Journal of Speech and Hearing Disorders, 51,* 291–299.

Yoder, P., Camarata, S., & Gardner, E. (in press). Treatment effects and predictors of speech intelligibility and length of utterance in children with specific language and intelligibility impairments. *Journal of Early Intervention.*

Yoder, P., Kaiser, A., & Alpert, C. (1991). An exploratory study of the interaction between language teaching methods and child characteristics. *Journal of Speech and Hearing Research, 34,* 155–167.

Yoder, P.J., Kaiser, A.P., Goldstein, H., Alpert, C., Mousetis, L., Kaczmarek, L., & Fischer, R. (1995). An exploratory comparison of milieu teaching and responsive interaction in the classroom. *Journal of Early Intervention, 19,* 218–242.

Yoder, P.J., & Molfese, D. (2002). *ERP correlates of behavioral predictors of response to BTR treatment.* Unpublished data, Vanderbilt University.

Yoder, P.J., & Warren, S.F. (1993). Can the prelinguistic intervention enhance the language development of children with developmental delays. In S.F. Warren & J. Reichle

(Series Eds.) & A.P. Kaiser & D. Gray (Vol. Eds.), *Communication and language intervention series: Vol. 2. Enhancing children's communication: Research foundations for early language intervention* (pp. 35–62). Baltimore: Paul H. Brookes Publishing Co.

Yoder, P.J., & Warren, S.F. (1998). Maternal responsivity predicts the prelinguistic communication intervention that facilitates generalized intentional communication. *Journal of Speech, Language, and Hearing Research, 41*(5), 1207–1219.

Yoder, P.J., & Warren, S.F. (2001a). Intentional communication elicits language-facilitating maternal responses in dyads with children who have developmental disabilities. *American Journal on Mental Retardation, 106*(4), 327–335.

Yoder, P.J., & Warren, S.F. (2001b). Relative treatment effects of two prelinguistic communication interventions on language development in toddlers with developmental delays vary by maternal characteristics. *Journal of Speech, Language, and Hearing Research, 44*(1), 224–237.

II

Interventions Targeting More Advanced Language and Literacy

11

Overview of Section II

Interventions Targeting More
Advanced Language and Literacy

REBECCA J. MCCAULEY AND MARC E. FEY

As authors in preceding sections have made clear and as many readers know firsthand, young children with language disorders usually experience considerable growth in their oral language skills through maturation and, it is hoped, effective early treatment. Despite these gains, however, they frequently go on to manifest additional and sometimes more persistent problems once confronted with the demands of learning to read and write. In fact, possibly one of the most replicated findings in research on language disorders in children is the substantial increase in risk such children face for difficulties in written language (Catts, Fey, Zhang, & Tomblin, 2001; Catts & Kamhi, 1999).

The chapters in this section introduce readers to four quite varied approaches to helping children with language impairments address their ongoing and changing needs in oral language as well as their emerging needs in literacy. Although most of the interventions share roots in methods designed for use with children without known impairments, considerable variability in the intent and focus across treatments is evident. The approaches vary from an intervention with the basic goal of preventing later literacy problems among children with identified communication disorders (Phonological Awareness Intervention, Chapter 12) to one aimed at skill enhancement not only in older children with language disorders, but their typically developing classmates as well (The Writing Lab Approach for Building Language, Literacy, and Communication Skills, Chapter 15). Targeted clients range from preschoolers to adults, with several strategies seen as applicable to persons of any age who demonstrate poorer literacy skills (Balanced Reading Intervention and Assessment in AAC, Chapter 13; Visual Strategies to Facilitate Written Language Development, Chapter 14; The Writing Lab Approach, Chapter 15). The use of technology was relatively modest in three of the approaches (Phonological Awareness Intervention, Chapter 12; Balanced Reading Intervention in AAC, Chapter 13; Visual Strategies, Chapter 14) yet extensive in the fourth

(The Writing Lab Approach, Chapter 15). Table 11.1 summarizes structural and content-related characteristics such as these for the four approaches described in this section. Although these characteristics are of practical and theoretical importance in the selection of a treatment approach, other equally and, in fact, several *more* important characteristics require greater elaboration, leading us to include the brief summaries of each intervention. We close our consideration of each approach on an evaluative note, with a brief discussion of its strengths, weaknesses, and future research needs.

PHONOLOGICAL AWARENESS INTERVENTION (CHAPTER 12)

In Chapter 12, Gillon describes a preventive framework for preschool children with specific communication problems. That framework might be characterized as targeting tertiary prevention efforts, in that efforts are made to limit the functional impact of children's earlier communication problems in the form of later deficits in reading, spelling, and writing. The term *tertiary prevention* contrasts with *primary prevention* in which efforts are made to reduce risk factors leading to initial diagnosis of communication disorders (e.g., neglect, prematurity), as well as with *secondary prevention* in which efforts focus on reducing the impact of the initial diagnosis (e.g., reduced communicative effectiveness, impaired comprehension; Dalton, Elias, & Wandersman, 2001). Although it is well established that children with early speech and/or language impairments are at risk for literacy deficits (e.g., Bird, Bishop, & Freeman, 1995; Larrivee & Catts, 1999; Lewis, Freebairn, Hansen, Iyengar, & Taylor, 2004), Gillon's work in this chapter and in a recent book (Gillon, 2004) is innovative because it applies methods developed for general population of school-age children as well as older children with *known* deficits in literacy and/or phonological awareness to this subgroup of at-risk children who are underrepresented in this area of treatment research.

Gillon selected and adapted the intervention goals and procedures she describes in Chapter 12 because they had emerged as best practice for the populations of older, impaired, and typically developing children used in the majority of previous studies of phonological interventions (Ehri et al., 2001). Specifically, her primary intermediate goal is to facilitate phonological awareness for phonemes (rather than for syllable or onset-rime awareness), using activities that involve subordinate intermediate goals of phoneme categorization and identification as well as matching and blending of phonemes and segmentation for short, familiar words. Knowledge of names of letters and sounds associated with individual letters is also targeted. The intervention is implemented within relatively intensive individual or small-group sessions. Chapter 12 offers guidance for developing intermediate and specific phonological awareness goals both as separate treatment goals and as goals that are embedded within other, preexisting speech and language goals that may be relevant for particular children. Assessment methods are designed to de-

Table 11.1. Characteristics of interventions featured in Section II

Treatment	Phonological awareness intervention	Balanced reading intervention and assessment in augmentative communication	Visual strategies to facilitate written language development abilities	The writing lab approach for building language, literacy, and communication
Chapter	12	13	14	15
Client age (chronological or developmental)	3–4 years old	Variable	School-age children	School-age children
Primary client populations	Children with specific speech or language impairments	Children with severe speech and physical impairments	Children identified as poor readers, including children with attention-deficit/hyperactivity disorder and with autism spectrum disorder	Children whose language and literacy learning difficulties have a negative impact on academic achievement and social interaction, including those who do not qualify for special services
General characterization of methods	Phonological awareness activities	Adaptation of a conventional reading approach for use with augmentative and alternative communication	Visual instruction strategies	Inclusive, computer-supported, classroom-based methods
Nature of goals	Prevention of written language difficulties in children who are at increased risk	Fostering of student learning of concepts about print, the alphabetic principle, phonological awareness, and oral language	Improvement of word recognition and comprehension in reading	Enhancement of complexity and appropriateness of oral and written communications as well as social interaction and self-regulation
Intervention agents	Speech-language pathologists (SLPs) working in collaboration with parents, preschool teachers, or child care workers	SLPs and reading specialists for areas of challenge; as well as parents, paraprofessionals, volunteers, and peers for areas of strength	SLPs	SLPs working in collaboration with general and special education teachers
Nature of sessions	Individuals and small groups	Individuals and small groups	Individual, small-group, and classroom activities	Classroom based
Demands for technology	Some use of computers	Use of the Internet and simple technologies	No computer use	Extensive computer use

scribe and track a child's level of phonological awareness during intervention and are expressly not diagnostic in nature because of the acknowledged inappropriateness of diagnosis of such difficulties in children ages 3–4 for whom wide variability in performance and exposure to text is the norm.

The empirical or research base for this intervention for children with speech and/or language disorders is largely indirect in the sense that it consists primarily of evidence regarding similar interventions studied for their effectiveness with related, but distinct, populations of children (e.g., children with identified reading and spelling problems and normally developing children exposed to the demands of learning an alphabetic system of written language; see Blachman, Ball, Black, & Tangel, 1994; Torgesen et al., 1999). Gillon offers more direct support in her discussion of several studies showing positive treatment effects for similar interventions when used with young children who demonstrate speech sound system disorders (e.g., Gillon, 2000, 2002, 2003), speech and/or language problems (van Kleeck, Gillam, & McFadden, 1998), as well as expressive and receptive language disorders (e.g., Korkman & Peltomma, 1993; van Kleeck, Gillam, & McFadden, 1998; Warrick, Rubin, & Rowe-Walsh, 1993)—groups included among the intended recipients of the present intervention. Although the practical significance of the observed treatment effects is somewhat difficult to gauge because of the absence of effect size information, these more direct reports include some attention to the persistence of effects (e.g., Gillon, 2002) and the examination of outcome measures related to reading and spelling. Indeed, we would join the author in describing the studies she reviews as providing "early evidence supporting the use of phonological awareness interventions for children with communication problems." (p. 289).

BALANCED READING INTERVENTION AND ASSESSMENT IN AUGMENTATIVE COMMUNICATION (CHAPTER 13)

This adaptation of an existing reading approach, the whole-to-part model of silent reading comprehension (Cunningham, 1993), was undertaken to meet the widely varying needs of a subgroup of individuals with developmental disabilities, namely those who use augmentative and/or alternative communication (AAC) to mitigate the obstacles to the acquisition of reading skills for children with severe speech and physical impairments (SSPIs). The balanced reading intervention described in this chapter was developed by Erickson, Koppenhaver, and Cunningham to improve outcomes for this population by combining several separate methods of reading instruction (e.g., reading comprehension as well as phonics and sight-word instruction) and allowing both teacher and learner to make choices that affect the specifics of instruction. Of additional importance to the authors' attribution of balance to their intervention is the attention it gives to what they term *whole-text print processes,* including some processes that appear to present special problems to individuals with severe speech and physical impairments. These include specific goals of developing eye movement strategies for tracking text, use of inner speech to support memory processes needed to process text, moving directly from print to meaning without an intervening use of sound information, reading with intonation as a support for meaning, and the integration of the numerous strategies normally used to access meaning during the reading process. Two additional assumptions behind the adaptation of the whole-to-part model for this population are that 1) although skills underlying literacy are likely to be the same for all readers, methods of instruction and modes of communication must be responsive to individual needs; and 2) past and present participation and access barriers to print-oriented experiences will require special efforts by the child's educational team.

Because the balanced reading intervention has as its primary basic goal beginning reading skills, including spelling, rather than emergent literacy, the authors suggest that it be used with individuals who are at least school-age. They advocate that the level of personnel involved and amount of time spent in focusing on specific skills reflect the severity of the deficit in the area. Thus, more highly trained or experienced individuals and more time are devoted to skills that are identified in assessment as posing greater barriers to the learner's more advanced performance in reading. Time spent in actual reading of connected text is stressed both because it has been shown to be associated with increases in reading skill among children without SSPIs and because it represents a particularly vulnerable requirement for children with SSPIs who use AAC.

Skill areas receiving the greatest attention in the balanced reading intervention are word identification, language or reading comprehension, and whole-text print processing. Within each skill area, the authors provide detailed descriptions of how to adapt methods developed for individuals who do not use AAC for children with SSPIs. For example, in a pre-reading activity meant to facilitate reading comprehension by exploring and building background knowledge, use of past personal experiences is facilitated for people who use AAC if a chronological organization has been implemented on their communication devices to store information for later use. Similarly, in a discussion of procedures related to the classroom "word wall," the authors describe how students using AAC can be helped to learn spelling by focusing on two procedures. These include subvocalizing needed words once they identify them on the display and then using a pencil or alphabet display to more actively indicate their spelling attempt. As these examples are intended to illustrate, throughout this chapter the authors wed established reading instruction procedures to the special demands placed on people who use AAC by their longer response access and preparation times and, frequently, by their unavoidable need to use writing or gesture to gain knowledge about reading and writing.

Most of the evidence provided by the authors in support of the balanced reading intervention involves studies of children without obvious learning and communication problems. In fact, direct evidence is restricted to three case studies (Blischak, 1995; Erickson, Koppenhaver, Yoder, & Nance, 1997; Gipe, Duffy, & Richards, 1993), of which only the Erickson et al. study specifically cited use of the whole-to-part model. The other two studies included elements consistent with this approach, however. Because of the paucity of direct evidence, readers' acceptance of this strategy depends on their acceptance of the theoretical argument that children with SSPIs need to master essentially the same skills as those being addressed in well-studied programs of reading instruction, with accommodations made to address their special difficulties in access and output.

VISUAL STRATEGIES TO FACILITATE
WRITTEN LANGUAGE DEVELOPMENT (CHAPTER 14)

This intervention focuses on procedures that make use of visual information to address the basic literacy learning goals of children who experience delays in oral language and/or the language processing skills, some of whom may be described as *visual learners*. The authors, Hoffman and Norris, note that children with autism spectrum disorders or attention-deficit/hyperactivity disorder may be somewhat more likely to be visual learners than children with language disorders with different etiologies. However, they also suggest that children who are failing to learn to read after some exposure may benefit from visual strategies, even in the absence of a visual learning style or evidence of language disorder. The visual strategies, or tools, developed by Hoffman and Norris are designed for use with individual children or small groups, or within classroom literacy activities.

In addition to its assumption that visual learning styles may contribute to language and literacy challenges for a significant number of children, the theoretical basis for the visual strategies approach is a theory of the verbal processes required in reading and language (Norris, 1998; Norris & Hoffman, 2002) that assumes simultaneous and interactive processing such as that characterized in connectionist models (e.g., Rumelhart & McClelland, 1986). Within this theory, nine specific processors are postulated as generating different types of mental representations and are used by the authors to explain both normal and disordered patterns of reading. These processors consist of a perceptual processor, a phonemic processor, a categorical processor, a canonical processor, a referential processor, a denotative processor, a connotative processor, a macrostructure processor, and a prior knowledge processor. The authors propose that children who have difficulty in single-word reading and sounding out words can be seen as having difficulties affecting processors that contribute to decoding, whereas children who have difficulties in reading connected text are thought to have difficulties with processors that contribute to comprehension.

The visual tools proposed by Hoffman and Norris can be categorized into those that address these two major sorts of basic difficulties: single-word reading (or decoding) and reading comprehension. In particular, the visually based procedures addressing single-word reading skills are Phonic Faces (Norris, 2002) and iconic words. Phonic Faces map visual features signifying *how* a sound is produced to provide phoneme knowledge as an overlay on the letter that is used to indicate an associated grapheme. Thus, for example, the Phonic Face for the letter *b* includes a drawing indicating a lower lip on the bottom of the grapheme to signal the labial place of articulation. These faces become more complex as the child begins to read digraphs and vowels; that is, graphemes with many associated sounds and sounds with many associated graphemes. Iconic words consist of words that are likely to appear as sight vocabulary which are overlaid with drawings meant to cue the meaning of the word. For example, pupils are drawn into the centers of the letter *o* in the word *look* to make its meaning more transparent. With more abstract words, explanations supplement the visual images.

The visually based procedures that Hoffman and Norris propose to address comprehension of connected text specifically provide visual support for the processing of figurative language, complex sentences, punctuation, and discourse structures. *Picture stories* are used to illustrate events within a sentence so that the child can understand the phrase and clause structures underlying longer sentences and problem punctuation is introduced within picture stories then applied to written texts. *Storyboards* are used to illustrate story structure elements.

Initial assessments used for this approach focus first on reading, with efforts to identify sources of reading difficulty in decoding versus comprehension, then on possible indications that the child is a visual learner (e.g., better nonverbal intelligence scores than reading test scores). Ongoing assessment consists of weekly probes in which the child is asked to read text that is similar to the level of difficulty of texts being used in treatment. Measures include reading time to track fluency of reading, number of miscues to track decoding accuracy, and comprehension questions to track understanding of what is being read.

As with the authors of the balanced reading intervention, the authors of this approach make no claims of efficacy evidence; rather, they appeal to readers on theoretical grounds. The theoretical components they describe are built on empirical studies of children who are developing written language skills normally and, to a far lesser extent, of children with oral and written language impairments whose visual learner status is unknown. Thus, as with other approaches within this volume, the authors suggest that readers consider implementing it in the cautious manner they outline, with several methods of examining progress used to guide decision making. In addition, they offer a very strong appeal to researchers whose efforts can provide the firmer empirical bases for its more widespread use.

THE WRITING LAB APPROACH FOR BUILDING LANGUAGE, LITERACY, AND COMMUNICATION SKILLS (CHAPTER 15)

Of the four approaches included in this section, the approach of Nelson and Van Meter reaches widest in terms of its intended populations and settings; it is proposed for use with children with identified problems in language learning and literacy, for their classmates who are without formally identified problems but who may present some concerns to their teachers, and for their classmates who are developing reading and writing skills typically. Put more eloquently, it is "designed to integrate language *intervention* for students with disabilities into writing process *instruction* for all students" (p. 383). The use of revision and ongoing attention to audience and purpose during the writing process—frequent characteristics of writing instruction for individuals without known deficits (Hayes & Flower, 1980)—are applied as an alternative to a traditional emphasis on word- and phrase-level exercises. In addition to a focus on improvements in the writing process as a central basic goal of the Writing Lab Approach, Nelson and Van Meter cite two additional procedural components they consider vital to this approach: the use of computer supports (e.g., graphic organizers and outliners, word prediction programs, and acoustic feedback to facilitate revisions), and inclusive instruction processes that ensure that writing tasks address authentic, curriculum-based assignments.

The suggested intervention context for this approach is a writing lab in which both general and special education teachers collaborate with speech-language pathologists to integrate written and spoken language goals within the context of curriculum-based writing projects. Children work alone or in small groups while the speech-language pathologist functions as an active participant in the classroom. Theoretically, this approach is based on a cognitive-neurolinguistic model of language learning disabilities and a social-constructionist theory of how children learn. From these foundations, the authors propose that children's challenges in literacy are best addressed through the provision of gradually diminishing supports for speaking and writing tasks undertaken within meaningful social contexts. The use of such scaffolding in conjunction with the use of highly meaningful tasks is seen as both helping children form connections between various brain regions involved in word pronunciation, word meaning, pattern recognition, and discourse and pragmatic skills, as well as helping them develop improved self-regulation and motivation for achievement.

In terms of dosage, writing labs are ideally held in 1-hour blocks, two to three times per week. They include a 10–15-minute minilesson taught to the entire class for purposes of introducing a new intermediate objective (e.g., how to think of story topics, how to respond to others' writing), with the remaining time used for individual or small-group practice of that skill during writing and other learning activities (often carried out using computers) that may address any curricular area (e.g., social sciences, language arts, science). Scaffolding that focuses on writing problems directly or on spoken language challenges that underlie them occurs during individualized minilessons and as children work on assigned tasks. Procedures consist of the adult providing "framing, selecting, focusing, and feedback environmental experiences" (Feuerstein, 1979, p. 179) to the child as a means of leading the child to more advanced performance. Revising is facilitated through the use of adult and, after peer training, peer feedback procedures in which appreciation about aspects of the written product is followed by questions designed to indicate areas where increased clarity is needed which then serve as prompts for revision. Use of an "author chair" group conference about a written product performs a similar function but also invokes celebration of the author's achievement. Improved organization of materials used in writing is fostered through author notebooks, which may contain written drafts, handouts, and personal dictionaries; posters that detail aspects of the writing process; and word walls.

Assessment for this approach is an integral aspect of the Writing Lab intervention because scaffolding grows out of dynamic assessment strategies in which the adult first provides and then fades the level of support being given as success is achieved. To track progress, writing samples of written narratives are transcribed and then analyzed via the Systematic Analysis of Language Transcripts software (Miller & Chapman, 2000) to produce measures at the level of discourse, sentence, word (including spelling), and writing conventions. Details regarding aspects of these measures are given in the section on empirical bases rather than in sections typically used for that purpose in other chapters because of the authors' need to describe the measures as part of their description of their most recent studies of the approach.

The empirical base described by Nelson and Van Meter resembles that of other interventions discussed in this section in that a considerable amount of indirect support from studies of discrete component intervention strategies is supplemented by more direct evidence from case studies and nonexperimental trials involving groups exposed to the entire intervention. Because of the complexity of the intervention and the diversity of children for which it is intended, the scope of the indirect evidence is quite extensive. For example, the introduction of students to a deliberate writing process that includes revision and careful attention to audience and purpose has been shown to produce better results for children without identified problems in a 1993 study conducted by the U.S. Department of Education (Office of Educational Research Improvement, 1996). Nelson and Van Meter also describe an extensive series of studies over more than 10 years in which a team of researchers (e.g., Danoff, Harris, & Graham, 1993; De La Paz & Graham, 2002; MacArthur, Graham, & Schwartz, 1993) provided support for the use of computers and an explicit focus on the writing process with groups of children with learning disabilities as well as with groups of typically developing peers. Selected studies within this body of work also expanded the use of computer supports beyond conventional word processing to include word prediction and synthesized speech feedback, with positive results (e.g., MacArthur, 1998). Nelson and Van Meter also describe numerous other studies that track the level of outcomes (e.g., discourse versus word-level effects) that may be expected from interventions that focus on the writing process (e.g., Vallecorsa & De-Bettencourt, 1992; Zaragoza & Vaughn, 1992). The authors interpret these studies as suggesting the need for direct instruction on target word- and sentence-level skills in addition to the need for activities conducted within a meaningful context to target discourse skills—features that are incorporated within the Writing Lab.

Nelson and Van Meter caution readers that the large variability in their data and the lack of control groups preclude any interpretation of the direct evidence for the Writing Lab approach that rules out possible contributions of maturation and related factors. Nonetheless, in their recent book (Nelson, Bahr, & Van Meter, 2004) and in this chapter, they offer readers a glimpse of positive, preliminary outcomes for an implementation of the Writing Lab approach for children in grades 1 through 5. Among reported outcomes are results for several measures, such as those related to word production fluency and story adequacy, that are associated with large effect sizes. Advances in spelling and sentence structure remained more elusive, consistent with previous findings. Nonetheless, although the authors recognize that research designs that make use of random assignment to groups and other refinements in treatment efficacy methodology need to be applied to achieve a greater understanding of the intervention, they view their existing evidence as support for the Writing Lab for children both with special needs and with typical development. We agree and conclude that, as with the other approaches discussed in this section, early exploratory and efficacy findings warrant intensified research activity and clinical implementation that is tempered by careful attention to clinical judgment and the needs, preferences, and values of intended clients.

REFERENCES

Bird, J., Bishop, D., & Freeman, N. (1995). Phonological awareness and literacy development in children with expressive phonological impairments. *Journal of Speech and Hearing Research, 36,* 446–462.

Blachman, B., Ball, E., Black, R., & Tangel, D. (1994). Kindergarten teachers develop phonological awareness in low-income, inner-city classroom. *Reading and Writing: An Interdisciplinary Journal, 6,* 1–18.

Blischak, D.M. (1995). Thomas the writer: Case study of a child with severe physical, speech, and visual impairments. *Language, Speech, and Hearing Services in Schools, 26*(1), 11–20.

Catts, H., Fey, M.E., Zhang, X., & Tomblin, B. (2001). Estimating the risk of future reading difficulties in kindergarten children: A research-based model and its clinical implementation. *Language, Speech, and Hearing Services in Schools, 32,* 38–51.

Catts, H., & Kamhi, A. (1999). Defining reading disabilities. In H. Catts & A. Kamhi (Eds.), *Language and reading disabilities* (pp. 50–72). Boston: Allyn & Bacon.

Cunningham, J.W. (1993). Whole-to-part reading diagnosis. *Reading and Writing Quarterly: Overcoming Learning Difficulties, 9,* 31–49.

Dalton, J.H., Elias, M.J., & Wandersman, A. (2001). Concepts for understanding prevention and promotion. *Community psychology: Linking individuals and communities* (pp. 266–269). Belmont, CA: Wadsworth.

Danoff, B., Harris, K.R., & Graham, S. (1993). Incorporating strategy instruction within the writing process in the regular classroom. Effects on the writing of students with and without learning disabilities. *Journal of Reading Behavior, 25,* 295–322.

De La Paz, S., & Graham, S. (2002). Strategy instruction in planning: Effects on the writing performance and behavior of students with learning disabilities. *Exceptional Children, 63,* 167–181.

Ehri, L.C., Nunes, S.R., Willows, D.M., Schuster, B.V., Yaghoub-Zadeh, Z., & Shanahan, T. (2001). Phonemic awareness instruction helps children learn to read: Evidence from the National Reading Panel's meta-analysis. *Reading Research Quarterly, 36*(3), 250–287.

Erickson, K.A., Koppenhaver, D.A., Yoder, D.E., & Nance, J. (1997). Integrated communication and literacy instruction for a child with multiple disabilities. *Focus on Autism and Other Developmental Disabilities, 12*(3), 142–150.

Feuerstein, R. (1979). *The dynamic assessment of retarded performers.* Baltimore: University Park Press.

Gillon, G. (2000). The efficacy of phonological awareness intervention for children with spoken language impairment. *Language, Speech, and Hearing Services in Schools, 31,* 126–141.

Gillon, G. (2002). Follow-up study investigating benefits of phonological awareness intervention for children with spoken language impairment. *International Journal of Language and Communication Disorders, 37*(4), 381–400.

Gillon, G. (2003, November). *Phonological awareness intervention for preschool children.* Paper presented at the American Speech-Language-Hearing Association annual convention, Chicago.

Gillon, G. (2004). *Phonological awareness: From research to practice.* New York: Guilford Press.

Gipe, J., Duffy, C.A., & Richards, J.C. (1993). Helping a non-speaking adult male with cerebral palsy achieve literacy. *Journal of Reading, 36*(5), 380–389.

Hayes, J., & Flower, L. (1980). Identifying the organization of the writing process. In L.W. Gregg & E.R. Steinberg (Eds.), *Cognitive processes in writing* (pp. 3–10). Hillsdale, NJ: Lawrence Erlbaum Associates.

Korkman, K., & Peltomma, A. (1993). Preventative treatment of dyslexia by a preschool training program for children with language impairments. *Journal of Clinical Child Psychology, 22,* 227–287.

Larrivee, L., & Catts, H. (1999). Early reading achievement in children with expressive phonological disorders. *American Journal of Speech-Language Pathology, 8,* 137–148.

Lewis, B.A., Freebairn, L.A., Hansen, A.J., Iyengar, S.K., & Taylor, H.G. (2004). School-age follow-up of children with childhood apraxia of speech. *Language, Speech, and Hearing Services in Schools, 35,* 122–140.

MacArthur, C. (1998). Word processing with speech synthesis and word prediction: Effects on the dialogue journal writing of students with learning disabilities. *Learning Disabilities Quarterly, 21,* 151–166.

MacArthur, C., Graham,, S., & Schwartz, S. (1993). Integrating strategy instruction and word processing into a process approach to writing instruction. *School Psychology Review, 22,* 671–681.

Miller, J., & Chapman, R. (2000). Systematic Analysis of Language Transcripts (SALT) [Computer software]. Madison, WI: Waisman Center, University of Wisconsin–Madison.

Nelson, N.W., Bahr, C., & Van Meter, A. (2004). *The Writing Lab approach to language instruction and intervention.* Baltimore: Paul H. Brookes Publishing Co.

Norris, J.A. (1998). "I could read if I had a little help": Facilitating reading in whole language contexts. In C. Weaver (Ed.), *Practicing what we know: Informed reading instruction* (pp. 513–553). Urbana, IL: National Council of Teachers of English.

Norris, J.A. (2002). *Phonic Faces.* Baton Rouge, LA: EleMentory.com.

Norris, J.A., & Hoffman, P.R. (2002). Language development and late talkers: A connectionist perspective. In R.G. Daniloff (Ed.), *Connectionist approaches to clinical problems in speech and language: Therapeutic and scientific applications* (pp. 1–110). Mahwah, NJ: Lawrence Erlbaum Associates.

Rummelhart, D.E., & McClelland, J.L. (1986). *Parallel distributed processing: Explorations in the microstructure of cognition. Volume 1: Foundations.* Cambridge, MA: The MIT Press.

Torgesen, J., Wagner, R., Rashotte, C., Lindamood, P., Rose, E., Conway, T., & Garvan, C. (1999). Preventing reading failure in young children with phonological processing disabilities: Group and individual responses to instruction. *Journal of Educational Psychology, 91,* 579–593.

U.S. Department of Education, Office of Educational Research and Improvement (OERI). (1996). Can students benefit from process writing? *NAEP Facts, 1*(3), 1–6.

Vallecorsa, A.L., & DeBettencourt, L.U. (1992). Teaching composing skills to learning disabled adolescents using a process-oriented strategy. *Journal of Developmental and Physical Disabilities, 4,* 277–297.

van Kleeck, A., Gillam, R., & McFadden, T. (1998). A study of classroom-based phonological awareness training for preschoolers with speech and/or language disorders. *American Journal of Speech-Language Pathology, 7*(3), 65–76.

Warrick, N., Rubin, H., & Rowe-Walsh, S. (1993). Phoneme awareness in language delayed children: Comparative studies and intervention. *Annals of Dyslexia, 43,* 153–173.

Zaragosa, N., & Vaughn, S. (1992). The effects of processing writing instruction on three 2nd grade students with different achievement profiles. *Learning Disabilities Research, 7,* 184–193.

12

Phonological Awareness Intervention

A Preventive Framework for Preschool Children
with Specific Speech and Language Impairments

GAIL T. GILLON

ABSTRACT

Children with speech and language impairments are at risk for persistent reading and spelling difficulties. In this chapter, a preventive intervention for these children is described in which phonological awareness skills that have proven critical for literacy success are stimulated from an early age. The rationale and framework for the integration of specific phonological awareness activities into therapy programs for 3- and 4-year-old children are presented. The phonological awareness intervention proposed is based on strong theoretical and empirical research and is innovative in its application to young children with communication disorders.

INTRODUCTION

Phonological awareness interventions have emerged from a strong research base that has examined factors associated with reading and spelling acquisition. Explicit awareness of the sound structure of a spoken word, referred to as *phonological awareness,* is critical to the process of recognizing and decoding words in print and is also important in learning to spell. The research evidence from a vast array of studies across differing alphabetic languages is very clear: Children who approach reading and spelling instruction with strong phonological awareness knowledge are likely to move from speaking their native language to reading and writing their native language with relative ease. In contrast, children with poor phonological awareness skills and difficulty in processing and holding phonological information in memory are more likely to experience early literacy difficulties and are at risk for persistent reading and spelling failure (see Gillon, 2004, and Stanovich, 2000, for reviews of this research). Children with diagnosed written language disorders such as dyslexia frequently display severe phonological awareness deficits. Indeed, difficulty in processing phonological information is considered a causative factor in reading disorder (Catts & Kamhi, 2005). Phonological awareness interventions have developed, therefore, as a method to resolve phonological awareness deficits that contribute to children's reading and spelling difficulties, as a method of preventing or limiting difficulties for children identified as being at risk for literacy disorder, or as a means to enhance all children's early reading and spelling success.

TARGET POPULATIONS AND ASSESSMENTS FOR DETERMINING TREATMENT RELEVANCE AND GOALS

This chapter focuses on phonological awareness interventions for young children with specific speech and/or language impairments. The particular targets for the intervention approach described are 3- and 4-year-old children who have speech and/or language difficulties in the absence of sensory, neurological, physical, or intellectual impairments, or behavioral and emotional disorders. Children with speech and language impairments frequently display poor phonological awareness knowledge compared with their peers (Gillon, 2000; Larrivee & Catts, 1999; Rvachew, Ohberg, Grawburg, & Heyding, 2003; Stothard, Snowling, Bishop, Chipchase, & Kaplan, 1998). As a group at kindergarten age, these children are 4–5 times more likely to experience reading difficulties than children from the general population (Catts, Fey, Zhang, & Tomblin, 2001). It is critical, therefore, to explore carefully interventions that may help prevent written language difficulties for these children.

Phonological awareness may be viewed as developing along a continuum with differing levels of difficulty (Anthony & Lonigan, 2004) Three levels of awareness commonly identified are

1. Awareness that words have a syllabic structure (syllable awareness). Tasks such as identifying the number of syllables in words or deleting syllables from words may be used to measure children's syllable awareness.

2. Awareness that a syllable has a beginning part, or an onset, and a rime unit (referred to as *onset-rime awareness*). Recognizing or producing rhyming words is an example of phonological awareness at this level.

3. Awareness that words are formed from individual speech sounds or phonemes (phoneme awareness). A range of tasks provides insight into a child's phoneme awareness. Identifying the beginning or ending sound in a spoken word (phoneme identity), segmenting a word into its individual sounds (phoneme segmentation), blending speech sounds together to form a word (phoneme blending), and deleting and manipulating sounds in words are all examples of phoneme awareness.

These tasks differ in complexity and the cognitive requirements necessary to complete the task, but they are generally considered to be closely related to each other (Anthony & Lonigan, 2004; Stanovich, Cunningham, & Cramer,

1984). Awareness that spoken words can be divided at the syllable, onset-rime and phoneme level helps children to understand the relationship between speech and print. Phoneme level awareness is particularly important in the early stages of spelling and word decoding and has been described as the best single predictor of reading performance (Liberman, Shankweiler, & Liberman, 1989; Lundberg, Olofsson, & Wall, 1980).

Assessment tools developed to measure young children's phonological awareness abilities frequently include measures of performance of syllable, onset-rime, and phoneme awareness. Two examples of such tests that contain normative data for children as young as age 3 or 4 years are 1) the Preschool and Primary Inventory of Phonological Awareness (PIPA; Dodd, Crosbie, MacIntosh, Teitzel, & Ozanne, 2000), designed for children ages 3 years to 6 years, 11 months; and 2) the Phonological Abilities Test (PAT; Muter, Hulme, & Snowling, 1997), containing normative data for children ages 4 years to 7 years, 11 months. The Phonological Awareness Literacy Screening Pre-Kindergarten test (PALS-PreK; Invernizzi, Sullivan, & Meier, 2002) is an example of a phonological awareness screening measure designed for 4-year-old children that measures both rhyme awareness and early phoneme awareness. A range of informal tasks has also been used in research studies to evaluate phonological awareness development in 3- and 4-year-old children. These include

- Detecting a word (from a series of three pictures) that does not rhyme

- Matching words that rhyme

- Detecting the word (from a series of three pictures) that starts with a different sound (phoneme detection)

- Detecting the word that starts with the same sound as a target word (phoneme matching)

- Blending syllables to form words

- Deleting a syllable from a word

Lonigan et al. (1998, p. 310) and MacLean et al. (1987, p. 261) provide lists of stimulus items used with very young children.

The focus of phonological awareness assessment with children as young as 3 and 4 years of age is not to identify and label children as having a phonological awareness deficit. Given the wide variability in phonological awareness performance of typically developing children in this age group (see discussion later in this chapter), such labeling would be inappropriate. Rather, assessment in this age group of children with speech and/or language impairment should be aimed at 1) observing a child's current level of phonological awareness development; and 2) monitoring early phonological awareness development to determine whether a child is gaining phonological awareness skills through the home language environment, an early childhood education program, or the speech and language intervention provided.

The assessment must be viewed in context with a range of other variables including environment, culture, biological and cognitive factors, and, in particular, the nature and severity of the child's speech and/or language impairment. All of these variables influence reading and spelling development in children with speech and language impairments. Phonological awareness assessment is just one part of a comprehensive evaluation these children require. It is also important to consider assessment data from the child's language assessment prior to phonological awareness intervention. Establishing the level of instruction and linguistic concepts the child will understand as well as analyzing the child's speech production abilities are important for planning stimulus items and activities.

Assessment of children's phonological awareness abilities prior to intervention is critical to determine the effectiveness of intervention. If a specific goal of an intervention period is to stimulate phonological awareness development, establishing preintervention baselines through the use of phonological awareness assessment probes is necessary to evaluate change postintervention (see Paul, 2001, for a discussion of assessment probes). Once a stable baseline of phonological awareness performance has been established, intervention can begin.

THEORETICAL BASIS

The goal of phonological awareness intervention is to enhance reading and writing performance. Activities that promote the explicit understanding of a word's sound structure are valuable primarily to the extent that they can develop a child's ability to recognize printed words or to spell words. In practical terms there is little value, for example, in being able to identify the number of phonemes in a spoken word (phoneme segmentation ability). However, if this ability leads to improved decoding of words in print, helps the child to instantly recognize words in print, enhances reading comprehension performance, and develops the child's ability to spell words, then the benefit of phoneme segmentation training becomes apparent.

Theoretical assumptions that underlie the goals of phonological awareness intervention include the following:

- Phonological awareness knowledge is critical to the processes involved in reading single words in isolation (referred to as *word recognition*) and in learning how to spell words.

- Word recognition performance contributes significantly to reading comprehension.

- Phonological awareness allows children to engage in a self-teaching process of acquiring new knowledge in reading and spelling.

- Reading is an interactive process that integrates information from a variety of sources including phonological knowledge.

- An interactive relationship between phonological awareness and experiences in reading and spelling, including early experiences with letter-name knowledge, is evident.

- Phonological awareness develops in children with age and exposure to print and is not complete when children begin to read.

Each of these theoretical assumptions is summarized in this section and the implications for phonological awareness intervention are presented.

Phonological Awareness Contributes to Word Recognition and Spelling

Early theories of word recognition known as *dual route theories* (e.g., Coltheart, 1978) proposed that words could be read out of context via a phonological route (e.g., sounding out regularly spelled words such as *bird: b-ir-d*) or a visual route (e.g., rote learning the visual image of irregularly spelled words such as *sword* at the whole-word level). Within this theory, phonological awareness knowledge contributes only to the recognition of phonologically regular words through the decoding process. Decoding an unknown word in print draws on awareness that multisyllabic words can be divided into syllables (syllable awareness), that syllables can be segmented into individual phonemes (phoneme segmentation), that particular speech sounds are associated with particular letters or letter combinations (phoneme–grapheme relationships), and that phonemes and syllables can be blended together to form a complete phonological form of a word (phoneme blending). Meaning is subsequently attached to the decoded word if the word is in the reader's vocabulary store.

More recent models of word recognition such as Ehri's modified dual route theory (Ehri, 1992) and connectionist models of word recognition (Seidenberg & McClelland, 1989) propose that the processing of phonological information is necessary to the recognition of all words in print—both words that are phonetically regular and words that are phonetically irregular. Ehri (1992) pointed out that most irregular words are only partially irregular. In the word *sword,* for example, only the *w* does not follow regular spelling patterns. Phonological awareness that promotes understanding of the grapheme–phoneme relationships for *s* or *d* may help cue recognition of the word. Ehri suggested that the reader may utilize the systemic relations between spelling and pronunciation that the word offers to aid memory and thus reduce memory demand, rather than learn the entire form visually by rote. Ehri argued that the rote learning required to access words via visual memory is inefficient because remembering the orthographic shape of each new word acquired in an arbitrary manner (e.g., based on the shape of the letter combinations and having no relationship to the phonemes associated with the letters) places heavy demands on memory. It is more plausible to hypothesize that once a child has acquired knowledge of connections between graphemes and phonemes, the child will partially use these cues in reading. Even by second grade, children who do not make use of phonological cues in reading but rely solely on whole-word visual recognition are likely to be the poorest readers (Stuart, 1995). These later theoretical models suggest that successful phonological awareness interventions should ultimately lead to improvements in the reading of all word types, both phonetically regularly and irregularly spelled words.

The importance of phonological awareness to early spelling development is also well recognized (Treiman & Bourassa, 2000). The utilization of a phonological strategy in spelling a word involves segmenting the target word into phonemes and applying knowledge of how individual sounds in words are represented in spelling. Teaching strategies that encourage children to listen for the first sound of word, to break down a word into parts, and to sound out the word when spelling are consistent with the phonological route theory of spelling. A phonological route provides an alternative to relying solely on rote learning of the visual image for each word in print and facilitates spelling attempts of new words not previously seen. Successful preventive models of phonological awareness should also provide strong foundation skills for early spelling attempts in addition to enhancing early word recognition performance.

Some aspects of phonological awareness intervention are based on an analogy theory of word recognition and spelling (Goswami & Bryant, 1992). This theory holds that children can decode and encode new words based on their knowledge of known words that have similar spelling and phonological patterns (referred to as *reading, or spelling, by analogy*). For example, a child may read a new word such as *fan* based on their knowledge of known words *man* and *can*. That is, they are using their knowledge of the rime unit in these words and how words can be segmented at an onset-rime level (*c - an; f - an*) rather than decoding the word phoneme by phoneme. Phonological awareness interventions that include teaching young children to understand and hear similar sound patterns within words, for example, by recognizing and producing rhyming words, may help children to develop knowledge necessary for utilizing an analogy method for word recognition and spelling.

Word Recognition Contributes to Reading Comprehension

Comprehension of written text is undoubtedly the desired outcome of reading. The ability to fluently decode words is only of importance as it relates to accessing the meaning of written words. A wide range of linguistic and metacognitive abilities contributes to a child's reading comprehension abilities (see Westby, 2005). Researchers have demonstrated, however, that a large proportion of the variance in children's reading comprehension performance can be explained by their level of word recognition (Stanovich, 1985). Inefficient and effortful decoding of text is likely to hamper an individual's ability to process the meaning of the text, and it is therefore predicted that poor word decoding skills are central to the comprehension problems of many poor readers (Stanovich, 1991b). Phonological awareness interventions aimed at enhancing word recognition skills should ultimately result in improvements in the child's ability to comprehend written text. Thus, phonological awareness may be viewed as contributing to reading comprehension via its importance to efficient word recognition.

Phonological Awareness Contributes to Self-Teaching

Phonological awareness intervention is consistent with a self-teaching model of word recognition development (Share, 1995). Share hypothesized that children develop efficiency in recognizing printed words through a self-teaching process. Early successful decoding attempts allow children to gain further knowledge about phoneme–grapheme relationships that in turn leads to increased decoding success. The development of the ability to immediately recognize words by sight (as opposed to decoding each word letter by letter) may be viewed as an accumulation of phonological and orthographic word knowledge developed in response to successful decoding attempts. Children who struggle in their early attempts to decode words will be exposed to far fewer decoding attempts than early successful readers, and they will become less likely to gain experiences in more complex phoneme–grapheme relationships. Thus, their opportunities to engage in a self-teaching process are severely restricted.

Phonological awareness interventions assume that by enhancing children's understanding of the sound structures of words and how phonemes relate to graphemes will enable them to engage in independent learning or self-teaching. Skills developed in phonological awareness interventions are expected to transfer to the decoding of novel words and, with frequent reading experiences, should then allow the child to accumulate knowledge to develop further efficiency in word recognition processes. Within a self-teaching model, phonological awareness intervention may be viewed as a method to stimulate the word recognition process, rather than as an intervention aimed at complete mastery of word recognition. The self-teaching hypothesis also provides a strong rationale for phonological awareness intervention at a young age to foster successful early decoding attempts for children at risk for reading difficulties.

Reading Is an Interactive Process

An interactive theory of connected text reading (e.g., Rumelhart, 1977) holds that phonological knowledge is integrated with a child's semantic, syntactic, and morphological knowledge. For example, knowledge of sentence structure, vocabulary knowledge, understanding words that are commonly associated with each other (semantic association knowledge), as well as phonological information all interact to help a child efficiently and fluently read connected text. Thus, although phonological awareness is critical to early reading and spelling acquisition, it must be viewed within the context of a range of other linguistic variables that contribute to written language development. Scarborough's (1998) meta-analysis of 61 research studies that investigated the correlations between kindergarten performance on a range of variables and later reading performance confirmed the importance of phonological awareness, but it also highlighted the contribution of other measures of language proficiency and print knowledge to the reading process. Phonological awareness as a preventive intervention for young children should also be viewed within the broader context of a comprehensive program to facilitate language development. Activities such as shared book reading, story telling, vocabulary enrichment, and involvement in a wide range of meaningful speaking, listening, reading, and writing activities will all help to foster written language acquisition. Phonological awareness intervention provides one aspect of a variety of language experiences that will contribute to written language success.

Phonological Awareness Development

Successful intervention planning depends on the interventionist's understanding of typical phonological awareness development and factors that influence this. (For a detailed review of phonological awareness development in English and in other alphabetic languages, refer to Gillon, 2004.) A general developmental progression in phonological awareness is evident, with the awareness of larger units in words developing prior to awareness of smaller units (Johnston, Anderson, & Holligan, 1996; Treiman & Zukowsky, 1991). We currently do not fully understand whether there is a smooth progression from one level of phonological awareness to the next and whether awareness of larger units is necessary to facilitate awareness of smaller units for all children (Duncan & Johnston, 1999). It is established, however, that many 4-year-old children can demonstrate syllable awareness and will show the emergence of rhyme awareness. Sensitivity to phonemes in words may be developing in 4- and 5-year-old children (Johnston et al., 1996), but more demanding phoneme awareness tasks such as phoneme manipulation only develop after exposure to literacy instruction. For example, 5–7-year-old children with typical language development can be expected to demonstrate some success on phoneme categorization, phoneme matching, and phoneme identity tasks, whereas they are likely to experience more difficulty with phoneme blending, phoneme deletion, phoneme segmentation, and phoneme manipulation tasks (Schatschneider, Francis, Foorman, Fletcher, & Mehta, 1999). This pattern of phonological awareness development evident in English is also apparent in other languages, such as Spanish (e.g., Denton, Hasbrouck, Weaver, & Riccio, 2000) and Italian (Cossu, Shankweiler, Liberman, Katz, & Tola, 1988).

There is wide variation in performance on phonological awareness tasks in young children. Although as a group, performance stability does not emerge until after 4 years of age, some children as young as 2 and 3 years old can demonstrate success on phonological awareness tasks (Lonigan et al., 1998). Many factors influence the wide variance in children's phonological awareness development prior to the onset of formal literacy instruction. These factors include

- Vocabulary development (Metsala, 1999)

- Knowledge of nursery rhymes (Bryant, Bradley, MacLean, & Crossland, 1989)

- Letter-name knowledge (Burgess & Lonigan, 1998; Johnston et al., 1996)

- The quality of the child's phonological representation of spoken words (Elbro, Borstrom, & Petersen, 1998; Swan & Goswami, 1997)

- Socioeconomic factors (Lonigan et al., 1998)

- Native language experiences (Cossu et al., 1988; Holm & Dodd, 1996)

With the onset of instruction in reading and spelling, a strong reciprocal relationship exists between advancing word recognition and spelling skills and development in phoneme awareness. Experiences in reading and spelling clearly influence later phoneme awareness development (e.g., Burgess & Lonigan, 1998; Read, Zhang, Nie, & Ding, 1986). The pattern of interactions that has emerged from the research is that a general awareness that words can be broken into smaller parts is a necessary base on which to build successful word recognition and spelling skills. Experiences in decoding and encoding print further develop knowledge about a word's sound structure, particularly at the phoneme level, and increased proficiency in word recognition allows children to successfully complete complex phonological tasks such as phoneme manipulation and phoneme deletion tasks. Thus, following an initial impetus from phonological awareness to reading and spelling, these relationships become mutually supportive (Perfetti, Beck, Ball, & Hughes, 1987). Phonological awareness intervention within a preventive model prior to literacy instruction is aimed, therefore, at ensuring that young children have the necessary base in phonological awareness skills to contribute to early reading development. It is not aimed at mastery of complex phoneme tasks that should develop as a result of successful reading and spelling experiences.

EMPIRICAL BASIS

One of the most exciting developments in understanding reading disorder in recent years is evidence supporting the benefits of phonological awareness interventions. Children with severe phonological awareness deficits who are at high risk for literacy difficulties or who have experienced years of reading failure can respond positively to specific phonological awareness interventions or programs that integrate phonological awareness activities (e.g., Blachman, Ball, Black, & Tangel, 1994; Castle, Riach, & Nicholson, 1994; Gillon, 2000; Gillon & Dodd, 1995, 1997; Lovett, Steinbach, & Frijters, 2000; Lovett et al., 1994; Torgesen et al., 1999). Indeed, some children have shown remarkable and sustained growth in literacy skills following instruction to enhance their phonological awareness skills and develop their understanding of how phonemes relate to graphemes in the reading and spelling process (e.g., Gillon & Dodd, 1997). Few areas of language instruction and intervention have been exposed to the rigorous meta-analyses, research methodology critiques, and dissection of treatment benefits as that of phonological awareness. A meta-analysis of 52 controlled research studies in phonological awareness training confirmed that phonological awareness instruction has a statistically significant impact on developing word recognition, reading comprehension, and spelling (Ehri et al., 2001). The positive effect of phonological awareness instruction for written language development was evident for children considered to be at risk for reading difficulties, children identified as having reading problems, as well as children with typical reading development.

The strong research base for phonological awareness intervention has provided valuable information for practitioners as to conditions that increase the efficiency of the treatment. For example, it is now generally accepted that phonological awareness intervention should focus on developing skills at a phoneme level, should provide small-group or individual instruction of a relatively intensive nature for children with severe phonological awareness deficits, and should include activities to make explicit the connections between speech and print (see Ehri et al., 2001).

Much of the research into phonological awareness intervention, however, has excluded children with diagnosed speech and language impairments. Unique challenges in the implementation of phonological awareness intervention are presented for these children. Unintelligible speech, limited language comprehension skills, difficulty following instructions, difficulty formulating sentences or asking questions to seek clarification from an instructor, or difficulty listening and attending to auditory information are common characteristics of children with speech and language disorders. The phonological awareness, reading, and spelling difficulties present in children with specific speech and language impairments are not readily resolved through classroom instruction. Interventions focused solely on resolving speech production difficulties or language impairment may also have limited impact on improving phoneme awareness and word recognition (Fey, Catts, & Larrivee, 1995; Gillon, 2000; and references therein). The research evidence suggests that without specific phonological awareness intervention, the phonological awareness deficits of many children with specific speech and language impairment persist over time (Bird, Bishop, & Freeman, 1995; Gillon, 2002; Korkman & Peltomma, 1993; Snowling, Bishop, & Stothard, 2000). These children have particular difficulty acquiring phonological awareness skills at the phoneme level (Gillon, 2002; Webster, Plante, & Couvillion, 1997). Even when the spoken language difficulties of children with specific language impairment are considered to have resolved in preschool or in the early school years, some of these children display weakness on complex phoneme awareness tasks and show weakness in aspects of reading and spelling during their adolescent years (Stothard et al., 1998).

Fortunately, studies provide early evidence supporting the use of phonological awareness interventions for children with communication problems. Warrick, Rubin, and Rowe-Walsh (1993) examined the efficacy of phonological awareness intervention for kindergarten-age children with specific language impairment. In this study, 28 children with specific expressive and or receptive language impairments (identified by poor performance on standardized language tests and average performance on nonverbal intelligence measures) were divided into two matched groups according to their language abilities. One group received phonological awareness training and the other group did not. A third group of children with typically developing language also participated as a control group. All of the participants were monolingual speakers of English.

Intervention comprised two 20-minute sessions (with groups of seven children) implemented over an 8-week period. The training activities included tasks to enhance syllable awareness (clapping and counting the syllables in children's names and names of animals), onset-rime awareness (rhyme recognition, onset-rime blending, and segmentation), and phoneme awareness (bringing children's attention to the initial phoneme in target words through repetition and prolongation of the phoneme, sound categorization activities, and phoneme segmentation with two and three phoneme words). Using a pretest/posttest design, the results provided clear evidence that the training was effective in developing the phonological awareness skills of children with delayed language who participated in the experimental group. This group showed accelerated growth in their phonological awareness skills and reached performance levels of children with typical development at the completion of the intervention. The children with language impairment who did not receive the training showed persistent difficulties in phonological awareness, and the gap between their performance level and that of typically developing children increased over time. Follow-up assessment 12 months after intervention using standardized measures of real word and nonword reading, nonword spelling, and previously administered experimental phonological awareness measures revealed that the treatment effects were maintained over time and that improved phonological awareness development transferred to the reading process.

van Kleeck, Gillam, and McFadden (1998) extended the work of Warrick et al. (1993) by demonstrating that phonological awareness intervention may be successfully implemented with children with differing types of specific language impairment as young as 4 years of age. In this study, children with specific speech impairments and/or language impairments received intervention that focused on developing rhyme awareness for 12 weeks followed by 12 weeks focused on phoneme awareness. Gains were compared with historical controls from the same classroom before the phonological processing interventions had been implemented. Interestingly, data analysis suggested that only the children's gains in phoneme awareness could be attributed to the intervention program. The improvements made in rhyme awareness were not significantly different from progress made by the historical control group. This outcome is consistent with other findings in the literature indicating that the syllable and or rhyme awareness of children with spoken language difficulties improve with other types of speech and language intervention, classroom curriculum, or improvements in speech production skills (Gillon, 2000; Webster et al., 1997).

In contrast to development in syllable and rhyme awareness, Gillon (2000) illustrated that development in these children's skills at the phoneme level requires more specific and direct training. This study examined the efficacy of phonological awareness training in enhancing word decoding, reading comprehension, and early spelling development for children with developmental speech impairments. The 61 children who participated in this study (ages between 5 years, 6 months and 7 years, 6 months) all had expressive phonological impairments, as demonstrated by the percentage of consonants correctly articulated on articulation measures. Twenty-three children participated in 20 hours of phonological awareness intervention; 23 received 20 hours of a control intervention targeting speech production and expressive language; and 15 children, who were unable to access more intensive therapy, were provided minimal intervention focusing on speech production. Prior to intervention, there were no group differences on a range of measures including speech production, phoneme awareness, and reading ability, and these groups showed significantly delayed development in these areas compared with a control group of children with typical spoken language development.

The phonological awareness intervention was implemented on an individual basis for two 1-hour sessions weekly until 20 hours of intervention had been completed. The program content included activities to develop onset-rime awareness, but predominantly focused on developing skills at the phoneme level (phoneme identity, phoneme blending, phoneme segmentation, phoneme manipulation, and tracking sound changes in words). Activities incorporated letter-sound knowledge and made explicit for the children the link between speech and print.

The results of the study indicated that the children in the phonological awareness intervention group made accelerated progress on phoneme awareness tasks, reaching levels similar to typically developing children at the post-intervention assessment. Transfer of skills to the reading process was clearly evident. The performance of the children in this group was significantly superior to both the speech treatment and minimal intervention control groups on two measures of word recognition ability, reading accuracy, reading comprehension of connected text, and nonword decoding ability. Importantly, the results revealed that improvements in phonological awareness were not at the expense of improvements in speech production. There was a nonsignificant trend for children who received the phonological awareness instruction to show more improvement in their spontaneous articulation of single words than children in other interventions that were aimed predominantly at resolving speech sound errors.

Follow-up assessment 11 months after phonological awareness intervention indicated sustained and continued growth in phoneme awareness, speech production, reading, and spelling development (Gillon, 2002). With continued classroom instruction and reading support, the majority of children who received phonological awareness intervention were reading at or above the expected level for their age at the follow-up assessment. In contrast, children who received speech production intervention and no direct phonological awareness intervention during their participation in the experiment made remarkably little progress in phoneme level skills after the project intervention was completed. This lack of progress was noted despite other forms of remedial reading and speech-language intervention that were part of their school programs after the end of their formal participation in the original study. The majority of these children remained poor readers at follow-up assessment.

This latter finding is consistent with previous research for non–English-speaking children. Korkman and Peltomma (1993) investigated phonological awareness treatment effects for 6-year-old boys in Finland who were classified as having a language impairment (as evidenced by receptive language deficits and expressive naming difficulties). In this study, an experimental group of 26 boys received weekly small-group instruction in syllable awareness, onset-rime phoneme awareness, and letter-sound knowledge training during their kindergarten year. Speech-language pathologists (SLPs), preschool teachers, or psychologists implemented the program following training by the researchers.

A control group of 20 boys matched to the experimental group at preintervention for age, intelligence, socioeconomic status, and spoken language abilities received other types of services (e.g., 17 of the boys in the control group received individual speech and language therapy), but they did not receive the structured experimental program in phonological awareness. Comprehensive follow-up testing of the children at the end of their first year at school indicated that the experimental group that had received phoneme awareness intervention had significantly superior abilities in reading comprehension, spelling, and phoneme awareness compared with the control group of children. The results of this study suggested that the inclusion of phonological awareness instruction for these 6-year-old Finnish boys with language impairment was a critical factor in determining their early literacy outcomes.

Additional research suggests that integrating structured phonological awareness activities into intervention for children with specific speech impairments as young as 3 and 4 years old is also beneficial (Gillon, 2005). Gillon followed a group of 11 children with moderate and severe speech impairment from 3 years of age through to the end of their first year at school. These children received speech and language therapy that included specific training in early developing phoneme awareness skills and letter-sound knowledge training. This training was integrated into phonological therapy to improve their speech production following Hodson and Paden's cycles approach to therapy (Hodson & Paden, 1991). Each block of training involved approximately 8–10 hours of therapy over a 4- or 5-week period, and all children received two blocks of therapy prior to school entry at 5 years of age. A few children with more severe impairments received three blocks of intervention. For ethical reasons, a retrospective design was used to obtain a control group. Eleven children were selected who closely matched the experimental group with regard to nature of speech difficulty at 3 or 4 years of age, the amount of speech and language therapy services received between 3 and 5 years, and socio-economic background. The control group had not received any formal training in phonological awareness. This retrospective matching was possible through inspection of detailed case records and assessment results that were available for the children in the control group. Children from both the experimental and control group were tested on the same battery of speech production, language, phonological awareness, and literacy tasks at approximately 6 years of age. Although there were no significant group differences in speech production and receptive language abilities, the children who had received phonological awareness instruction performed significantly better on phoneme awareness and word recognition tasks. These findings were consistent with other results (Major & Bernhardt, 1998) that have indicated significant benefits from including phonological awareness activities into early intervention for preschool children with severe expressive phonological and syntactic disorders.

Research by O'Connor, Jenkins, Leister, and Slocum (1993) indicated that it is possible to develop the phonological awareness skills of 4–6-year-old children who have more pervasive language and cognitive delays. The 47 children who participated in their study were enrolled in a special education preschool facility. Most of these children had significant language impairments and some had additional physical and cognitive impairments or behavioral disorders. The study indicated that the children responded positively to short periods of phonological awareness intervention (10 minutes, 4 times weekly, for a 7-week period). However, testing using experimental assessment tasks showed the children only improved on the phonological task taught (i.e., rhyming, or blending, or segmentation tasks) and little transfer was evident from one type of phonological awareness tasks to another. Transfer to reading and spelling skills was not examined and remains to be studied in this population.

There is strong evidence, then, that children with specific speech and/or language impairments frequently exhibit poor phonological awareness particularly at the phoneme level. Yet evidence also suggests that these children can acquire age-appropriate phoneme awareness if they receive specific intervention to develop such skills. Given the importance of phonological awareness to successful early literacy acquisition, it is critical that early interventions for children with speech and/or language impairments also serve to stimulate phonological awareness development. Ensuring that these children approach formal reading and spelling instruction with strong phonological awareness knowledge and an initial understanding of the links between speech and print will help toward the prevention of written language difficulties that many of these children will otherwise face. The next sections detail an intervention framework to foster the development of phonological awareness skills in preschool children at risk.

PRACTICAL REQUIREMENTS

This section describes a preventive framework for phonological awareness development in 3- and 4-year-old children that have speech and language impairment. The framework proposed is based on the following clinical assumptions:

1. The children have already been identified as having a specific speech and/or language impairment that places them at risk for literacy difficulties such as receptive or expressive language impairment, delayed or disordered expressive phonological impairment, or childhood apraxia of speech.

2. The children are receiving, or will receive, periods of regular intervention by an SLP.

SLPs' expertise in spoken language development is necessary to direct the planning and intervention framework for these children. Collaboration between the child's parents, preschool teachers, or child care workers and the child's SLP should be encouraged. Such collaboration is likely to increase opportunities for children to engage in purposeful activities aimed at facilitating phonological awareness development.

KEY COMPONENTS

The aim of phonological awareness intervention at this young age is to stimulate the development of phonological awareness skills that will influence literacy development. The developmental progression of phonological awareness and an understanding of the difficulty level of specific phonological awareness tasks should guide the planning of phonological awareness intervention. Typically, phonological awareness interventions in this age group would develop skills at the syllable level (e.g., tapping out syllables in words), the onset-rime level (e.g., listening to rhyming words and beginning to identify rhyming words), and early phoneme awareness (e.g., developing awareness of initial sounds in words). However, because research suggests that syllable awareness and rhyme awareness develop more readily from general speech and language stimulation than does phoneme awareness, it is important for SLPs to directly target the stimulation of early phoneme awareness. Engaging children in activities such as phoneme categorization, phoneme identity, and phoneme matching will encourage this development. Blending and segmentation tasks at the onset-rime (e.g., *c -at*) and phoneme level (for common two- and three-phoneme words) are useful as the child draws closer to formal literacy instruction.

It is strongly recommended that clinicians plan activities that introduce letter-name and letter-sound knowledge for a small group of letters into therapy. Selecting letters that are visually distinct and may be associated with speech production goals or the child and family members' names is suggested. Table 12.1 provides examples of how a clinician may stimulate some key components of phonological awareness intervention (i.e., activities to promote early awareness at the phoneme level) and to draw a child's attention to sound-to-print matching.

Intervention Approaches

Two approaches to phonological awareness intervention in this young age group may be useful. One approach is to plan phonological awareness activities around the child's speech and oral language goals. For example, a child who deletes initial or final consonant sounds in words can focus on the phonological awareness goal of identifying initial and final phonemes in words. A child whose language goals include developing vocabulary knowledge using a thematic approach can include the phonological awareness goal of phoneme categorization. This would involve tasks such as finding pictures related to the theme topic that start with a target sound.

A second approach to intervention is to plan phonological awareness activities at the syllable, onset-rime, and/or phoneme level that are independent of other spoken language goals. A defined period of time at the beginning or end of each intervention session may be set for these activities or they may be interspersed among activities targeting other speech and language goals.

The instructor directs both approaches. That is, the SLP plans predetermined goals, implements prescribed activities for achieving these goals, and carefully plans the stimulus items to ensure they are appropriate to the child's speech and vocabulary development. Children's interests must also be considered, particularly in terms of game activities and props used in the interventions. Engaging a 3- or 4-year-old child in an instructor-directed activity is likely to be easier if the activity involves a child's favorite toy or a toy that will quickly capture the child's attention.

Table 12.1. Examples of key components for 3- and 4-year-old children

Key component	Phoneme awareness: phoneme categorization
Aim	To identify words that start with a target phoneme
Activity 1	Sort toys and "animal friends" by the initial phoneme of their name
	Clinician: "This is my friend turtle. *Turtle* starts with a /t/ sound. This letter is *t,* and it makes a /t/ sound (referring to a large poster-size letter *t*). Turtle wants to find a friend that starts with /t/." The clinician asks the children to name other soft toys such as *teddy, mouse,* and *seal* and helps the children find the toy that starts with /t/.
Teaching hint	Choose toys whose names have wide initial phoneme contrasts, and encourage the children to look at the clinician's mouth as he or she articulates the word carefully, or to "feel" the first phoneme as they articulate the words.
Activity 2	Find pictures or toy objects that start with a target sound with the assistance of a puppet.
	"Here is the letter *m*; it makes an /m/ sound (large poster-size letter of an *m*). Can you help me make the /m/ sound? My friend, 'Munching Monkey' is going to eat the pictures that start with an /m/ sound. Let's help him find the pictures that start with an /m/ sound."
	At the end of the activity, place all the pictures that start with an /m/ sound beside the letter *m* for review. "Listen to all these pictures that start with an /m/ sound: *meat, milk, man, mouse.*"
Teaching hint	Choose pictures with wide initial sound contrasts, and place pictures out in pairs for the child to select the one that starts with the target sound (e.g., *meat/corn, mouse/dog, milk/soda*). These pictures can be used for other language goals such as semantic category (e.g., find all the animals, food, or drinks).
Key component	Phoneme awareness: phoneme isolation
	Speech-to-print matching
Aim	To bring the child's attention to the initial phoneme in a word and to recognize the grapheme associated with the phoneme
Activity	Selecting toy objects or picture cards from a mystery bag
	"Let's see what you can find in the mystery bag. (Child selects an object). Tell me what you've found. Yes, you've found a car in the mystery bag. (Encourage the child to articulate the word correctly as appropriate to speech production goals). *Car* starts with a /k/ sound and this letter can make a /k/ sound. (pointing to a large poster-size letter *c*). Drive the car to the letter *c*" (child has a choice of *c* or *m*).
Teaching hint	Place toys or picture cards of objects into the mystery bag that start with one of only two phonemes that are represented by letters that are visually distinct (e.g., *m* and *c*). Write the letters in very large print on poster-size cardboard.
Key component	Introduction to the alphabetic principle
Aim	To bring children's attention to the connections between an alphabetic letter, its letter name, and the sound(s) we commonly associate with the letter
Activity	Use of computer software
	Computer software, designed for young children, that teaches the alphabet letters and speech-to-print concepts can provide a novel activity. For example, The "Owl's Word Shop" activity from Winnie the Pooh Kindergarten (Disney Interactive, 1999) teaches children to identify words that start with a target grapheme and phoneme.
Teaching hint	With the use of a small data projector in a group therapy session, the clinician can project the computer image (e.g., Winnie the Pooh characters) onto a blank wall and engage children in running up to touch the target words or letters. Dimming the lights in the therapy room to ensure a strong projected image on the wall helps to capture young children's attention and focuses them on the projected computer image. The clinician can use the mute sound button on the computer to teach an activity at a slower pace or reinforce ideas presented by the computer image.

A variety of game activities that involve children's active participation should be planned. The activities need to provide the maximal opportunities to achieve a target goal in a short period of time (e.g., a 5- or 10-minute period) but ensure the child's interest and enjoyment in the activity are maintained. Young children often enjoy the familiarity of known activities. Structuring sessions to reintroduce favorite activities in a similar sequence during each session may help manage young children's behavior and cooperation.

Research has not established that it is necessary to master one level of phonological awareness before developing skills in another. Thus a vertical approach to implementation, such as teaching syllable awareness to 90% success before introducing onset-rime awareness, and in turn teaching these skills to 90% success before introducing early developing phoneme awareness tasks, does not seem justified. Such a method for young children with speech and language impairment is likely to require lengthy periods of intervention. If the goal of phonological awareness intervention during this preschool period is to ensure that children are developing the skills they require for word decoding when they approach literacy instruction, then exposure to a range of early-developing phonological awareness skills is important.

Different phonological awareness goals may be implemented in a variety of learning environments simultaneously. For example, if an SLP is working collaboratively with early child care teachers and the child's parents, the goal of improving the child's rhyme knowledge may be implemented in the home or preschool context. Reciting nursery rhymes, chanting stories and poems to a rhythmic beat, reading rhyming stories, and playing rhyming games are fun activities that preschool teachers and parents may readily engage in with the child (or training to develop the parents' skills in these activities can be provided). Early child care centers often include rhyming activities in their early education programs. Thus, ensuring that children with spoken language impairment actively participate in these activities may be an important goal in the child care setting.

Whereas parents and childcare workers focus on developing syllable and rhyme knowledge, an SLP may focus on stimulating the emergence of early phoneme awareness during individual or group intervention sessions. This level of phonological awareness is likely to require more structured scaffolding techniques, prompting, and adapting to ensure learning success in young children. The next section describes how task difficulty can be adapted to suit an individual child's needs.

Adapting Phonological Awareness Task Difficulty

It is important for an SLP or early intervention teacher to understand how to adjust the difficulty level of phonological awareness tasks. Table 12.2 (adapted from Gillon, 2004) focuses specifically on activities suitable for preschool children with spoken language impairments. Examples of how stimulus items can be integrated into other speech and language activities are also provided.

Table 12.2. Examples for adjusting difficulty level and task integration

Phonological awareness level	Easier level	More challenging level	Example of integration with other speech/language goals
Syllable awareness	Segmenting two-syllable familiar words: e.g., *teddy,* ted-dy	Segmenting three- and four-syllable familiar words: e.g., *elephant*	Correct articulation of medial consonants in words
	Clapping simple sentences in a rhythmic pattern based on syllabic structure: e.g., "He is walking" = 4 claps	Increasing sentence length or introducing words with three syllables	Correct production of target sentence structures
Onset-rime awareness	Rhyme recognition: e.g., "Do these words rhyme? *car, tar.*"	Odd one out: e.g., "Which one does not rhyme?"	Engage child in shared book reading using a story with rhyming words.
	Blending and segmenting at onset-rime level with picture cues: e.g., c- at = cat (choice of *cat* or *car*)	Blending and segmenting words without picture prompts	Select words to segment and blend from a favorite story that has been read to the child.
Phoneme awareness			
Phoneme identity	Identifying phonemes in the initial position of single-syllable familiar words: e.g., "*Sun* starts with /s/"	Odd one out: e.g., "Let's find the word that starts with a different sound (two- and three-phoneme words): *car, key, core, mat.*"	Use words in the phoneme identity tasks from vocabulary extension work. Select target phonemes associated with speech production goals.
Phoneme matching	Matching words with a target phoneme using pictures and words with wide sound contrasts: e.g., "Find the picture that starts with /s/: *sea, car.*"	Stimulus words containing three or more phonemes: e.g., "Help me find the word that starts with /d/: *man, sock, dog.*"	Use the target words as conversational or narrative topics: e.g., "Do you have a *dog*? Tell me about your *dog.*"
Phoneme isolation	Articulate the first sound in words with consonant-vowel structure: e.g., "Tell me the first sound in *four.*"	Articulate the first sound in a range of words with two and three phonemes.	Select words for phoneme isolation games that are target words for the child's speech production practice.
Grapheme–phoneme	Identify the named letter from a choice of two or three letters: e.g., "Throw the bean bag onto the letter s." (Large poster-size letters of *s* and *m* are placed on the floor.)	Name a letter from a small group of trained letters: e.g., child blows some bubbles and says the name of the letter the bubbles land on.	Teach letter names and sounds associated with speech production targets. Use alphabet books to extend vocabulary.

Source: Gillon, 2004.

ASSESSMENT METHODS TO SUPPORT ONGOING DECISION MAKING

Evaluation of phonological awareness intervention at 3 and 4 years of age must be seen in context with the child's primary speech and language goals and in context with typical development. It would be unrealistic to expect phonological awareness intervention at this age to result in a child with very limited awareness of sound structure in words to master a range of phoneme level tasks within a short period of time (as we may expect with older children already engaged in literacy instruction). In children with typical development, these skills are only beginning to emerge at 3 and 4 years of age. What must be determined is whether these skills are also emerging in children with speech and language impairment as a result of the intervention. Short assessment probes are valuable to ensure that the specific skills (e.g., see Tables 12.1 and 12.2) targeted are being acquired and transferring to novel test items. Records also should be kept concerning the level of prompting or scaffolding required to complete a task successfully. Parental and preschool teacher observations and anecdotal assessments of the child's ability to engage in syllable, rhyme, and early phoneme awareness games also provide valuable data in evaluating the effectiveness of the intervention to enhance phonological awareness knowledge.

Ongoing monitoring of the phonological awareness development of children with spoken language impairment in relation to their emerging literacy skills is essential. Formal evaluation of phonological awareness skills prior to starting school and following 6 months and 12 months of schooling is recommended. A preventive model of phonological awareness intervention can only be considered successful if the skills taught transfer to early word recognition and spelling development. If a child makes the expected progress with grade 1 classroom reading and spelling instruction and shows evidence that he or she can efficiently use phonological cues in the reading and spelling process, then further phonological awareness intervention may not be required. In contrast, if children with speech and language impairment struggle with early reading and spelling and are not developing more complex phoneme awareness in response to classroom literacy instruction, then small-group or individual intervention directly aimed at enhancing phoneme awareness and knowledge of phoneme grapheme relationships should be implemented (Gillon, 2000, 2002).

CHILDREN FROM CULTURALLY AND LINGUISTICALLY DIVERSE BACKGROUNDS

The development of phonological awareness is not strictly language specific. Rather, the cognitive processes involved in developing an awareness of the sound structure of words in one alphabetic language can be applied to other alphabetic languages the child acquires (Comeau, Cormier, Grandmaison, &

Lacroix, 1999). Bilingual children who learn English as their second language after previous exposure to an alphabetic written language are able to demonstrate phonological awareness skills in both languages after a relatively short period of learning English (Chiappe & Siegel, 1999). Children can also display comparable phonological awareness skills across two languages such as English and French (Comeau et al., 1999). Language experiences, however, may influence some aspects of phonological awareness such as the use of phonological knowledge in reading and spelling (Holm & Dodd, 1996).

Based on this evidence, for children who are learning two or more alphabetic languages, clinicians may consider targeting phonological awareness in the differing languages. For example, the child's parents and family may be encouraged to develop the child's rhyme awareness and bring the child's attention to beginning sounds in words in the language spoken in the home environment. If English is the language of instruction in preschool or speech-language pathology intervention sessions (and the teachers and SLPs have some vocabulary knowledge of the child's first language), then words from both languages may be used as stimulus targets for phoneme awareness activities.

APPLICATION TO AN INDIVIDUAL CHILD

A case example of a child who participated in an early intervention study (Gillon, 2005) is presented to provide insights into the potential benefits of a preventive framework for phonological awareness intervention. The child, Joe, was 3 years of age when first assessed for the study. He presented with severe speech disorder. Phonological assessment revealed only 4% consonants correct in single-word elicitation. His speech attempts were characterized by nasalized vowel productions with only [h, n,] and [m] consonants used in his spontaneous speech. He used gesturing and speech attempts with appropriate intonation patterns in attempting to communicate his needs. His anterior nose, oral cavity, oropharynx, and palate were all normal. Examination of oral motor functioning revealed some weaknesses in volitional tongue movements, but no major fine motor or physical abnormalities were evident. In addition to his severe speech disorder, factors placing Joe at risk for later literacy difficulties included familial history of speech difficulties and hearing difficulties. (Joe had a low-frequency conductive hearing loss in his left ear and normal hearing in the right ear.) Positive prognostic signs for literacy development and progress in intervention included average intellectual and receptive language abilities (low-average range), appropriate pragmatic language skills such as appropriate eye contact and play interactions, cooperative behavior, and a supportive home environment; apart from issues with hearing, including lengthy waiting periods for pressure-equalization tube insertion, Joe presented with no other health problems.

Following assessment and establishment of stable baselines on assessment probe tasks (see below), Joe received 8 weeks of therapy between the ages of 3 years, 2 months and 3 years, 5 months. This involved one group session per week for 45 minutes with two other 3-year-old children and one individual 45-minute session per week. A qualified SLP administered the therapy at a university clinic and a sound-field system was used in all group sessions to provide optimal listening conditions. The first 4 weeks focused on improving speech production only, and the second 4 weeks continued to focus on improving speech production but introduced letter-name training and phonological awareness intervention focused at the initial phoneme level (phoneme identity, phoneme matching, phoneme categorization). Rhyme and syllable awareness were not directly targeted in the therapy sessions, but Joe was exposed to rhyming activities in the home environment.

Assessment probe data using colorful pictures for a rhyme oddity task ("Which word doesn't rhyme: *pig, hat, bat?*") and a phoneme matching task (target /m/ for mouse: "Which word starts with /m/: *doll, milk, bear?*") were collected to monitor phonological awareness development and transfer of skills from therapy activities at the phoneme level to novel tasks with untrained stimulus items. Letter recognition assessment probe data assessed a group of letters including letters in his name and some speech production targets (*b, f, m, h, k, j, c, v, g, l, t, s*). Joe was required to point to the letter named by the examiner. Figures 12.1 and 12.2 show the results of the probe assessments. Figure 12.1 suggests that phase 2 of treatment, during which phoneme and letter knowledge were introduced, had a positive effect in stimulating the skills being targeted (i.e., early phoneme awareness). Observational record keeping and intervention data collected indicated that Joe progressed well during clinical sessions on the phoneme identity tasks. Transfer of skills to untrained tasks was not clearly established, however, during this first block of therapy. Figure 12.2 shows that Joe was able to rapidly learn the names of the letters presented during the intervention sessions.

Joe received two further blocks of therapy (commencing at ages 3 years, 8 months and 4 years, 5 months) before starting school at 5 years of age. Each block consisted of the same model of two sessions per week, one group session and one individual session, for a 6-week period. The aim of these therapy blocks focused on improving speech intelligibility (using a cycles approach to therapy; Hodson & Paden, 1991), and all of these therapy sessions included structured phoneme awareness intervention involving phoneme categorization, phoneme identity, phoneme isolation, and phoneme matching; segmentation at the onset-rime level, and letter-name and letter-sound knowledge training. From 4 years of age, the PIPA (Dodd et al., 2000) was introduced as a formal measure of phonological awareness development in addition to assessment probe data and observational record keeping. The PIPA was administered at approximately 8-month intervals until Joe was 6 years

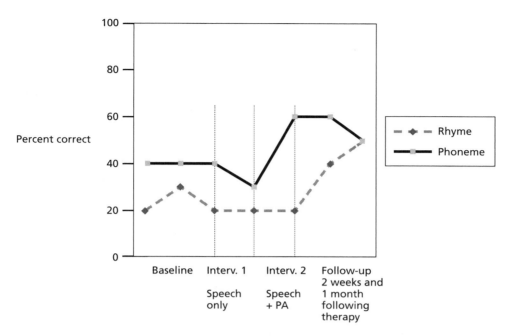

Figure 12.1. Transfer of skills to novel stimulus items and task type. Assessment probes data for rhyme and phoneme matching tasks.

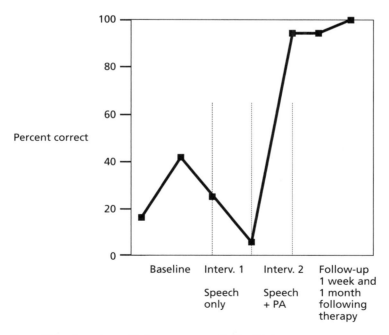

Figure 12.2. Percentage of letter names correctly identified.

of age. The percentage correct on the PIPA tasks of rhyme awareness ("Which one doesn't belong: *wall, fall, ball, cat*?"), phoneme awareness ("Which one doesn't belong: *duck, door, dog, cake*?"), phoneme isolation ("Tell me the first sound in *ball*"), and syllable awareness of unfamiliar words ("Tap out the parts to *originator*") were calculated and the percentage correct scores are shown in Figure 12.3. A period of rapid development in phonological awareness coincided with the third block of intervention provided. Joe started school at 5 years with age-appropriate rhyme and syllable awareness and showed particular strength in phoneme awareness. Joe's speech production steadily improved over time, although he started school with a moderate speech difficulty. Percent consonants correct scores from 75 words elicited in isolation are shown in Table 12.3.

Joe made rapid progress in early reading and spelling development during his first year at school. Teachers remarked on his strength in reading. At 6 years of age, Joe's reading development was assessed as well above average for both word recognition and reading comprehension. Joe's progress was in sharp contrast to a control group of 11 children with specific speech impairment who did not receive phonological awareness intervention in their preschool speech intervention (Gillon, 2005). The majority of these children showed delayed development in early reading skills and were identified as needing remedial reading programs at 6 years of age.

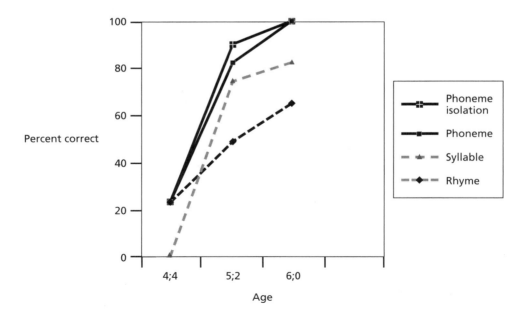

Figure 12.3. Growth over time in phoneme syllable and rhyme awareness as indicated by performance on the Preschool and Primary Inventory of Phonological Awareness (PIPA; Dodd et al., 2000).

Table 12.3. Percentage of consonants correctly articulated (PCC) at each assessment trial

Age of assessment	PCC
3;01	3
3;08	38
3;11	54
5;02 (school entry)	71
6;0	89

FUTURE DIRECTIONS

The prevention of reading difficulty for any young child identified as being at risk is indeed an important and valuable pursuit. Evidence demonstrating the negative spiralling effects of early reading failure (Stanovich, 1986) demands that continued research and resources are focused toward preventive interventions. It is critical to conduct further research into methods that are both efficient and effective in ensuring young children begin their school life with knowledge and skills necessary for success in literacy experiences. Understanding the interactions between phonological awareness development and speech and language development in the preschool years requires ongoing research. Understanding, for example, how phonological awareness intervention may positively influence a child's speech production through the development of more distinct underlying phonological representations is an important area for future study. Continued research efforts in identifying the effectiveness of differing intervention models, content structure, and implementation methods will enhance our knowledge of effective practices for ensuring that children reach their potential in both spoken and written language development. Programs that integrate phonological awareness interventions into management plans for children with speech and language impairments, particularly interventions that stimulate awareness that words are comprised of individual sounds and how these sounds may be represented in print, hold much promise.

RECOMMENDED READINGS

Catts, H., & Kamhi, A. (2005). *Language and reading disabilities* (2nd ed.). Upper Saddle River, NJ: Pearson Education.

Ehri, L.C., Nunes, S.R., Willows, D.M., Schuster, B.V., Yaghoub-Zadeh, Z., & Shanahan, T. (2001). Phonemic awareness instruction helps children learn to read: Evidence from the National Reading Panel's meta-analysis. *Reading Research Quarterly, 36*(3), 250–287.

Gillon, G. (2004). *Phonological awareness: From research to practice.* New York: Guilford Press.

Lonigan, C., Burgess, S., Anthony, J.L., & Barker, T.A. (1998). Development of phonological sensitivity in 2- to 5-year-old children. *Journal of Educational Psychology, 90*(2), 294–311.

REFERENCES

Anthony, J., & Lonigan, C. (2004). The nature of phonological awareness: Converging evidence from four studies of preschool and early grade school children. *Journal of Educational Psychology, 96*(1), 43–55.

Bird, J., Bishop, D., & Freeman, N. (1995). Phonological awareness and literacy development in children with expressive phonological impairments. *Journal of Speech and Hearing Research, 36,* 446–462.

Blachman, B., Ball, E., Black, R., & Tangel, D. (1994). Kindergarten teachers develop phoneme awareness in low-income, inner-city classrooms. *Reading and Writing: An Interdisciplinary Journal, 6,* 1–18.

Bryant, P., Bradley, L., MacLean, M., & Crossland, J. (1989). Nursery rhymes, phonological skills and reading. *Journal of Child Language, 16,* 407–428.

Burgess, S.R., & Lonigan, C.J. (1998). Bidirectional relations of phonological sensitivity and prereading abilities: Evidence from a preschool sample. *Journal of Experimental Child Psychology, 70*(2), 117–141.

Castle, J.M., Riach, J., & Nicholson, T. (1994). Getting off to a better start in reading and spelling: The effects of phonemic awareness instruction within a whole language program. *Journal of Educational Psychology, 86,* 350–359.

Catts, H., Fey, M., Zhang, X., & Tomblin, B. (2001). Estimating the risk of future reading difficulties in kindergarten children: A research-based model and its clinical implementation. *Language, Speech, and Hearing Services in Schools, 32,* 38–51.

Catts, H., & Kamhi, A. (2005). Defining reading disabilities. In H. Catts & A. Kamhi (Eds.), *Language and reading disabilities* (2nd ed., pp. 50–71). Upper Saddle River, NJ: Pearson Education.

Chiappe, P., & Siegel, L.S. (1999). Phonological awareness and reading acquisition in English- and Punjabi-speaking Canadian children. *Journal of Educational Psychology, 91*(1), 20–28.

Coltheart, M. (1978). Lexical access in simple reading tasks. In G. Underwood (Ed.), *Strategies of information processing* (pp. 151–216). London: Academic Press.

Comeau, L., Cormier, P., Grandmaison, E., & Lacroix, D. (1999). A longitudinal study of phonological processing skills in children learning to read in a second language. *Journal of Educational Psychology, 91*(1), 29–43.

Cossu, G., Shankweiler, D., Liberman, I., Katz, L., & Tola, G. (1988). Awareness of phonological segments and reading ability in Italian children. *Applied Psycholinguistics, 9,* 1–16.

Denton, C.A., Hasbrouck, J.E., Weaver, L.R., & Riccio, C.A. (2000). What do we know about phonological awareness in Spanish? *Reading Psychology, 21*(4), 335–352.

Disney Interactive. (1999). Winnie the Pooh Kindergarten: Owl's Word Shop [Computer software]. Burbank, CA: Author.

Dodd, B., Crosbie, S., MacIntosh, B., Teitzel, T., & Ozanne, A. (2000). *Preschool and Primary Inventory of Phonological Awareness (PIPA).* London: Psychological Corporation.

Duncan, L.G., & Johnston, R.S. (1999). How does phonological awareness relate to nonword reading amongst poor readers? *Reading and Writing: An Interdisciplinary Journal, 11,* 405–439.

Ehri, L. (1992). Reconceptualizing the development of sight word reading and its relationship to recoding. In L. Gough & R. Treiman (Eds.), *Reading acquisition.* Hillsdale, NJ: Lawrence Erlbaum Associates.

Ehri, L.C., Nunes, S.R., Willows, D.M., Schuster, B.V., Yaghoub-Zadeh, Z., & Shanahan, T. (2001). Phonemic awareness instruction helps children learn to read: Evidence from the National Reading Panel's meta-analysis. *Reading Research Quarterly, 36*(3), 250–287.

Elbro, C., Borstrom, I., & Petersen, D.K. (1998). Predicting dyslexia from kindergarten: The importance of distinctness of phonological representations of lexical items. *Reading Research Quarterly, 33*(1), 36–60.

Fey, M.E., Catts, H.W., & Larrivee, L.S. (1995). Preparing preschoolers for the academic and social challenges of school. In S.F. Warren & J. Reichle (Series Eds.) & M.E. Fey, J. Windsor, & S.F. Warren (Vol. Eds.), *Communication and language intervention series: Vol. 5. Language intervention: Preschool through the elementary years* (pp. 3–37). Baltimore: Paul H. Brookes Publishing Co.

Gillon, G. (2000). The efficacy of phonological awareness intervention for children with spoken language impairment. *Language, Speech, and Hearing Services in Schools, 31,* 126–141.

Gillon, G. (2002). Follow-up study investigating benefits of phonological awareness intervention for children with spoken language impairment. *International Journal of Language and Communication Disorders, 37*(4), 381–400.

Gillon, G. (2004). *Phonological awareness: From research to practice.* New York: Guilford Press.

Gillon, G. (2005). Facilitating phoneme awareness development in 3- and 4-year-old children with speech impairment. *Language, Speech, and Hearing Services in Schools, 36,* 308–324.

Gillon, G., & Dodd, B. (1995). The effects of training phonological, semantic and syntactic processing skills in spoken language on reading ability. *Language, Speech, and Hearing Services in Schools, 26,* 58–68.

Gillon, G., & Dodd, B. (1997). Enhancing the phonological processing skills of children with specific reading disability. *European Journal of Disorders of Communication, 32,* 67–90.

Goswami, U., & Bryant, P. (1992). Rhyme, analogy, and children's reading. In L. Gough, L. Ehri, & R. Treiman (Eds.), *Reading acquisition* (pp. 49–63). Hillsdale, NJ: Lawrence Erlbaum Associates.

Hodson, B., & Paden, E. (1991). *A phonological approach to targeting intelligible speech* (2nd ed.). Austin, TX: PRO-ED.

Holm, A., & Dodd, B. (1996). The effect of first written language on the acquisition of literacy. *Cognition, 59,* 119–147.

Invernizzi, M., Sullivan, A., & Meier, J. (2002). *PALS-PreK Phonological Awareness Literacy Screening.* Charlottesville, VA: The Virginia State Department of Education, The University of Virginia.

Johnston, R.S., Anderson, M., & Holligan, C. (1996). Knowledge of the alphabet and explicit awareness of phonemes in pre-readers: The nature of the relationship. *Reading and Writing: An Interdisciplinary Journal, 8*(3), 217–234.

Korkman, K., & Peltomma, A. (1993). Preventative treatment of dyslexia by a preschool training program for children with language impairments. *Journal of Clinical Child Psychology, 22,* 227–287.

Larrivee, L., & Catts, H. (1999). Early reading achievement in children with expressive phonological disorders. *American Journal of Speech-Language Pathology, 8,* 137–148.

Liberman, I.Y., Shankweiler, D., & Liberman, A.M. (1989). The alphabetic principle and learning to read. In D. Shankweiler & I.Y. Liberman (Eds.), *Phonology and reading disability: Solving the reading puzzle* (Research Monograph Series). Ann Arbor, MI: University of Michigan Press.

Lonigan, C., Burgess, S., Anthony, J.L., & Barker, T.A. (1998). Development of phonological sensitivity in 2- to 5-year-old children. *Journal of Educational Psychology, 90*(2), 294–311.

Lovett, M.W., Borden, S., Deluca, T., Lacerenza, L., Benson, N., & Brackstone, D. (1994). Treating the core deficits of developmental dyslexia: Evidence of transfer of learning after phonologically- and strategy-based reading training programs. *Developmental Psychology, 30,* 805–822.

Lovett, M., Steinbach, K., & Frijters, J. (2000). Remediating the core deficits of developmental reading disability: A double deficit hypothesis. *Journal of Learning Disabilities, 33,* 334–358.

Lundberg, I., Olofsson, A., & Wall, S. (1980). Reading and spelling skills in the first years predicted from phonemic awareness skills in kindergarten. *Scandinavian Journal of Psychology, 21,* 159–173.

MacLean, M., Bryant, P., & Bradley, L. (1987). Rhymes, nursery rhymes, and reading in early childhood. *Merrill-Palmer Quarterly, 33,* 255–281.

Major, E.M., & Bernhardt, B.H. (1998). Metaphonological skills of children with phonological disorders before and after phonological and metaphonological intervention. *International Journal of Language & Communication Disorders, 33*(4), 413–444.

Metsala, J.L. (1999). Young children's phonological awareness and nonword repetition as a function of vocabulary development. *Journal of Educational Psychology, 91*(1), 3–19.

Muter, V., Hulme, C., & Snowling, M. (1997). *Phonological Abilities Test.* London: Psychological Corporation.

O'Connor, R., Jenkins, J., Leicester, N., & Slocum, T. (1993). Teaching phonological awareness to young children with learning disabilities. *Exceptional Children, 59,* 532–546

Paul, R. (2001). *Language disorders from infancy through adolescence.* St. Louis: Mosby.

Perfetti, C.A., Beck, I., Ball, L.C., & Hughes, C. (1987). Phonemic knowledge and learning to read are reciprocal: A longitudinal study of first grade children. *Merrill-Palmer Quarterly, 33,* 283–319.

Read, C., Zhang, Y., Nie, H., & Ding, B. (1986). The ability to manipulate speech sounds depends on knowing alphabetic writing. *Cognition, 24,* 31–44.

Rumelhart, D. (1977). Toward an interactive model of reading. In S. Dornic (Ed.), *Attention and performance V1* (pp. 573–603). Hillsdale, NJ: Lawrence Erlbaum Associates.

Rvachew, S., Ohberg, A., Grawburg, M., & Heyding, J. (2003). Phonological awareness and phonemic perception in 4-year-old children with delayed expressive phonology skills. *Language, Speech, and Hearing Services in Schools, 12,* 463–471.

Scarborough, H. (1998). Early identification of children at risk for reading disabilities: Phonological awareness and some other promising predictors. In B.K. Shapiro, P.J. Accardo, & A.J. Capute (Eds.), *Specific reading disabilities: A view of the spectrum* (pp. 75–119). Timonium, MD: York Press.

Schatschneider, C., Francis, D.J., Foorman, B.R., Fletcher, J.M., & Mehta, P. (1999). The dimensionality of phonological awareness: An application of item response theory. *Journal of Educational Psychology, 91*(3), 439–449.

Seidenberg, M., & McClelland, J. (1989). A distributed, developmental model of word recognition and naming. *Psychological Review, 96,* 523–568.

Share, D. (1995). Phonological recoding and self-teaching: Sine qua non of reading acquisition. *Cognition, 55,* 151–218.

Snowling, M., Bishop, D.V.M., & Stothard, S.E. (2000). Is preschool language impairment a risk factor for dyslexia in adolescence? *Journal of Child Psychology and Psychiatry and Allied Disciplines, 41*(5), 587–600.

Stanovich, K.E. (1985). Explaining the variance in reading ability in terms of psychological processes. What have we learned? *Annals of Dyslexia, 35,* 67–69.

Stanovich, K.E. (1986). Matthew effects in reading: Some consequences of individual differences in the acquisition of literacy. *Reading Research Quarterly, 21,* 360–407.

Stanovich, K.E. (1991b). Word recognition: Changing perspectives. In R. Barr, M. Kamil, P. Mosenthal, & P. Pearson (Eds.), *Handbook of reading research, Vol. 2* (pp. 418–452). New York: Longman.

Stanovich, K.E. (2000). *Progress in understanding reading: Scientific foundations and new frontiers*. New York: Guilford Press.

Stanovich, K.E., Cunningham, A., & Cramer, B. (1984). Assessing phonological awareness in kindergarten children: Issues of task comparability. *Journal of Experimental Child Psychology, 38,* 175–190.

Stothard, S.E., Snowling, M.J., Bishop, D.V.M., Chipchase, B.B., & Kaplan, C.A. (1998). Language-impaired preschoolers: A follow-up into adolescence. *Journal of Speech, Language, and Hearing Research, 41*(2), 407–418.

Stuart, M. (1995). Prediction and qualitative assessment of five-and six-year-old children's reading: A longitudinal study. *British Journal of Educational Psychology, 65,* 287–296.

Swan, D., & Goswami, U. (1997). Phonological awareness deficits in developmental dyslexia and the phonological representations hypothesis. *Journal of Experimental Child Psychology, 66*(1), 18–41.

Torgesen, J., Wagner, R., Rashotte, C., Lindamood, P., Rose, E., Conway, T., & Garvan, C. (1999). Preventing reading failure in young children with phonological processing disabilities: Group and individual responses to instruction. *Journal of Educational Psychology, 91,* 579–593.

Treiman, R., & Bourassa, D.C. (2000). The development of spelling skill. *Topics in Language Disorders, 20*(3), 1–18.

Treiman, R., & Zukowsky, A. (1991). Levels of phonological awareness. In S.A. Brady & D.P. Shankweiler (Eds.), *Phonological processes in literacy: A tribute to Isabelle Y. Liberman* (pp. 67–83). Hillsdale, NJ: Lawrence Erlbaum Associates.

van Kleeck, A., Gillam, R., & McFadden, T. (1998). A study of classroom-based phonological awareness training for preschoolers with speech and/or language disorders. *American Journal of Speech-Language Pathology, 7*(3), 65–76.

Warrick, N., Rubin, H., & Rowe-Walsh, S. (1993). Phoneme awareness in language delayed children: Comparative studies and intervention. *Annals of Dyslexia, 43,* 153–173.

Webster, P., Plante, A., & Couvillion, L. (1997). Phonologic impairment and pre-reading: Update on a longitudinal study. *Journal of Learning Disabilities, 30,* 365–375.

Westby, C. (2005). Assessing and remediating text comprehension problems. In H. Catts & A. Kamhi (Eds.), *Language and reading disabilities* (2nd ed., pp. 157–232). Upper Saddle River, NJ: Pearson Education.

13

Balanced Reading Intervention and Assessment in Augmentative Communication

KAREN A. ERICKSON, DAVID A. KOPPENHAVER, AND JAMES W. CUNNINGHAM

ABSTRACT

The purpose of this chapter is to demonstrate how the techniques of a conventional reading instructional approach can be modified for children with severe speech and physical impairments (SSPIs). No single reading program addresses the needs of all readers, particularly those as individually different as children with SSPIs. Instead, successful reading intervention carefully considers the student's instructional needs, skills, and experiences. In this chapter, we will use the whole-to-part model (WTP) of silent reading comprehension (Cunningham, 1993) as a basis for a balanced approach to reading intervention. We will describe specific approaches that meet the needs of students who use augmentative and alternative communication (AAC) and have successfully developed understandings of concepts about print, the alphabetic principle, phonological awareness, and oral language.

TARGET POPULATIONS AND ASSESSMENTS FOR DETERMINING TREATMENT RELEVANCE AND GOALS

The learners to be addressed specifically in this chapter are students with SSPIs who use AAC. SSPI refers to "individuals who have a severe speech problem that is due primarily to physical, neuromuscular, cognitive, or emotional deficits and not to hearing impairment, and who cannot, at the present time, use speech independently as their primary means of communication . . . [and who also have] congenital or acquired motor impairment[s] which may also impair speech, nonverbal communication, and writing as a result of problems with muscle tone, posture, and involuntary movements" (Koppenhaver & Yoder, 1992, p. 157). As a subset of individuals with developmental disabilities (DD), individuals with SSPIs have impairments that manifest before age 22, are likely to persist, require special types of intervention, and result in

functional limitations in language, learning, self-direction, independent living, and employment (Developmental Disabilities Assistance and Bill of Rights
Act of 2000, PL 106-402). Within the population of students with SSPIs who
use AAC, 70%–90% lag significantly behind peers without disabilities in their
literacy learning, even when intelligence is controlled for statistically (Koppenhaver & Yoder, 1992). These difficulties appear to persist across the life span.
For example, 79% of adults with varying degrees of speech impairment and
74% of adults with varying degrees of physical impairment perform at the
lowest levels on national surveys, and less than 1% of either population reads
at the most sophisticated survey task levels (Kirsch, Jungeblut, Jenkins, &
Kolstad, 1993). At the same time, however, there are highly literate university graduates who use AAC, and there is a growing body of evidence suggesting that even individuals who use AAC and have concomitant language and
cognitive impairments can be taught to read and write (e.g., Blischak, 1995;
Erickson & Koppenhaver, 1998; Erickson, Koppenhaver, Yoder, & Nance, 1997;
Gipe, Duffy, & Richards, 1993; Koppenhaver, Evans, & Yoder, 1991). Across
these success stories, effective instructional strategies consistently have been
based on best practices in general education, with accommodations that make
these practices accessible, interactive, and intensive (e.g., Cousin, Weekly,
& Gerard, 1993; Erickson & Koppenhaver, 1995; Erickson et al., 1997; Gipe
et al., 1993; Mike, 1995; Worthy & Invernizzi, 1995).

Likewise, the balanced intervention described in this chapter derives
from best practice in general education (Cunningham, 1999; Cunningham &
Allington, 2003). The intervention is balanced in three ways. First, it is balanced in combining four distinct approaches to reading instruction emphasizing instruction in phonics and sight words, reading comprehension, writing, and self-direction in reading. Second, it is balanced in addressing all of
the principal cognitive processes necessary for successful silent reading with
comprehension to be described below. Third, it is balanced in being both
teacher and student centered. Teachers control selection of materials and
activities to support student learning of phonics, words, and reading with
comprehension. Students control selection of writing topics, content, and
forms as well as materials in self-directed reading.

Balanced intervention is appropriately employed as a beginning reading
approach at any time in the life span. Although there is no clear line of de-
marcation, an important distinction must be made here between emergent
literacy and beginning reading. Emergent literacy interventions are designed
to provide learners with a wide range of oral and written language experiences to increase their awareness of print forms, uses, and content. Beginning reading programs are designed to move children from awareness to independent use of written language for their own personal and interactive
purposes. The strategies described in this chapter are inappropriate before
first grade. During preschool and kindergarten, children should be provided
with a language- and print-rich learning environment that focuses on build-

ing interaction, communication, and language skills (IRA/NAEYC, 1998). As children come to value written language and see themselves as learners, they also establish a solid foundation in oral language, concepts about print, the alphabetic principle, and phonological awareness necessary for success with formal beginning reading instruction (Adams, 1990). Although the evidence regarding the development of these emergent literacy understandings for individuals who use AAC is limited and mixed, it does suggest that this same foundation is important (Dahlgren Sandberg & Hjelmquist, 1996; Vandervelden & Siegel, 1999) and can be promoted (Gillon et al., 2003; Koppenhaver & Erickson, 2003; Skotko, Koppenhaver, & Erickson, 2004). There is no upper age limit for implementation of this approach. Balanced intervention success has been reported in students with SSPIs in upper elementary grades (Blischak, 1995; Erickson et al., 1997), high school (Hogan & Wolf, 2002; Wershing & Hughes, 2002), and adulthood (Gipe et al., 1993).

Although the need for language- and print-rich learning environments is recognized most readily for young, typically developing children, it is no less critical to any student who has yet to be provided sufficient opportunities to develop foundational understandings and skills. There is no defined set of prerequisite skills that must be mastered; however, several informal measures can be used to determine whether a student has had sufficient emergent literacy learning opportunities (for a complete discussion, see Erickson, 2000). No standardized measures or formal criteria are available that are specific to individuals who use AAC. Informally, it is useful to measure students' developing skills and understandings of 1) concepts about print (e.g., knowledge of book orientation, left-to-right, top-to-bottom nature of English print, one-to-one correspondence between the written and spoken word); 2) letter identification; 3) word generation (i.e., numbers of words student can spell independently given 10 minutes); 4) phonological and phonemic awareness (i.e., ability to hear and manipulate words and individual phonemes within words); and 5) receptive language (i.e., background knowledge and experiences). Measures of developing skills in these areas provide an important means to monitor the individual student's growing understandings and to ensure that opportunities for learning are provided across these areas so that conventional intervention can be initiated with greater confidence.

THEORETICAL BASIS

The whole-to-part model of the constructs underlying silent reading comprehension (Cunningham, 1993) serves as the theoretical basis for the approaches described in this chapter. The whole-to-part (WTP) model begins with the assertion that reading comprehension requires word identification, language comprehension, and whole-text print processing (e.g., sentences, paragraphs, pages). Each of these integrated abilities is part of silent read-

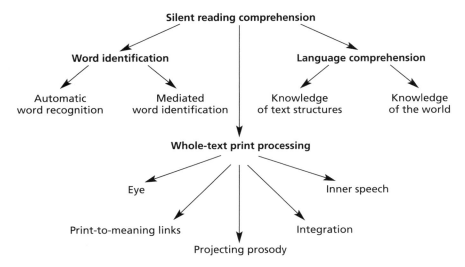

Figure 13.1. Model of the constructs underlying the whole-to-part model of silent reading comprehension.

ing comprehension ability, yet each is an ability that can be considered an independent whole that also is composed of its own parts. Each of these integrated abilities, presented in Figure 13.1, will be discussed in more detail in this chapter.

The overall ability represented in the model is silent reading comprehension. As the ultimate goal of reading intervention, successful silent reading comprehension is targeted by every strategy included in a comprehensive reading intervention program. In order to achieve the goal of reading silently with comprehension, each of the whole-parts must be addressed.

Word Identification

In silent reading comprehension, word identification is the cognitive process of making print-to-sound links in order to translate both familiar and unfamiliar printed words into pronunciations (Cunningham & Cunningham, 1978; Perfetti, Bell, & Delaney, 1988; Van Orden, Johnston, & Hale, 1988). Printed words may be turned into pronounced words vocally (during oral reading), subvocally (during silent reading), or neurologically (during silent reading without subvocalization). Word identification, the internal or external process of turning print into sound, helps readers use working memory to remember words and word order and assign prosody (Rayner & Pollatsek, 1989). Good readers pronounce almost every word they encounter when reading silently. Notable exceptions to this are described in the following section on whole-text print processing.

The WTP model assumes that word identification is necessary for and strongly related to silent reading comprehension ability (LaBerge & Samuels, 1974; Perfetti & Hogaboam, 1975; Perfetti & Lesgold, 1977). The WTP model also recognizes the relationship between phonological coding, a part of word identification, and silent reading comprehension (Garrity, 1977; Hardyck & Petrinovich, 1969, 1970; Hardyck, Petrinovich, & Ellsworth, 1966; Locke, 1971, 1978; McCutchen, Bell, France, & Perfetti, 1991; McGuigan, 1970, 1971; Slowiaczek & Clifton, 1980). Word identification is integral to silent reading comprehension.

Although the WTP model recognizes the relationship between word identification and silent reading comprehension, it does so with the assertion that word identification refers to reading words by print cues alone. Reading words through the use of context or context cues is not word identification; instead, it is an application of the language comprehension whole-part (described in the next section) that allows the reader or listener to fill in a missing word without identifying the individual word itself. In other words, context allows a reader to guess at a word based on knowledge of language rather than use of word identification strategies or skills. Word identification, or reading words by making print-to-sound links, can occur automatically or by mediation.

Automatic word recognition occurs when a reader accesses the phonological representation of a word effortlessly. The more words a reader can identify without conscious attention, the better silent reading will be (Daneman, 1991; Hogaboam & Perfetti, 1978; Levy, Abello, & Lysynchuk, 1997; Perfetti, Finger, & Hogaboam, 1978; Perfetti & Hogaboam, 1975; Stanovich, Cunningham, & Feeman, 1984). *Mediated word identification* involves decoding words and is depended on when a reader cannot identify a word with automaticity. Decoding typically involves accessing knowledge of letter–sound correspondences in order to form a phonological representation for a printed word (Daneman, 1991; Wagner & Torgesen, 1987). Decoding ability is associated with relative ease in learning to read words with automaticity (Cunningham, 1993; Share, 1999; Shepard & Uhry, 1997).

Language Comprehension

With respect to the WTP model, language comprehension is composed of two constructs: knowledge of the world and processing of text structures. It represents the crossover between an individual's ability to comprehend written language when listening and when reading. *Knowledge of the world* is defined as background knowledge or experience related to the topics assumed by a text's author. Readers must have this knowledge and be able to access it when needed in order for successful language comprehension to occur, either while listening or reading. Furthermore, comprehension through listening or reading requires access to knowledge of *text structures* including syntax, cohesion, conventions, and organizational or genre patterns. Without experience and familiarity with a variety of text structures, readers or listeners may not be able to process written language even if their knowledge of the world is such that one would anticipate success.

Whole-Text Print Processing

Everything that silent reading with comprehension requires beyond word identification and language comprehension is considered whole-text print processing. This whole-part is the component that makes the WTP model particularly appropriate as the theoretical basis for use with persons who use AAC. There are other models of silent reading comprehension that include both word identification and language comprehension as described earlier (e.g., Dreyer & Katz, 1992; Gough & Tunmer, 1986; Hoover & Gough, 1990), but these models provide insufficient explanations for the reading difficulties many AAC users experience. For example, many AAC users are able to learn to read words in isolation (i.e., *automatic or mediated word identification*) and can understand written language when others read it to them (i.e., *language comprehension including knowledge of the world and knowledge of text structures*), yet they are unable to independently read text with comprehension. This profile can be explained by the third whole-part of the WTP model, whole-text print processing. At least five parts compose the construct of whole-text print processing: 1) eye movement strategies, 2) inner speech use, 3) print-to-meaning links, 4) prosody projection, and 5) integration.

Eye Movement Strategies

The eye movements required for the processing of connected text in silent reading involve rapid, intermittent movements (i.e., saccades) with split-second fixations and metacognitively controlled regressions. The movements are not merely motoric or behavioral, and there is evidence that eye movement behavioral training does not improve reading comprehension (Rayner, 1985). In fact, training readers to make accurate and efficient eye movements is widely viewed as one way to make learning to read very difficult (Flippo, 1998). The eye movements required for mediated word identification (i.e., decoding of individual words in print) do not appear to be the same as those required for successful reading of connected text (Rayner & Pollatsek, 1989).

Inner Speech

The ability to phonologically recode words in silent reading requires the use of *inner speech.* Whether the reader is using inner speech to monitor comprehension or to mediate the identification of words, inner speech allows the reader to hold ideas in memory and integrate them across connected text (Daneman & Newson, 1992). When readers are reading silently and their inner speech is suppressed, it does not interfere with memory of individual words in the text, but it does inhibit the integration of ideas across the text (Daneman & Newson, 1992; Slowiaczek & Clifton, 1980).

Growing evidence suggests that individuals who use AAC have difficulty with inner speech. In particular, they are believed to have difficulty creating stable phonological representations, which could possibly explain why so many individuals who use AAC have difficulty when learning to read and write (Dahlgren Sandberg, 2001; Dahlgren Sandberg & Hjelmquist, 1996, 1997; Vandervelden & Siegel, 2001). Two studies with the same group of seven children with SSPIs were conducted 3 years apart. The children who used AAC in these studies had significantly more difficulty spelling and identifying words when given visual stimuli (i.e., photographs) than when given auditory stimuli (Dahlgren Sandberg, 2001). In the second study, for example, the subjects were able to correctly respond to 80% of the items when given auditory stimuli and to only 25% with visual stimuli. Similar results were achieved with a group of 32 students who used AAC (Vandervelden & Siegel, 1999). Despite these difficulties with phonological recoding and inner speech at beginning reading levels, there is evidence that AAC users can and do develop inner speech as they learn to read and can complete a variety of phonological and phonemic tasks that demonstrate their ability to form stable phonological representations over time (Dahlgren Sandberg, 2001; Foley, 1993; Foley & Pollatsek, 1999; Gillon et al., 2003).

Print-to-Meaning Links

As suggested above, good readers phonologically recode almost every word they encounter when reading silently. An exception occurs when readers encounter words they can identify automatically and go directly from print to meaning without first translating the print to sound. Skilled readers continue to access sound for low-frequency words when they are reading connected text, but they move directly from print to meaning for high-frequency words (Van Orden, 1991). As long as comprehension proceeds unimpeded, highly skilled readers rely on their ability to make direct print-to-meaning links while reading. As soon as comprehension breaks down or unfamiliar words are encountered, skilled readers revert to recoding of individual words to support successful text comprehension. Using a direct print-to-meaning link for some words during reading does not preclude using a parallel indirect print-to-sound-to-meaning link for most of the words.

Projecting Prosody

Reading with intonation and expression, whether done orally or subvocally, supports comprehension. The ability to attend to the structural aspects of the individual words and the words in whole texts supports a reader in holding information in memory long enough to comprehend beyond the individual sentence. Although reading with prosody is not sufficient to ensure comprehension of meaning (Koriat, Greenberg, & Kreiner, 2002), the ability to project prosody, as measured in oral reading, does correlate with more sophisticated levels of comprehension (Cowie, Douglas-Cowie, & Wichmann, 2002). In silent reading, prosody is projected via inner speech and is consequently difficult to measure directly.

Integration

The final process within whole-text print processing is integration. In order to read silently with comprehension, a reader must orchestrate all of these processes simultaneously while also identifying the individual words and attending to meaning through language comprehension.

Assumptions Underlying the Whole-to-Part Model as a Theoretical Basis

The WTP model provides a framework for understanding why intervention approaches that target specific skill areas (e.g., phonics, sight word learning, or literal-level comprehension) are insufficient as general reading intervention programs. The multiple whole-parts in the model support the assumption that successful reading intervention programs must be multifaceted and address the integration of all of the whole-parts represented in the WTP model. Furthermore, the model provides a more hopeful view of reading intervention for persons who use AAC by suggesting that no single explanation can account for all reading difficulties. It assumes that the cognitive processing involved in reading successfully with comprehension is the same for all readers but not that the instructional, assistive technology, or routes to success will be the same for all readers. That is, no narrowly focused intervention approach can possibly meet the needs of all learners, whether or not they use AAC.

Finally, successful application of the WTP model to reading intervention for AAC users assumes that participation and access barriers have been addressed. Students who use AAC often experience restrictions on their reading-related activity and participation that result from their functional limitations or teacher and caregiver assumptions about those limitations. For example, there is evidence to suggest that although most individuals who use AAC grow up in environments that may restrict literacy learning access and opportunities (e.g., Koppenhaver & Yoder, 1992; Light & Kelford Smith, 1993; Mike, 1995), those who grow up in supportive physical, social, and attitudinal environments are successful in learning to read (Koppenhaver et al., 1991). Such individuals are provided with frequent access to print-based experiences and are active participants in those experiences. So, while these individuals exhibit the same functional limitations as others who use AAC, they have fewer restrictions placed on their activities and participation which results in improved reading outcomes.

Children who use AAC begin to experience reading-related activity and participation restrictions when they are very young. They are less likely to engage in writing and drawing activities than peers without disabilities, less likely to be read with daily, and more likely to be relatively passive participants in storybook interactions (e.g., answering yes/no questions or pointing in response to "show me" directives rather than open-ended or child-initiated conversations) (Coleman, 1991; Light, Binger, & Kelford Smith, 1994; Light & Kelford Smith, 1993). Evidence continues to accumulate suggesting that reading outcomes for individuals who use AAC are less related to the severity of their disabilities (Berninger & Gans, 1986) than the nature of the activity and participation restrictions placed on them, especially those that affect literacy experiences (e.g., Coleman, 1991; Erickson et al., 1997; Koppenhaver & Yoder, 1992; Skotko et al., 2004).

For the reading instruction described in this chapter to be effective, the activity and participation restrictions that apply to reading experiences of people who use AAC must be removed. In the absence of opportunity to actively participate in appropriate reading instruction, the intervention cannot be successful. Numerous resources are available to support clinicians, educators, families, and individuals in their attempts to address the activity and participation restrictions that face many people who use AAC (see, e.g., Giangreco, Cloninger, & Iverson, 1998). The WTP model assumes that these restrictions have been addressed and specifically targets instruction in word identification, language comprehension, whole-text print processing, and all of the whole-parts that underlie them.

EMPIRICAL BASIS

The balanced intervention approach described in this chapter is consistent with balanced, mainstream, primary classroom approaches to beginning reading instruction (see, e.g., Au, Carroll, & Scheu, 2001; Cunningham & Allington, 2003; Pressley, 2002). One of the most widely known and researched classroom applications of a balanced approach is the Four Blocks® literacy framework (Cunningham, 1999; Cunningham & Hall, 1998a). The instruction in the Four Blocks is literally divided into four equal segments of time devoted to four distinct approaches to reading instruction: guided reading, working with words, self-selected reading, and writing. Similar to the balanced approach described in this chapter, the Four Blocks addresses all of the whole-parts in the WTP model. In a report of 8 years of evidence gathered from schools and school systems across the country, the authors of the Four Blocks approach report on the success of the balanced approach for children with a broad range of socioeconomic backgrounds and literacy levels (Cunningham, Hall, & Defee, 1998). Specifically, the authors report on results from two relatively large, suburban school systems (both reporting about 25% of students receiving free and reduced-cost lunch) and one small rural district (84% qualify for free or reduced-cost lunch) all in the southeast region of the United States. Data for the two suburban school systems were gathered through individual reading inventories, whereas the rural school used standardized measures. The schools generated all of the data as part of their typical schoolwide assessment procedures. Whether the schools compared the results of classrooms implementing the Four Blocks program with other reading instructional programs or compared children across years, the results consistently demonstrated higher scores for the groups receiving the balanced, Four Blocks instruction.

A number of empirical investigations have illustrated the usefulness of the Four Blocks balanced literacy approach under conditions that allowed for some level of experimental control but did not include students who use AAC. In a comparison of the Four Blocks and a basal reader approach across four classrooms housed in two separate schools, the Four Blocks approach resulted in superior results (Popplewell & Doty, 2001). Differences in subject performance on a pretest measure of instructional reading level were controlled using analysis of covariance. Univariate analysis of variance on posttest retelling and comprehension measures indicated that students in the Four Blocks school performed significantly higher than students in the basal reader school.

In Toronto, Canada, 480 children in kindergarten and first grade were followed longitudinally as their teachers implemented balanced literacy instruction that was modeled after the Four Blocks approach (French, Morgan, Vanayan, & White, 2001). Compared with normative data, the students demonstrated better than expected progress on seven of eight standardized measures.

In studies of other forms of balanced instruction, similar results have been found. In an intensive summer program for children who were struggling to learn to read, a balanced approach led to accelerated progress across standardized measures of word identification, comprehension, attitudes, and overall reading instructional levels (Duffy, 2001). Investigations of exemplary first-grade teachers find that teachers judged to be "most-effective-for-locale" balance the teaching of skills such as decoding or writing conventions with an emphasis on literature and language comprehension (Pressley et al., 2002). These exemplary teachers carefully integrate a balance of strategies to meet the diverse needs of the students they teach each year.

In a year-long ethnographic investigation of literacy learning in a first-grade classroom serving the needs of children with diverse linguistic and ethnic backgrounds, a balanced approach was deemed to be a key component of reading achievement (Fitzgerald & Noblit, 2000). In a longitudinal investigation of the implementation of a balanced approach, 298 students from six elementary schools in a suburban school district in the midwestern United States were studied across 3 years (McCarthy, 1999). Across the sample, student achievement was positively correlated with implementation of the balanced approach being studied. All subjects reached expected standard levels of performance on measures of word reading and comprehension by the end of second grade and maintained that level of performance through the end of grade 3 when the study was completed. Correlation analysis indicated that increased teacher training led to more consistent implementation of the balanced instruction, and years of training was positively correlated with student performance.

In a large-scale study of the impact of a balanced approach to reading instruction, a multistage sampling design was used to select 577 students that represented the entire population of grade 4 students in the state of Maryland (Guthrie, 2001). Using a hierarchical linear modeling procedure, the effects of balanced reading instruction on student reading achievement, as measured by the National Assessment of Educational Progress (NAEP), was tested. When compared with students who received instruction that focused on particular areas of reading instruction, students who received the greatest balance of instruction demonstrated the highest levels of achievement.

One final study supports the effectiveness of the balanced reading approach described in this chapter with students who have developmental disabilities. Hedrick, Katims, and Carr (1999) conducted a descriptive study of the effectiveness of a Four Blocks program on the reading achievement of nine elementary school students with mild to moderate mental retardation (mean IQ = 58; range 40−76). Their results indicate that a balanced approach to reading intervention led to improved student achievement across two formal measures (BRIGANCE Diagnostic Comprehensive Inventory of Basic Skills [Brigance, 1983] and the Test of Early Reading Ability-2 [TERA-2; Reid, Hresko, & Hammill, 1989]) and five informal measures (concepts about print, story retellings, writing, word decoding, and the Analytical Reading Inventory [ARI; Woods & Moe, 1995]). The students received balanced literacy instruction for a total of 3 hours each day across an entire school year, with 45 minutes devoted to each of the Four Blocks described previously. The results are limited by the small sample size and lack of experimental control; nonetheless, the combination of intervention targeting language comprehension, word identification, and whole-text print processing led to measurable gains for students who traditionally have difficulty learning to read with understanding.

Studies that specifically address the balanced approach with persons who use AAC are largely exploratory. Three published single-subject case studies report on the success of intervention approaches that provided a balance of strategies across the components of the WTP model (Blischak, 1995; Erickson et al., 1998; Gipe et al., 1993), but only the study conducted by the authors of this chapter explicitly referenced the WTP model. The subjects of the three case studies all demonstrated growth in reading across a variety of naturalistic probes and work samples including writing samples, developmental spelling probes, and informal word identification measures. The specific intervention strategies employed in each case differed, but all systematically combined strategies to promote learning across the components represented in the WTP model.

In summary, there is a broad base of evidence for the balanced reading approach described in this chapter for children without obvious learning and communication difficulties. Although there is scant research that specifically addresses the application of the approach or any other with students who use AAC, there is case study evidence (see, e.g., Erickson et al., 1997; Gipe et al., 1993) to support its application with the students who are the target of this chapter.

PRACTICAL REQUIREMENTS

Effective reading intervention requires time. Whether the students are 6-year-olds experiencing their first conventional reading instruction, 13-year-olds continuing to struggle with reading, or individuals of any age who use AAC, beginning readers require a combination of direct instruction, guided practice, and independent experience to progress in learning to read with comprehension. Mainstream beginning reading programs devote 1.5–2 hours to reading and language arts instruction per day (Allington & Cunningham, 2001; Cunningham & Allington, 2003). However, substantial increases in reading achievement have been correlated with increased time engaged in reading connected text for children without physical challenges (Anderson, Wilson, & Fielding, 1988; Leinhardt, Zigmond, & Cooley, 1981; Reutzel & Hollingsworth, 1991). It is reasonable to expect that learners with SSPIs who use AAC would require at least this amount of time, if not more, to make progress. In addition to the slow rates of communication and composition of people who use AAC (Higginbotham, Lesher, & Moulton, 2000), learners with SSPIs may find it challenging to hold a book, to turn the pages, and to see the words on the computer screen, and they may find fewer accessible reading materials in more limited locations (e.g., a shelf or two in the library as opposed to the entire collection available to children without access issues). When 2 or more hours of instructional time cannot be devoted to literacy instruction for students with SSPIs, especially older students, reading intervention can be combined with content area classes, related services, or other areas of instruction and intervention.

The WTP model serves also as a framework for assessment that guides instructional decision making as to what to teach, how much time to devote to particular interventions, and which personnel might best address particular reading needs. When used as a guide to instructional decision making, the WTP model supports comparison of a student's abilities in word identification, listening comprehension, and silent reading comprehension. Comparing abilities in these three areas answers the question, *What is preventing this student from reading silently with comprehension one grade level higher?* The answer to this question is determined by finding the weakest of the three areas (i.e., word identification, listening comprehension, or silent reading comprehension). This area is defined as the area of greatest instructional need. Consequently, it receives the greatest proportion of available time and intervention, and intervention is delivered by the most highly qualified personnel available at the school. Areas of strength, however, receive less instructional emphasis and are often addressed by personnel who may lack specific training in language and reading (e.g., paraprofessionals or volunteers) or even peer tutoring or cooperative group arrangements. This division of labor among primary clinicians, educators, classmates, and other participants also allows each individual to learn a particular instructional strategy or approach rather than requiring that each individual learn all there is to know about successful reading instruction. This division of labor places a premium on regular communication among instructional team members to ensure optimal student progress. More information on the use of the WTP model as a guide to assessment is available on videotape and in a variety of written materials from the Center for Literacy and Disability Studies at the University of North Carolina at Chapel Hill (http://www.med.unc.edu/ahs/clds).

Clinicians, educators, and parents looking for education that will support their implementation of the balanced approach described in this chapter should seek instructional opportunities that are intended to build greater understanding of the skills and processes required for successful reading. This type of education is often difficult to find in a time when much continuing education is conceived of as "training" and focuses on particular commercial reading programs and their implementation. These program-specific training opportunities typically fail to provide sufficient background information to problem solve when the programs are unsuccessful or require modifications to make them accessible to individuals who use AAC. Broader education of this nature is available through the Center for Literacy and Disability Studies (for more information, see http://www.med.unc.edu/ahs/clds). An increasing number of university speech-language and communication disorders programs are also including literacy coursework in their educational offerings. University-based graduate-level programs in reading are another source of broad education in a variety of instructional and assessment strategies, although they typically do not address considerations of students who use AAC in coursework or field experiences.

Further support in implementing the balanced instruction described in this chapter can be provided when educational teams include educational reading specialists. Although most reading specialists are unfamiliar with the particular access and communication needs of students who use AAC, they can work with a team to provide important information about the reading strategies they would use to address particular instructional needs, and the team can make the appropriate modifications for access, communication, and participation.

The materials required to implement the reading intervention strategies described in this chapter are already available in most schools and clinics in the United States and Canada. A good librarian, access to the Internet, understanding of appropriate text difficulty, and access to some simple technologies can allow clinicians and educators to get started with the suggestions without waiting for requisition approvals, new budget years, or a new computer or communication device. The specific materials described below might make the clinician's job easier or make the intervention more engaging for a particular student, but these specific materials are not required.

KEY COMPONENTS

The specific intervention described here is intended to help individuals who use AAC learn to read silently with comprehension. Although we cannot begin to address all of the strategies that would be involved in a comprehensive reading intervention program in a chapter of this length, we can offer starting places and resources. In particular, we will address starting places in the three whole-parts needed according to the WTP model in order to foster successful silent reading comprehension: language comprehension, word identification, and whole-text print processing.

Language Comprehension Intervention

As described above, the WTP model defines language comprehension as the combination of knowledge of text structures and knowledge of the world. Intervention intended to teach children to read with comprehension must address both of these aspects. Language comprehension intervention to improve silent reading comprehension ability rests on two principles. First, simply asking a student to read and respond to comprehension questions serves to *assess* how well the student understands the passage, but it does not *teach* comprehension. If we are to teach comprehension, we must guide students to read for a wide variety of purposes while simultaneously drawing on their own relevant background knowledge and experience and doing so in a wide variety of text genres (e.g., narratives, informational texts, poetry, drama, or directions). To do so requires that our intervention include instructional supports before, during, and after students read texts.

Second, language comprehension instruction to improve silent reading comprehension should ordinarily be done through reading rather than listening. Although language comprehension ability can be improved through listening comprehension instruction, it is less likely to transfer to reading than is reading comprehension instruction. When a student learns to comprehend the language of texts better while reading, that student simultaneously is learning to coordinate these language comprehension improvements with word identification and whole-text print processing. Learning to comprehend better while listening does not help the student learn to coordinate comprehension improvement with the other whole-parts of reading, and so this skill is much less likely to transfer to reading.

Before-Reading Instruction

As described in the WTP model, successful silent reading comprehension involves knowledge of the world and knowledge of text structures. Knowledge of the world is a language-based ability to recall and apply background knowledge, an essential component of successful comprehension and effective comprehension instruction. Before reading, it is important to build or activate the students' background knowledge. It is also important that students have an understanding of the structure of the type of text they are about to encounter. In other words, successful intervention helps a learner understand, recall, and apply understanding of the type of text about to be read. Building or activating background knowledge, knowledge of text structures, and setting a clear purpose for reading or listening are all important before-reading intervention activities. The first two activities are directly instructional, assisting students in developing the understandings they will need to read texts of increasing difficulty with increasing comprehension and increasing independence. The last activity, setting a purpose for reading, is indirectly instructional because it assists developing readers in focusing their attention and increases the chance that they will successfully apply what has been taught in reading with comprehension, and it sensitizes them to the text structures that are targeted by the specific purpose given.

Background Knowledge For some texts and purposes, we must teach the requisite background knowledge; for others, our task is merely to help the readers recall what they already know. In either case, our before-reading instruction can easily incorporate a brief assessment of students' existing background knowledge. A clinician might ask students to brainstorm a list of vocabulary related to a topic or select vocabulary from the text and ask the student to identify, define, or provide examples of each. The students might be asked to recall their own experiences related to the topic at hand. Many teachers of students with SSPIs begin units of instruction with direct experiences (e.g., field trips, experiments, simulations, video footage) in order to ensure that experiential limitations are not the cause of a student's difficulty with a particular text. Aaron's fourth-grade teacher, for example, learning from his mother that he had never read myths of any kind, engaged the class in the following activities before reading Hercules. First, she questioned the class about what myths were and how the content and structure of myths compared with the legends the class had read the previous week. Next, she showed a short clip of the Disney animated movie of Hercules (which Aaron and many of his classmates had seen previously in movie theaters). Then, she asked the students to tell her what they remembered about the events of the movie, organizing their comments with reference to structural elements they had just discussed. At each step of the instruction, her questions to the class and Aaron allowed her to assess gaps in knowledge or understanding of myth structure and background knowledge relevant to the Hercules myth, and to adjust her own comments and questions accordingly. These before-reading background assessment activities are particularly important for students who use AAC for another reason: their background knowledge demands are intensified by the need to recall symbols, icon sequences, and messages they have that are related to a particular area of knowledge. The following example illustrates the type of difficulties many students who use AAC encounter with this type of before reading activity:

> The teacher begins, "Today we're going to read the next chapter of our book, *The Bridge to Terabithia*. Before we begin, let's spend a few minutes talking about the friends you have in your life. I'll write on the board while you tell me all of the words you can that describe a friend." As the children in the class begin calling out words and relating stories about the friends in their lives and the words that describe them, one girl is busy navigating through her AAC device. She knows that she has lots of messages about friends. There was the time her mom programmed a message about her good friend, Alyssa, who had gone with her on vacation. There was another time when she had a message about a friend who worked with her on her merit badge. She could think of lots of things she wanted to say about her friends, but she couldn't find any of those messages. Finally, she resorted to contributing a few words. By the time she selected *like* and *nice*, they had been contributed by multiple children in the class and a learning opportunity had been lost.

While this type of before-reading activity is exactly the type of discussion that can help all children activate background knowledge, most AAC systems are not programmed with the intent of supporting students in accessing their memories and experiences for more than a few weeks. Like the student in the previous example, without careful attention to developing a system through which old news can be meaningfully stored for retrieval at any time, students who use AAC often struggle in participating actively in background knowledge intervention. Two critical problems associated with passive student lesson involvement are that 1) students may not be as cognitively engaged in the instruction as those who are more actively involved, and 2) teachers lose a valuable means of assessing student understandings (or lack thereof).

It is possible, however, to organize AAC systems to support access to memories and background experiences. One adolescent girl uses a calendar system to organize the messages that convey her life experiences. An adolescent boy uses categories to organize his. Another young girl has a scrapbook, much like the memory books used by adult clients with Alzheimer disease, to represent the events in her life in a chronological order. In each case, these students can potentially access any message or memory to share with others and support their own silent reading comprehension.

Vocabulary learning plays an important role in before-reading activities. For AAC users, it is common to find text-specific vocabulary programmed for these activities. One student's team programmed vocabulary words and definitions into the child's device for before-reading activities. Like many teams, his went to great lengths to make sure that new vocabulary words were programmed into his AAC device for use before, during, and after reading. Unfortunately, the content-specific vocabulary often was of little conversational use outside of the instructional experience for which it was programmed.

The team worked to find an alternative means to involve this child in vocabulary learning that would generalize across contexts and activities. They eventually decided to stop the practice of programming all new vocabulary words into his device. Instead, they worked with him to use the existing, comprehensive set of vocabulary items he already had, to demonstrate his understanding of new vocabulary that was taught in class. For example, some vocabulary words from a social text were: transcontinental railroad, urbanization, and tenement. Rather than programming these very low-frequency words, he called on existing vocabulary to demonstrate his understanding. He combined *across-land-train* for transcontinental railroad. He combined *city-grow-make-job-change* for urbanization and *old-apartment-crowd* for tenement. This method also allowed him to connect new words with his existing vocabulary, a process that led to an ever-increasing semantic network to which new vocabulary could be added meaningfully. The new method also moved him away from the daily and weekly process of memorizing vocabulary words and definitions and moved him toward a more active and generative learning process.

Knowledge of Text Structures   In addition to building or accessing language-based knowledge that will support comprehension of the text, intervention must help students build an increasingly complex understanding of the structures of written language. This is often interpreted narrowly as being able to label parts of a story grammar (i.e., character, setting, and so forth) and other text-related jargon. However, in order to read with comprehension, students need to know how information is organized in different types of texts rather than to be able to label and identify parts of a story or types of transitions and text features.

Before reading, knowledge of text structures can be strengthened by helping students recall and discuss other texts they have read that were like the one they are about to read. Previewing the text and searching for specific text features is another effective strategy for building knowledge of text structure and also focuses the readers' attention by enabling them to anticipate text events or content. For example, assume a student is being asked to read a book about baseball. Before beginning to read, the clinician asks the student what she knows about baseball. Because the student's brother plays little league and her dad plays softball, she has been to many baseball and softball games. The student recalls a few messages that were programmed into her device, finds them with the other "old family news" messages, and shares them with the clinician. The clinician builds on that knowledge and experience by introducing a few additional key vocabulary words. Next, the clinician reminds the student of the story they read together the previous week about a girl who played soccer. She asks the student to think about that story as they preview today's text about baseball. As they examine the text, the clinician points out the photographs and captions as well as the underlined, bold, and italicized words throughout the text. After exploring several pages, the clinician asks the student if she thinks this text about baseball is going to be like the story about soccer. The student responds, "different," and the clinician asks her if she can point to something in the text that supports her answer. The student points to an underlined heading and some bold words in the text of a paragraph.

Without ever introducing text structure jargon, the clinician has helped the student prepare to successfully read the baseball text. She has helped the girl compare her existing knowledge of a soccer text with this new sports text, to think about the features of the text that let her know she'd be learning information about baseball rather than reading a story about baseball, and provided the student with an opportunity to demonstrate her understanding of the differences.

Setting Purposes   The final before-reading activity requires the clinician or teacher to clearly state a purpose for reading. More than once we have heard a clinician or educator comment, "I can't always give him a purpose. He needs to be able to do that on his own." We agree that students need to be able to set their own purposes, but giving students a purpose before they read is what focuses the lesson on one or a few of the structural elements or aspects of the text. Without a purpose, the teacher really isn't teaching the student how to comprehend better. In our own undergraduate and graduate courses, we continue to set purposes for reading for our students, although the vast majority of them are able to set their own purposes for reading. However, we have instructional objectives that drive the purposes we provide the students; the purposes they set on their own are unlikely to match our instructional objectives. If students are not given a clear purpose for comprehending, they are essentially left to one of two difficult tasks: reading to remember everything or reading to guess what the instructor will ask them (to do) after reading. If we as interventionists know why we have selected a particular text, we can support student learning by stating that as clearly as possible before texts are read. Giving students a good purpose for reading is our main tool for focusing today's lesson on the aspect of text comprehension we want to teach the students how to do better.

Effective purposes can be quite varied but they share three important characteristics: 1) they help the reader focus attention on what is relevant to the day's lesson; 2) they lead the reader to construct inferences or main ideas; and 3) they require processing of (nearly) the entire text, at least on initial reading of a text. However, the same text can, and should, be read on multiple occasions for different purposes. Through repeated experiences with a single text, beginning readers gain increased understanding of text structure and vocabulary, are better able to apply their relevant background knowledge and use their augmentative communication systems, and increase their silent reading fluency.

During Reading

Reading should take the majority of time in a reading comprehension lesson. The before- and after-reading lessons are important, but the amount of time spent reading whole texts is the best predictor of achievement in reading (Anderson et al., 1988; Cipielwski & Stanovich, 1992). Intervention is necessary to support student application of relevant background knowledge and strategies and to focus student attention, but the goal of this instruction (i.e., independent silent reading with comprehension) should not be withheld from students. Comprehension can be improved whether students read texts themselves or whether they listen to others read them aloud. However, if we want to assist students in reaching the goal of independent reading, they must have regular and frequent opportunities to read texts themselves. There are two primary strategies that clinicians can apply in supporting comprehension during text reading: guiding student application of the purpose that has been set and selecting texts for reading or listening at a level that the student can understand.

Guiding student application of the purpose during reading is most easily accomplished by engaging the students in a task that enables them, and the clinician, to monitor the use of the purpose. For example, a clinician was working with a mixed ability group of students, including a student who uses AAC, to improve their questioning and monitoring. The students were to read the fourth chapter of *Holes* (Sachar, 2000) in order to explain the significance of five short phrases: *two tall trees; Well, duh; Mr. Sir; dig one hole;* and *electric fence.* The clinician gave each pair of children five sticky notes and had the student who uses AAC and her partner complete the same task using a simple word processor on the computer. The student who uses AAC had her communication device interfaced with the computer so that her words would be typed in the word processor while the partner typed using the standard keyboard. As the students came across these phrases, they were to discuss and then write down why the phrases were significant enough for the author, Louis Sachar, to include them in the chapter. The clinician was able to listen in on the student conversations, read their notes as the reading progressed, and build on their (mis)understandings to strengthen student comprehension.

One of the main goals of reading comprehension instruction is to help students learn to make meaning from an increasingly complex and broad array of texts. Skills must be practiced successfully in order to improve, but if the text is too difficult for the student, the goal cannot be met. In general, texts selected for use in reading comprehension instruction should be at the student's lowest level of ability across word identification, listening comprehension, and silent reading comprehension. In other words, a student who can read words at the third-grade level, understand through listening to text at the fifth-grade level, but read text silently with comprehension at the first-grade level should use first-grade-level texts or easier during reading comprehension instruction. A student who can read words at the fourth-grade level, understand through listening at second-grade level, and read silently with comprehension at the third-grade level should have second-grade-level texts or easier during reading comprehension instruction.

After Reading

Once students have read a text successfully for a given purpose, they must engage in a task that allows them to demonstrate their understanding (or misunderstanding). This enables students to check their understanding and educators to intervene as necessary to support learning. It can be challenging to generate meaningful purposes and tasks that reflect completion of the purpose but do not require more time than the reading of the text. In fact, aside from the process of selecting materials to use in comprehension instruction, generating a purpose and task are the most challenging aspects of successful reading comprehension intervention.

Once the purpose and task have been generated, it becomes clear what background knowledge and knowledge of text structures must be addressed before reading. The following are examples of combinations of background knowledge, purposes, and tasks that can be completed even if a student does not use a complex communication system:

1. Purpose (before reading): *Read so that you can put the story events in order.*

Task (after reading): The teacher writes the events on sentence strips, and the student points to put them in the correct order after reading.

Background (before reading): The teacher must make sure the student can successfully sequence events—not a skill most students learn without instruction. Teach sequencing by using content that is *very* familiar to the student, such as days of the week, meals in the day, or the schedule students follow at school. Use both examples and nonexamples of events to ensure that students have the required background knowledge.

2. Purpose (before reading): *Read so that you can show me which of the five words I have written on index cards best describe the main character, setting, climax, problem,* or *resolution.* (The teacher selects only one and returns to the text on another day if it seems important to find the words that best describe another feature of the text.)

Task (after reading): The student selects from the words that are written on index cards (either generated by the student or selected by the student from the choices provided by the teacher).

Background (before reading): If the student uses a comprehensive AAC system, ask the student to generate words that could be used to describe a person, place, event, or whatever is appropriate given the exact purpose you have set. Take any describing words the student can generate and write them on index cards. If the student does not have a comprehensive system, prepare examples and nonexamples on index cards ahead of time and ask the student to indicate whether the word fits the purpose. Use any inaccurate responses as teaching opportunities but do not simply correct the error.

3. Purpose (before reading): *Read so that you can compare and contrast the two main characters in the story.*

Task (after reading): Students place, or guide placement of, the descriptive words in the right location on the Venn diagram.

Background (before reading): Begin by making sure the student understands a Venn diagram. Create one with the student comparing and contrasting two very familiar people (e.g., mom and teacher). Once the Venn diagram structure is understood, ask the student either to generate descriptive words or to select from the examples and nonexamples you have prepared (as in Example 2).

The final step in a successful reading comprehension lesson is the provision of informative feedback. The primary purpose of informative feedback is building cognitive clarity; that is, helping the student understand what he or she did that led to success or what might be done differently next time to increase success. Informative feedback is very different from reinforcement or correction. Informative feedback focuses on helping the student understand what he or she did, how information was found, remembered, or processed, and how the strategy or strategies employed would work with other texts.

Word Identification Intervention

Instruction on how to pronounce printed words during silent reading must have a dual emphasis on building automatic word recognition and phonics (i.e., decoding skills) for mediated word identification. As described in the WTP model, the combination of the two is required for successful silent reading comprehension. Readers must be able to recognize most of the words they encounter effortlessly while simultaneously possessing the skills to figure out unfamiliar words. Silent reading comprehension will probably suffer if intervention emphasizes only one or the other. When students are not taught skills to figure out unfamiliar words, they have no choice but to skip them or depend solely on context, and their ability to learn words automatically suffers. Alternatively, when students are taught to stop and sound out or consciously think about every word they encounter, they are expending cognitive resources that would otherwise be devoted to comprehension (LaBerge, 1974; Perfetti, 1977, 1985).

Here, we describe a few strategies that we use to teach word identification. Of all components of the WTP model, our intervention in word reading is most systematic and adult directed. The clinician or teacher determines which words to teach, in which order, by which methods. Furthermore, intervention in this area is most successful when all of the members of the educational team are aware of the words and word identification strategies being taught, so that they can support the student across learning environments.

Word Wall

At the core of the word identification intervention is a specific application of a *word wall* (for a comprehensive description, see Cunningham, 1999). The word wall is a large display to which words are added slowly and systematically during a school year or intervention period. Words added to the wall should be those that the student is expected to read with automaticity and spell with accuracy at the end of the intervention period. For these two reasons, no more than five new words are added each week. Successful word walls are always available and easy to see. The words on them are practiced every day through a variety of activities, and students are expected to spell every word on the wall correctly in all of their writing.

Creating a word wall requires some initial problem solving. The display must have all 26 letters of the alphabet as headers and room to add words printed large enough for the student to see easily. All of the letters and words must be on a single display rather than separated on pages of a notebook, programmed on separate pages in a communication device, or otherwise presented in a dictionary-type alphabetical format. In general education class-rooms, the displays are quite literally posted on a wall in the classroom. When created for individual students, word walls might be displayed on an open file folder, a trifold science display, or a large piece of chart paper. The key is to select a format that will accommodate the 120-plus words that will be added during the year in a size that can be read easily by the student.

We used to recommend that word walls be programmed in students' AAC devices to facilitate communication about those words during word wall lessons. Our experience and a wise speech-language pathologist helped us understand that we were negating the potential added benefits of our instruction to face-to-face communication when we didn't expect students to access word wall words from the logical arrangement of vocabulary already in their devices. In other terms, we want students either to spell the word wall words or have them integrated into the general vocabulary so that they can be used across reading, writing, and communication contexts. Combined with a light-tech display of all of the words, we are beginning to see our strategy pay off.

For all beginning readers, the words that go on a word wall come from two primary sources: high-frequency words (e.g., *I, the, every*) and words that contain a useful spelling pattern (e.g., *hat, sit, can*). A handful of words on the wall might be words that have great utility in the student's life (e.g., name of school, favorite TV show) and are likely to be encountered regularly in the texts the student reads and writes. Word wall words do not come from content-area vocabulary lists (e.g., *porpoise, myth, settlers*) because these words have only temporary utility during a particular unit of instruction. Such words, however, might be displayed on a bulletin board, or thematic vocabulary wall, during the unit. Word walls also do not include student names because these names rarely support reading of other words and rarely appear in written texts. However, in primary-grade classrooms, such words might be placed on a name wall to support children's attempts to write and communicate with one another. In general, the rule to remember is that each word displayed should be one that you expect the student to read with automaticity and spell with accuracy by the end of the year.

As five new words are added to the wall each week, the word meanings are taught and the words are used in complete sentences. Students who use AAC are then guided in spelling each of those words by repeating the letters subvocally, or "in their heads." As the words are spelled, students clap for each letter. Students with significant motor impairments might rock, tap their trays, vocalize, or participate in another clapping alternative. Finally, each of the five new words is spelled, letter-by-letter, using a complete alphabet display if writing with a pencil is not possible. It is critical that students actually spell the words letter by letter at this point. If the student is merely selecting a whole word from a display, a key to this powerful learning opportunity is lost.

Once the new words have been added to the wall, they are never removed. During the ensuing weeks, the student is guided in practicing new words as well as words that were added previously. The goal is not mastery of the words the first week they are posted, but learning all of the words and how to use them to read and write other words over time. In addition to practicing the words on the wall using a variety of activities that emphasize their spelling, students are referred to the wall to support their reading and writing attempts across the day. For example, when the student looks for help reading an unfamiliar word encountered in a text, an adult directs the student to use the word wall. The conversation might go as follows:

Student: Looks up at the adult and vocalizes while gesturing for help and pointing to the word *might*.

Adult: "You need help with that word?"

Student: Indicates *yes* by looking up.

Adult: "Okay. There is a word on your word wall that might help. Did you look?"

Student: Indicates *yes* by looking up then looks down for *no*.

Adult: "You looked but couldn't find one. Okay, look under the letter *N*. Can you find the word?"

Student: Looks at word wall and the words under the letter *N*. After a few seconds, the student sits upright and smiles.

Teacher: "You found it? Say that word in your head. Now, look at this one. How is it the same and how is it different? Is the beginning the same?"

Student: Looks down to indicate *no*.

Teacher: "You're right. The beginning is different. Say the sound that this word begins with (pointing to *might*) and then use that word from your word wall to help you. Can you do it?"

Student: Looks intently at the word, vocalizes some, and then looks up at the teacher, smiling.

The word wall is a powerful intervention tool when combined with other strategies that support the student in learning to use known words to read and spell unfamiliar words. One easy-to-implement strategy is compare/contrast. In this strategy, the student is given three known words on index cards (e.g., *care, best, find*). The words are reviewed briefly with the student and then a sentence is written with one word underlined (e.g., Is there something in that *nest*?). The underlined word shares a spelling pattern with one of the three known words. The adult reads the sentence aloud without saying the underlined word. The student then selects the word that will "help them read the underlined word." Once the student has made a selection, the adult guides the student in comparing and contrasting the selected word with the underlined word.

Making Words

Making Words (Cunningham & Hall, 1994, 1997b) is an activity designed to teach students to look for and use spelling patterns in words. Making Words was designed as a multilevel, whole-class instructional activity. We have used a variation of the strategy to provide individualized, targeted phonics instruction for students who use AAC. Because the strategy works with a limited letter set, it decreases access demands and leads to more efficient intervention. The original strategy requires no speaking but provides continuous evidence of student understanding, so it is particularly useful with AAC users.

In the basic strategy, students are given access to letters that can be unscrambled to make a single word (e.g., *e, i, k, n, t, t* [*kitten*]). The six to eight letters include only a single vowel to increase student success when the strategy is first used, but soon the letters include more than one vowel. Students are guided in using the letters to make words of varying length beginning with one-letter words and progressing to words that use all of the letters. In planning the lesson, the adult sequences the target words so that minimal changes are made as the student progresses from one word to the next. This, too, increases student success but also enables students to recognize and understand within-word spelling patterns more efficiently. At each point in the lesson, the student first attempts to use the letters to make a word that the adult has indicated. After the attempt has been made, a model of the correct spelling printed on an index card or piece of paper is provided. The attempt is then compared with the correct version, and the student makes corrections as needed. To best support careful student examination of within-word spelling patterns, it is important that students be guided in comparing their words letter by letter with the target word rather than merely copying the model.

Once all of the words have been made, students are guided in sorting the word cards. This sorting encourages them to explore once again the spelling patterns within each word. Initially, the adult suggests the rules for sorting (e.g., number of letters, same first letter, same vowel, same ending), but gradually students are encouraged to identify and sort by their own rules. Finally, the students are directed to use the words they have made to try to spell words using letters not available in the lesson. For example, assume the students have made the words *take, make*, and *sake*. In this final transfer activity, they might be asked to spell *fake* and *rake*.

The word wall and Making Words are only two of many intervention activities that are required to help students learn to identify and spell words. They are excellent examples of intervention strategies that can be made accessible to students who use AAC without changing the cognitive process required by students without disabilities for whom they were designed. For more information about instructional strategies like these that are accessible to students who use AAC, refer to the series of Month-by-Month phonics books (Cunningham & Hall, 1997a, 1998b, 1998c; Hall & Cunningham, 1998).

Whole-Text Print Processing

The most important thing when building students' skills in whole-text print processing is to provide multiple opportunities to read easy, connected text every day. This wide reading of easy text is required to help students learn to integrate all of the processes required when reading connected text. Across each of the whole-parts in whole-text print processing, there are activities that can help students become more aware of the processes required, but finding text that the students can read independently and providing many opportunities to read text at that level is most important.

The two whole-parts within whole-text print processing that appear to present the greatest challenge to students who use AAC are inner speech and eye movements. Difficulties with projecting prosody onto print seem to be influenced by problems with reading in inner speech. Once students become aware of and are able to use their inner speech during reading, projecting prosody can become less problematic. Some of the specific ways in which we are trying to assist students with inner speech and eye movements are described below.

Inner Speech

We are learning that we must first help students who use AAC become aware of their inner voice. Research with speaking children suggests that they are not conscious of their inner voice until age 7 or 8 years, although there is research evidence that they are engaging in subvocal rehearsal by the age of 4 (Flavell, Green, Flavell, & Grossman, 1997). In other words, years before children without disabilities are aware that they have an inner voice, they are using it. In similar but delayed fashion, beginning readers who use AAC indicate that they are not aware of an inner voice, but literate adults who use AAC report that they are aware of an inner voice.

We are teaching some students who use AAC to become aware of their inner speech in a number of ways including 1) encouraging them to rehearse subvocally (i.e., say it in your head) for their face-to-face communication; 2) singing songs, such as B-I-N-G-O, that pair a hand clap or other available volitional movement with subvocal letter naming; and 3) using their favorite songs on the radio or CD player to show them how they can keep singing the song subvocally when the volume is turned all the way down and come in right on track when the volume is returned to normal. Based on research that suggests it is beneficial, we also use talking word processors and AAC devices with voice output to assist students in pairing their ideas with sound

(Foley & Pollatsek, 1999; Koppenhaver et al., 1991; Vandervelden & Siegel, 1999). These last two strategies are meant to assist students in recognizing and controlling the outer speech that we would like them to internalize for reading. All of the strategies are meant to help students who use AAC understand what we mean when we asked them to use their inner speech while reading. Once they are aware of their inner speech, we must then provide a great deal of practice with easy-to-read, meaningful text so they can use that inner speech in reading.

Eye Movement

Eye movements seem to present a challenge for people who use AAC, particularly those who also experience severe physical impairments. As with all of the processes in whole-text print processing, the eye movements needed for silent reading comprehension can only be developed through successful reading of connected text. The challenges are 1) finding a text layout and font size that students with eye-movement difficulties can read successfully and then 2) incrementally changing that presentation to make it more and more like standard text. We found early on in our clinical work, for example, that we were making eye movements more difficult by simply enlarging text because, we believe, words no longer looked like words but strings of letters. However, when we added spaces between words and increased the space between lines of text from double to quadruple spacing, we were able to create text that the students who used AAC could read. Given opportunities to read dozens of texts presented in this way, we were then able to decrease the spacing between words and lines to triple. Over time, we systematically supported the students in building the eye-movement strategies they required to process standard text.

ASSESSMENT METHODS TO SUPPORT ONGOING DECISION MAKING

On an annual basis, it is helpful to complete an informal reading inventory based on the WTP model as referenced earlier. This assessment identifies an individual student's strengths and weaknesses and is helpful in guiding instructional decision making. In our work with school systems that have adopted this informal assessment process at the beginning and end of each academic year, we have discovered the power of understanding and teaching to these individual profiles. Students are showing us that their needs change on a year-to-year basis as the instruction they are provided supports their relative strengths and addresses their relative weaknesses, resulting in a new profile. In addition to this annual assessment, there are several indicators of progress that clinicians and educators can look for during the course of the year.

One important indicator is improvement in written composition as readers improve in word identification, language comprehension, and whole-text print processing. For example, increased automatic word recognition skill is usually accompanied by improved spelling of high-frequency words when students write connected text. Improved skills in mediated word identification are typically reflected in more accurate attempts at spelling unfamiliar words. Improved language comprehension, particularly knowledge of text structures, should be reflected in more conventional and complex syntax in writing, a more logical sequence of events in narratives, and eventually a clear beginning, middle, and end. Increased knowledge of the world may result in a broader selection of topics or improved use of details and support for arguments during self-directed writing activities. Improvements in whole-text print processing, particularly print-to-meaning links, are often accompanied by more accurate use of homophones and punctuation in writing.

Other indicators of improvements in reading that might be observed include

- Engagement with increasingly complex texts during self-selected reading
- More complex interactions about the meaning of texts after reading or listening to them
- Increased levels of success with word identification and comprehension instructional tasks

One specific strategy that can be used to monitor progress in an ongoing manner is the modified cloze procedure called *maze* (Guthrie, 1973):

- Select a passage about 100–125 words in length.
- Leave the first two sentences intact.
- Beginning with the fifth word in the third sentence, delete every fifth word and insert a blank.
- Prepare three choices for each blank. One will be the original word that fits in the blank. The second choice will be a word that is the same part of speech as the target word. The final choice can be any word that is structurally similar to the target word.

Ask the student to begin reading the modified text. If the student has adequate motor and visual skills, it is appropriate to present the three choices either in or under the blank. If the student cannot motorically or visually select from three choices presented in that manner, ask the student look up at each blank and select from three choices presented in an eye-gaze display or another appropriate three-item choice display. If the original passage is to be used to increase the student's reading fluency, a score of 50%–60% or higher should be achieved before reading the complete text. After three or four repeated readings of the complete text without the maze modifications, an accuracy of 80% would be anticipated. By 6–10 repetitions, if the passage is of appropriate difficulty, students usually demonstrate 90% accuracy and it is time to introduce a new passage to sustain engagement.

CONSIDERATIONS FOR CHILDREN FROM
CULTURALLY AND LINGUISTICALLY DIVERSE BACKGROUNDS

The WTP model provides a means for understanding the particular needs and challenges presented by children who use AAC and who are culturally and linguistically diverse. A primary consideration is the English language knowledge that the child brings to learning to read. Children who understand language within normal limits in their first language often have a difficult time in learning to read in English because they don't have sufficient knowledge of how to encode that knowledge in English. We can accommodate these differences in a number of ways through the background knowledge instruction we provide as part of our listening and reading comprehension instruction. Although this before-reading activity is important for all readers, it is critical to the reading success of children who are from linguistically and culturally diverse backgrounds.

Specifically, it is important to link the new learning to existing knowledge and experience. If students are learning new vocabulary or information, and teachers do not help them carefully connect that learning to existing knowledge, the children might be successful with the text at hand but will be unlikely to be able to apply that newly acquired information in other texts. For children from nonmainstream cultures who use AAC, this may mean a communication system that integrates their first language with the second. The specific before-, during-, and after-reading instructional structure described in this chapter is particularly considerate of the different knowledge and experience that children who are from culturally and linguistically diverse backgrounds. Every attempt to teach comprehension is initiated with instruction that builds on or activates the existing background knowledge that children bring to the reading event. The strategy helps clinicians and teachers have a framework for evaluating and teaching the background knowledge the children require to be successful with the reading task at hand. It makes it clear that the children do not have to know everything to be successful with the current text and task. If there is more to learn from a particular text than a single purpose and task can accomplish, then rereading for another purpose with new background knowledge learning or activation supports the readers' success.

The choice of text can also help linguistically diverse children, especially at first. So-called *predictable books* often have repetitive syntactic structures that vary content words. Because linguistically diverse children usually lack facility with English syntax, having them read predictable books with syntactic repetition and concrete pictures that reflect the meanings of the content vocabulary can help them improve their sentence comprehension ability. Unfortunately, these texts often lack the whole-passage meaning necessary for good comprehension instruction, so they should probably only be used early on and for a brief period.

APPLICATION TO AN INDIVIDUAL CHILD

Julianne is a 12-year-old girl who uses a DynaVox to support her face-to-face communication, but she rarely uses it except when asked a direct question during content area instruction. Instead, Julianne depends on her limited repertoire of signs and verbal approximations to interact successfully with familiar others. Prior to the introduction of the approach described in this chapter, her progress in reading across her school career had been extremely limited. Best estimates suggested that her receptive single-word vocabulary was within normal limits, and her parents had been told repeatedly that she could read at the third-grade level. Despite this information, Julianne continued to struggle as a reader, writer, and communicator.

Our initial interactions with and informal assessment of Julianne revealed that she could listen with comprehension at the third-grade level, but she could only identify words at the primer level and could not read any connected text with comprehension. Given the information we collected, her educational team made a commitment to address Julianne's reading needs with greater intensity during the course of an entire school year. They understood that measurable progress in the overall ability to read silently with comprehension was going to take time to achieve.

Prior to her seventh-grade year, many changes were made in Julianne's school day. The team looked carefully at the interventions they had employed during previous years. The team continued to use strategies that had proven to support Julianne's success in content area classes. The team discontinued all interventions that demonstrated they were not supporting Julianne's success (e.g., weekly spelling lists that Julianne memorized to receive high scores on tests but could not spell or read a few days later). Organizationally, Julianne was supported by a paraprofessional who worked with her for two periods each day directly on reading, a speech-language pathologist and occupational therapist who saw her for two separate 30-minute sessions each week during this reading intervention time, and a resource room teacher who was available to support planning and problem solving on a daily basis.

Intervention for word identification included both the word wall and Making Words approaches described previously. Across content areas, the paraprofessional used the before-, during-, and after-reading comprehension format described earlier. She learned to build or activate background knowledge, set a clear purpose, and engage Julianne in completing an after-reading task that was directly related to the purpose that had been set. In these comprehension lessons and across the day, the paraprofessional also learned to provide Julianne with informative feedback that focused on what she had done effectively and what she might do next time to experience more success. In addition to these word identification and reading comprehension lessons, Julianne engaged in self-selected reading of primer level texts on a daily basis. Sources of reading materials included children's poetry (e.g., Jack Prelutsky's *A Pizza the Size of the Sun* [1996] and Shel Silverstein's *Falling Up* [1996]), small books made by cutting apart old basal readers, notes from her paraprofessional and others, and song lyrics. Finally, Julianne was provided with daily writing intervention. The intervention combined opportunities to write without standards (i.e., readers responded to the content and not the form of her writing) using her DynaVox as a keyboard, with writing experiences directed by the paraprofessional.

After 1 year of this balanced intervention, Julianne was able to read first-grade-level materials with comprehension as measured with an adapted form of the Qualitative Reading Inventory-3 (Leslie & Caldwell, 2000). She was able to comprehend fifth-grade materials when they were read to her, and she was identifying words at the first-grade level. Julianne continued to lag significantly behind same-age peers, but she made almost a full year of progress in a school year after making almost no progress as a reader during 7 previous years.

FUTURE DIRECTIONS

The balanced intervention approach and the assessment procedures described in this chapter are the result of a decade of research and development by an interdisciplinary team at the Center for Literacy and Disability Studies. Currently, efforts are being directed at the development of a reliable and valid standardized reading assessment battery that is specifically designed for children who use AAC. Careful attention is being paid to issues of construct validity, because the focus has been on developing theoretically sound measures from the ground up instead of modifying existing measures to make them accessible to individuals who use AAC. Guided by the WTP model, these development efforts will yield a comprehensive assessment battery that extends beyond probes of individual skills and processes to all of the components of the WTP model. For example, theoretically sound measures that differentiate between difficulties with automatic versus mediated word identification, the processes within whole-text print processing, as well as reliable measures of language comprehension must be developed and researched. Beyond the whole-parts described in the WTP model, measures must also be developed and validated that assess student ability in underlying skills and processes such as phonemic awareness, working memory, and other cognitive and linguistic processes related to reading. Although each of these is currently available for students who use speech to communicate, none is currently available for use with people who use AAC.

The preliminary development of appropriate standardized assessment measures is only the first step toward the future. As the measures are developed, their efficacy as guides to intervention must be investigated through more controlled studies. Furthermore, future research is required to validate each of the approaches described in this chapter for students who use AAC.

Currently, our evidence for their application with students who use AAC is limited to case studies and anecdotal descriptions. Carefully designed single-subject studies as well as group studies are required to establish efficacy and effectiveness within this group of students. Until we have a reliable and valid means to measure progress across the whole-parts described in the WTP model, it is difficult to design research that goes beyond curriculum-based measures of growth.

RECOMMENDED READINGS

Allington, R.L. (2001). *What really matters for struggling readers.* New York: Longman.

Cunningham, P.M., Hall, D.P., & Sigmon, C.M. (1999). *The teacher's guide to the Four Blocks.* Greensboro, NC: Carson-Dellosa.

Erickson, K.A., & Koppenhaver, D.A. (1998). Using the "write talk-nology" with Patrik. *Teaching Exceptional Children, 31*(1), 58–64.

Erickson, K.A., Koppenhaver, D.A., & Yoder, D.E. (Eds.). (2002). *Waves of words: Augmented communicators read and write.* Toronto: ISAAC Press.

Koppenhaver, D.A., Spadorcia, S., & Erickson, K.A. (1998). Inclusive early literacy instruction for children with disabilities. In S.B. Neuman & K. Roskos (Eds.), *Children achieving: Instructional practices in early literacy* (pp. 77–97). Newark, DE: International Reading Association.

Koppenhaver, D.A., & Erickson, K.A. (2002). Quick-Guide #12: Supporting literacy learning in all children. In M.F. Giangreco (Ed.), *Quick-Guides to Inclusion 3: Ideas for educating students with disabilities* (pp. 29–56). Baltimore: Paul H. Brookes Publishing Co.

Sturm, J., & Koppenhaver, D.A. (2000). Supporting writing development in adolescents with developmental disabilities. *Topics in Language Disorders, 20*(2), 73–92.

REFERENCES

Adams, M.J. (1990). *Beginning to read: Thinking and learning about print.* Cambridge, MA: The MIT Press.

Allington, R.L., & Cunningham, P.M. (2001). *Schools that work: Where all children read and write* (2nd ed.). Upper Saddle River, NJ: Pearson Allyn & Bacon.

Anderson, R.C., Wilson, P.T., & Fielding, L.G. (1988). Growth in reading and how children spend them time outside of school. *Reading Research Quarterly, 23,* 285–303.

Au, K.H., Carroll, J.H., & Scheu, J.A. (2001). *Balanced literacy instruction: A teacher's resource book* (2nd ed.). Norwood, MA: Christopher-Gordon.

Berninger, V., & Gans, B. (1986). Assessing word processing capability of the nonvocal, nonwriting. *Augmentative and Alternative Communication, 2,* 56–63.

Blischak, D.M. (1995). Thomas the writer: Case study of a child with severe physical, speech, and visual impairments. *Language, Speech, and Hearing Services in the Schools, 26*(1), 11–20.

Brigance, A. (1983). *BRIGANCE Diagnostic Comprehensive Inventory of Basic Skills.* North Billerica, MA: Curriculum Associates.

Cipielwski, J., & Stanovich, K.E. (1992). Predicting growth in reading ability from children's exposure to print. *Journal of Experimental Child Psychology, 54,* 74–89.

Coleman, P.P. (1991). *Literacy lost: A qualitative analysis of the early literacy experiences of preschool children with severe speech and physical impairments.* Doctoral dissertation, University of North Carolina at Chapel Hill.

Cousin, P.T., Weekly, T., & Gerard, J. (1993). The functional uses of language and literacy by students with severe language and learning problems. *Language Arts, 70,* 548–556.

Cowie, R., Douglas-Cowie, E., & Wichmann, A. (2002). Fluency and expressiveness in 8–10-year-old readers. *Language and Speech, 45*(1), 47–82.

Cunningham, J.W. (1993). Whole-to-part reading diagnosis. *Reading and Writing Quarterly: Overcoming Learning Difficulties, 9,* 31–49.

Cunningham, J.W. (1999). How we can achieve best practices in literacy instruction. In L.B. Gambrell, L.M. Morrow, S.B. Neuman, & M. Pressley (Eds.), *Best practices in literacy instruction* (pp. 34–45). New York: Guilford Press.

Cunningham, P.M. (1999). *The teacher's guide to the Four Blocks.* Winston-Salem, NC: Carson-Dellosa.

Cunningham, P.M., & Allington, R.L. (2003). *Classrooms that work: They can all read and write* (3rd ed.). Upper Saddle River, NJ: Pearson Allyn & Bacon.

Cunningham, P.M., & Cunningham, J.W. (1978). Investigating the "print-to-meaning" hypothesis. In P.D. Pearson & J. Hansen (Eds.), *Reading: Disciplined inquiry in process and practice. 27th Yearbook of the National Reading Conference* (pp. 116–120). Clemson, SC: National Reading Conference.

Cunningham, P.M., & Hall, D.P. (1994). *Making words.* Greensboro, NC: Carson-Dellosa.

Cunningham, P.M., & Hall, D.P. (1997a). *Month-by-month phonics for first grade.* Greensboro, NC: Carson-Dellosa.

Cunningham, P.M., & Hall, D.P. (1997b). *More making words.* Greensboro, NC: Carson-Dellosa.

Cunningham, P.M., & Hall, D.P. (1998a). The Four Blocks: A balanced framework for literacy in primary classrooms. In K.R. Harris, S. Graham, & M. Pressley (Series Eds.) & K.R. Harris, S. Graham, & D. Deshler (Vol. Eds.), *Advances in teaching and learning series: Teaching every child every day: Learning in diverse schools and classrooms* (pp. 32–76). Cambridge, MA: Brookline.

Cunningham, P.M., & Hall, D.P. (1998b). *Month-by-month phonics for third grade.* Greensboro, NC: Carson-Dellosa.

Cunningham, P.M., & Hall, D.P. (1998c). *Month-by-month phonics for upper grades.* Greensboro, NC: Carson-Dellosa.

Cunningham, P.M., Hall, D.P., & Defee, M. (1998). Nonability grouped, multilevel instruction: Eight years later. *The Reading Teacher, 51,* 652–664.

Dahlgren Sandberg, A. (2001). Reading and spelling, phonological awareness, and working memory in children with severe speech impairments: A longitudinal study. *Augmentative and Alternative Communication, 17*(1), 11–26.

Dahlgren Sandberg, A. & Hjelmquist, E. (1996). Phonologic awareness and literacy abilities in nonspeaking preschool children with cerebral palsy. *Augmentative and Alternative Communication, 12,* 138–153.

Dahlgren Sandberg, A. & Hjelmquist, E. (1997). Language and literacy in nonvocal children with cerebral palsy. *Reading and Writing: An Interdisciplinary Journal, 9,* 107–133.

Daneman, M. (1991). Working memory as a predictor of verbal fluency. *Journal of Psycholinguistic Research, 20,* 445–464.

Daneman, M., & Newson, M. (1992). Assessing the importance of subvocalization during normal silent reading. *Reading and Writing: An Interdisciplinary Journal, 4*(1), 55–77.

Developmental Disabilities Assistance and Bill of Rights Act (DD Act) of 2000, PL 106-402, 42 U.S.C. §§ 6061–6066 *et seq.*

Dreyer, L.G., & Katz, L. (1992). An examination of "the simple view of reading." In C.K. Kinzer & D.J. Leu (Eds.), *Literacy research, theory, and practice: Views from many perspectives* (pp. 169–175). Washington, DC: The National Reading Conference, Inc.

Duffy, A.M. (2001). Balanced, literacy, acceleration, and responsive teaching in a summer school literacy program for elementary school struggling readers. *Reading Research and Instruction, 40*(2), 67–100.

Erickson, K.A. (2000). All children are ready to learn: An emergent versus readiness perspective in early literacy assessment. *Seminars in Speech and Language, 21*(3), 193–203.

Erickson, K.A., & Koppenhaver, D.A. (1995). Developing a literacy program for children with severe disabilities. *Reading Teacher, 48*(8), 676–684.

Erickson, K.A., & Koppenhaver, D. A. (1998). Using the "write talk-nology" with Patrik. *Teaching Exceptional Children, 31*, 58–64.

Erickson, K.A., Koppenhaver, D.A., Yoder, D.E., & Nance, J. (1997). Integrated communication and literacy instruction for a child with multiple disabilities. *Focus on Autism and Other Developmental Disabilities, 12*(3), 142–150.

Fitzgerald, J., & Noblit, G. (2000). Balance in the making: Learning to read in an ethnically diverse first-grade classroom. *Journal of Educational Psychology, 92*(1), 3–22.

Flavell, J.H., Green, F.L., Flavell, E.R., & Grossman, J.B. (1997). The development of preschool children's knowledge about inner speech. *Child Development, 68*(1), 39–45.

Flippo, R.F. (1998). Points of agreement: A display of professional unity in our field. *The Reading Teacher, 52*(1), 30–40.

Foley, B. (1993). The development of literacy in individuals with congenital speech and motor impairments. *Topics in Language Disorders, 13*, 16–32.

Foley, B., & Pollatsek, A. (1999). Phonological processing and reading abilities in adolescents and adult with severe congenital speech impairments. *Augmentative and Alternative Communication, 15*, 156–174.

French, C., Morgan, J., Vanayan, M., & White, N. (2001). Balanced literacy: Implementation and evaluation. *Education Canada, 40*(4). Retrieved June 5, 2003, from http://www.acea.ca/english/edcan_dec2000_01.phtml

Garrity, L.I. (1977). Electromyography: A review of the current status of subvocal speech research. *Memory & Cognition, 5*, 615–622.

Giangreco, M.F., Cloninger, C.J., & Iverson, V.S. (1998). *Choosing Outcomes and Accommodations for Children (COACH): A guide to educational planning for students with disabilities* (2nd ed.). Baltimore: Paul H. Brookes Publishing Co.

Gillon, G. (with Clendon, S., Cupples, L., Flynn, M., Iacono, T., Schmidtkie, T., Yoder, D., & Young, A.). (2003). Phonological awareness development in children with physical, sensory, or intellectual impairment. In G. Gillon (Ed.), *Phonological awareness: From research to practice* (pp. 183–223). New York: Guilford Press.

Gipe, J., Duffy, C.A., & Richards, J.C. (1993). Helping a non-speaking adult male with cerebral palsy achieve literacy. *Journal of Reading, 36*(5), 380–389.

Gough, P.B., & Tunmer, W.E. (1986). Decoding, reading, and reading disability. *Remedial and Special Education, 7*, 6–10.

Guthrie, J.T. (1973). Reading comprehension and syntactic responses in good and poor readers. *Journal of Educational Psychology, 65*, 294–300.

Guthrie, J.T., Schafer, W.D., & Chun-Wei, H. (2001). Benefits of opportunity to read and balanced literacy instruction on the NAEP. *Journal of Educational Research, 94*(3), 145–162.

Hall, D.P., & Cunningham, P.M. (1998). *Month-by-month phonics for second grade.* Greensboro, NC: Carson-Dellosa.

Hardyck, C.D., & Petrinovich, L.F. (1969). Treatment of subvocal speech during reading. *Journal of Reading, 12*, 361–368.

Hardyck, C.D., & Petrinovich, L.F. (1970). Subvocal speech and comprehension level as a function of the difficulty level of reading material. *Journal of Verbal Learning and Verbal Behavior, 9*, 647–652.

Hardyck, C.D., Petrinovich, L.F., & Ellsworth, D.W. (1966). Feedback of speech muscle activity during silent reading: Rapid extinction. *Science, 154,* 1467–1468.

Hedrick, W.B., Katims, D.S., & Carr, N.J. (1999). Implementing a multimethod, multilevel literacy program for students with mental retardation. *Focus on Autism and Other Developmental Disabilities, 14*(4), 231–239.

Higginbotham, D.J., Lesher, G., & Moulton, B. (2000). *Communication enhancement center: Research project #4: Evaluating and enhancing communication rate, efficiency, and effectiveness.* Retrieved February 9, 2004, from University of Buffalo, Department of Communication Disorders Web site: http://www.cadl.buffalo.edu/download/Rate.pdf

Hogaboam, T.W., & Perfetti, C.A. (1978). Reading skill and the role of verbal experience in decoding. *Journal of Educational Psychology, 70*(5), 717–729.

Hogan, N., & Wolf, L. (2002). "I am a writer": Literacy, strategic thinking and meta-cognitive awareness. In K. Erickson, D. Koppenhaver, & D. Yoder (Eds.), *Waves of words: Augmentative communicators read and write* (pp. 21–40). Toronto: ISAAC Press.

Hoover, W.A., & Gough, P.B. (1990). The simple view of reading. *Reading and Writing: An Interdisciplinary Journal, 2,* 127–160.

International Reading Association and the National Association for the Education of Young Children (IRA/NAEYC). (1998). Overview of learning to read and write: Developmentally appropriate practices for young children. A joint position statement of the International Reading Association (IRA) and the National Association for the Education of Young Children (NAEYC). *Young Children, 53*(4), 30–46.

Kirsch, I.S., Jungeblut, A., Jenkins, L., & Kolstad, A. (1993). *Executive summary from adult literacy in America.* Princeton, NJ: Educational Testing Service.

Koppenhaver, D.A., & Erickson, K.A. (2003). Natural emergent literacy supports for preschoolers with autism and severe communication impairments. *Topics in Language Disorders, 23*(4), 283–292.

Koppenhaver, D.A., Evans, D.A., & Yoder, D.E. (1991). Childhood reading and writing experiences of literate adults with severe speech and motor impairments. *Augmentative and Alternative Communication, 7*(1), 20–23.

Koppenhaver, D.A., & Yoder, D.E. (1992). Literacy issues in persons with severe speech and physical impairments. In R. Gaylord-Ross (Ed.), *Issues and research in special education* (Vol. 2, pp. 156–201). New York: Teachers College Press.

Koriat, A., Greenberg, S.N., & Kreiner, H. (2002). The extraction of structure during reading: Evidence from reading prosody. *Memory & Cognition, 30*(2), 270–280.

LaBerge, D., & Samuels, S. (1974). Toward a theory of automatic information processing in reading. *Cognitive Psychology, 6,* 292–323.

Leinhardt, G., Zigmond, N., & Cooley, W. (1981). Reading instruction and its effects. *American Educational Research Journal, 18,* 343–361.

Leslie, L., & Caldwell, J. (2000). *Qualitative Reading Inventory-3* (3rd ed.). Boston: Allyn & Bacon.

Levy, B.A., Abello, B., & Lysynchuk, L (1997). Transfer from word training to reading in context: Gains in reading fluency and comprehension. *Learning Disability Quarterly, 20*(3), 173–188.

Light, J.C., Binger, C., & Kelford Smith, A. (1994). Story reading interactions between preschoolers who use AAC and their mothers. *Augmentative and Alternative Communication, 10,* 255–268.

Light, J.C., & Kelford Smith, A. (1993). The home literacy experiences of preschoolers who use augmentative communication systems and their nondisabled peers. *Augmentative and Alternative Communication, 9,* 10–25.

Locke, J.L. (1971). Phonemic processing in silent reading. *Perceptual and Motor Skills, 32,* 905–906.

Locke, J.L. (1978). Phonemic effects in the silent reading of hearing and deaf children. *Cognition, 6,* 173–187.

McCarthy, P.A. (1999). *The effects of balanced literacy instructional training: A longitudinal study of reading performance in the primary grades.* Unpublished doctoral dissertation, Marquette University, Milwaukee.

McCutchen, D., Bell, L.C., France, I.M., & Perfetti, C.A. (1991). Phoneme-specific interference in reading: The tongue-twister effect revisited. *Reading Research Quarterly, 26*, 87–103.

McGuigan, F.J. (1970). Covert oral behavior during silent performance of language tasks. *Psychological Bulletin, 74*, 3409–3426.

McGuigan, F.J. (1971). External auditory feedback from covert oral behavior during silent reading. *Psychonomic Science, 25*, 212–214.

Mike, D.G. (1995). Literacy and cerebral palsy: Factors influencing literacy learning in a self-contained setting. *Journal of Reading Behavior, 27*(4), 627–642.

Perfetti, C.A. (1977). Language comprehension and fast decoding: Some psycholinguistic prerequisites for skilled reading comprehension. In J.T. Guthrie (Ed.), *Cognition, curriculum, and comprehension* (pp. 20–41). Newark, DE: International Reading Association.

Perfetti, C.A. (1985). *Reading ability.* New York: Oxford University Press.

Perfetti, C.A., Bell, L.C., & Delaney, S.M. (1988). Automatic (prelexical) phonetic activation in silent word reading: Evidence from backward masking. *Journal of Memory and Language, 27*(1), 59–70.

Perfetti, C., Finger, E., & Hogaboam, T. (1978). Sources of vocalization latency differences between skilled and less skilled young readers. *Journal of Educational Psychology, 70*(5), 730–739.

Perfetti, C.A., & Hogaboam, T. (1975). Relationship between single word decoding and reading comprehension skill. *Journal of Educational Psychology, 67*(4), 461–469.

Perfetti, C.A., & Lesgold, A.M. (1977). *Coding and comprehension in skilled reading and implications for reading instruction.* Washington, DC: National Institute of Education.

Popplewell, S.R., & Doty, D.E. (2001). Classroom instruction and reading comprehension: A comparison of one basal reader approach and the Four Blocks framework. *Reading Psychology, 22*, 83–94.

Prelutsky, J. (1996). *A pizza the size of the sun.* West Caldwell, NJ: Greenwillow Books.

Pressley, M. (2002). *Reading instruction that works: The case for balanced teaching* (2nd ed.). New York: Guilford Press.

Pressley, M., Allington, R.L., Wharton-McDonald, R., Block, C.C., & Morrow, L.M. (2001). *Learning to read: Lessons from exemplary first-grade classrooms. Solving problems in the teaching of literacy.* New York: Guilford Press.

Rayner, K. (1985). The role of eye movements in learning to read and reading disability. *Remedial and Special Education, 6*(6), 53–60.

Rayner, K., & Pollatsek, A. (1989). *The psychology of reading.* Upper Saddle River, NJ: Prentice Hall.

Reutzel, D.R., & Hollingsworth, P.M. (1991). Reading time in school: Effect on fourth graders' performance on a criterion-referenced comprehension test. *Journal of Educational Research, 84*(3), 170–176.

Reid, D.K., Hresko, W.P., & Hammill, D.D. (1989). *Test of Early Reading Ability-2.* Austin, TX: PRO-ED.

Sachar, L. (2000). *Holes.* Yearling Books: New York.

Share, D.L. (1999). Phonological recoding and orthographic learning: A direct test of the self-teaching hypothesis. *Journal of Experimental Child Psychology, 72*(2), 95–129.

Shepard, M.J., & Uhry, J.K. (1997). Teaching phonological recoding to young children with phonological processing deficits: The effect on sight-vocabulary acquisition. *Learning Disability Quarterly, 20*(2), 104–125.

Silverstein, S. (1996). *Falling up.* New York: HarperCollins.

Skotko, B., Koppenhaver, D., & Erickson, K. (2004). Parent reading behaviors and communication outcomes in girls with Rett syndrome. *Exceptional Children, 70*(2), 145–166.

Slowiaczek, M.L., & Clifton, C. (1980). Subvocalization and reading for meaning. *Journal of Verbal Learning and Verbal Behavior, 19*(5), 573–582.

Stanovich, K.E., Cunningham, A.E., & Feeman, D.J. (1984). Intelligence, cognitive skills, and early reading progress. *Reading Research Quarterly, 19,* 278–303.

Vandervelden, M., & Siegel, L. (1999). Phonological processing and literacy in AAC users and students with motor speech impairments. *Augmentative and Alternative Communication, 15,* 191–209.

Vandervelden, M., & Siegel, L. (2001). Phonological processing in written word learning: Assessment for children who use augmentative and alternative communication. *Augmentative and Alternative Communication, 17*(1), 37–51.

Van Orden, G.C. (1991). Phonological mediation is fundamental to reading. In D. Besner & G.W. Humphreys (Eds.), *Basic processes in reading: Visual word recognition* (pp. 77–103). Hillsdale, NJ: Lawrence Erlbaum Associates.

Van Orden, G.C., Johnston, J.C., & Hale, B.L. (1988). Word identification in reading proceeds from spelling to sound to meaning. *Journal of Experimental Psychology: Learning, Memory and Cognition, 14*(3), 371–386.

Wagner, R.K., & Torgesen, J.K. (1987). The nature of phonological processing and its causal role in the acquisition of reading skills. *Psychological Bulletin, 101,* 192–212.

Wershing, A., & Hughes, C. (2002). Just give me words. In K. Erickson, D. Koppenhaver, & D. Yoder (Eds.), *Waves of words: Augmentative communicators read and write* (pp. 45–56). Toronto: ISAAC Press.

Woods, M.L., & Moe, A. (1995). *Analytical Reading Inventory, Fifth Edition.* Upper Saddle River, NJ: Prentice Hall.

Worthy, M.J., & Invernizzi, M.A. (1995). Linking reading with meaning: A case study of a hyperlexic reader. *Journal of Reading Behavior, 27*(4), 585–603.

14

Visual Strategies to Facilitate Written Language Development

PAUL R. HOFFMAN AND JANET A. NORRIS

ABSTRACT

School-age children who are failing to develop written language skills often have delays in oral language development, and they may be dependent on visual learning strategies that are maladaptive when applied to reading and writing. Their reading and writing difficulties may stem from underdeveloped language processing, including the perception of auditory characteristics of speech, categorization of phonemes, orthographic relationships, syntax, and use of language macrostructures. These processing deficits may lead to a slowed rate of acquisition of knowledge, resulting in school failure. This chapter presents a variety of visual tools that can be used in individual, small-group, or classroom reading and writing activities to accommodate many of these types of deficits. These tools enable children to visualize the abstract relationships depicted in text as they develop the mental processing structures needed to support future learning.

INTRODUCTION

The visual tools described in this chapter are currently being developed for use with children identified as poor readers in the early elementary grades. Poor reading has been associated with a variety of potential etiologies including general cognitive delay, attention-deficit/hyperactivity disorder (ADHD), oral language impairment, auditory processing disorder, and delayed development of phonological awareness (Beitchman & Young, 1997). Our current interest in visual reading instruction tools is based on the premise that many of these children fail to learn to read because they are predominantly visual thinkers, whereas reading and the methods used to teach reading are based predominantly on an auditory mode of thought (Freed & Parsons, 1997; Vygotsky, 1978; West, 1991). We hypothesize that there is a normal distribution of learning styles, with visual thinkers at one end of the distribution and auditory thinkers at the other, and more balanced thinkers between. In addition, many children with reading disability may be visual thinkers because they have auditory processing difficulties. Children who conceptualize primarily in a visual mode will demonstrate delays in oral language development, development of phonological awareness, and written language development. Visual thinking also appears to co-occur with ADHD (West, 1991) and autism spectrum disorder (Grandin, 1995).

Our current assessment procedures focus primarily on the child's reading and secondarily on potential indicators of visual learning style. We assess children's reading abilities using reading inventories such as the Stieglitz Informal Reading Inventory (1992). These are informal assessment devices that require children to read graded lists of individual words and story passages orally and to answer comprehension questions regarding the passages. Figure 14.1 displays a model of the processes involved in reading that we use as a guide in describing an individual child's reading abilities. Failure to read individual words indicates that the processes on the left side of the model in Figure 14.1 need to be supported with visual tools that aid the child's acqui-

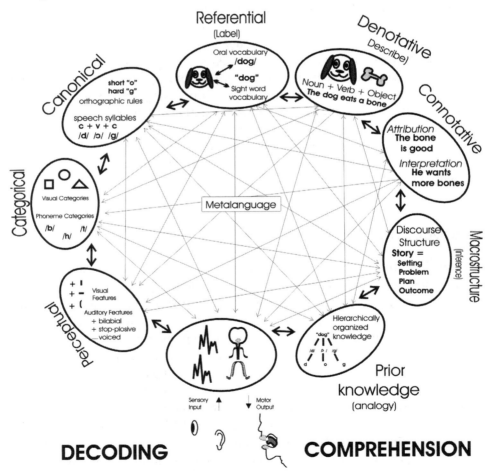

Figure 14.1. Constellation model of language abilities coordinated during reading. (From Norris, J.A. [2001]. *Phonic Faces* [p. 29]. Baton Rouge, LA: EleMentory. Copyright © 2001 J.A. Norris. Reprinted by permission.)

sition of phonemic awareness and orthography. An increase in miscues (i.e., aspects of an oral reading that deviate from the printed text) during passage reading indicates that the processes on the right side of the model need to be supported with visual tools that make vocabulary knowledge, syntactic structure, and discourse structure understandable. Failure to answer comprehension questions indicates a need to support the development of text macrostructure, to aid in derivation of connotative meaning, and to acquire knowledge from the text.

A variety of visual representations described in this chapter can be used to help visual learners develop the abilities represented by the processors in this model. Phonic Faces (Norris, 2001) is an alphabet in which each letter incorporates visual cues to the speech sounds represented by the letters. These are used to develop the processors on the left side of the model that are involved in speech sound perception, production, categorization, and sequencing. Iconic words are printed words that contain visual cues to the word's meaning. These are used to help develop the processing that occurs in the upper half of the model as the meanings of printed words are recognized. Picture sentences represent the relationships between grammatical structure, punctuation, and meaning of complex sentences. These are used to help develop the processing that occurs in the upper right quarter of the model. Storyboards are visual representations of the components of story structure, one aspect of the macrostructure component of the model. These are used to help the child develop the comprehension processes on the right side of the model.

TARGET POPULATIONS AND ASSESSMENTS FOR DETERMINING TREATMENT RELEVANCE AND GOALS

Individuals appear to be normally distributed with respect to their learning style: approximately 15% of the population are predominantly auditory learners, 15% are visual learners, and the remaining 70% are relatively balanced learners. Visual learners predominantly use the visual processing centers of the right side of the brain to solve problems. They often learn new concepts by combining and reordering visual images, are delayed in oral language development, and have difficulty learning to process print as a language system. Auditory learners use the language centers on the left side of the brain to solve problems verbally. They learn new concepts easily from verbal definitions, learn to read without effort, are good at organizing logical sequences, but may not excel in creatively applying mathematical concepts. Individuals at the far end of the auditory learning spectrum may be identified as having a nonverbal learning disability characterized by early success in reading, poor visuospatial abilities, significant problems in mathematical reasoning, and limited social competence (Rourke, 1995).

We are currently using a variety of indicators that a child is predominantly a visual learner. One indicator, borrowed from definitions of language learning disabilities, is a pattern of remarkably better nonverbal intelligence compared with reading ability. Tests of nonverbal intelligence (e.g., Brown, Sherbenou, & Johnsen, 1997) typically require analysis and evaluation of visual patterns while attempting to reduce the use of language processing. Children with better scores on such nonverbal tests compared with their oral or written language abilities appear to be more capable in visual than in verbal processing. A second indicator of a visual learning style is a right-brained score from Freed and Parsons's (1997) learning styles inventory. This is a parent questionnaire that includes items related to visuospatial abilities, hyperactivity, distractibility, and social interactions. A third indicator is good performance on visual memory tasks such as recalling a visual sequence of colors or letters (Freed & Parsons, 1997). A final indicator is poor performance in auditory decoding and integration abilities (Bellis, 1996). As a starting point, we have been using the SCAN screening test (Keith, 2000), which supplies measures of the degree to which a person uses the right or left hemispheres in dichotic listening tasks as well as a measures of the ability to fill in verbal information that has been filtered out of speech signals.

The more an individual child appears to be a visual learner, the more visual support we use in intervention. However, we have also found that provision of visual information may be useful in teaching reading skills to children who appear to be balanced learners but who have failed to develop reading abilities in the early grades.

THEORETICAL BASIS

West (1991) used biographical accounts of individuals known for their scientific or technical achievements who also had difficulty learning to read (e.g., Albert Einstein, Thomas Edison) to describe the differences between visual and auditory thinking and to suggest an explanation for the reading difficulties of visual thinkers. His definition of visual thinking involves the application of processes such as pattern recognition, transformation, and generation to visual forms and nonphysical abstract concepts. This type of thought is most directly applicable to understanding the physical world in artistic, scientific, or mathematical terms. Development of this type of thought is described in Piaget's work as occurring when objects and actions are studied and manipulated to form concepts and conceptual relationships (Piaget & Inhelder, 1973). Visual learning is most closely associated with right hemispheric processing and contrasts with auditory processing occurring in the left hemisphere. Auditory thinking employs processes such as logic, language, and sequential time. This type of thought is needed to understand the social world, including the actions, language, and thoughts of others within socially constructed events (Nelson, 1996). This type of thought is constructed with the help of more knowledgeable individuals within social interactions, as described by Vygotsky (1978). The potential for visual thinking to be a root cause of reading difficulty is supported by studies demonstrating that children with reading disability tend to demonstrate higher abilities on measures of performance IQ and visual perception than they do on verbal IQ and auditory perception, whereas many children with arithmetic disability show the opposite pattern (Badian, 1999).

The task facing young children reading a storybook is to use the visual images provided by the print to reconstruct the sequential actions represented by the language of a narrative. This is primarily an auditory/language task in which letter sequences such as *b-a-d* represent a sequence of phonemes. The phoneme sequences are organized within the sequentially organized syllables of words. The words are parts of larger sequences such as phrases, sentences, and the story elements that make up narratives. Children who apply visual thinking to the letter sequence *b-a-d* may have difficulty because they may think that *b* and *d* represent a single visual pattern that rotates to produce these different patterns rather than conceptualizing these as different letters (Vygotsky, 1978).

The visual tools described in this chapter are designed to give visual thinkers images they can use to learn about the verbal processes in the constellation model of reading and language shown in Figure 14.1 (Norris, 1998; Norris & Hoffman, 2002). This model is based on principles of connectionist models (Rumelhart & McClelland, 1986; Seidenberg & McClelland, 1989). It contains a set of nine processors that act simultaneously and interactively. Each processor employs different types of basic units to create different varieties of mental representations of patterns related to patterns in the environment. The patterns being developed in one processor both affect and are affected by the patterns being developed in the other processors. The following sections describe the functioning of each of the processors in normal and disordered reading.

Perceptual Processor

The *perceptual processor* recognizes relationships among features of the various forms of energy detected by the sensory systems. Visual stimuli are represented via relationships among lines, arcs, and other visual features. Auditory stimuli are represented as time-varying patterns of the amplitudes of various frequencies of sound. Interconnections among auditory and visual features represent relationships between sound sources and the sounds they produce. Speech perception involves recognition of some relatively direct relationships among visual and gestural features of speech sound production and the resulting auditory features of speech sounds. Some of these relationships appear to be present in the system near birth as demonstrated by infants' ability to associate the visual appearance of lip rounding and lip spreading with the auditory patterns for the vowels [u] and [i], respectively (Kuhl & Meltzoff, 1982).

Auditory processing deficits that decrease a child's ability to make these associations have been hypothesized to underlie both oral language and reading disabilities (Wright, Bowen, & Zecker, 2000). The decreased ability to attend to auditory stimuli exhibited by children with ADHD results in their performing poorly on a wide variety of auditory processing tasks (Breier, Fletcher, Foorman, Klass, & Gray, 2003). Difficulty in processing auditory features may cause children to prefer to focus on visual information. However, some children with ADHD and dyslexia appear to have a hypersensitivity to light, causing them to have trouble focusing in school because they perceive normal lighting as having an almost painful glare (Freed & Parsons, 1997). The process of gaining information during visual fixations on letter sequences during reading is disrupted and agitation occurs.

Categorical Processor

The *categorical processor* recognizes and generates phonemic patterns in the auditory, gestural, and visual features of speech production and letters in the visual features of print. The phenomenon of categorical perception is one example of an interaction among processors. The categorical processor uses auditory features detected by the perceptual processor to decide what phonemes are represented in speech. But, the categorical processor also shapes the features that the perceptual processor can detect. This results in adults being able to detect auditory features that are used to distinguish phonemes in their own language with considerable ease, whereas they frequently find it difficult or, in some cases, impossible to distinguish phonemes from other languages (Miyawaki et al., 1975). Moreover, the phonemic categories established in the categorical processor are shaped by the words learned in the referential processor to make distinctions between words forming minimal pairs.

In visual logic, the features of objects overlap with their meaning and function. The visual features of the flat, horizontal surface of a chair elevated by the chair's legs look like a fit for the shape of a person's legs when in a seated position. This combination of visual features is categorized as being a chair regardless of whether it is oriented to the right or left. It is natural to mentally view objects from multiple dimensions and orientations, and visual thinkers primarily create thoughts by reorienting and altering features of objects (Davis & Braun, 1997; Grandin, 1995; Vygotsky, 1978). A creative visual thinker might mentally consider alternative orientations of a chair's components to make the chair easier to get into or more comfortable.

However, letters are symbols for speech sounds and are not intended to follow the rules of visual logic. Letters bear no visual resemblance to the sounds they represent. The categorization of the letters *p, b, d,* and *q* requires that their orientation remain fixed in visual perception while the reader considers the auditory features that are associated with the letter. When a child applies visual logic to printed words and tries to abstract meaning by reorienting the letters to capture a meaningful view, the words may appear to move on the page, lines may be skipped, words may be altered, or letters may appear to grow or shrink (Davis & Braun, 1997). These transformations, which are adaptive and highly useful to other problems such as drawing or building with blocks, are nonproductive when reading, leaving the visual thinker confused and without useful strategies for understanding print.

Canonical Processor

The *canonical* processor organizes structured combinations of categories. In visual logic, categorical units are combined in space and reorganized across time. These are useful mental manipulation processes for the architect considering the effects of stress on the components of a complex structure. However, these manipulations fail in oral and written language, in which auditory logic dictates that categories be arranged into temporal sequences that cannot be reorganized across time without changing identities. Phonemes are organized into temporally sequenced syllables that include onsets preceding rimes. Letters are organized into orthographic units like *ph* and *gh*. Complex relationships are developed among phonemes and graphemes that depend on syllabic position. For example, the phoneme /f/ can be represented by the orthographic units *f, ff, gh,* and *ph.* Some of these units may occur at the beginning and end of syllables, and others may occur only at the end of a syllable.

Difficulty producing phoneme sequences to represent concepts during language acquisition, as demonstrated in phonological disorders, is associated with written language development problems. Longitudinal studies of preschool children who were delayed in speech sound development show they were also delayed in development of written language abilities (Felsenfeld, Broen, & McGue, 1992). Poor readers may have subtle inabilities to organize sensory-motor features in difficult speech tasks (Catts, 1989). Moreover, spelling errors often follow the patterns of phonological processes that describe the course of normal and delayed phonological development. Poor spellers display more phonological process errors in their spelling than do their peers. Again, an interaction among processors occurs inasmuch as children may eliminate the use of phonological process patterns from the spellings of words with simple consonant–vowel–consonant (CVC) structure, only to have them reappear in words with multiple syllables (Hoffman & Norris, 1989).

Referential Processor

The *referential* processor constructs meaningful units of oral language, including words and morphemes, by making arbitrary associations between particular sequences of phonemes and concepts in the *prior knowledge* processor. Reading requires learning arbitrary associations between oral words and sight words that then may be rapidly recognized in print. Skilled readers recognize simple words in print faster than they recognize the letters representing the word (Smith, 1971), indicating the development of sight words in the referential processor that enable word recognition before processing in the categorical and canonical processors is complete.

Difficulties in attending simultaneously to visual and auditory features of written language stimuli may contribute to oral language delays during the preschool years. As with letters, words are arbitrary symbols that bear no relationship to the visual objects and actions they represent. Therefore, it is difficult to overlap the phonetic features of words with the visual features of objects. Even in normal development, the words that emerge early in development represent objects and actions that can be seen, and only later do words representing abstract concepts and grammatical functions emerge. Function words are learned from mental representations of the *macrostructures* of events, as children begin to become aware of words in sentences for which they recognize no meaning (Nelson, 1996). This causes a need to attach meaning to these word forms, so context is used to abstract subtle meaningful contrasts in time (verb tense), number (plurals, pronouns, and auxiliary verbs designating noun–verb agreement), or subordination (subordinating conjunctions, relative pronouns). Visual thinkers may take longer to map words to even the most concrete objects, thus creating delayed oral language development, with a prolonged period of acquisition of grammatical morphemes.

Problems in referential development of oral and sight words are reciprocal. It has been estimated that the first-grade child knows 26,000 words and will gain an additional 3000–5000 words per year, with 50% being acquired through reading (Nagy & Herman, 1987; White, Graves, & Slater, 1989). Children who enter the reading process with smaller oral vocabularies soon find themselves attempting to sound out words that have no representation in the referential processor, contributing to their delays in reading. In turn, poor reading results in greater difficulty in determining the meaning of unknown words from the context, so vocabulary development lags further and further behind peers. The underlying different learning system remains to cause difficulties in the acquisition of written language. Tools and strategies that enable these types of children to visualize aspects of language as they are manifested in print would be useful and will be the focus of the interventions suggested in this chapter.

Denotative Processor

The *denotative* processor develops representations among cognitive event structures and linguistic grammatical structures. Event structures are basic units of experience (Nelson, 1996). Children participate in events in which objects are used by people to accomplish functional goals. Children display increasing knowledge of these event structures through self-help behaviors and in play. As language is acquired, words are used to refer to these events, initially using single words to reference the entire event (i.e., *juice* refers to the entire eating event) and gradually using complete sentences. The grammatical structures of these sentences express the relationships of meaning held between agents, actions, and objects within and across event structures. During reading, the printed words must activate appropriate event structures to derive the appropriate meaning in context. The more complex the sentence, the greater the number of events that must be coordinated to derive meaning.

Children exhibiting delayed syntactic development in kindergarten attain lower levels of reading in second and fourth grades than children exhibiting normal oral language development, especially if their language disabilities continue into the elementary grades (Catts, Fey, Tomblin, & Zhang, 2002). Unfortunately, reading involves mapping graphic symbols to oral language symbols (two arbitrary systems with no intermediary visual objects), a daunting task, which may contribute to the high percentage of reading disorders among children with early oral language delays, even when the language delay appears to be resolved.

Before a word is in focus during reading, it is being predicted by the grammatical units that have already been activated in the denotative processor. For example, having read the phrase *The wolf* at the start of a sentence, a reader has activated denotative units for a noun phrase that is most likely functioning as the grammatical subject of a sentence. This grammatical subject is also likely to be the agent of an action. This information is fed back to the referential processor to predict that the next word is likely to be a verb that expresses an action that a wolf might execute next in the sequence of actions being constructed in the macrostructure of the text. For example, if the text were referring to the Big Bad Wolf approaching the third little pig's house, the macrostructure of the story and denotative structure of the sentence to this point would be activating words like *huffed* and *puffed* in the referential processor. If this activation has accurately predicted the words in the text, reading one of these words based on partial processing by the phonemic and categorical processors will be rapid and effortless.

When information is incorrectly processed by the reader, the words primed for word recognition will be incorrect, resulting in reading miscues (Seidenberg & McClelland, 1989; Smith, 1971). An important source of inappropriate denotative predictions by poor readers is their relatively poor development of morphology and syntax. In a longitudinal study, Loban (1976) showed that poor readers reach school producing language that is syntactically less complex than that of better readers and that they fall increasingly further behind their average-reading peers from kindergarten through the twelfth grade in both oral and written language. They produce fewer words per communication unit, more mazes, fewer and less complex elaborations of adjective and adverbial clauses, and fewer dependent clauses. Their oral and written sentences are less elaborated in all aspects of grammar. As the texts being read in school become increasingly more complex from grade to grade, both word recognition and comprehension difficulties increase as a result of inadequate development of denotative structures. Consider the sentence, *The wolf who was very hungry huffed and puffed.* If the child's denotative system does not have strong representations for complex sentences with embedded clauses of this type, a miscue may occur. Reading *The wolf* may activate only possible verb phrases to complete a simple sentence structure rather than the word *who* that must be recognized in print.

Connotative Processor

The *connotative* processor uses information from the prior knowledge and macrostructure processors to create and interpret implied, inferred, and figurative meaning. A child reading the sentence *The wolf licked his lips when he saw the three pigs through the window of the brick house* is supposed to derive the connotation that the wolf is looking forward to eating the pigs. This involves accessing prior knowledge that wolves hunt and eat other animals and that pigs are considered a food source by wolves. The derivation of this inference is also supported by the child's knowledge of the story's macrostructure. As the wolf approaches the brick house, the child knows that the wolf is hungry, has not eaten anything, and has already made two attempts to eat pigs. However, when school-age children identified as having a language learning disability read and retell stories, they include fewer inferences to the mental states of characters and fail to answer comprehension questions that require inferences (Wright & Newhoff, 2001). Thus, they are likely to exhibit miscues in reading the more complex text that is typical of third- and fourth-grade reading.

Literate language and humor make use of nonliteral language forms including idioms (e.g., *He got carried away*), ambiguity (e.g., *What's black and white and read all over?*), metaphor (e.g., *She was a rock*), and simile (*She was like a rock*). Knowledge of these forms develops throughout the school years (Nippold, 1998) and presents challenges to children with language learning disabilities (Wallach & Butler, 1994). The child who interprets language visually will make a strong interpretation of the literal picture but will be less able to translate that into the implied meaning.

Macrostructure Processor

Macrostructures can be nonverbal event structures, as in knowing how to play baseball or how to dine in a restaurant, or verbal discourse structures that tell a story or explain a process. There are many types of discourse structure including poetry, exposition, conversation, and narrative. Children's early language development occurs within social interactions and is aided by the child's developing knowledge of the structure of events (Nelson, 1996). Within everyday events such as eating meals, the child is repeatedly exposed to a sequence of actions in which people play particular roles and objects are related to one another through goal-directed actions. The child is exposed to and uses language forms to talk about these repeated actions and objects. As a result, the child's developing mental representation for the event and the sensory stimulation from the event aid in the child's learning to talk within and about the event. Children as young as age 3 talk about events such as eating meals, shopping in stores, and eating in restaurants with an appropriate sequence of actions. Younger children mention the more important goal-directed actions of the event, whereas older children add details in their descriptions.

Narratives are organized around problems created when there are departures from the normal structure of an event. Stories that are patterned after traditional Western European folk tales include a setting, initiating event or problem, plan, attempts, outcomes, and evaluations (Stein & Glenn, 1979). The *setting* includes information about the time and location of the story, the main characters, and the habitual events that make up the characters' daily lives. The *initiating event* or *problem* is some change in the normal setting that poses a problem for the main characters that causes an *internal reaction and plan*. The initial internal reaction may be emotional but it also causes the main characters to think about the problem and to formulate plans to deal with the problem. The *attempt* includes the characters' actions that are organized to achieve the goals of the plan. An attempt will have an *outcome* or resolution that describes whether the character attained the goal. A failure to achieve the original goal may lead to abandoning the goal or creating a new plan. Children's stories that include larger numbers of these constituents and that include a higher number of problems with resolutions are rated as having better narrative quality by adults (McFadden & Gillam, 1996).

The stories told by school-age children with language learning disability often include a less coherent sequence of actions that omits the characters' internal reaction to the initiating event (Merritt & Liles, 1987, 1989; Ripich & Griffith, 1988; Wright & Newhoff, 2001). Their relative lack of narrative organization may also be seen in their production of more communicative disfluencies (i.e., stalls, repairs, and abandoned utterances) than their peers in story generation (MacLachlan & Chapman, 1988).

Creation and understanding of coherent narratives require the use of a variety of denotative structures, many of which function as cohesive ties. Cohesive ties signal that information needs to be interpreted by referring to information occurring earlier or later in the story. For example, pronouns are used to indicate that the current actions or states are attributed to earlier mentioned characters and objects. Complex sentence structures with and without conjunctions are used to specifically state temporal and causal relationships among actions. Mental verbs are used in complex sentences to explicitly state character internal responses and plans. Elementary school children identified with reading or language learning disabilities tend to retell stories with a higher percentage of pronouns without clear referents (Feagans & Short, 1984; Liles, 1985; Norris & Bruning, 1988). They may use fewer temporal and causative conjunctions, instead using *and* to combine clauses and sentences (Greenhalgh & Strong, 2001; Norris & Bruning, 1988). Furthermore, children with typically developing language may be more likely to repair their cohesion errors than are children with language learning disabilities (Purcell & Liles, 1992).

Prior Knowledge

Academic success entails creating organized hierarchies of information regarding content areas such as social studies, literature, and science. Readers with more background knowledge on a topic comprehend a passage more rapidly and easily because they have activated organized structures of referential, denotative, and connotative information as they start to read. They can more easily incorporate information acquired from the text into their well-formed knowledge structures. In addition, active readers are constantly evaluating the information presented in texts with respect to their current hierarchical understandings of the world. When the propositions found in a text and current knowledge are not similar, readers may adjust their hierarchical knowledge to include the new information or may reject the author's information as inaccurate.

Poor readers read less and comprehend less of what they do read. Therefore, they have created less background knowledge. Their lack of background knowledge makes it more difficult to read new material. Thus, a negative cycle continues in which poor readers learn less and less compared with their peers.

EMPIRICAL BASIS

Clinical use of the visual strategies described in this chapter is currently supported indirectly by data from studies of similar, but not identical, strategies being used for similar types of outcomes (Gillon, 2000; Idol, 1978; Idol & Croll, 1987; Lindamood-Bell Learning Processes, 2002; McFadden, 1998; Pokorni, Worthington, & Evans-Joyce, 2001; Torgesen, 1999). These studies typically have been conducted as efficacy studies in which the intent is to show that the use of a particular visual strategy is responsible for a particular behavioral change under relatively well-controlled conditions. The results of these studies suggest that visual strategies are useful in fostering some aspects of oral and written language. However, studies reported to date generally do not have a high degree of internal validity showing that it was the strategy itself that was responsible for a change in client behavior, rather than uncontrolled variables outside of the experiments.

Visual Representations of Letter–Speech Sound Relationships

A meta-analysis of 52 studies demonstrated that phonemic awareness training improved reading and spelling scores for children in preschool through first grade who were characterized as typically developing, at-risk, and having a reading disability (Ehri et al., 2001). This review also found that phonemic awareness training was more effective when conducted with reference to visual representations of the letters. The visual representations for letter–sound relationships described in this chapter, Phonic Faces (Norris, 2001), provide both the letter associated with particular sounds and a cue to the speech sound associated with the letter.

Our use of Phonic Faces (Norris, 2001) as a visual representation in support of decoding print into words is similar to part of the approach taken in Lindamood-Bell Learning Processes (2002) programs, which teach discrimination of speech sounds and sound–letter relationships using photographs of speakers producing the sounds as one set of teaching materials. The photographs are used as cues to the recognition of the articulatory placements of speech sounds. Practice is then provided in recognizing the sounds in words, the number of sounds in words, and the ordering of sounds in words using colored blocks. Practice is also provided in letter–sound correspondences and decoding of individual words and words within texts. Exploratory clinical data for large groups of children taught with this method in an intensive manner show increased reading accuracy for words and paragraphs, spelling, and improved comprehension of orally read paragraphs from pre-intervention to postintervention (Lindamood-Bell Learning Processes, 2002).

An exploratory study reported by Torgesen (1999) showed that eight 10-year-old children diagnosed with learning disabilities who received 80 hours of intensive instruction using the Lindamood-Bell method dramatically increased their rate of change on periodic administrations of word reading tests. Results of Torgesen's study also showed that a less intensive program that embedded phonics instruction within meaningful reading and writing activities showed similar improvements in word identification skills. This use would be similar to the use of Phonic Faces, a major component of the intervention described in this chapter, within meaningful reading and writing activities.

Although the preceding studies suggest that the Lindamood-Bell programs are effective, they have not isolated the visual aspects of the training program to demonstrate that they are responsible for the changes. Pokorni, and colleagues (2001) found that use of the Lindamood-Bell program produced improvements in phonemic awareness abilities for children with language impairments during an intensive 4-week summer program; however, these improvements were not greater than those produced by two other programs that did not use this type of visual stimuli.

Stick-Figure Drawings of Conceptual Relationships and Complex Syntax

The intervention described here uses stick-figure drawings to enhance the development of abstract language such as metaphors, similes, and complex sentence structure. The goal of our use of stick figures is to provide visual representations of how grammatical structures refer to the temporal, causal, and intentional relationships among actions. McFadden (1998) tested the efficacy of teaching 7–9-year-old children to make pictographic representations of story events within an exploratory study. The study included 61 children, 17 of whom were classified by their teachers as low achieving in language arts. The representations used were schematic pictures of events that signified temporal order from left to right. Story structure was represented in three pictures, one each for the setting, initiating event, and resolution. The children's oral stories told from the three-part pictographic representations were compared with stories told using written notes and single pictures drawn by the children. The children's stories told from pictographic representations were longer than stories constructed from written notes (effect size = .42) or a drawing (effect size = .27) and included more temporal conjunctions compared with stories constructed from written notes (effect size = .90) or picture drawings (effect size = .41).

Story Boards Representing Macrostructure

Two studies have shown the efficacy of instruction in story mapping on reading comprehension of children with learning disabilities in elementary grades (Idol, 1978; Idol & Croll, 1987). Idol (1978) taught small groups of third- and fourth-grade children to use story maps as an aid to reading comprehension within an effectiveness study. The study design incorporated multiple baselines across subject groups in which 22 children receiving classroom instruction in reading were randomly assigned to one of two groups. One group of children ($n = 11$) remained in the control condition, whereas the experimental group of 11 children received story map instruction. Two of the children in the first group had been classified as having a language learning disability. One child in the second group had been classified as having a language learning disability and two had been classified as low achieving. In the baseline condition, the teacher displayed a set of comprehension questions on an overhead projector while the children silently read a passage. The children handed in the passages prior to writing answers to the questions from memory.

The story map intervention was conducted in three phases: teacher modeling of map construction, teacher summarization of child maps, and student independent map construction. In the teacher modeling phase, the teacher displayed a story map outline on the overhead projector and gave children copies of the story map outline to be filled in as they silently read the story. The teacher modeled the use of story mapping by periodically asking individuals in the group to supply information to be filled in on the overhead version of the story map as they read. Students added information from the group story map to their individual maps. In the teacher summarization condition, the students read silently and filled in their own story maps, followed by the teacher leading construction of a group map on the overhead projector as the children made corrections to their individual maps. In the final phase of intervention, students independently constructed story maps as they read. Comprehension measurement was made in each phase by having students write answers to comprehension questions after they handed in their maps.

The visual format for the story maps contained five boxes arranged from top to bottom on a page. The first box was labeled *The Setting,* with lower level headings for *Characters, Time,* and *Place.* The second box was labeled *The Problem* and was used to record information regarding the initiating event. The third box, *The Goal,* included information regarding the characters' reactions to the initiating event and the characters' goals. The fourth and largest box, *Action,* provided a place to record the characters' actions that are their attempts to reach their goal. The last box, *The Outcome,* was used to record results of the attempts and the characters' reactions to these results.

Results showed that the two children with language learning disabilities in the first group displayed an increase in comprehension at a time when the three children in the second group, who were still in the baseline phase, did not show an improvement. After receiving intervention, the scores of the three children in the second group also improved. These results suggest that it was the intervention that caused improvements in comprehension. In addition, all of the children continued to improve in their comprehension in the remaining phases of intervention, and all of the children showed better comprehension test scores in a maintenance phase (mean = 80%, range = 55%–98%) compared with the baseline phase (mean = 44%, range = 33%–69%).

Idol and Croll (1987) conducted a single-subject design study for five children with reading comprehension problems whose intervention was similar to that described above but was provided individually in daily 20-minute sessions. With these children, the teachers also directed attention to where in the text the child could find information to make inferences that were problematic for the child. All of the children showed gains in comprehension from the baseline to treatment phases, and four of the five children maintained their gains in a maintenance phase. These four children also showed an increase in the number of story grammar components produced in retellings of the stories from baseline to intervention. These gains were maintained in the maintenance phase. In sum, these studies intimate that using pictorial representations of elements of story structure results in children producing more of these elements in their retellings of stories and better comprehension of story events.

PRACTICAL REQUIREMENTS

Successfully keeping visually oriented children with reading problems in the regular classroom must be a team effort. The speech-language pathologist (SLP) can play a central role through both direct intervention and consultation. Consultation with classroom teachers can help the teachers understand the learning differences of nonverbal learners and illustrate how they can supplement their teaching with visual input. Parent involvement can be crucial, because parents are the individuals who help with homework and frequently must re-teach information not understood in the classroom. Parents who understand how their child learns and how to compensate using visual input can provide continuity and help their children to deal with many difficulties encountered across grade levels. SLPs may be the best-trained professionals to provide intervention when needed and to serve as a consultant to teachers and parents. Our training in language is unique and provides the tools needed to understand each of the spoken and written language problems encountered across all processing clusters of the constellation. With this understanding, appropriate intervention can be planned.

The person using these visual tools needs to understand the underlying processes that are represented by the tool, strategies for visualizing information, and strategies for incorporating the tool into literacy-based activities such as storybook reading and writing. Similar visual strategies have been incorporated into commercially available products that may serve as models for the interventionist seeking to develop and use visual strategies (Isaacson, 2002; Norris, 2001).

The use of Phonic Faces requires a familiarity with the concept of phonemes, the nature of the relationship between phonemes and letters, and methods for facilitating the development of phonemic awareness and print knowledge. These topics are elaborated on in the Phonic Faces manual (Norris, 2001) which is available commercially at http://www.elementory.com.

The visual representation of sight words requires the intervention provider to quickly think of a visual representation of a word's meaning that is simple to sketch onto part of the printed word; for example, the word *reading* could incorporate a face inside the circle of the letter *d* that is reading a book (Isaacson, 2002). Sets of sight words with visual representations are available commercially at http://www.picturemereading.com.

Visual representations of sentence structure and punctuation require that the interventionist recognize major syntactic units in a sentence and understand how punctuation signifies the boundaries of these units. The use of storyboards requires the service provider to understand the components of story structure and be able to recognize them in the texts being read with children. Many visual teaching tools for these levels of language organization are commercially available from companies that market to SLPs, including Make Your Own Pictographs (http://www.picturemereading.com). Phonic Faces and Storyboards (http://www.elementory.com), Simple Sentence Structure (http://www.laureatelearning.com), Connect-a-Card (http://www.proedinc.com), and The Learning Ladder (http://www.thinkingpublications.com).

We have conducted parent training in the use of visual strategies in the following steps. First, the parent reads a description of a particular technique and asks questions to clarify any apparent misunderstandings. Next, the parent observes the facilitator modeling the technique or views a short video clip of the technique being utilized. The parent is then videotaped attempting the technique with the child. The parent and clinician then review the tape, and the clinician supplies feedback regarding the use of the technique. The parent tries the technique a second time. If this attempt is successful, a new technique may be added; if unsuccessful, the clinician provides more feedback and another chance to practice. Our exploratory use of this technique suggests parents can learn to utilize one or two techniques in a session.

KEY COMPONENTS

Children who perform poorly on single-word reading or who struggle to sound out words during their paragraph reading are demonstrating difficulties with the processes on the left half of the constellation model. We use two visual strategies, Phonic Faces (Norris, 2001) and iconic words, to aid in their development of these processes. Children whose miscues occur primarily in contextual reading are demonstrating difficulty with the processes on the right side of the model. For these children, we include visual tools that provide visual representations of figurative language, complex sentence structure, punctuation, and discourse structure.

Visual Representation of Sound–Letter Relationships

Phonic Faces (Norris, 2001) is a visual tool designed to aid learning of the relationships between the visual graphemes and auditory phonemes in the categorical processor. This tool incorporates a visual representation of some aspect of the phoneme's perceptual features into the shape of the letter so that the child receives simultaneous visual cues to both the grapheme and the phoneme. As seen in Figure 14.2, the *p, b,* and *d* Phonic Faces provide cues to the place of articulation of the sounds /p/, /b/, and /d/. In the Phonic Face *p,* the curve of the letter *p* forms the upper lip on a face, with lines representing the burst of air that pops out of the mouth during /p/ production. The adult instructs the child to touch the upper lip to feel the burst of air during /p/ production. The curve of the letter *b* forms the lower lip on the Phonic Face, and is introduced by touching the lower lip while producing the /b/ sound and feeling the lip move down. The circle of the letter *d* appears as a drum placed inside the mouth, the vertical line of the *d* is a drumstick affixed to the tongue to visually conceptualize the tongue movement that produces /d/.

During storybook reading the cards can be used to provide visual cues to aid in the repair of a miscue. If a child reads the word *dig* as "big," the adult lays the *d* card next to the word on the page and explains that the letter *d* tells the reader to raise the tongue tip to make the drumming sound. Or she

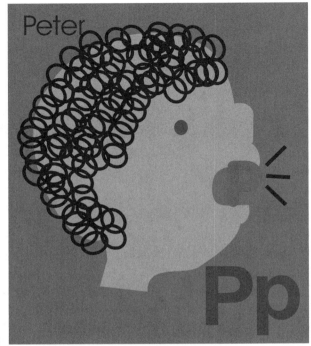

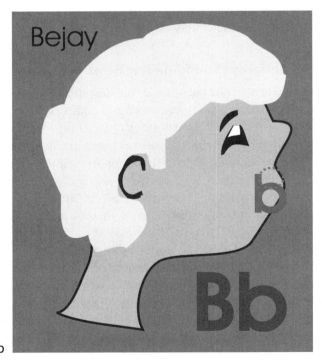

Figure 14.2. Phonic Faces depicting the letters *p, b,* and *d.* (From Norris, J.A. [2001]. *Phonic Faces* [pp. 64, 74, 104]. Baton Rouge, LA: EleMentory. Copyright © 2001 J.A. Norris. Reprinted by permission.)

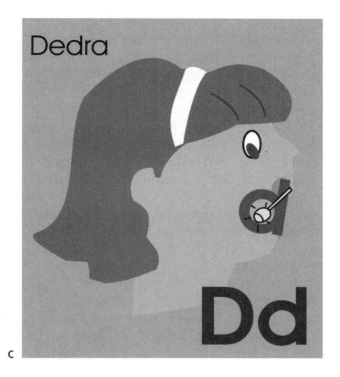

C

could place both the *b* and *d* cards next to the word while explaining the contrast in words created by the change from one letter to the other. The adult could say, "When the *b* starts the word, the reader puts his lips together and makes the [b] sound to start the word *big*. When the *d* starts the word, the reader lifts his tongue tip to make the drumming sound to start the word *dig*." SLPs will recognize this procedure as a case of using the contrast between a minimal pair of words to establish the contrast between two phonemes. It is also a procedure that helps the child establish phonemic awareness for the separation of a syllable into phonemes and recognition of rhyme. In this case, the /b/, /d/, and /p/ are syllable onsets that are being contrasted in combination with the syllable rime [ɪg] to produce a set of rhyming words: *big, dig, pig*. The child is provided a visual method of seeing that the phonemes /p/, /b/, and /d/ can be separated from the word and recombined to form new words. Reading the various combinations also supplies the child with practice in sound blending.

The cards may also be used in separate activities, to teach particular aspects of phonemic awareness and spelling. The child could listen to words and syllables and then choose the card that represents the initial sound or the final sound, or the set of cards that represents the whole syllable. The adult could lay out sound sequences for the child to blend together into fluent readings of syllables or words.

Explicit recognition of the relationship between the meaning of the word at the referential level and the print representation of the word can be enhanced by creating spellings for the labels of pictures. Given a picture of a dog, for example, a child would use a limited set of Phonic Faces to represent the sequence of sounds in the word. The cards also supply the spelling of the word that is sounded out. Within storybook reading, an adult can use the Phonic Faces to spell out words in the text that are also depicted in pictures on the page; for example, using the faces to create the sound sequence for the printed word *dog* while also showing a dog in a picture on the page.

By using the techniques described above, beginning readers are introduced to words with simple CVC structures in which regular graphophonemic relationships are maintained (e.g., *cat, dog, big*). These simple patterns are used to introduce the concept of sound blending, or pronouncing the sounds in sequence, until the words are recognized. Thus, interactive connections must be activated within the network for sensory, perceptual, categorical, canonical, and referential units.

By early first grade, more complex orthographic relationships are needed to read digraphs, long and short vowels, and words affected by the many orthographic patterns used in English so that five vowel letters can represent 14 vowel phonemes. The concept of long versus short vowels is represented in the Phonic Faces by two sets of vowels, a set of babies depicting the short vowels and a set of adults depicting the long vowels. Because vowel production does not involve places of articulation that are as easy to identify as the consonants, the vowel Phonic Faces involve visual cues that refer to nonverbal sounds or to words suggested by facial expression. For example, the baby *a* is depicted as an infant who is crying an [æ] sound, whereas baby *i* is grimacing to make the [ɪ] sound. A short story is associated with each character to explain their sounds. Baby *a* is unhappy so she cries all the time, and Baby *i* doesn't like carrots so she says [ɪ] as in "ick." The adult *a* is a cheerful, smiling character who says the long "a" sound, [eɪ], when she smiles and says, "Hooray! It's a good day." The explanation is that the sad Baby *a* grew up to be a happy adult. The adult *i* is pictured with prominent eyeglasses to cue production of the sound [aɪ]. Her story is that because Baby *i* didn't eat her carrots, she grew up to need eyeglasses.

Similar short stories are used to explain orthographic patterns for the vowel sounds, as in the double-vowel rule; that is, the phoneme represented by two vowel letters in one syllable is usually the long vowel sound of the first vowel. To explain this rule, the adult first spells the word with two baby vowels, then explains, "It's not a good idea to leave two babies alone, so usually the grown-up of the first baby comes in to take care of both of them." The "adult" long vowel face could be selected by the child and placed on top of the two babies, so that the sound blending attempt now uses the long vowel production (see Figure 14.3).

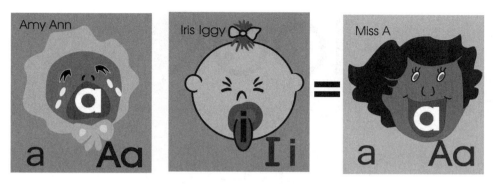

Figure 14.3. Use of Phonic Faces to show the phonic rule for double vowels. (From Norris, J.A. [2001]. *Phonic Faces* [p. 285]. Baton Rouge, LA: EleMentory. Copyright © 2001 J.A. Norris. Reprinted by permission.)

Visual Representations of Sight Words: Iconic Words

In first grade, students are often expected to learn several new sight words each week. Typical teaching strategies include worksheets that place the print under a picture of the word, or flash cards with the print on one side and a picture on the other. These strategies may fail with visual learners because there is too much separation between the print and pictorial representations of a concept. An alternative strategy, which we refer to as *iconic words,* is to create more visual overlap between the print and pictorial representations of words by drawing visual cues to the concept on the printed word as in Figure 14.4. The meaning of the word *look* is suggested by making the two *o* letters appear to be eyes that are looking at something. The word *run* could be enhanced by adding a simple stick figure head to the top of the *r* with running legs at the bottom. The letter *t* in the word *tree* could be drawn with a tree trunk and two branches.

More abstract concepts may require that the drawing be accompanied by a verbal explanation. Fortunately, at least some visual learners are happy to create these explanations. The drawing for *else* in Figure 14.4 was created by a first grader who explained it as follows: "The *l* is tall, and everyone else is short."

This strategy can be used into middle school when students learn complex abstract words made up of multiple morphemes as part of science and social studies. The child who reads about the concepts in a chapter is aided in developing visual additions to the letters that cue some aspect of the word's meaning. Figure 14.5 shows the cues to meaning and sound production that a child added to the word *photosynthesis*. He sketched the sun's rays on an *o* to symbolize the sun's energy that triggers the process. He drew the frosting and a candle of a birthday cake on the top of the *n* to remind himself that photosynthesis produces sugar. He called the cake a "sin" food (because it has too many calories) to cue the decoding of the syllable *syn.* Finally,

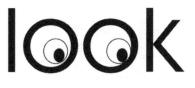

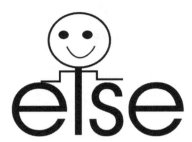

Figure 14.4. Iconic words used to picture both meaning and orthographic structure of written words. (From Norris, J.A. [2001]. *Phonic Faces* [p. 267]. Baton Rouge, LA: EleMentory. Copyright © 2001 J.A. Norris. Reprinted by permission.)

he added eyes to the *i* in the final syllable as a cue to read this syllable like the name he uses for his sister, *sis*.

One of the indicators of visual learning style is an ability to stare at a complex word for 10–15 seconds, then close the eyes and mentally read off the spelling of the word forward and backward (Freed & Parsons, 1997). We use this as a study technique in which the child visualizes the iconic words to get a simultaneous visual picture of the spelling, phonemic sequence, and meaning of the word. These word drawings, as well as drawings of concept relationships, become the child's study notes.

Visual Representations of Sentence Structure and Punctuation: Picture Sentences

The poor reader's development of denotative structure is often inadequate, leading to difficulties in understanding both the basic and implied meanings of a passage. The written sentences of a reading passage provide an ideal context to employ visual strategies to benefit development of both written and more advanced oral language. Unlike spoken sentences, which are momentary and rapid, written sentences are permanent and can be repeatedly examined, parsed into component phrases, reordered to establish the basic relationships, visualized in picture phrases, and in other ways explored until a child understands how the complex sentence works. By working through each of the sentences in a reading passage on which a child miscues or reads with inappropriate phrasing and intonation, competence can be acquired for

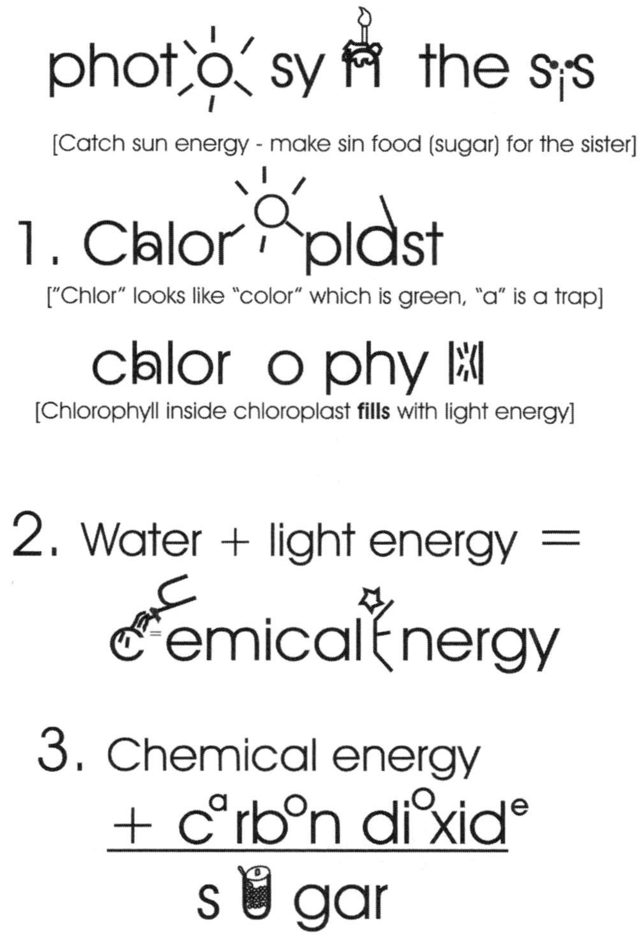

phot o sy the s i s

[Catch sun energy - make sin food (sugar) for the sister]

1. Chlor plast

["Chlor" looks like "color" which is green, "a" is a trap]

chlor o phy

[Chlorophyll inside chloroplast **fills** with light energy]

2. Water + light energy =

chemical energy

3. Chemical energy
+ carbon dioxide
sugar

Figure 14.5. Use of iconic words for science vocabulary and study guide. (From Norris, J.A. [2001]. *Phonic Faces* [p. 305]. Baton Rouge, LA: Ele-Mentory. Copyright © 2002 J.A. Norris. Reprinted by permission.)

grammatical structures more complex than those comprehended or used in oral and/or written language (Norris, 1998).

The sentence, *She ran up four flights of stairs to the bedroom that she and her sisters shared,* for example, can be understood if parsed into three parts: 1) she raced up four flights of stairs, 2) to the bedroom, 3) that she and her sisters shared. Children who do not understand the language of such texts read them with flat intonation without pausing at appropriate clause and phrase boundaries. The adult can aid the children in visualizing the events of the sentence by sketching a representation of the events and their linkages as seen in Figure 14.6—a strategy we refer to as *picture sentences.*

Visual learners tend to have great difficulty with function words that are not easy to represent visually. The meaning of these forms can be made ex-

She raced up four flights of stairs to the bedroom that she
and her sisters shared

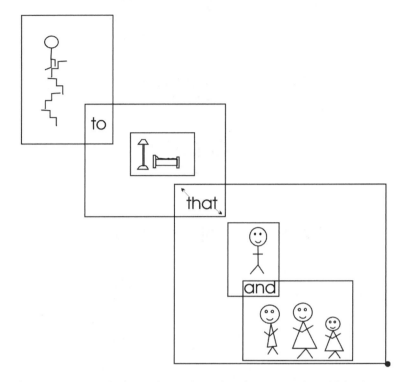

Figure 14.6. Picture sentences demonstrating how function words establish relationships of meaning between component phrases.

plicit by drawing the content information inside picture frames that indicate
information that must be read and understood as a unit, and then placing
the function or relational words in the overlapping corners of these frames.
The words in the sentence could then be read while pointing to the corresponding elements in the picture: *She ran up* [pointing to the stick figure]
four flights [count the four flights] *of stairs to* [pointing to the connecting
word] *the bedroom* [pointing to the middle picture] *that* [pointing to the
connecting word and showing how the arrows indicate that the pronoun
refers in both directions] *she* [pointing to the girl] *and* [pointing to the connecting word] *her sisters* [pointing to the sisters] *shared*. When we reach
the end of the picture sentence, the final picture frame is "nailed shut" with
a period in the lower right-hand corner to indicate that is the final element
of the scene that must be pictured. The child is then asked to reread the
word sentence. If the structure and meaning are clear, the sentence should
be read with appropriate intonation and phrasing. Any place in the sentence
where intonation or phrasing is still incorrect means that something in the
language is still not understood. We know exactly what to picture further.

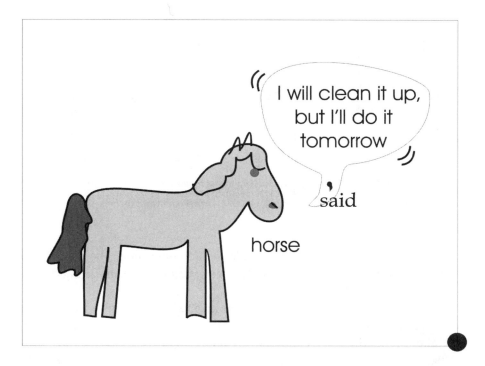

I will clean it up but I will do it tomorrow said horse

Figure 14.7. Picture strategy used for demonstrating the meaning and function of quotation marks. (From Norris, J.A. [2002]. *Learn to punctuate visually* [p. 36]. Baton Rouge, LA. EleMentory.com. Copyright © 2002 Norris. Reprinted by permission.)

Punctuation is used to cue many aspects of sentence structure and meaning. The following sentence shows many of these difficulties: "'I will clean it up, but I will do it tomorrow,' said horse." The quotation marks indicate there is a speaker who is talking, the first comma connects two clauses, the second comma shifts meaning to the narrator who tells who is talking, and the period designates when the idea is complete. Figure 14.7 shows a pictorial representation of the meaning of these types of punctuation. The speaker, in this case the horse, was drawn along with his spoken words in a talking bubble like those used in cartoons. The unpunctuated sentence is written below the picture. The adult explains that the child needs to figure out a way to put everything from the picture sentence into the word sentence, including the talking bubble, the pointer on the talking bubble, and the picture frame. The children suggest a few strategies. The adult suggests drawing a corner at the beginning of the talking bubble, using the open quotation marks. The child is asked to put the same marks in the word sentence. This is repeated for the closed parentheses. The adult points out that the part of the speech bubble that points to the speaker looks like a comma. It is found on the pic-

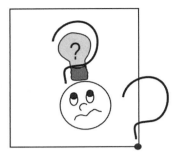 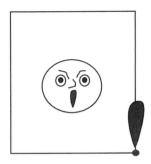

Figure 14.8. Picture strategy used for demonstrating the meaning and function of punctuation. (From Norris, J.A. [2002]. *Learn to punctuate visually* [p. 28]. Baton Rouge, LA. EleMentory.com. Copyright © 2002 Norris. Reprinted by permission.)

ture before the right end of the bubble, so a comma should be placed before the closing quotation marks. All of the picture sentences are framed, and all are nailed shut with a period.

Exclamation marks are explained as having a period plus a "yelling" mark. Question marks have a period plus a light bulb, meaning that someone is asking about something they don't know, as in Figure 14.8. If commas are not understood within a sentence, the two clauses are pictured as in Figure 14.6, and the comma is placed in the corner of the overlapping frames.

Visual Representation of Macrostructure: Storyboards

Visual thinkers combine pictures to recall events. They can accomplish this with amazing speed, but the pictures that are most salient to them may not fit traditional story structure. To help structure stories for better comprehension, or for drafts of writing, a storyboard can be used. The storyboard depicted in Figure 14.9 uses pictures paired with words to cue elements of story structure. Story setting is represented by time (a clock face), character (stick figures), and setting (a house). A problem is depicted by a chagrined facial expression. The plan is represented by a light bulb indicating an idea. The attempt is represented by a hand that would perform some action. The outcome of the story is represented by a face that has two sides, one for a positive outcome and one for a negative outcome. Finally, the evaluation includes a thought bubble to capture the reader's evaluation of the story's events.

Place the storyboard next to a white board, or draw a similar representation on a white board and review the events of the story that have been read on previous days to set the context for the day's reading. As the story is read, the children are asked to identify where new information fits in the story structure, writing next to the icon for *character* or *problem,* and so forth. The explanations of the characters' reactions and plans provide op-

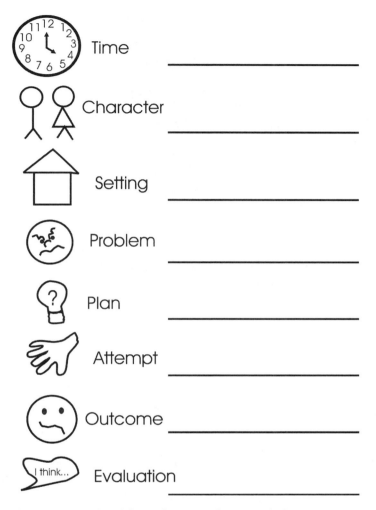

Time _____

Character _____

Setting _____

Problem _____

Plan _____

Attempt _____

Outcome _____

Evaluation _____

Figure 14.9. Storyboard for reading comprehension and planning narrative writing. (From Norris, J.A. [2002]. *Storyboard stickers* [p. 2]. Baton Rouge, LA. EleMentory.com. Copyright © 2002 Norris. Reprinted by permission.)

portunities to practice the construction of complex syntactic structures. Most stories have multiple episodes, some of them interrupting or embedded within others, so often there are several developing episodes plotted across the board. At the end of a day's reading, the children use the storyboard to summarize the reading either orally or in writing. The storyboard is also used to provide children with feedback when they are talking about personal experiences to cue when they are not supplying enough information for the listener to understand what they are saying.

Expository texts use a variety of macrostructures to represent relationships among denotative and connotative meanings regarding a topic. Figure

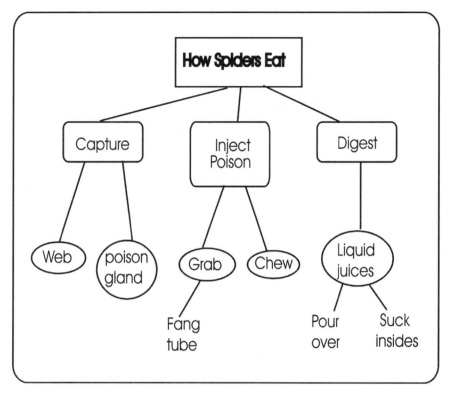

Figure 14.10.   Graphic organizer picturing hierarchical relationships among concepts. (Copyright ©
2002 Norris. Reprinted by permission.)

14.10 shows a graphic organizer developed to represent a science textbook
description of how spiders eat. It shows a temporal sequence of three main
stages: capturing prey, injecting poison, and digestion. Each stage includes
key concepts (i.e., agents, actions, objects) involved in that particular process. The adult aids in the children's development of these graphic organizers
during oral reading of the text. The children use them when they summarize
information from the text and when they study for tests.

ASSESSMENT METHODS TO SUPPORT ONGOING DECISION MAKING

Assessments at the beginning of intervention should include an evaluation of
oral and written language to determine strengths and weaknesses in vocabulary, semantics, syntax, morphology, phonemic awareness, and oral reading
and writing. The reading test should include passage reading where miscues
are marked, indicating where errors are occurring. We mark for specific sub-
stitutions, missed punctuation, intonation contours, poor phrasing, and other
subtle errors that yield clues to the language the child is failing to process.
The test also should include comprehension questions that ask for a range of

questions including those that require inferencing. Most reading inventories and a few standardized tests, such as the Gray Oral Reading Test (Wiederholt & Bryant, 1992) provide this format. The writing test should ask for a sample of writing, scored according to a rubric; for example, the Test of Written Language (Hammill & Larsen, 1999).

During intervention, we conduct weekly probes. A probe is created by selecting a story with the same level of readability as the intervention text that has never been read in intervention. The probe story is segmented into episodes, usually about one to three pages of text. An episode is randomly selected out of order at the end of each week for reading. The child reads from the book while miscues are marked on a photocopy. The passage reading is timed as a measure of fluency. Word-by-word reading, stopping to decode words, or rereading phrases to reestablish meaning all add seconds to the reading time. Following the reading, we ask 10 comprehension questions, two each at the increasingly more difficult semantic levels of description (e.g., questions about character actions), attributes (e.g., questions about the observable characteristics of characters and objects), interpretations (e.g., questions about character emotions and intentions), inferences (e.g., questions about possible future events in the story), and analogies (e.g., relationships between story events and events in the child's life). For beginning readers we substitute questions regarding labels instead of analogies. We then plot the results on three graphs. If a child is improving, miscues should decrease over time, reading time should decrease, and the number of comprehension questions correctly answered should increase. If these changes are not seen, then the miscue profile will indicate what is not understood and where greater emphasis should be placed. The following are two different profiles of miscues for the same sentence.

Text: He felt confused, unsure whether the sound was coming from some place in the room or if it was in his head.

Reader 1: He was confused and unsure if the sound was coming from some place in the room or in his head.

Reader 2: He felt confuse unsure? When the sound was coming from some place in the room. Or __it was in his head.

The first reader understood the meaning but simplified the surface structure of the grammar as he read. This reading resulted in four miscues with an appropriate reading rate and good comprehension, because the miscues did not significantly change the meaning.

The second reader shows both semantic and syntactic confusions. He either does not have the word *confused* as a vocabulary word, or he does not understand the connotative meaning in this sentence. *Unsure* is not interpreted as a relational word within the sentence. Sentences are revised and shortened, indicating difficulty with syntactic complexities. This reading resulted in six miscues, a longer reading time because of pauses and attempts to recognize words, and a loss of comprehension because key concepts and relationships of meaning were missed.

These errors guide intervention. Picturing how the phrases of the sentences are combined as in Figure 14.6 would increase accuracy for Reader 1. Reader 2 shows multiple sources of error. In this case, a picture showing a confused face that could be used to focus an explanation would provide the needed visual referent. Other elements of the sentence could be added to the picture phrase by phrase, such as adding lines to indicate a noise in the room, and lines in a thought bubble to indicate noise in his head. The word *unsure* would then be written between the two noise sources. Following an explanation of the picture, the sentence should be reread by the child without error and with appropriate intonation and phrasing. If errors occur, other elements of the language are still not understood and need to be clarified. For example, the spelling patterns of *unsure* might be confusing, in which case Phonic Faces could be used to model how the sounds and syllables are interpreted.

Posttesting could involve repetition of any or all of the tests in the original battery. Because increases in readability reflect increases in syntactic complexity and semantic abstraction of words in a text, scores on measures of these language abilities should improve as fluency and accuracy of reading increase.

CONSIDERATIONS FOR CHILDREN FROM CULTURALLY AND LINGUISTICALLY DIVERSE BACKGROUNDS

Children whose linguistic backgrounds are different from the language of the teacher and the texts that are read in the classroom will have created different connections among various levels of the model compared with children whose language experiences have been more similar to the language of the classroom. The child whose African American, Spanish, or Cajun dialect does not distinguish [d] and [ð] at the phoneme level (Lowe, 1994) may relate the letter sequences *th, d,* and *dd* to a phonemic /d/, resulting in miscues in reading and misspelled words in writing. Children from lower socioeconomic status homes with little exposure to storybooks or social interactions in which the events of the day are recounted in personal narratives may not have developed story macrostructures that include all of the story structure elements (Battle, 2002). Fortunately, the model described in this chapter is able to help people who work with such children develop a flexible and therefore individually tailored understanding of their difficulties with written language that has standard forms different from those of the child.

Teaching language through literacy is an excellent approach for working with culturally and linguistically diverse populations seeking to develop knowledge of standard English forms. It provides a context in which standard English is modeled and used without negative comment on a child's dialect or acquisition of English as a Second Language. The opportunity to repeatedly read the same passage provides the time and exposure needed to process many of the complexities of English. Books can be selected according to readability, which controls for syntactic and semantic complexity, thus providing a continuum of language that can be increased systematically as a child gains competence and is ready to move on to more complex structures. Books at the emergent end of this continuum have pictures and text that overlap, so that whatever is in the text is also in the picture, providing ideal visual support for learning vocabulary, syntax, narrative structure, and phoneme and print knowledge.

Reading and writing activities supported by Phonic Faces can help children gain phonemic awareness, print awareness, and an appreciation for the pronunciations of words in the dialect of the author. Iconic words are modeled by the facilitator but are ultimately developed by the child who will utilize associations from their own background to cue meaning relationships. The sentence picturing strategy first divides utterances into meaning units that should be relatively unaffected by dialect and then frames linguistic units. It can be used to compare the language forms that the child would choose based on his or her dialect with those that would be used by speakers of other dialects. Similarly, the storyboard representation could be used to analyze stories written by authors using both standard and nonstandard story structures.

APPLICATION TO AN INDIVIDUAL CHILD

Austin's case history reads like the description of the visual learner in the first section of this chapter. On the positive side, he is a visually gifted child who drew his first representational picture of a human character at 18 months: a skater complete with facial features, a trunk, arms, fingers, and ice skates. His testing for admission into an elementary school for gifted students in the visual and performing arts revealed a nonverbal IQ of 145, average oral language abilities, and some scattered speech sound production errors. On the negative side, Austin has a history of chronic otitis media that was first treated with pressure-equalization tubes at age 11 months. In kindergarten, he became inattentive whenever the topic involved letters and sounds. He would learn the letter–sound relationships introduced in the classroom only with great effort in school and at home; they would be forgotten the next week. Tests of phonemic awareness given during his kindergarten year revealed that he could segment sentences into words, but he could not divide words into phonemic units. In first grade, Austin was diagnosed with ADHD and drug therapy was started. Tests of auditory processing abilities at age 10 revealed that Austin did not integrate auditory information presented simultaneously to both ears.

Within the first month of kindergarten, Austin's failure to learn letter–sound relationships prompted his family to seek a referral to an SLP who included him in a small group of children having similar difficulties. She used Phonic Faces to simultaneously teach the sound–letter relationships addressed in the classroom as well as phonemic awareness skills such as recognizing the first sound of a word and creating rhyming words. Austin quickly caught up with the other members of his class in these abilities. In the spring of his kindergarten year, his teacher used the Phonic Faces to help him learn sound blending and spelling of simple CVC words with short vowels. His speech sound errors were eliminated by the end of the school year.

Austin fell behind again in first grade when the contrast between short and long vowels and the various vowel orthographic rules became important in the curriculum. The SLP addressed these with Phonic Faces while reading the storybooks used in the classroom. She also helped Austin use iconic words to master the spelling words that were assigned each week. He learned to make up his own iconic words in preparation for the weekly test.

In second grade, Austin's reading fluency failed to develop. He read through the punctuation in a monotone, with numerous miscues. Both his passage reading and reading comprehension scores on the Gray Oral Reading Test were below average. He was unable to retell stories that were read in class. The SLP again included him in a small group in which she used sentence drawing strategies to improve his understanding of complex sentence structures and the use of punctuation. Storyboards were created to scaffold his writing assignments. By the end of the year, his reading test scores were in the average range.

In third and fourth grades, Austin struggled with figurative language. The mental pictures he created in response to the texts' implied meanings and metaphors were often not the same as those intended by the author. For example, in a story he read, the text stated that an Alaskan pilot "covered 500 miles each day." He knew it sounded improbable, but his description of this event was that the pilot covered the ground with snow from his plane for 500 miles. The SLP helped Austin by having him draw quick sketches of the meaning of the language based on his real-world knowledge. In this case, Austin knew that pilots fly planes and that Alaska is a very large state. To make the appropriate interpretation of the text, the SLP helped him draw a sketch of a pilot flying a plane across 500 miles on an outline map of Alaska.

In Austin's time in fifth grade, the SLP continued to use the strategy of creating iconic words for subjects such as science in which larger numbers of new abstract words and their meanings need to be learned and remembered. She helped Austin learn to develop his own iconic words, as well as drawings of concept maps that became the notes from which he studied. The goal is for Austin and children like him to develop cognitive structures supporting language use and to develop the ability to generate their own visual cues as tools to be used in support of their studies.

FUTURE DIRECTIONS

Currently, almost all of the techniques described in the preceding sections are potential independent variables in need of empirical verification to demonstrate whether they can be used effectively to facilitate development of the various levels of the constellation model. During a summer program, we used a combination of Phonic Faces, iconic words, stick-figure drawing, and storyboards with small groups of second- and third-grade children with delayed reading development. The children were referred by teachers who identified children who were failing to keep up with the written language demands of the classroom. Pretesting with standardized reading and writing tests showed delays of at least two grade levels for all of the children. After a 6-week (12-hour) group intervention program in reading narrative texts, these children improved an average of 1.23 grade levels (range, 0–3 grades) in both word recognition and comprehension during paragraph reading. These results need to be replicated with appropriate controls, with a wider variety of dependent variables that can assess changes around the constellation model, and with attention to child characteristics that may predict which children will show success.

We are also focusing on early reading development using storybooks that incorporate Phonic Faces characters as a means to develop phonemic awareness and sound–letter relationship knowledge. Preliminary results from our first study suggest that parents of preschool children are more likely to talk about speech sounds and sound–letter relationships in storybooks that incorporate the Phonic Face characters than in more typical storybooks. A brief parent training component was followed by an increase in focus on speech sounds and sound–letter relationships. We will be expanding this study to measure effects of these storybooks on instruction in Head Start classrooms and the potential effects on the children's development of phonemic awareness and early literacy skills.

RECOMMENDED READINGS

Davis, R.D., & Braun, E.M. (1997). *The gift of dyslexia: Why some of the smartest people can't read and how they can learn.* East Rutherford, NJ: Perigee Press.

Freed, J., & Parsons, L. (1997). *Right-brained children in a left-brained world.* New York: Fireside.

West, T.G. (1991). *In the mind's eye: Visual thinkers, gifted people with dyslexia and other learning difficulties, computer images and the ironies of creativity.* Amherst, NY: Prometheus Books.

REFERENCES

Badian, N.A. (1999). Persistent arithmetic, reading, or arithmetic and reading disability. *Annals of Dyslexia, 49,* 45–70.

Battle, D.E. (2002). Language development and disorders in culturally and linguistically diverse children. In Bernstein, D.K., & Tiegerman-Farber, E.M. (Eds.), *Language and communication disorders in children* (5th ed., pp. 354–386). Boston: Allyn & Bacon.

Beitchman, J.H., & Young, A.R. (1997). Learning disorders with a special emphasis on reading disorders: A review of the past 10 years. *Journal of the American Academy of Child and Adolescent Psychiatry, 36,* 1020–1035.

Bellis, T.J. (1996). *Central auditory processing disorders in the educational setting: From science to practice.* San Diego: Singular Publishing Group.

Breier, J.I., Fletcher, J.K., Foorman, B.R., Klass, P., & Gray, L.C. (2003). Auditory temporal processing in children with specific reading disability with and without attention deficit/hyperactivity disorder. *Journal of Speech, Language, and Hearing Research, 46,* 31–42.

Brown, L., Sherbenou, R., & Johnsen, S. (1997). *Test of Nonverbal Intelligence (TONI-3).* Austin, TX: PRO-ED.

Catts, H.W. (1989). Speech production deficits in developmental dyslexia. *Journal of Speech and Hearing Research, 36,* 422–428.

Catts, H.W., Fey, M.E., Tomblin, J.B., & Zhang, X. (2002). A longitudinal investigation of reading outcomes in children with language impairments. *Journal of Speech, Language, and Hearing Research, 45,* 1142–1157.

Davis, R.D., & Braun, E.M. (1997). *The gift of dyslexia: Why some of the smartest people can't read and how they can learn.* East Rutherford, NJ: Perigee Press.

Ehri, L.C., Nunes, S.R., Willows, D.M., Schuster, B.V., Yaghoub-Zadeh, Z., & Shanahan, T. (2001). Phonemic awareness instruction helps children learn to read: Evidence from the National Panel's meta-analysis. *Reading Research Quarterly, 36*(3), 250–287.

Feagans, L., & Short, E. (1984). Developmental differences in the comprehension and production of narratives by reading disabled and normally achieving children. *Child Development, 55,* 1727–1736.

Felsenfeld, S., Broen, P.A., & McGue, M. (1992). A 28-year follow-up of adults with a history of moderate phonological disorder: Linguistic and personality results. *Journal of Speech and Hearing Research, 35,* 1114–1125.

Freed, J., & Parsons, L. (1997). *Right-brained children in a left-brained world.* New York: Fireside.

Gillon, G.T. (2000). The efficacy of phonological awareness intervention for children with spoken language impairment. *Language, Speech, and Hearing Services in Schools, 31,* 126–141.

Grandin, T. (1995). *Thinking in pictures and other reports from my life with autism.* New York: Doubleday.

Greenhalgh, K.S., & Strong, C.J. (2001). Literate language features in spoken narratives of children with typical language and children with language impairments. *Language, Speech, and Hearing Services in Schools, 32,* 114–125.

Hammill, D.D. & Larsen, S.C. (1999). *Test of Written Language (TOWL-3).* Austin, TX: PRO-ED.

Hoffman, P.R., & Norris, J.A. (1989). On the nature of phonological processes: Evidence from normal children's spelling errors. *Journal of Speech and Hearing Research, 32,* 787–794.

Idol, L. (1978). Group story mapping: A comprehension strategy for both skilled and unskilled readers. *Journal of Learning Disabilities, 20,* 196–205.

Idol, L., & Croll, V.J. (1987). Story-mapping training as a means of improving reading comprehension. *Learning Disabilities Quarterly, 10,* 214–229.

Isaacson, M.I. (2002). *Make your own pictographs.* Spring Valley, CA: Picture Me Reading.

Keith, R.W. (2000). *SCAN-C Test for Auditory Processing Disorders–Revised.* San Antonio, TX: Harcourt Assessment.

Kuhl, P.K., & Meltzoff, A. (1982). The bimodal perception of speech in infancy. *Science, 218,* 1138–1144.

Liles, B.Z. (1985). Cohesion in the narratives of normal and language-disordered children. *Journal of Speech and Hearing Research, 28,* 123–133.

Lindamood-Bell Learning Processes. (2002). *2001 clinical statistics.* San Luis Obispo, CA: Author.

Loban, W. (1976). *Language development: Kindergarten through grade twelve.* Urbana, IL: National Council of Teachers of English.

Lowe, R.J. (1994). *Phonology: Assessment and intervention applications in speech pathology.* Baltimore: Lippincott Williams & Wilkins.

MacLachlan, B.G., & Chapman, R.S. (1988). Communication breakdowns in normal and language-learning disabled children's conversation and narration. *Journal of Speech and Hearing Disorders, 53,* 2–7.

McFadden, T.U. (1998). The immediate effects of pictographic representation on children's narratives. *Child Language Teaching and Therapy, 14,* 51–67.

McFadden, T.U., & Gillam, R.B. (1996). An examination of the quality of narratives produced by children with language disorders. *Language, Speech, and Hearing Services in Schools, 27,* 48–56.

Merritt, D.D., & Liles, B.Z. (1987). Story grammar ability in children with and without language disorder: Story generation, story retelling, and story comprehension. *Journal of Speech and Hearing Research, 30,* 539–552.

Merritt, D.D., & Liles, B.Z. (1989). Narrative analysis, clinical applications of story generation and story retelling. *Journal of Speech and Hearing Disorders, 54,* 438–447.

Miyawaki, K., Strange, W., Verbrugge, R., Liberman, A.M., Jenkins, J.J., & Fujimura, O. (1975). An effect of linguistic experience: The discrimination of [r] and [l] by native speakers of Japanese and English. *Perception & Psychophysics, 18,* 331–340.

Nagy, W.E., & Herman, P.A. (1987). Breadth and depth of vocabulary knowledge: Implications for acquisition and instruction. In M.G. McKeown & M.E. Curtiss (Eds.), *The nature of vocabulary acquisition* (pp. 19–35). Hillsdale, NJ: Lawrence Erlbaum Associates.

Nelson, K. (1996). *Language in cognitive development: The emergence of the mediated mind.* New York: Cambridge University Press.

Nippold, M.A. (1998). *Later language.* Austin, TX: PRO-ED.

Norris, J.A. (1998). "I could read if I had a little help": Facilitating reading in whole language contexts. In C. Weaver (Ed.), *Practicing what we know: Informed reading instruction* (pp. 513–553). Urbana, IL: National Council of Teachers of English.

Norris, J.A. (2001). *Phonic Faces.* Baton Rouge, LA: EleMentory.

Norris, J.A., & Bruning, R.H. (1988) Cohesion in narratives of good and poor readers. *Journal of Speech and Hearing Disorders, 53,* 416–423.

Norris, J.A., & Hoffman, P.R. (2002). Language development and late talkers: A connectionist perspective. In R.G. Daniloff (Ed.), *Connectionist approaches to clinical problems in speech and language: Therapeutic and scientific applications* (pp. 1–110). Mahwah, NJ: Lawrence Erlbaum Associates.

Piaget, J., & Inhelder, B. (1973). *Memory and intelligence.* New York: Basic Books.

Pokorni, J.L., Worthington, C.K., & Evans-Joyce, M. (2001, November). Fast ForWord, Earobics, and LiPS: A comparison of three programs. Paper presented at the annual meeting of the American Speech-Language-Hearing Association, New Orleans.

Purcell, S.L., & Liles, B.Z. (1992). Cohesion repairs in the narratives of normal-language and language-disordered school-age children. *Journal of Speech and Hearing Research, 35,* 354–362.

Ripich, D.N., & Griffith, P.L. (1988). Narrative abilities of children with learning disabilities and nondisabled children: Story structure, cohesion and propositions. *Journal of Learning Disabilities, 21*(3), 165–173.

Rourke, B.P. (1995). *Syndrome of nonverbal leaning disabilities.* New York: Guilford Press.

Rumelhart, D.E., & McClelland, J.L. (1986). *Parallel distributed processing: Explorations in the microstructure of cognition. Vol. 1: Foundations.* Cambridge, MA: The MIT Press.

Seidenberg, M.S., & McClelland, J.L. (1989). A distributed, developmental model of word recognition and naming. *Psychological Review, 96*(4), 523–568.

Smith, F. (1971). *Understanding reading.* Hillsdale, NJ: Lawrence Erlbaum Associates.

Steiglitz, E.L. (1992). *The Stieglitz Informal Reading Inventory: Assessing reading behaviors from emergent to advanced levels.* Boston: Allyn & Bacon.

Stein, N.L., & Glenn, C.G. (1979). An analysis of story comprehension in elementary school children. In R.O. Freedle (Ed.), *New directions in discourse processing, Vol. II. Advances in discourse processes* (pp. 53–120). Norwood, NJ: Ablex.

Torgesen, J.K. (1999). Assessment and instruction for phonemic awareness and word recognition skills. In H.W. Catts & A.G. Kamhi (Eds.), *Language and reading disabilities* (pp. 128–153). Boston: Allyn & Bacon.

Vygotsky, L.S. (1978). *Mind in society: The development of higher psychological processes.* Cambridge, MA: The MIT Press.

Wallach, G.P., & Butler, K.G. (1994). *Language learning disabilities in school-age children and adolescents.* Upper Saddle River, NJ: Prentice Hall.

West, T.G. (1991). *In the mind's eye: Visual thinkers, gifted people with dyslexia and other learning difficulties, computer images and the ironies of creativity.* Amherst, NY: Prometheus Books.

White, T.G., Graves, M.F., & Slater, W.H. (1989). Growth of reading vocabulary in diverse elementary schools. *Journal of Educational Psychology, 82,* 281–290.

Wiederholt, J.L., & Bryant, B. (1992). *Gray Oral Reading Test–Fourth Edition (GORT-4).* Austin, TX: PRO-ED.

Wright, B.A., Bowen, R.W., & Zecker, S.G. (2000). Nonlinguistic perceptual deficits associated with reading and language disorders. *Current Opinions in Neurobiology, 10,* 482–486.

Wright, H.H., & Newhoff, M. (2001). Narration abilities of children with language-learning disabilities in response to oral and written stimuli. *American Journal of Speech-Language Pathology, 10,* 308–319.

15

The Writing Lab Approach for Building Language, Literacy, and Communication Abilities

NICKOLA WOLF NELSON AND ADELIA M. VAN METER

ABSTRACT

The writing lab approach is an inclusive, computer-supported, classroom-based approach for building language and literacy abilities. The three major components are writing process instruction, computer supports, and inclusive instructional practices. In writing labs, speech-language pathologists (SLPs) collaborate with general and special education teachers to target reciprocal spoken and written language in curriculum-based writing projects. Through instructor-mediated scaffolding, students learn to use increasingly elaborated and pragmatically tuned language to communicate ideas to interested audiences of peers, instructors, and parents. Evidence is reviewed supporting the effectiveness of a writing lab approach at the discourse, sentence, and word levels, with broader outcomes in areas of social interaction and self-regulation.

INTRODUCTION

The writing lab approach (Nelson, Bahr, & Van Meter, 2004) is designed to integrate language *intervention* for students with disabilities into writing process *instruction* for all students. It is this combination of intervention with instruction that allows SLPs and other special educators to work collaboratively with general education teachers to influence growth for individual students while promoting systemic change. The model for the writing lab

The funded projects whose results are reported in this chapter were co-directed by Dr. Christine Bahr, our longtime colleague and co-author. This work was supported by U.S. Department of Education Office of Special Education Programs research Grants H180G20005 and H324R980120. Engagement of graduate students in the activities also was supported by training Grants HO29B10245, HO29B40183, and H325H010023.

We are grateful to the teachers, administrators, and parents, and particularly to the students, who agreed to collaborate with us in this work and to grant their permission to share the results of our joint efforts.

Computer-Supported Writing Lab Model

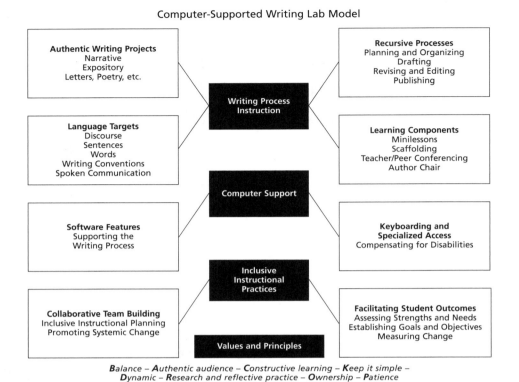

Balance – *A*uthentic audience – *C*onstructive learning – *K*eep it simple –
*D*ynamic – *R*esearch and reflective practice – *O*wnership – Patience

Figure 15.1. Model of the writing lab approach. (From Nelson, N.W., Van Meter, A.M., Chamberlain, D., & Bahr, C.M. [2001]. The speech-language pathologist's role in a writing lab approach. *Seminars in Speech and Language, 22*[3], 211; adapted by permission.)

approach (see Figure 15.1) features three components—writing process instruction, computer supports, and inclusive instructional practices.

Writing process instruction involves encouraging students to use recursive writing processes (Hayes & Flower, 1980), to write extensively, and to produce authentic products for a real audience. This contrasts with writing at the word and phrase level, mostly on worksheets and primarily for the purpose of measuring correctness, which has been the tradition for many special education students (Allington & McGill-Franzen, 1989). Writing processes include topic selection, planning, organizing, drafting, revising, editing, publishing, and presenting. Students learn to use these processes while working on authentic, curriculum-based projects. Instructional activities include group and individual minilessons, peer and teacher conferencing, and author chair exchanges. Environmental supports include word walls and author notebooks. Therapeutic scaffolding is the primary means for delivering individualized language intervention. It targets language skills (spoken and written) at the levels of discourse, sentences, words, and sounds, and also it targets self-regulatory and social interaction skills.

Computer supports, the second major component of the writing lab approach, can facilitate all stages of the writing process (Nelson et al., 2004). Although features of children's word processing programs allow students with disabilities to produce written products that look as good as those of their classmates, they support *all* stages of the writing process (not just publishing). Examples include graphic organizers or outliners for planning (Bahr, Nelson, & Van Meter, 1996), word prediction for drafting, synthetic speech feedback for revising and editing, and multimedia programs for publishing (Bahr, Nelson, Van Meter, & Yanna, 1996).

The third major component involves both collaborative team building and inclusive, individualized service delivery. In the writing lab approach, language specialists use their specialized knowledge of language and communication systems to assess language systems, establish benchmarks, scaffold skills, evaluate improvements, and continually update plans. SLPs are well prepared to assume this role of language specialist (Nelson, Van Meter, Chamberlain, & Bahr, 2001), but the approach is transdisciplinary in that team members actively assist each other to develop new skills and share roles.

TARGET POPULATIONS AND ASSESSMENTS FOR DETERMINING TREATMENT RELEVANCE AND GOALS

The writing lab approach aims at keeping students with disabilities in the general education curriculum by situating language intervention services in general education projects and classrooms. Assessments lead directly to intervention targets relevant to school success, making it possible for a wide range of students with and without disabilities to benefit.

Target Populations

As a therapeutic method, the writing lab approach is designed to meet the needs of any school-age student whose language and literacy learning difficulties have a negative impact on academic achievement and social interaction. The approach also addresses the needs of "gray area" students who do not qualify for special services despite teachers' concerns about language and literacy learning difficulties.

Language and literacy difficulties stem from a variety of known, suspected, and unknown causes, including specific language impairments and learning disabilities, as well as a wide range of other disabilities such as cognitive impairment, autism spectrum disorders, hearing impairment, emotional impairment, neuromotor impairment, and traumatic brain injury. English-language learners (students in families in which a language other than English is spoken) also may benefit, whether or not they have disabilities.

Relating Assessed Difficulties to Treatment Relevance

When working side-by-side with language specialists, teachers can improve their knowledge of language and literacy components (Moats & Foorman, 2003) and scaffolding techniques for students with disabilities and other challenges. At the same time, SLPs can improve their group management skills and calibrate their intervention objectives, techniques, and intervention discourse to the demands of the general education curriculum. In the process, the language and literacy needs of a broader range of students can be addressed without labeling them or pulling them away from the general curriculum and the positive models of typically developing peers.

It has long been understood that literacy learning (both reading and writing) depends on a foundation of general language ability (Snow, Burns, & Griffin, 1998; Snow & Tabors, 1993). Children with inadequate language knowledge are at high risk for literacy learning difficulties (e.g., Catts, Fey, Tomblin, & Zhang, 2002; Catts & Kamhi, 1999; Kamhi & Catts, 2002; Lewis, O'Donnell, Freebairn, & Taylor, 1998; Scarborough, 2002; Tomblin et al., 1997) and for academic difficulties across the general curriculum (ASHA Committee on Reading and Writing, 2001; Catts & Kamhi, 1999; Wallach & Butler, 1994). To add to the problem, language difficulties often have a domino effect, such that difficulty in language learning leads to difficulty in literacy learning which, in turn, makes it difficult to function successfully in other areas of academic learning and social interaction (Juel, 1988; Stanovich, 1986).

The writing lab context is ideal for promoting reciprocal relationships between spoken and written language. Students work individually and in small groups, constructing increasingly elaborate written discourse for curriculum-related communicative purposes. SLPs can avoid the undesirable classroom-based intervention scenario in which they stand at the back of a classroom watching the teacher teach, unable to work with caseload students for fear of disrupting the class.

THEORETICAL BASIS

The writing lab approach is consistent with current views of language-learning disabilities as the product of such *intrinsic* factors as genetically linked neurobiological predisposition to disability (Lyon, Shaywitz, & Shaywitz, 2003; Pennington, 2003) interacting with such *extrinsic* factors as the sociocultural expectations of familial and educational systems (e.g., Englert, 1992; Englert & Palincsar, 1991). Cognitive-neurolinguistic theory provides the theoretical underpinnings for using writing lab interventions to help students organize and connect intrinsic neurobiological language and literacy processing systems. Social-constructionist theory provides the theoretical rationale for using scaffolding to provide extrinsic supports to help students make intrinsic neurolinguistic changes and activate their sense of self-efficacy for attempting higher-level challenges.

Cognitive-Neurolinguistic Theory

A growing body of evidence suggests there are neurobiological differences in the brains of individuals with language and learning disabilities (e.g., Lyon et al., 2003; Paulesu et al., 1996; Pennington, 2003). Thus, it would seem that efforts to reduce impairment and improve functional activity must target modifications in those intrinsic underlying systems. That is, improvements in students' language and literacy competence and processing skills should reflect improved coordination and connection among the neurobiologically situated language, literacy, social-communicative, and executive control systems within students' brains. We also believe that knowledge about the internal workings of the brain brings insights to the on-line decisions language specialists make while providing assessment and intervention services.

According to cognitive-neurolinguistic theory, key areas of the brain are recruited in a connected and coordinated fashion when a person is involved actively in processing language and constructing meaning. In normal development, the activation of neural networks strengthens dendritic connections, which in turn support the automatic and rapid (i.e., fluent) processing of spoken and written words and their constituent units. According to this theory, when lower level functions occur automatically, greater attentional and cognitive resources become available for performing higher-level cognitive-linguistic functions, including sentence-level and discourse-level comprehension, formulation, and critical analysis. By extension, this theory suggests that neural connections and integrated systems needed for performing complex tasks are less likely to develop if students' brains are engaged mostly in tasks that activate discrete skills in isolation from one another.

Complex and interactive language-processing systems can be represented with a "pinball wizardry" model (Nelson, 1998), which represents parallel encoding of language and world knowledge across cerebral hemispheres, ranging from cortical to subcortical structures of the brain. Phonological-graphemic, morphological-orthographic, semantic, and syntactic systems are represented on the left side of the model (see Figure 15.1). Discourse and pragmatic knowledge, audience sensitivity, and capabilities for using world knowledge to draw inferences are represented on the right side of the model. Input-output connections between subcortical and external sensory and motor pathways are illustrated with an arrow at the base of the model interfacing with external linguistic and nonlinguistic information. Executive control and self-regulatory functions are represented with an arrow at the top of the model. Smaller arrows represent white matter pathways for supporting neural networks, working memory, and connections to stored language and world knowledge. Collectively, the model represents the complex neural-based systems and mechanisms that competent language users draw on selectively and with strategic coordination (hence the pinball wizardry metaphor) when engaging in spoken- and written-language tasks. The central focus of language processing in this model is the construction of meaning.

Lyon and colleagues (2003) summarized converging evidence for a neurobiological basis of dyslexia, indicating anterior regions of the left hemisphere working in isolation from posterior brain regions, a phenomenon that led Paulesu et al. (1996) to hypothesize dyslexia as a disconnection syndrome. At least three areas are recruited and coordinated by typical brains attempting word-analysis tasks involving associations among phonological, semantic, and orthographic systems (Lyon et al., 2003). Brain activation maps show that readers without impairment activate a coordinated system of three primary areas: 1) an anterior system in the left inferior frontal region for analyzing words into phonologic segments for rhyming, reading, speaking, or spelling; 2) a dorsal parietotemporal system for analyzing the auditory components of words and connecting them to their meanings; and 3) a ventral occipitotemporal system that predominates "when a reader has become skilled, and has bound together as a unit the orthographic, phonologic, and semantic features of the word" (p. 5). The lesser-known right hemisphere appears to add contributions to social-pragmatic skills, figurative language, and cognitive-linguistic inferencing (Ratey, 2001).

Interventions should be designed to help students form neurolinguistic connections between anterior (word pronunciation) and posterior (word meaning, pattern recognition) processing, and to connect across hemispheres to discourse and pragmatic abilities. The outcome should be integrated and contextualized processing and enhanced social-communication abilities.

Social-Constructionist Theory

Although research evidence increasingly supports a physical reality for something like a pinball wizardry model, its importance at present stems primarily from its implications for guiding effective scaffolding aimed at changing how students represent language in their brains. The theory is that scaffolding can lead brains to "light up" in strategically organized and effective patterns, forming enhanced neural associations. The explicit therapeutic intention is to help students become more competent and independent "pinball wizards" in the process.

The theoretical foundation for scaffolding is social-constructionism. This theory forms the basis for motivational and instructional elements, emphasizing the value of authentic writing projects and an interested audience to stimulate change (Englert, 1992; Englert & Palincsar, 1991). It taps into the natural desire of students to belong to their peer group and receive affirmation from parents and others. When students are scaffolded to realize that they *need* more organized discourse structures, complex syntax, interesting word choices, accurate spelling, appropriate writing conventions, intelligible articulation, fluent speech, and adequate vocal intensity to communicate their ideas, they become open to growth.

Scaffolding, as a concept, owes its foundations to Russian psychologist Lev Vygotsky's description of dialogic mediation. Vygotsky first wrote about the importance of inner speech for regulating thought and behavior in *Thought and Language* (1962 translation). In his later book, *Mind in Society: The Development of Higher Psychological Processes* (1978 translation), Vygotsky expanded on the role of social mediation to describe how interpersonal communication can become intrapersonal thought, noting, "Any function in the child's cultural development appears twice, or on two planes. First, it appears on the social plane, and then on the psychological plane . . . Social relations among people genetically underlie all higher functions and their relationships" (1978, pp. 163–164).

According to social-constructionist theory, learning takes place when a child is in an environment that provides assistance at a point when the child needs it and can benefit from it. Pressley indicated that critical developmental interactions occur "between the two extremes of tasks, the ones children can do autonomously and those they could never do" (2002, p. 97). We call this the *developing edge of competence.* Vygotsky (1978) called it the *zone of proximal development.* It is in this zone that a scaffolding bridge can be constructed from current perceptions and associations to those that otherwise would be beyond the student's reach. The goal is to push individual zones of proximal development continuously upward. The test is whether higher-level competence remains when scaffolds are removed.

EMPIRICAL BASIS

The overarching goal of the writing lab approach is for students with language disorders and other special needs to take increasingly larger steps toward the language development standards of typically developing peers. The levels of proficiency should be growing for all students, which constantly raises the bar.

Other researchers have investigated many components of writing process instruction, yielding positive evidence that it can improve the quality of written compositions. We also have gathered preliminary evidence of the effectiveness of a writing lab approach in our own work, based both on data from group probes and individual case studies.

General Support for Effectiveness of Writing Process Instruction

An early study by the National Center for Educational Statistics (U.S. Department of Education, OERI, 1996) provided support for the effectiveness of process approaches to writing based on the National Assessment of Educational Progress (NAEP) results for fourth-, eighth-, and twelfth-grade students who took the exam in 1992. Students who reported that their teachers frequently asked them to plan and do prewriting, to define their purpose and audience, and to produce more than one draft earned the highest average writing scores on the NAEP. Those who did prewriting using lists, outlines, or diagrams on the actual national writing sample also had higher average proficiency scores. Students who used unrelated notes or drawings, or who wrote different versions or first drafts, performed about the same as those who did no prewriting.

The constructivist elements of writing process instruction also were the subject of a number of early reports. Englert (1992) and Englert and Palincsar (1991) described the sociocultural framework for writing process instruction, which they dubbed *cognitive strategy instruction in writing* (CSIW; Englert & Raphael, 1989). CSIW is guided by four assumptions, including that 1) writing is a holistic cognitive activity, 2) cognitive processes are learned in dialogic interactions with others, 3) cognitive development occurs in students' zones of proximal development, and 4) knowledge construction is a social and cultural phenomenon. This team's research on the implementation of the approach by teachers of fourth- and fifth-grade students in general and special education provided support for its effectiveness in improving both writing performance and metacognitive knowledge of students with learning disabilities (Englert, Raphael, & Anderson, 1992; Englert, Raphael, Anderson, Anthony, & Stevens, 1991).

An Extensive Research Program

An extensive body of research has been conducted on writing process and self-regulatory strategy instruction by the team of Steve Graham, Karen Harris, Charles MacArthur, Shirley Schwartz, and their colleagues. Much of this research has been conducted with students with learning disabilities at upper elementary and middle school ages. For example, Graham, Harris, MacArthur, and Schwartz (1991) summarized the writing difficulties of students with learning disabilities and the effectiveness of writing process instruction for addressing them. The team's preliminary evidence supported the promise of a writing process approach involving strategy instruction, procedural facilitation, word processing, and basic skills instruction.

Focusing on self-regulation, Graham and Harris (1989) taught a self-organizing strategy with the mnemonic: *W-W-W, What = 2, How = 2*. They measured effects on composition skills and self-efficacy for 22 students with learning disabilities and 11 typically achieving students in fifth and sixth grades. Mnemonic components were modeled as a "think-aloud" and were supported with controlled practice. Self-talk questions included the following:

Who *is the main character in my story and who else is in it?*

When *does the story take place?*

Where *does it take place?*

What *does the main character want to do?*

What *happens when he or she tries to do it?*

How *does the story end?*

How *does the main character feel?* (p. 357)

At posttest, students with learning disabilities produced stories with as many story grammar elements as students without learning disabilities. They also demonstrated a significantly heightened sense of self-efficacy but continued to produce shorter compositions rated lower in quality than their typical classmates.

MacArthur, Schwartz, and Graham (1991) and MacArthur, Graham, and Schwartz (1993) published evaluation results from a 2-year Computers and Writing Instruction Project (CWIP). In this intervention, teachers in self-contained classrooms for students with learning disabilities implemented a program consisting of three main components: a process approach to writing, word processing, and strategy instruction. The curriculum was based on the principles that "students need to engage in authentic writing tasks for real audiences, progress toward skilled writing requires development of cognitive and metacognitive strategies, and teachers guide students' development through extensive interaction with individuals and groups" (1993, p. 672). This form of computer-supported writing process instruction (with daily access to computers for drafting) was implemented in 18 self-contained classrooms for students with learning disabilities ($N = 180$) at elementary through middle school levels. Pre/post data came from probes taken in October and April in which students wrote both personal narratives and informative letters describing their school. Students from 15 control classrooms ($N = 125$) who did not receive the intervention also produced probe samples. In the first year, CWIP students achieved significantly higher gains in qualitative ratings of narrative and informative writing quality. They also wrote longer compositions with a lower proportion of misspelled words than control students. In the second year, holistic quality ratings also improved significantly from pre- to posttest for both narrative and informative writing, but only the narrative writing gains were greater than control group gains.

Subsequently, Danoff, Harris, and Graham (1993) studied strategy instruction in writing workshops in general education classrooms. They used a multiple-baseline design to measure effects on the schematic structure of stories for two fourth-grade and four fifth-grade students and documented maintenance of higher-level skills for all but one of them with a new teacher. By introducing instructional components in staggered fashion, these researchers found evidence for the additive effects of multiple instructional components and for addressing all stages of the writing process.

Graham, MacArthur, and Schwartz (1995) investigated the effects of procedural assistance aimed at revising for fifth- and sixth-grade students with learning disabilities ($N = 70$). These students received writing process instruction in six self-contained classrooms four times per week. Students were assigned randomly to one of three revising conditions: 1) general goal to improve the composition, 2) goal to add information, and 3) goal to add information plus procedural facilitation. Pre- and postintervention narratives were compared for number of words, evidence of revisions, and holistic scores (based on an 8-point quality scale). The goal to add information significantly affected text quality over the general goal condition. Procedural facilitation did not appreciably raise ratings further.

Troia, Graham, and Harris (1999) measured the effects of intervention on planning. They used a single-subject case-study design replicated across three fifth-grade students with learning disabilities to investigate the effectiveness of self-regulatory strategy instruction for teaching students to mindfully plan stories and essays. In a series of seven 60–90-minute instructional sessions taught over a 3-week period, students learned self-regulatory strategies for setting goals, brainstorming ideas, and sequencing ideas. Improvements over baseline were found for all three students in story grammar scores and numbers of functional essay elements, and they were maintained 3 weeks later.

Ferretti, MacArthur, and Dowdy (2000) studied the effects of elaborated goal setting on persuasive essays written by fourth- and fifth-grade students with and without learning disabilities. The general goal was for students to write a letter to persuade others to agree with their position (e.g., to persuade teachers to give less homework). Students in the experimental condition received additional explicit subgoals to include not only reasons and evidence for their position, but also rebuttal for opposing positions. The results showed that students with learning disabilities included fewer persuasive arguments. Additionally, sixth-grade students in the elaborated goal condition produced more persuasive arguments than sixth graders in the simple goal condition or fourth-grade students in either condition. The authors concluded that some higher-level skills are beyond the zone of proximal development for students of a particular age, even with procedural facilitation.

De La Paz and Graham (2002) used random assignment to experimental and control classrooms to investigate the effectiveness of writing process instruction for middle school students with learning disabilities in general education classrooms. Results showed that essays written by 30 students receiving instruction aimed at planning, drafting, and revising were longer, contained more mature vocabulary, and were rated qualitatively better than essays written by 28 students randomly assigned to the control condition.

MacArthur (1998), concentrating on the effectiveness of computer supports for writing, studied speech synthesis and word prediction. He compared the writing that five students with learning disabilities (ages 9 and 10) produced with and without computer supports. When using software features, four of the five students produced written dialog journal entries for which legibility and correct spelling increased from baseline rates as low as 55% to 90%–100% legible words, and from 42% to 75% correctly spelled words.

MacArthur, Ferretti, Okolo, and Cavalier (2001) summarized other studies that provided evidence that computer-assisted instruction, particularly synthesized speech feedback, could improve phonemic awareness, decoding skills, and written-language abilities at the word level.

Other Contributions Across Age Levels, Language Levels, and Modalities

As critical as the information is on the success of writing process instruction on discourse production by older elementary and middle school students with learning disabilities, language specialists also need evidence for the effectiveness of a writing lab approach for children with disorders of spoken language, for changes at the sentence and word level (as well as at the discourse level), and in the early elementary years. Evidence also is needed for the effectiveness of intervention on what Berninger (1999) termed *transcription skills* (i.e., spelling and handwriting abilities) and for students with disorders in general education classrooms (as well as in special education classrooms; Baker, Gersten, & Graham, 2003).

Studies measuring the effectiveness of writing process instruction on sentence-level skills have provided only sketchy evidence thus far. Vallecorsa and deBettencourt (1992) studied implementation of a writing process approach first in isolation, and then in combination with computerized word processing. They found improved length and overall quality of compositions, but less evidence for improved sentence structure. Their results also suggested that the computer supports were beneficial for some but not all students.

Berninger (1999) studied the influence of instruction both on word-level transcription (handwriting and spelling) and sentence and discourse levels of text generation. She described a model of internal processing requiring coordination in time of multilevel processes through working memory (much like the pinball wizardry model described previously). Berninger noted that levels of processing "may develop at different rates in different children" (1999, p. 100). She added that spelling is relatively harder to remediate than word recognition, handwriting, or composing, but reported initial success with an approach aimed at helping students appreciate the functional unit for mapping sound onto writing as larger than the single letter.

Gillam and Johnston (1992) also emphasized the multilevel mechanical and cognitive demands of producing narratives in more than one modality. They analyzed spoken and written narratives produced by 10 children with spoken-language disorders between 9 and 12 years of age, compared with those produced by age-, language-, and reading-matched controls (7 boys and 3 girls in each group, for a total of 40 students). Students with spoken-language disorders demonstrated less proficiency with complex linguistic forms in spoken and written narratives than students in any of the other groups. They produced more grammatical errors in both modalities, but particularly in written stories. Spoken narratives for all students tended to be stronger at the sentence level in that they included longer sentences and more connectives; written narratives tended to be stronger at the discourse level, in that they included more elaborate plots, a higher proportion of linked episode components, and better story coherence.

Gillam, McFadden, and van Kleeck (1995) compared spoken and written narratives from students with spoken-language disorders and learning disabilities after 2 years of treatment in either a special education program with a *whole-language* (content-oriented) approach or with a *language skills* (form-oriented) approach to intervention. In this study, posttest results were compared for the four students in each program, who ranged in age from 9 to 12 years ($M = 10;10$) during final data collection. The two groups were made up of students matched for verbal intelligence and reading and writing abilities when they began the instruction, and for nonverbal intelligence and degree of language disorder at the time of data collection. As the authors cautioned in their discussion, this was not a pre/post comparison study, but a comparison of abilities at posttesting for similar students who had participated in two types of language education. Results showed that those who had received the form-oriented direct instruction in the language skills program had relatively better skills at the sentence level on both spoken and written narratives, whereas those who had received the content-oriented instruction in the whole-language program received higher values on content measures and holistic judgments of quality, especially for their spoken narratives. This small study is important not only for its comparison of two approaches, but also because it suggests that intervention influences abilities differentially depending on the nature of the targeted abilities and the methods used for intervention. The writing lab approach encourages focusing greater or lesser attention on word-, sentence-, and discourse-level skills, depending on the baseline assessment of individual students' needs and intermittent probes, but maintaining a balance across all levels of language learning.

Zaragoza and Vaughn (1992) also studied the effects of process writing instruction on word-level and sentence-level writing convention skills. They provided evidence in the form of case studies for three second-grade students with varied achievement profiles—one with learning disabilities, one low achieving, and one gifted. All three demonstrated growth in punctuation, spelling, capitalization, and fluency in sample pieces written every 3 weeks over a 6-month period of classroom-based instruction.

Chapman (1994) offered evidence of the effectiveness of a writing process approach for even younger students, but at the discourse level only. She studied the emergence of features of different genres among first graders. Her results highlighted the beneficial contextual aspects of writing workshops, with social-interaction features involving talking, reading, and writing.

Starting even younger and emphasizing the phonological makeup of words, Craig (2003) studied the effectiveness of interactive writing plus word-level instruction for kindergarten students. She compared this approach with a phonemic awareness intervention that did not include a writing component. Craig's study involved 87 children in four half-day kindergarten classrooms who were randomly assigned to conditions. Her "interactive writing-plus treatment" provided text-based reading experiences, response to texts using interactive writing, similar to the whole-language approach studied previously by Gillam and colleagues (1995), but with supplemental direct instruction in letter–sound association. Craig's comparison group students were more like those in the "language skills" group studied by Gillam et al. in that they received "metalinguistic games-plus treatment" that involved listening, rhyming, synthesis, and analysis games. Craig measured phonological awareness, alphabetic knowledge, and early reading abilities. Her results indicated that the students in the interactive writing-plus group matched or exceeded the students in the metalinguistic games group on each word-level measure, including phonological awareness, spelling, and pseudo-word reading. They also scored higher on the three reading measures. Craig reported ability-group effect sizes for word identification, computed as Cohen's d (1988), as 0.34 for the low, 0.50 for the middle, and 0.77 for the high group. Passage comprehension effect sizes were 0.49 for the low, 0.65 for the middle, and 1.03 for the high group.

Taken together, these studies suggest that word- and sentence-level abilities, particularly for students with disordered language development, are more likely to change if they are the target of some relatively direct instruction. At the same time, coherence and creativity of qualitative discourse-level features seem to be nurtured best in an environment that encourages focus on meaning and audience effect. Language specialists cannot afford to abandon either area—content or form. The writing lab approach is designed to allow a shift of focus between content and form, with opportunity for tilting the balance depending on the needs of individual students.

Meta-analysis of Process Writing Instruction

Hierarchies for judging levels of evidence generally place meta-analysis studies with clear and stringent selection criteria at the highest level. Gersten and Baker's (2001) comprehensive review of the literature identified 13 studies that had 1) at least one dependent measure of expressive writing, 2) an independent variable pertaining to written expression instruction, 3) intervention lasting at least 45 minutes across 3 days per week, 4) students with officially identified learning disabilities making up at least 66% of the sample, and 5) a comparison group that also included students with learning disabilities. Three of the 13 studies (De La Paz & Graham, 1997; Jaben, 1983, 1987) used random assignment to condition.

Gersten and Baker (2001) used effect size as the index for judging intervention effectiveness, computed as the standardized difference between means, the version of Cohen's d (1988) in which differences between treatment and comparison group means are divided by the pooled standard deviation. The inclusion of a comparison group in these 13 studies added a control for maturation, regression to the mean, and other influences on outcome measures. Summed across all 13 studies, the authors found a mean effect size on the aggregate writing measure of 0.81, which met Cohen's recommended criterion as a strong effect. They noted that positive effect sizes were found for all 13 studies, ranging in magnitude from 0.30 (MacArthur, Graham, Schwartz, & Shafer, 1995) to 1.73 (Wong, Butler, Ficzere, & Kuperis, 1996). Gersten and Baker further suggested that their meta-analysis identified three components that should be part of explicit instruction in any comprehensive program: 1) writing processes, 2) instruction regarding critical dimensions for different writing genres (both narrative and expository writing genres were investigated in the 13 studies), and 3) structures for giving students extensive peer and/or teacher feedback on the quality of their writing.

Preliminary Results from Our Research on the Writing Lab Approach

Our research thus far has concentrated on documenting written-language abilities for students at different grade levels, measuring change in language levels (discourse, sentence, and word) in written probes gathered at the beginning, middle, and end of the school year (Nelson & Van Meter, 2003; Nelson, Van Meter, & Bahr, 2003). These multiple probes have allowed us to assess outcome measures and to conduct pre/post comparisons. We also have computed the standardized difference mean (Meline & Schmitt, 1997) by dividing the difference between pre/post means by the standard deviation of the pre/post difference scores. Effect sizes computed this way allow us to compare levels of change for a variety of measures and for students with and without language disorders. The lack of an untreated group for comparison, however, permits no control for factors other than the treatment that might account for gains (e.g., maturation and regression to the mean). As the standard deviations suggest in the tables of data reported in this chapter, some of the measures we use also have wide variability. Thus, at this point, our results must be interpreted with caution. More comprehensive questions about efficacy and effectiveness await studies using randomized controlled trials.

We first reported case study and group data for students with speech-language impairments and related disabilities in relationship to their typically learning peers in Chapter 17 of our book (Nelson et al., 2004). These were students in three third-grade classrooms who were receiving writing lab instruction and intervention in their classroom or the school's computer laboratory 3 days per week for 45–60 minutes per session. Two SLPs worked collaboratively with the general education teachers in each classroom to provide instruction. Some of the students with special needs spent part of the school day in a special education room, and services were coordinated with that teacher as well (Nelson et al., 2001). The classrooms were in a school in an impoverished neighborhood in a moderately sized, ethnically diverse Midwestern U.S. city. Of the 53 students in these classrooms, 24 were African American, 24 were European American, 4 were Latino, and 1 was Asian American. The nine students who provided group data for the special needs group included three with speech-language impairments only, four with learning disabilities and/or emotional impairments, and two identified as having both speech-language impairment and other disabilities (including one student with a learning disability and one with an autism spectrum disorder). Two additional students with cognitive impairments (one mild and one moderate) participated in the program but were not able to write independently enough to contribute to the group data. In Chapter 17 of our book (Nelson et al., 2004), we provide case study data and examples of dictated work showing growth in spoken communication abilities for these students, as well as qualitative changes for them and others.

In the current chapter, we report the quantifiable outcomes of treatment using measures tested in a variety of outreach schools when implementing the writing lab approach at varied elementary grade levels from first through fifth (Nelson & Van Meter, 2003; Nelson et al., 2003). For all analyses, narrative probes were transcribed and coded using the computer software Systematic Analysis of Language Transcripts (SALT; Miller & Chapman, 2000). This yielded counts of such variables as the number of different words, conjunction types, and coded sentence types. We used paired t-tests and related effect sizes to report pre/post changes for typical and special needs students in the three third-grade classrooms. These results are important because they provide preliminary evidence that a writing lab approach can assist students with special needs to achieve language growth rates that approximate, and even exceed, those of their typically developing peers. The data tables in this chapter summarize results for the quantitative measures we have developed at the discourse, sentence, and word level. In the text, we discuss those that we have found to be most discriminative of age and language disorder (Nelson & Van Meter, 2003; Nelson et al., 2003).

To analyze abilities at the discourse level (see Table 15.1), we used a fluency measure of total words produced during 1-hour probes, counting only words students wrote independently. A second discourse-level measure consisted of story grammar scores crediting the addition of features leading up to mature narratives, starting with isolated descriptions and culminating in complex or multiple episodes. The results summarized in Table 15.1 indicated significant improvement and strong effect sizes (although with wide variability) according to both measures for students with special needs and students who are developing typically.

At the sentence level, we are still seeking the best measures for analyzing abilities and capturing growth. As Gillam and his colleagues (1995) indicated, it is important to have a sentence-level (form) measure as well as dis-

Table 15.1. Story scores and total words before and after instruction for children with special needs and with typical language

Variable	Group	Sept 3 probe		May 4 probe		Paired difference			Sig. (2-tailed)	Effect size
		M	SD	M	SD	M	SD	t-test		
Story scores	S	1.40	0.84	3.50	1.08	2.10	0.74	9.00	0.00	2.85
	T	2.47	0.86	4.23	1.04	1.77	0.90	10.78	0.00	1.97
Total words	S	21.78	11.76	121.90	128.28	100.12	122.03	2.46	0.04	0.82
	T	42.94	20.52	119.75	90.51	76.81	92.69	4.69	0.00	0.83

Key: S, students with special needs ($n = 9$); T, students who were typically developing ($n = 32$); Sig., significance. Effect size was computed as Cohen's d, by dividing the difference between pre/posttest means (M) by the pooled standard deviation (SD).

course-level measures of content and quality. Our multigrade cross-sectional analyses (Nelson & Van Meter, 2003; Nelson et al., 2003) indicate that a commonly reported measure, mean length of T-unit (MLTU), is not sensitive enough to document differences associated with disabilities, normal development, or changes with intervention. A better measure for documenting advancing syntactic maturity may be the total number of conjunctions or types of conjunctions. These counts, which reflect sentence-combining skill (similar to the "percent of marked relationships" measure used by Gillam et al., 1995, p. 167), can be made fairly easily with SALT software (Miller & Chapman, 2000). The data in Table 15.2 show large effect sizes for students with special needs both for total conjunctions ($d = 0.90$) and types of conjunctions ($d = 1.56$).

Another sentence-level measure that we use clinically is similar to two measures reported by Gillam et al. (1995) as "propositions per T-unit" and "percent of acceptable T-units" (p. 167). Our measure involves analysis of proportions of simple incorrect [si], simple correct [sc], complex incorrect [ci], and complex correct [cc] sentences. Sentences are coded as complex when they are made up of 1) a single T-unit that combines more than one verb phrase (finite or nonfinite) through such processes as subordination or embedding, or 2) a maximum of two T-units joined with a coordinating conjunction (as recommended by Lee, 1974). If more than two T-units are joined as coordinated clauses, the third in sequence is coded as "run-on" and treated as the beginning of a new sentence. As Table 15.2 shows, our third-grade students with special needs showed a medium effect size of .56 decrease for simple incorrect sentences, but at the same time, a large effect size of .98 increase for complex incorrect sentences. This suggests that the students were experimenting, although not always successfully, with more complex sentence structures. This finding is consistent with descriptions of students with language disorders as having particular difficulty with grammatical correctness in both their spoken and written narratives (Gillam & Johnston, 1992). In contrast, the typically developing students showed higher proportions of correct sentences in both categories, at the same time they were reducing proportions of incorrect sentences in both categories.

Word diversity can be measured by using the SALT software (Miller & Chapman, 2000) to provide a count of the number of different words (NDW). This measure is highly influenced, of course, by the total number of words the student produces in the time allotted (i.e., fluency). Nevertheless, we do not adjust it by counting the NDW in a specified number of words (e.g., in the first 50 or 100 words) as sometimes recommended, because of the high variability in children's ability to produce written words. Many children with special needs cannot produce even a 50-word story in the early stages of development, regardless of grade level. Thus, the NDW measure is highly confounded with the fluency measure. The data in Table 15.3 show large pre/post

Table 15.2. Sentence-level changes for third-grade students with special needs and with typical development

Variable	Group	Sept 3 probe		May 4 probe		Paired difference				Effect size
		M	SD	M	SD	M	SD	t-test	Sig. (2-tailed)	
MLTU	S	6.73	2.63	7.26	1.35	0.53	3.36	0.470	0.651	0.16
	T	7.47	2.63	7.96	1.68	0.49	3.03	0.921	0.364	0.16
Tot conj	S	1.67	2.50	16.22	17.25	14.56	16.24	2.689	0.028	0.90
	T	5.16	3.48	8.81	8.16	3.65	9.30	2.181	0.037	0.39
Type conj	S	1.11	1.27	3.44	2.01	2.33	1.50	4.667	0.001	1.56
	T	2.13	1.09	3.10	1.68	0.97	2.02	2.661	0.012	0.48
% simp incorr	S	21.30	27.36	4.52	9.77	−16.78	29.74	−1.693	0.129	−0.56
% simp corr	S	32.41	32.39	31.34	17.21	−1.07	36.36	−0.088	0.932	−0.03
% comp incorr	S	2.78	8.33	33.52	30.63	30.74	31.35	2.942	0.019	0.98
% comp corr	S	43.52	40.35	30.27	22.27	−13.25	47.45	−0.838	0.426	−0.28
% simp incorr	T	13.30	13.63	6.81	9.98	−6.49	17.31	−2.088	0.045	−0.38
% simp corr	T	23.86	23.40	36.01	20.73	12.15	23.30	2.903	0.007	0.52
% comp incorr	T	25.67	25.14	14.27	12.28	−11.41	26.27	−2.417	0.022	−0.43
% comp corr	T	37.17	26.68	42.92	21.09	5.75	25.18	1.271	0.214	0.23

Key: MLTU, mean length of T-unit; S, students with special needs (*n* = 9); T, students who were typically developing (*n* = 32); Tot conj, total conjunctions; Type conj, type of conjunction; simp, simple; comp, complex; incorr, incorrect; corr, correct. Effect size was computed as Cohen's *d*, by dividing the difference between pre/posttest means (*M*) by the pooled standard deviation (*SD*).

Table 15.3. Word-level changes for third-grade students with special needs and with typical development

Variable	Group	Sept 3 probe M	Sept 3 probe SD	May 4 probe M	May 4 probe SD	Paired difference M	Paired difference SD	t-test	Sig. (2-tailed)	Effect size
% corr spelling	S	79.78	13.53	82.74	13.02	2.96	15.93	0.525	0.616	0.19
	T	79.03	18.55	85.79	9.50	6.77	18.32	2.090	0.045	0.37
Number diff wds	S	13.79	6.42	54.67	40.06	40.88	35.64	3.441	0.009	1.15
	T	27.70	10.74	62.37	32.65	34.68	34.29	5.720	0.000	1.01

Key: S, students with special needs (*n* = 9); T, students who were typically developing (*n* = 32). Effect size was computed as Cohen's *d*, by dividing the difference between pre/posttest means (*M*) by the pooled standard deviation (*SD*).

effect sizes for increases in number of different words both for special needs ($d = 1.15$) and typically developing students ($d = 1.01$).

Our writing lab assessment model incorporates spelling as a word-level linguistic skill. The percentage of words spelled correctly is easy to compute by hand. As Table 15.3 shows, the data for changes in percentage of words spelled correctly showed no significant growth either for students with special needs or for those who are typically developing. An alternative approach for capturing growth in spelling development, and one with clinical implications for guiding scaffolding, is to analyze a corpus for evidence of maturing spelling strategies using a system suggested by Beers and Henderson (1977) and Gentry (1982). Earlier in development, most children demonstrate prephonetic strategies for generating spellings of unknown words. Gradually, they demonstrate increasing facility with phonetic analysis and sound–symbol association. As they become more mature, their generated spellings show evidence of transitional skills in the form of orthographic awareness relating multiletter patterns with morphological components and spelling "word families." When spelling conventionally, students demonstrate the ability to draw on a variety of linguistically consistent patterns stored in long-term memory and to use analogical as well as phonetic strategies to spell novel words. The long-term goal is for students to have a direct and automatic route to spelling, without needing to resort to generative processes.

Although we use spelling categories clinically to guide scaffolding decisions, we are only beginning to incorporate them into our analyses of probes for research purposes. We have coded all spellings in our SALT (Miller & Chapman, 2000) transcripts with correct spellings followed by the students' misspellings in square brackets. This makes it possible for the software to count the number of different word roots accurately and print an array of patterns. At this point, one graduate thesis (Ansell, 2004) has demonstrated this measure's potential to capture growth of spelling ability with treatment.

In summary, our own preliminary data show that growth at the word, sentence, and discourse levels can be documented for special needs students as well as for typically developing students in a writing lab approach. Effect sizes for changes in word production fluency and story scores are large. Growth in sentence structure is not as easy to achieve in a classroom-based, contextualized intervention program. This is consistent with results reported by others (e.g., Gillam et al., 1995; Vallecorsa & deBettencourt, 1992), but our students with special needs did demonstrate growth in their use of conjunctions and complex sentences, even though their more complex sentences often included grammatical errors. At the word level, growth in the number of different words provides evidence of improvements in vocabulary diversity along with greater fluency. As Berninger (1999) observed as well, spelling development also comes more slowly. Although it is difficult to document in contextualized samples, Ansell's (2004) results have shown that students receiving treatment use significantly more later-developing strategies than those in a group for whom treatment stopped.

PRACTICAL REQUIREMENTS

Setting up a writing lab requires an initial set of logistic decisions and arrangements. Practical requirements include collaborating with classroom and special education teachers to 1) find a time to plan, 2) schedule a mutual time for writing lab activities, 3) arrange access to computer supports, and 4) select curriculum-based writing projects with a real purpose and audience.

Once a decision is made to collaborate, the team must find a mutual time to plan. At the beginning of a collaborative effort, regularly scheduled and longer times are needed. We have met during lunchtime, before and after school, and during teachers' planning time. After members get to know each other and begin to work well as a team, they can plan for longer periods in advance (requiring less frequent meetings) and meet only briefly in the doorway, while students are working, or through email. Later meetings often focus on ways to adjust instruction to achieve improved outcomes and on how to gather evidence for answering action research questions formulated jointly.

A Schedule for Implementing Lab Activities

Perhaps the most critical practical concern is to schedule a mutually agreeable writing lab time at least twice per week, preferably three times, when the SLP can come into the classroom for a portion of the session. One-hour sessions are preferred because it is difficult to conduct a minilesson and provide extended writing and learning opportunities in less than 60 minutes, particularly if students are working on computers and need time to save and print drafts.

When attempting to integrate language intervention into general education instruction many SLPs face the practical difficulties of meeting the demands of itinerant service delivery and overburdened caseloads. Moving among multiple schools makes it difficult to satisfy curriculum-relevant language and literacy needs of students and teachers. Creative ways to serve students are needed to accommodate the increasing demands on the SLP's time. One possibility is to cluster students with special needs in a single classroom with a willing teacher. Another is for all teachers at a particular grade to form a team with the SLP and special educator responsible for serving mutual students. The larger team plans curriculum-based projects. Then, the SLP either moves among the multiple classrooms to work with students on the caseload, or the students are regrouped during writing lab activities in a particular location, creating opportunity to interact with typically developing peers as well.

Alternative Service Delivery Settings

Although the writing lab approach is designed for collaborative implementation in inclusive classrooms, we have implemented it in a variety of contexts. When it is not feasible to work in general education classrooms, SLPs may collaborate with special education teachers to provide writing lab intervention in special education classrooms. At the middle and high school levels, in particular, educators may gain policy approval for a special class to qualify as the students' language arts academic credit (Anderson & Nelson, 1988). We also have implemented several variations of after-school service delivery in a university computer lab and in community schools, as well as implementing components within more traditional small-group settings.

Curriculum-Based Projects That Involve Writing

An important aspect of this therapeutic *intervention* approach is its relationship to *instruction* in the general education curriculum. This means that the approach must be adaptable to curricular domains as diverse as language arts, social studies, and science. The choice of curriculum projects often is based on the part of the curriculum a teacher has planned to teach during the portion of the school day when a mutual schedule can be coordinated.

Access to Computer Supports

Computer supports are a key component of writing lab instruction and intervention. If the school has access to computers, scheduling should take advantage of computer availability. Even now, it is rare for a school to have enough computers for each student to have continued access. As long as drafts can be printed after each session, students can work actively on their plans and compositions, using such instructional activities as peer conferencing, revising, editing, or author chair activities, even on noncomputer days. Teaching students routines for independent management of their disks and for opening files, saving, printing, and closing can make the process more efficient.

KEY COMPONENTS

As stated in the introduction, the model for the writing lab approach, which was shown in Figure 15.1, includes the three primary components—writing process instruction, computer supports, and inclusive instructional practice. These are grounded in the values of respect and trust and the "backdrop" principles—balance, authentic audience, constructive learning, keep it simple, dynamic, research and reflection, ownership, and patience. In this section, we describe key instructional components—minilessons, scaffolding, teacher or peer conferencing, author chair, and author notebooks.

A typical day in the writing lab starts with a brief minilesson, followed by work on an ongoing project in which students put into practice new skills targeted in the minilesson. A major portion of the sessions is devoted to writing, and some days have no minilessons in order to extend the writing time. SLPs divide their time among the several students with identified special needs, scaffolding language skills to meet their goals and objectives.

Minilessons

Within 1-hour class sessions, large-group minilessons are used to introduce stages of the writing process and specialized topics aimed at helping students become better writers and language users. Minilessons also are used to introduce each new instructional component and to respond to emergent classroom concerns. Many speech-language intervention goals, including listening and large-group contributions, can be addressed in these group discussions.

Although it is difficult to keep the "mini" in minilessons, they should take no more than 10–15 minutes. Most start with introduction of the topic, modeling new skills, and related self-talk. The introduction also offers opportunities for brainstorming so that there is no one right answer. This opens the discussion for multiple contributions and provides an opportunity to work on goals for contributing to class discussions; for example, about what good listeners do, how to think of story topics, or things an author should look for while editing. After brainstorming, students practice the targeted skill. Generally, a handout is provided and added to a section of author notebooks. These supports then remain available to remind students of the lesson and guide them toward independent application.

Scaffolding During Individual Minilessons and Extended Writing Times

As introduced previously, scaffolding is the primary therapeutic technique of the writing lab approach. In some cases, scaffolding is embedded in pre-planned individual minilessons aimed at specific objectives and identified areas of weakness. Scaffolding also is embedded in everyday interactions with students as they work through the writing process. The skilled SLP and teacher partners make balanced choices at any point in time about which language abilities to scaffold and which to leave alone for the moment. Examples include judging what intervention would stifle a fragile learner, impede growing fluency, or set back emerging independence. One advantage of classroom-based intervention is that a language specialist can scaffold a student to set a goal for independent production of several sentences, words, or research notes, then work with other students across the room, returning as promised to appreciate the accomplishment of the goal or to set a new one, thus working on therapy objectives even while interacting with other students.

Scaffolding differs from casual assistance to students in its deliberate, intentional focus on specific objectives based on individualized assessment of students' strengths and needs. We base our scaffolding on Feuerstein's description of instructional "mediation," in which an intentioned adult uses "framing, selecting, focusing, and feeding back environmental experiences" to produce in a child "appropriate learning sets and habits" (1979, p. 179). Scaffolding starts at a level where the student can be successful so that the language specialist can bring the student in touch with a base of knowledge he or she can build on.

For example, many students go through a stage of confusing *in* with *and,* hearing the two words as homophones. Drawing on their oral-language experience, they might write, for example, *My sister in me is going.* Scaffolding in this case might start with comments framing the fact that the student is hearing the similarity in how the two words usually sound when spoken. The specialist might then conduct an individual minilesson by opening a page in the student's author notebook, writing the two words across from each other on a blank page to show that they are actually different, framing the distinctive features in the two spellings, and focusing the student on differences in pronunciation and meaning. Several example phrases might be listed in a column under each word, starting with the language specialist providing full support, and gradually scaffolding the student to construct new examples independently. Then the process returns to the contextualized activity, with the specialist framing contexts for use of *in* and *and* when they occur in the student's composition on this and subsequent days, and praising the student for differentiating the two words and contexts. The intention is for the student to learn more than how to differentiate two specific words. It also is a broader lesson in how to learn new words and pronounce them in a literate manner. If the student needs further instruction, he or she can be redirected to the minilesson in the author notebook as a personal support for enhancing independence and generalization of the new knowledge.

Teacher and Peer Conferencing

Revising rarely is a favorite activity of students. They need audience feedback in order to want to make their written products better. Peer or teacher conferences or author–group interactions can generate strategic questions that lead authors to fill in missing information for their audience or to add more descriptive language.

A minilesson can introduce the concepts and roles of peer conferencing. It is helpful to label roles clearly, such as *author* and *audience*, so that students can be clear about what they do in the role of author when they read their stories and seek feedback from peers. This contrasts with the role of audience when they listen closely to a peer's story, offer comments about what they like and ask questions in areas where they wish they knew more or to clarify confusions.

Teacher conferences can be structured in a similar manner. Students with disabilities need conferences with general education teachers as well as with special service providers. Teacher conferences should be used to express the authentic audience appreciation for the student's ideas first and then scaffold the student toward revisions. Following a minilesson on editing symbols, teachers can help students mark drafts while discussing need for edits in spelling, capitalization, and punctuation.

Author Chair

The author chair experience adds a formal and celebratory element to peer and teacher conferencing. It sets the tone for a community of writers. In author chair activities, students take turns sitting in a special chair, perhaps using a microphone, sharing drafts and final products, and providing feedback to each other. This provides the opportunity for all students to listen and to offer input, as well as to receive it. Interactions encourage higher-order thinking and develop an enhanced sense of audience and joy of communicating. When time permits, a usual routine is for students to read their work, and then to call on one or two students to make a comment and one or two to ask a question. This provides opportunity for metapragmatic understanding of varied speech acts of commenting and questioning, as well as opportunity to scaffold higher-quality input and the ability to use it to make revisions. This, in turn, leads to personal goals and ownership for attempting higher levels of accomplishment.

Author Notebooks, Computer Software Features, and Other Environmental Supports

Author notebooks are used to organize materials for writing projects. Students can make labels for the various sections of their notebooks, such as writing lab schedules, works in progress, minilesson handouts, personal minilessons, and personal dictionaries. Notebooks can help students learn self-regulatory strategies and provide opportunities to work on directional vocabulary (e.g., *before, after, behind, first, last*). Other environmental supports include posters outlining the writing process, for example, and "word walls," which are large-print displays of frequently used words, to which students can refer while writing.

Computer software features are a key component of the writing lab approach. In our book (Nelson et al., 2004), we provide a taxonomy, example software programs, and teaching tips for helping students use computer software features to support all stages of the writing process. These include graphic organizers to assist planning; word prediction and speech synthesis features to assist drafting, reviewing, and revising; standard word processing features to assist editing; and graphic and formatting features to prepare works for publication or multimedia presentation.

ASSESSMENT METHODS TO SUPPORT ONGOING DECISION MAKING

Writing assessment in the writing lab approach combines curriculum-based assessment and dynamic assessment methods. Its purposes are to identify individual profiles of spoken and written-language strengths and weaknesses, gather measures that can be repeated at intervals over time, investigate strategies that may be most effective in intervention, and yield meaningful and relevant goals and benchmarks.

The assessment procedure we have developed involves gathering a written-language probe and analyzing it systematically. We have described this procedure in greater depth in two previous works (Nelson & Van Meter, 2002; Nelson et al., 2004). In the current discussion, we offer a brief overview of the assessment framework.

The first step in the assessment process is collecting a written-language sample in a writing lab context. Decisions regarding genre are best made in collaboration with the classroom teacher, who is familiar with targeted grade-level outcomes. The sampling probe can be repeated later under similar conditions to check for growth over time. The story found in Figure 15.2 was written by Grant, a third-grade boy identified with language-learning disability in response to this prompt: *We are interested in the stories students write. Your story should tell about a problem and what happens. It can be real or imaginary.* The emphasis on the role of the "problem" element is designed to elicit a true narrative with a high point (Labov, 1972), if the child is capable of one.

Some students produce little text independently during the writing period. In these cases, SLPs use dynamic assessment techniques to explore the type and amount of support needed to assist the student to be more successful. For example, asking for a dictated story might present a starting point in understanding the student's spoken language at the discourse, sentence, and word levels. The purposes are to understand the student's developing edge of competence and to collect a sample of language performance leading to intervention targets aimed at next steps of development in three areas: 1) writing processes and self-regulation; 2) written-language products at the discourse, sentence, and word levels; and 3) spoken-language skills.

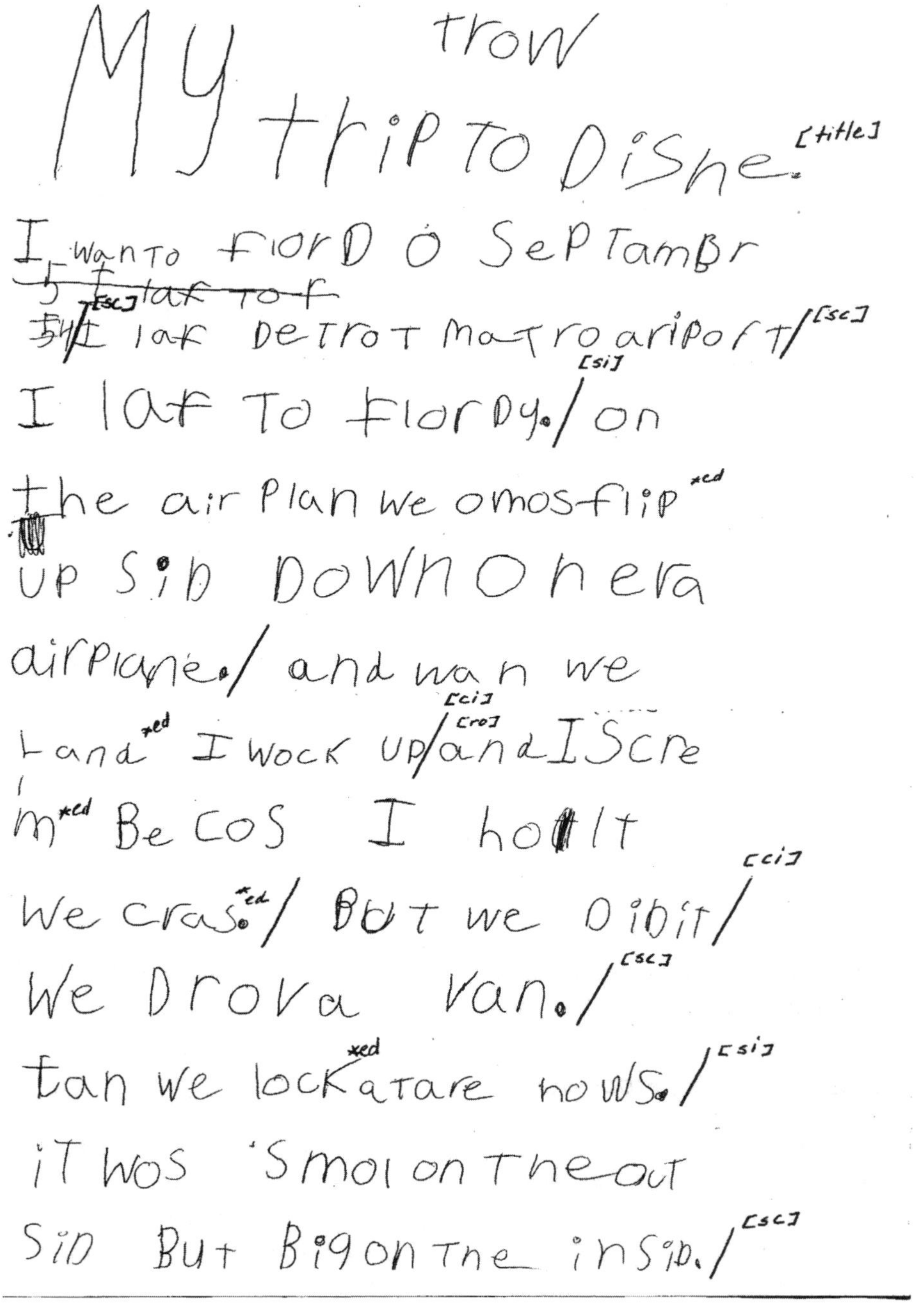

My trow
trip TO Dishe [title]

I want o fiorD o SePTamBr
[sc] laf To f
BuT I lak DETroT maTro ariPorT / [sc]

I laf To fiorDy. / [si] on

the air Plan we omos fliP xed

uP Sib DOWN o n eva

airPlane. / and wan we

Land xed I wock uP / [ci] and I Scre [ro]

m xed Be coS I hollt

We cras xed. / But we Dibit / [ci]

We Drova van. / [sc]

tan we lock a Tare xed no wS. / [si]

iT woS 'Smol on The out

Sib But Big on The insib. / [sc]

a

Figure 15.2. Grant's mid-third-grade probe.

(continued)

Figure 15.2.   *(continued)*

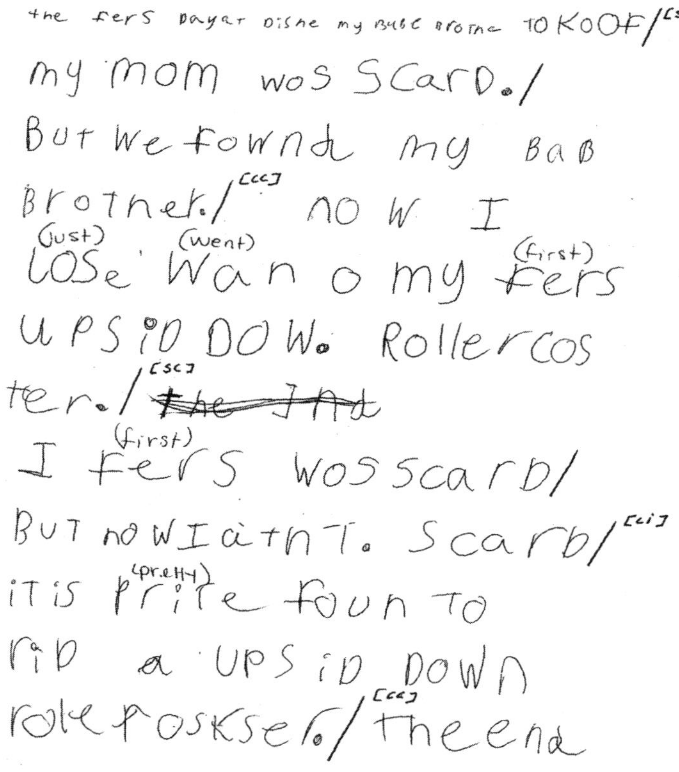

the fers payer oisne my Babe broThe TO KOOF/[sc]

my mom wos ScarD./

But We fownd my BaB

Brotnek./[cc] no W I

(just)   (went)

lose Wan o my fers (first)

u PS iD DO W. Rollercos

ter./[sc] ~~the Ind~~

I fers wos scarb/ (first)

But no W I a tn T. Scarb/[ci]

it is prite foun To (pretty)

riD a UPS iD DoWn

role fosksef./[cc] the end

b

The completed writing process and product worksheet for Grant in Figure 15.3 illustrates our analysis methods.

Assessing Writing Processes

Observation of the degree to which students use recursive writing processes strategically can reveal strengths and needs that may not be reflected in written end products. In the area of planning and organizing, we observe to see if a student approaches writing willingly, produces a topic independently and uses a written or oral method of planning. In the area of drafting, we observe to see if a student proceeds easily from beginning to end, refers to planning guides, and the type of support needed to generate text. In observing for revising and editing processes, we look to see if the student appears to reread his or her work and make changes that make the work clearer or more interesting to the audience. Examples of revising might include adding information, rewording ideas, clarifying references, and reorganizing con-

WRITING PROCESS AND PRODUCT WORKSHEET

Student Name _Grant_ Teacher _Smith_ School _____ Grade _3_ Birthdate _____ Age _8_

Date of Sample _____ Sampling Activity _Narrative Probe_ Observer _T.a._

ASSESSING WRITING PROCESSES

Planning and Organizing

- + Approaches writing tasks willingly
- + Arrives at topic independently
- + Picture - _illustration_
- ~ Graphic organizer Type _(grant)_
- − Notes
- + Dictates

Drafting

- − Refers to planning
- − Proceeds quickly from start to finish
- + Pauses periodically
- ~ Revises along the way
- ~ Dependent on others for spelling

Revising and Editing

- − Rereads work   − Corrects grammar
- + Adds information − Corrects spelling
- − Rewords ideas   − Corrects punctuation
- − Clarifies references 0 # edits
- − Reorganizes content

ASSESSING WRITTEN PRODUCTS

Discourse Level

Fluency
- 121 Total # words
- 6.8 # words/t-unit

Structural Organization
- + True to genre: _narrative_
- Maturity level: _causal sequence_

Cohesion
- + Clarity within sentences
- ~ Clarity across text—_repeats idea_
- ~ Pronoun reference cohesion
- ~ Verb tense cohesion

Sense of Audience
- + Title ~ End _"the end"_
- ~ Creative and original
- + Relevant information
- ~ Adequate information
- − Dialogue/ Other literary devices

Sentence Level

T-units
- 17 Total # T-units
- 4-11 range of T-unit length

Types of Sentences
- 2 # Simple incorrect
- 6 # Simple correct
- 3 # Complex incorrect
- 2 # Complex correct
- 1 # run-on clauses (after 2 coord.)

Variability
- ~ Varied sentence types
- − Over-reliance on a particular construction

— word omissions

— past tense- ed
  omissions-4/4

Word Level

Word Choice
- ~ Mature and interesting choices –_upside- down_
- al Over-reliance on particular words
- yes Usage errors

Spelling Accuracy
- 49 % incorrect

Spelling developmental Stage
- — Pre-phonetic
- — Semi-phonetic
- ~ Phonetic   b/d reversals
- — Transitional
- — Conventional

Examples
- wun/want, went, when
- o/on   work/woke
- laf/left   lock/look
- rid/ride   tan/then
- was/was   crite/pretty
- fers/first   buks/bab/baby
                    + separates words

Conventions

Capitalization
- ~ Initial letter of sentence
- ~ Titles ~ Proper nouns

End punctuation
- ~ Periods ___ Question marks

Commas
- ___ Divide series ___ Divide clauses

Apostrophes
- ___ Contractions ___ Possessives

Quotation marks
- ___ Direct quotes

Formatting
- ___ Paragraphs
- ___ Poetry/other

ASSESSING SPOKEN LANGUAGE IN WRITING PROCESS CONTEXTS

Listening and Comprehension
- + Makes eye contact with speaker
- ~ Listens without interrupting
- ~ Seeks clarification when needed
- + Follows directions

Manner
- + Articulates clearly
- + Speaks fluently
- + Uses natural prosody
- + Appropriate eye gaze
- ~ Appropriate loudness - _quiet_

Topic Maintenance
- + Situationally appropriate
- ~ Provides adequate information
- + Asks relevant questions
- + Shares opinions
- ~ Reflects on own work and others'
- + Engages in conversational turn-taking

Linguistic Skill
- ~ Organizes ideas adequately
- + Completes utterances
- ~ Uses specific vocabulary

Figure 15.3. Writing process and product worksheet completed for Grant's probe. *Key:* +, clearly evident, independent; ~, partially evident, still needs scaffolding; −, not yet emerging.

tent. For editing, we look at the number and type of edits made in correcting grammar, spelling, punctuation, and formatting.

Assessing Written Products

To analyze written products, as illustrated in Figure 15.3, we describe language using a variety of measurement strategies at the discourse, sentence, word, and writing conventions levels. At the *discourse level,* the number of written words a student produces within the 45–50-minute probe can be used as a measure of fluency. Although longer does not always equate with better, increasing levels of fluency reflect greater command over written language, especially for beginning authors. Discourse organization and maturity also are evaluated using progressions that specify features that tend to be added with each new level of development (Glenn & Stein, 1980; Hedberg & Westby, 1993; Hughes, McGillivray, & Schmidek, 1997; Westby & Clauser 1999). These scales and rubrics are used to identify "next steps" to target in intervention. Also at the discourse level, the student's sense of audience is considered by rating success in providing readers with relevant, adequate, and well-organized information and judging the student's use of language to have an apparent intended effect (e.g., for humor, drama, or persuasion).

At the *sentence level,* we employ measures to capture increasing syntactic maturity and variety. First, samples are divided into T-units, defined as independent clauses and any embedded or subordinated syntactic elements. MLTU is calculated by counting the number of words in each "utterance" and dividing by the total number of T-units. This measure is useful in tracking growth in sentence elaboration and complexity when students initially produce very short sentences. Other sentence-level measures provide information about syntactic variety and accuracy. We code sentences as simple or complex based on the number of verb phrases and judge each sentence as correct or incorrect based on the rules of standard edited English. Constructions correct within a student's dialect of heritage also may be noted. Frequency counts across the spectrum from simple incorrect [si], to simple correct [sc], to complex incorrect [ci], to complex correct [cc] are then used to plan objectives and measure change. As demonstrated in Table 15.2, clinicians should not be surprised to see the percentage of incorrect T-units actually increase, at least for complex sentences. This may reflect increased growth and risk taking in formulating complex sentences and lead the SLP to place greater focus on the form of the child's increasingly complex grammatical structures.

At the *word level,* word choice is analyzed with a focus on elements of maturity, interest, variety, and specificity. Word knowledge also is reflected in a student's spelling attempts; therefore, spelling is addressed at the word level. We compute the ratio of correctly to incorrectly spelled words and analyze the spelling patterns found in the student's correct and incorrect spellings or miscues. Although spelling stages (Gentry, 1982) are somewhat controversial (Bourassa & Trieman, 2001; Masterson & Apel, 2000), they can assist SLPs to identify patterns that characterize a student's developing use of spelling strategies. Scaffolding targets for spelling are based on strategies needed to advance to the next spelling level. Additional probes to assess sound–symbol repertoires more systematically are conducted for students functioning at a pre- or semiphonetic level.

In the area of *writing conventions,* written products are assessed for patterns of use for capitalization, punctuation, and formatting. Dynamic assessment procedures help to clarify what students know about conventions and related concepts of words and sentences.

When assessing spoken-language abilities in writing lab activities, SLPs make observations of student's interactions in the formal presentations as well as in small- and large-group discussions. These observations address a student's listening behaviors and ability to comprehend spoken language. Also noted are social-pragmatic skills and the student's manner of spoken communication, including articulation, eye gaze, loudness, fluency, and prosody. Topic initiation and maintenance are additional areas to consider.

Summarizing Observations and Writing Goals

The writing assessment summary and goals form for Grant in Figure 15.4 provides a way to summarize and integrate assessment impressions and associated goals and benchmarks. This example also shows how writing process (self-regulatory) goals may be integrated with language product goals at the discourse, sentence, word, and writing convention levels.

CONSIDERATIONS FOR CHILDREN FROM CULTURALLY AND LINGUISTICALLY DIVERSE BACKGROUNDS

The writing lab approach is particularly suited to the needs of students from culturally and linguistically diverse backgrounds. The narrative genre, in particular, sets the context for individuals to express personal and cultural meanings. Teachers and SLPs can respond easily to messages students convey in their writing in a positive and accepting manner while also encouraging their growing fluency with Standard English forms and conventions.

At each language level addressed in our assessment framework, cultural and linguistic differences may contribute to variations in written-language use. At the discourse level, students who are socialized to tell stories that vary in organization from the dominant European-tradition culture may produce narratives that cannot be scored fairly using assessment tools designed to evaluate topic-centered structures. At the sentence level, students may produce grammatical forms that differ from Standard English. At the word level, choices may vary with cultural differences, and early phonetic spell-

WRITING ASSESSMENT SUMMARY AND GOALS

Student _____ *Grant* _____ Grade _*3*_ Teacher _____ *Smith* _____
Assessment sources _*mid-year probe*_ Genre _*narrative*_ Date _*Jan*_

OBSERVATIONS AND IMPRESSIONS	GOALS AND BENCHMARKS

Writing Processes
Planning and organizing
• *Chose topic independently*
• *Planned orally by sequencing ideas*
• *Started story web, but did not use*
 	
Drafting
• *Proceeds from start to finish with occasional pauses*
 	
Revising and editing
• *Crossed out "the end" and added information*
• *No evidence of editing*
	In end-of-semester probe, Grant will independently demonstrate the following:
	
	1. Move from oral to written planning by completing a graphic organizer prior to drafting
	
	2. Re-read work aloud to revise and edit for
	  a. Missing words and morphemes
	  b. Tense agreement across story

Written Products
Discourse level
Told vacation story in "what next" sequence with causal links. Some problems stated, but no goal setting or planning to resolve
 	
Cohesion problems with pronouns and verb tense
 	
Sentence level
Incorrect sentences characterized by missing words and morphemes; past tense –ed missing 4/4 times
 	
Word level
49% of words misspelled
Reliance on phonetic spelling strategies
 	
Conventions
Inconsistent sentence capitalization and punctuation
	3. Develop story ideas by adding goal setting and planning to resolve problems.
	
	4. Identify characters by proper names, prior to using pronouns.
	
	5. Improve sentence level skills by
	  a. Rereading work and adding omitted words
	  b. Using past tense markers when required
	
	6. Increase spelling accuracy by:
	  a. Using end morpheme –ed
	  b. Learning visual orthographic patterns for at least 5 high-frequency words, e.g., was, on, look
	  c. Learning and applying "silent e" spelling pattern with minimal scaffolding
	  d. Using a personal dictionary to record and access difficult-to-spell words and spelling minilessons.

Oral Language **Writing process oral contexts** • *Fluent speech* • *Contributes good ideas* **Genre specific** • *Likes to tell family stories*	*7. Revise with a peer and independently recognize two opportunities for revision in his own work.*

Figure 15.4. Writing assessment summary and goals for Grant.

ings may reflect dialectal pronunciations. Therefore, assessment tools must be sensitive to cultural differences and modified to avoid inappropriate penalties for cultural-linguistic variants.

The balance principle in our backdrop acronym applies here. We believe that it is important to respect and honor communication differences as legitimate variations and, particularly, to celebrate ethnically rich stylistic creativity (Smitherman, 1994). We also believe that to be successful in school and to maximize vocational and economic potential, all students need to know how and when to use standard language forms (Delpit, 1995). Students must develop proficiency in use of literate language forms to be successful in school and have prospects for higher education and well-paying employment. Explicit instruction comparing and contrasting influences of students' heritage languages or dialects and the formal language of schooling may be conducted during group minilessons or using one-on-one scaffolding when revising. The goal is to create a classroom culture where differences are respected, valued, and shared, while advancing the formal language learning of all students.

APPLICATION TO AN INDIVIDUAL CHILD

To illustrate how the writing lab approach can lead to individual growth, we draw on our work with Grant, the third grader with a language-learning disability whose written work and associated assessment pieces are illustrated in Figures 15.2–15.4.

Assessment

Grant approached writing willingly, independently choosing to write about his family's trip to Disney World. Observation of writing processes showed that he first planned his story by drawing a picture with a story title, then turned to a peer and orally dictated his story, ticking off on his fingers the events of his trip. While drafting his story, Grant paused along the way periodically. He asked for support with spelling several times but made generative attempts with minimal encouragement. Grant made one revision in his story. He crossed out his first *The end* and extended his story by describing his feelings related to rollercoaster rides. No edits were observed in Grant's story.

Grant wrote a 121-word story with a discourse structure that is characterized by a "What next?" style of relating actions and events. Although it is a temporal sequence, causal relationships are implied, and some internal responses by the main characters are stated. Grant introduced two problems that occurred on the trip, but he did not include goal setting and planning to solve the problems. Information was sufficient; however, the story lacked description or detail. Grant's story is relatively easy to follow, although he shows some difficulty in maintaining verb tense cohesion across the story. In addition he never clearly identified the *we* that is repeated multiple times.

At the sentence level, Grant produced both correct and incorrect simple and complex sentences. He omitted the past tense morpheme *–ed* several times. At the word level, Grant primarily chose simple but appropriate vocabulary for his story. He added some detail when specifying the name of the airport and an interesting descriptor, *upside-down*. Spelling was an area of major difficulty for Grant. He correctly spelled only 47% of his words, and spelling pattern analysis showed a strong reliance on phonetic strategies, although his phonetic knowledge was incomplete. Grant inconsistently used capital letters and end punctuation to mark sentence boundaries. In the area of spoken language, Grant was a quiet speaker who demonstrated strong listening skills, but he needed scaffolding support to identify and clarify some confusions.

Goals and Benchmarks

Process, product, and spoken-language goals for Grant are listed in Figure 15.4. One focus was to move from oral to written planning strategies by completing a graphic organizer prior to drafting. To build on his oral-language strengths, one goal was for Grant to use peer-conferencing activities to recognize the need for revisions and to make at least two changes in his current draft. A second goal was to use self-talk to recognize comprehension breakdowns and to ask questions to seek clarification of misunderstandings.

A next step in the area of spelling was for Grant was to represent all phonemes, learn final morphemes, such as *-ed*, and acquire several new word root patterns. A self-regulatory goal was to use a personal dictionary to assist with spelling.

Projects and Scaffolding

An early classroom project was writing science reports on animals. Classroom instruction focused on using questions to guide information gathering, note taking, and writing a three-paragraph report with an introduction, a middle, and a conclusion. Grant chose to write on zebras, a topic of strong affinity for him. The SLP provided individual support for reading books and on-line resources. Grant was taught to state ideas in his own words, then write them. With support, Grant successfully completed a planning sheet.

In early drafts, Grant showed difficulty organizing information logically and listed his notes rather than formulating complete sentences. The SLP used scaffolding questions to help Grant to organize information by related subtopics and to supply missing information where needed. He was guided to produce full sentences, first orally and then in writing.

During revising and editing, Grant recognized missing words and morphemes when others read his work aloud; however, he needed support to read slowly and to check for missing words or word parts on his own. Peers also scaffolded Grant by asking questions when they were confused by a fact or by telling him what they wanted to know more about.

A second activity focused on writing stories. Grant was guided to use a graphic organizer to plan ideas, including goals for problem solving and clear conclusions. From his plan, he drafted his work. During revising and editing, the SLP read Grant's work aloud with pronunciation reflecting Grant's incomplete phonetic spellings so that the feedback could help him to identify misspelled words. Each session, a few word families with patterns represented in the words of his story were taught and entered in his personal dictionary. This section of the author notebook included new words, word families, morphemes, and guides for frequently confused words such as *want*, *went*, and *when*.

Progress

In a repeat story probe taken 3 months later, Grant wrote a pretend story about rescuing a friend from a monster. He planned his story by writing a rough draft with main ideas. He copied his plan but elaborated on some ideas. Analysis of language levels in Grant's story showed improved story maturity. His story contained features of a clear problem with internal response and planning to solve the problem. Grant also added dialogue to this story and idiomatic temporal links, *just in time* and *fell right to sleep*. Grant continued to experience significant difficulty with spelling, with 45% spelling accuracy. His spelling errors showed evidence of phonetic spelling (*frand* for friend, *rit* for right), as well as attempts to recall visual patterns (*shaid* for said, *wher* for where). Grant used end morpheme –*ed* in three of four opportunities. He did not use his personal dictionary spontaneously to generate spelling or edit his work. In author chair following the probe, Grant shared his work with peers, reading the suspense elements with some excitement. Next steps for Grant should be continuing to focus on spelling patterns and use of spelling supports, as well as developing his ideas in writing.

FUTURE DIRECTIONS

Our understanding of the potential of the writing lab approach grows with each new experience. We continue to hone our skills at scaffolding, particularly in inner city schools where students face many social-emotional challenges and discouragement often gets in the way of learning. We engage our graduate students in these experiences as well, so that the next generation of SLPs can learn how to be relevant to students' needs to acquire language and literacy abilities and participate successfully in regular curricular activities.

We believe that we have taken some important strides in studying the effectiveness of the writing lab approach, but more well-designed research is sorely needed. Our preliminary results of these school-based interventions are promising, and the writing lab methods and results appear to be transferred relatively easily across grade levels and settings. The approach is not only rewarding in terms of students' progress, but also entertaining and heartwarming for instructional teams. No 20-item drill can hold even a drop of the mutual joy that comes when a student takes the author chair for the first time and delights peers and adults by reading his or her own original ideas in writing.

RECOMMENDED READINGS

Atwell, N. (1987). *In the middle: Writing, reading, and learning with adolescents.* Portsmouth, NH: Heinemann.

Calkins, L. (1990). *Living between the lines.* Portsmouth, NH: Heinemann.

Calkins, L. (1994). *The art of teaching writing* (2nd ed.). Portsmouth, NH: Heinemann.

Graves, D.H. (1983). *Writing: Teachers and children at work.* Portsmouth, NH: Heinemann.

Nelson, N.W., Bahr, C.M., & Van Meter, A.M. (2004). *The writing lab approach to language instruction and intervention.* Baltimore: Paul H. Brookes Publishing Co.

Swoger, P.A. (1989). Scott's gift. *English Journal, 78,* 61–65.

REFERENCES

Allington, R.L., & McGill-Franzen, A. (1989). School response to reading failure: Instruction to Chapter I and special education students in grades two, four, and eight. *Elementary School Journal, 89,* 529–542.

American Speech-Language-Hearing Association (ASHA) Committee on Reading and Writing. (2001). *Roles and responsibilities of speech-language pathologists with respect to reading and writing in children and adolescents: Position statement, technical report, and guidelines.* Rockville, MD: Author.

Anderson, G.M., & Nelson, N.W. (1988). Integrating language intervention and education in an alternate adolescent language classroom. *Seminars in Speech and Language, 9*(4), 341–353.

Ansell, P. (2004). *Measuring spelling growth over time in elementary school writing samples.* Unpublished master's thesis, Western Michigan University, Kalamazoo, MI.

Bahr, C.M., Nelson, N.W., & Van Meter, A.M. (1996). The effects of text-based and graphics-based software tools on planning and organizing of stories. *Journal of Learning Disabilities, 29,* 355–370. This article also appears in a monograph, *Technology for students with learning disabilities: Educational applications,* with a print version and additional annotative text in a digital version. Austin, TX: PRO-ED.

Bahr, C.M., Nelson, N.W., Van Meter, A.M., & Yanna, J.V. (1996). Children's use of desktop publishing features: Process and product. *Journal of Computing in Childhood Education, 7*(3/4), 149–177.

Baker, S., Gersten, R., & Graham, S. (2003). Teaching expressive writing to students with learning disabilities: Research-based applications and examples. *Journal of Learning Disabilities, 36,* 109–123.

Beers, J., & Henderson, E.H. (1977). A study of developing orthographic concepts among first graders. *Research on Teaching of English, 11,* 133–148.

Berninger, V.W. (1999). Coordinating transcription and text generation in working memory during composing: Automatic and constructive processes. *Learning Disability Quarterly, 22,* 99–112.

Bourassa, D.C., & Trieman, R. (2001). Spelling development and disability: The importance of linguistic factors. *Language, Speech, and Hearing in Schools, 32,* 172–181.

Catts, H.W., Fey, M.E., Tomblin, J.B., & Zhang, X. (2002). A longitudinal investigation of reading outcomes in children with language impairments. *Journal of Speech, Language, and Hearing Research, 45,* 1142–1157.

Catts, H.W., & Kamhi, A.G. (1999). Defining reading disabilities. In H.W. Catts & A.G. Kamhi (Eds.), *Language and reading disabilities* (pp. 50–72). Boston: Allyn & Bacon.

Chapman, M.L. (1994). The emergence of genres: Some findings from an examination of first-grade writing. *Written Communication, 11*, 348–380.

Cohen, J. (1988). *Statistical power analysis for the behavioral sciences.* Hillsdale, NJ: Lawrence Erlbaum Associates.

Craig, S.A. (2003). The effects of an adapted interactive writing intervention on kindergarten children's phonological awareness, spelling, and early reading development [IRA Outstanding Dissertation Award for 2003]. *Reading Research Quarterly, 38*, 438–440.

Danoff, B., Harris, K.R., & Graham, S. (1993). Incorporating strategy instruction within the writing process in the regular classroom: Effects on the writing of students with and without learning disabilities. *Journal of Reading Behavior, 25*, 295–322.

De La Paz, S., & Graham, S. (1997). Strategy instruction in planning: Effects on the writing performance and behavior of students with learning disabilities. *Exceptional Children, 63*, 167–181.

De La Paz, S., & Graham, S. (2002). Explicitly teaching strategies, skills, and knowledge: Writing instruction in middle school classrooms. *Journal of Educational Psychology, 94*, 687–698.

Delpit, L. (1995). *Other people's children: Cultural conflict in the classroom.* New York: New Press.

Englert, C.S. (1992). Writing instruction from a sociocultural perspective: The holistic, dialogic, and social enterprise of writing. *Journal of Learning Disabilities, 25*(3), 153–172.

Englert, C.S., & Palincsar, A.S. (1991). Reconsidering instructional research in literacy from a sociocultural perspective. *Learning Disabilities Research & Practice, 6,* 225–229.

Englert, C.S., & Raphael, T.E. (1989). Developing successful writers through cognitive strategy instruction. In J.E. Brophy (Ed.), *Advances in research on teaching* (Vol. 1, pp. 105–151). Greenwich, CT: JAI Press.

Englert, C.S., Raphael, T.E., & Anderson, L.M. (1992). Socially-mediated instruction: Students' knowledge and talk about writing. *Elementary School Journal, 92,* 411–449.

Englert, C.S., Raphael, T.E., Anderson, L.M., Anthony, H.M., & Stevens, D.D. (1991). Making writing strategies and self-talk visible: Strategy instruction in regular and special education classrooms. *American Educational Research Journal, 28*, 337–372.

Ferretti, R.P., MacArthur, C.A., & Dowdy, N.S. (2000). The effects of an elaborated goal on the persuasive writing of students with learning disabilities and their normally achieving peers. *Journal of Educational Psychology, 92*, 694–702.

Feuerstein, R. (1979). *The dynamic assessment of retarded performers.* Baltimore: University Park Press.

Gentry, J.R. (1982). An analysis of developmental spelling in GNYS AT WRK. *The Reading Teacher, 36,* 192–201.

Gersten, R., & Baker, S. (2001). Teaching expressive writing to students with learning disabilities: A meta-analysis. *Elementary School Journal, 101*, 251–272.

Gillam, R., & Johnston, J.R. (1992). Spoken and written language relationships in language/learning-impaired and normally achieving school-age children. *Journal of Speech and Hearing Research, 35*, 1303–1315.

Gillam, R., McFadden, T., & van Kleeck, A. (1995). Improving narrative abilities: Whole language and language skills approaches. In S.F. Warren & J. Reichle (Series Eds.) & M.E. Fey, J. Windsor, & S.F. Warren (Vol. Eds.), *Communication and language intervention series: Vol. 5.* Language intervention: Preschool through the elementary years (pp. 145–182). Baltimore: Paul H. Brookes Publishing Co.

Glenn, C.G., & Stein, N. (1980). *Syntactic structures and real world themes in stories generated by children.* Urbana, IL: University of Illinois Center for the Study of Reading.

Graham, S., & Harris, K.R. (1989). Component analysis of cognitive strategy instruction: Effects on learning disabled students' compositions and self-efficacy. *Journal of Educational Psychology, 81*, 353–361.

Graham, S., Harris, K., MacArthur, C.A., & Schwartz, S.S. (1991). Writing and writing instruction with students with learning disabilities: A review of a program of research. *Learning Disability Quarterly, 14,* 18–114.

Graham, S., MacArthur, C.A., & Schwartz, S. (1995). Effects of goal setting and procedural facilitation on the revising behavior and writing performance of students with writing and learning problems. *Journal of Educational Psychology, 87,* 230–240.

Hayes, J., & Flower, L. (1980). Identifying the organization of the writing process. In L.W. Gregg & E.R. Steinberg (Eds.), *Cognitive processes in writing* (pp. 3–10). Hillsdale, NJ: Lawrence Erlbaum Associates.

Hedberg, N.L., & Westby, C.E. (1993). *Analyzing story telling skills: Theory to practice.* Austin, TX: PRO-ED.

Hughes, D., McGillivray, L., & Schmidek, M. (1997). *Guide to narrative language.* Eau Claire, WI: Thinking Publications.

Jaben, T.H. (1983). The effects of creativity training on learning disabled students' creative written expression. *Journal of Learning Disabilities, 16,* 264–265.

Jaben, T.H. (1987). Effects of training on learning disabled students' creative written expression. *Psychological Reports, 60,* 23–26.

Juel, C. (1988). Learning to read and write: A longitudinal study of 54 children from first through fourth grades. *Journal of Educational Psychology, 80,* 437–447.

Kamhi, A.G., & Catts, H.W. (2002). The language basis of reading: Implications for classification and treatment of children with reading disabilities. In K.G. Butler & E.R. Silliman (Eds.), *Speaking, reading, and writing in children with language learning disabilities* (pp. 45–72). Mahwah, NJ: Lawrence Erlbaum Associates.

Labov, W. (1972). *Language in the inner city.* Philadelphia: University of Pennsylvania Press.

Lee, L.L. (1974). *Developmental sentence analysis.* Evanston, IL: Northwestern University Press.

Lewis, B.A., O'Donnell, B., Freebairn, L.A., & Taylor, H.G. (1998). Spoken language and written expression: Interplay of delays. *American Journal of Speech-Language Pathology, 7*(3), 77–84.

Lyon, G.R., Shaywitz, S.E., & Shaywitz, B.A. (2003). A definition of dyslexia. *Annals of Dyslexia, 53,* 1–14.

MacArthur, C.A. (1998). Word processing with speech synthesis and word prediction: Effects on the dialogue journal writing of students with learning disabilities. *Learning Disability Quarterly, 21,* 151–166.

MacArthur, C.A., Ferretti, R.P., Okolo, C.M., & Cavalier, A.R. (2001). Technology applications for students with literacy problems: A critical review. *The Elementary School Journal, 101,* 273–301.

MacArthur, C., Graham, S., & Schwartz, S. (1993). Integrating strategy instruction and word processing into a process approach to writing instruction. *School Psychology Review, 22,* 671–681.

MacArthur, C., Graham, S., Schwartz, S., & Shafer, W.D. (1995). Evaluation of a writing instruction model that integrated a process approach, strategy instruction, and word processing. *Learning Disability Quarterly, 18,* 278–291.

MacArthur, C., Schwartz, S., & Graham, S. (1991). Effects of a reciprocal peer revision strategy in special education classrooms. *Learning Disabilities Research and Practice, 6,* 201–210.

Masterson, J.J., & Apel, K. (2000). Spelling assessment: Charting a path to optimal intervention. *Topics in Language Disorders, 20*(3), 50–65.

Meline, T., & Schmitt, J.F. (1997). Case studies for evaluating statistical significance in group designs. *American Journal of Speech-Language Pathology, 6*(1), 33–41.

Miller, J., & Chapman, R. (2000). *Systematic analysis of language transcripts* (SALT) [Computer program]. Madison, WI: Waisman Center, University of Wisconsin–Madison.

Moats, L.C., & Foorman, B.R. (2003). Measuring teachers' content knowledge of language and reading. *Annals of Dyslexia, 53,* 23–45.

Nelson, N.W. (1998). *Childhood language disorders in context: Infancy through adolescence* (2nd ed.). Boston: Allyn & Bacon.

Nelson, N.W., Bahr, C.M., & Van Meter, A.M. (2004). *The writing lab approach to language instruction and intervention.* Baltimore: Paul H. Brookes Publishing Co.

Nelson, N.W., & Van Meter, A.M. (2002). Assessing curriculum-based reading and writing samples. *Topics in Language Disorders, 22*(2), 35–59.

Nelson, N.W., & Van Meter, A.M. (2003, June). *Measuring written language abilities and change through the elementary years.* Poster presented at the Symposium for Research in Child Language Disorders, University of Wisconsin–Madison.

Nelson, N.W., Van Meter, A.M., & Bahr, C.M. (2003, July). *Written language development and writing lab instruction: Growth for students with and without language-learning difficulties.* Poster presented at the International Academy of Learning Disabilities, University of Wales, Bangor.

Nelson, N.W., Van Meter, A.M., Chamberlain, D., & Bahr, C.M. (2001). The speech-language pathologist's role in a writing lab approach. *Seminars in Speech and Language, 22*(3), 209–220.

Paulesu, E., Frith, U., Snowling, M., Gallagher, A., Morton, J., Frackowiak, R.S.J., & Frith, C.D. (1996). Is developmental dyslexia a disconnection syndrome? Evidence from PET scanning. *Brain, 119,* 143–157.

Pennington, B.F. (2003). Understanding the comorbidity of dyslexia. *Annals of Dyslexia, 53,* 15–14–22.

Pressley, M. (2002). *Reading instruction that works: The case for balanced teaching* (2nd ed.). New York: Guilford Press.

Ratey, J.J. (2001). *A user's guide to the brain: Perception, attention, and the four theatres of the brain.* New York: Pantheon.

Scarborough, H.S. (2002). Connecting early language and literacy to later reading (dis)abilities: Evidence, theory, and practice. In S.B. Neuman & D.K. Dickinson (Eds.), *Handbook of early literacy research* (pp. 97–110). New York: Guilford Press.

Smitherman, G. (1994). "The blacker the berry, the sweeter the juice": African American student writers. In A.H. Dyson & C. Genishi (Eds.), *The need for story: Cultural diversity in classroom and community* (pp. 80–101). Urbana, IL: National Council of Teachers of English.

Snow, C., Burns, S., & Griffin, M. (Eds.). (1998). *Preventing reading difficulties in young children.* Washington, DC: National Academy Press.

Snow, C.E., & Tabors, P.O. (1993). Language skills that relate to literacy development. In P. Spodek & O.N. Saracho (Eds.), *Language and literacy in early childhood education* (pp. 1–20). New York: Teachers College Press.

Stanovich, K.E. (1986). Matthew effects in reading: Some consequences of individual differences in the acquisition of literacy. *Reading Research Quarterly, 21,* 360–407.

Tomblin, J.B., Records, N., Buckwalter, P., Zhang, X., Smith, E., & O'Brien, M. (1997). Prevalence of specific language impairment in kindergarten children. *Journal of Speech, Language, and Hearing Research, 40,* 1245–1260.

Troia, G.A., Graham, S., & Harris, K.R. (1999). Teaching students with learning disabilities to mindfully plan when writing. *Exceptional Children, 65,* 235–252.

U.S. Department of Education, Office of Educational Research and Improvement (OERI). (1996). Can students benefit from process writing? *NAEP Facts* (a news publication of the National Center for Education Statistics), *1*(3), 1–6.

Vallecorsa, A.L., & deBettencourt, L.U. (1992). Teaching composing skills to learning disabled adolescents using a process-oriented strategy. *Journal of Developmental and Physical Disabilities, 4,* 277–297.

Vygotsky, L.S. (1962). *Thought and language.* Cambridge, MA: The MIT Press.

Vygotsky, L.S. (1978). *Mind in society: The development of higher psychological processes*. Cambridge, MA: Harvard University Press.

Wallach, G.P., & Butler, K.G. (1994). (Eds.). *Language and learning disabilities in schoolage children and adolescents: Some principles and applications*. Boston: Allyn & Bacon.

Westby, C.E., & Clauser, P.S. (1999). The right stuff for writing: Assessing and facilitating written language. In H.W. Catts & A.G. Kamhi (Eds.), *Language and reading disabilities* (pp. 259–324). Boston: Allyn & Bacon.

Wong, B.Y.L., Butler, D.L., Ficzere, S.A., & Kuperis, S. (1996). Teaching low achieving students with learning disabilities to plan, write, and revise opinion essays. *Journal of Learning Disabilities, 29,* 197–212.

Zaragoza, N., & Vaughn, S. (1992). The effects of process writing instruction on three 2nd-grade students with different achievement profiles. *Learning Disabilities Research, 7,* 184–193.

16

Overview of Section III

*Interventions Targeting Multiple Levels of
Language Development and Nonlanguage Goals*

REBECCA J. MCCAULEY AND MARC E. FEY

In previous sections, interventions have generally addressed basic and intermediate-level goals (e.g., those affecting phonological awareness, oral expression of vocabulary and grammar, reading, written expression) among particular groups of children, distinguished largely by age and/or general developmental level. For the most part, these interventions are designed to compensate for the child's language-learning deficits by modifying the environment or instructional materials in ways that will make learning maximally efficient. For example, responsivity education/prelinguistic milieu teaching (Chapter 3) and It Takes Two to Talk—The Hanen Program (Chapter 4) aim to facilitate first nonverbal and then verbal communication by creating an optimally responsive environment in which child acts are carefully observed, interpreted, and responded to in ways that are sensitive to the child's perceived intentions. Focused stimulation (Chapter 8) and conversational recasting (Chapter 10) require clinicians to select specific lexical, phonological, and grammatical targets. Intervention agents then modify the input to the child by increasing the frequency and saliency of targeted language forms, thus making them more learnable by children with inefficient learning mechanisms. Similarly, the visual tools provided in the chapter by Hoffman and Norris (visual strategies to facilitate written language development, Chapter 14) are designed to increase the visual cues available to students, thereby reducing the dependence on or otherwise enhancing the processing of phonological features during reading. The System for Augmenting Language (Chapter 6) and the balanced reading intervention for AAC users (Chapter 13) are perhaps the best examples of these efforts to help children learn despite their communication and language-learning difficulties.

In this final section, three interventions are described that have fundamentally different basic goals than those described in the first two sections. Consequently, they are fundamentally different approaches than those described earlier. For example, rather than compensating for children's language learning difficulties through management of the environment, these approaches are designed to treat the underlying obstacles to high-level performance directly. In fact, because the goals of each intervention represented in this section vary so greatly, on the surface they appear to represent an "apples and oranges" aggregation: one targets sensory processing deficits across one or more sensory modalities (sensory integration, Chapter 17); the second targets problem behaviors that are seen as arising because they serve communicative functions, although maladaptively (functional communication training, Chapter 19); and the third targets hypothesized auditory processing deficits as well as language skills that are viewed as contributing to impairments of both language and literacy (Fast ForWord Language, Chapter 18). Despite the variety of goals, however, we believe that these interventions distinguish themselves by their efforts to change the children themselves in ways that will influence their ability to learn language even outside of a therapy context (e.g., as in sensory integration and Fast ForWord) or to eliminate challenging behaviors (e.g., as in functional communication training).

Table 16.1 describes a few structural and content-related characteristics of the three interventions. A brief perusal of this table further confirms an impression of great variety. Unlike the interventions discussed in the preceding sections, all of these interventions may be delivered by professionals other than speech-language pathologists (SLPs). Occupational therapists are designated as the principal professionals planning and implementing sensory integration intervention (Chapter 17). In addition, although functional communication training (Chapter 19) may be implemented by an SLP, because the primary basic goal is to eliminate challenging behaviors by providing communication alternatives, it may just as frequently be implemented by a psychologist or educator who has been trained in behavioral methodology. Fast ForWord Language can be implemented by a variety of professionals or even parents who have received specific training in its use.

One of the interventions (functional communication training, Chapter 19) makes little use of specialized materials. In contrast, the other two are material intensive, with one making generous use of a variety of moveable objects (e.g., blocks, weighted vests) and permanent structures (e.g., suspended hammocks) designed to facilitate therapeutic sensory experiences (sensory integration, Chapter 17), and the other making intensive use of computer-based exercises (Fast ForWord Language, Chapter 18). Recommended ages for these three interventions are similarly variable. In the sections that follow, more information is provided that will highlight principal features as well as the theoretical and empirical foundations of each intervention.

SENSORY INTEGRATION (CHAPTER 17)

Sensory integration (SI) interventions are designed to target learning and behavior difficulties arising from a presumed difficulty in organizing sensory information. In Chapter 17, Cermak and Mitchell immediately dispense with

Table 16.1.   Summary characteristics of three interventions targeting multiple levels of language development and nonlanguage goals

Treatment	Sensory integration (SI)	Fast ForWord Language	Functional communication training (FCT)
Chapter	17	18	19
Client age (chronological or developmental)	Children of all ages	Four years old to adults	Children and adults
Primary client populations	Children with mild to moderate learning and/or behavior problems associated with sensory processing deficits, including children with co-existing communication disorders	Children with specific language impairment, children with temporal auditory processing disorders, as well as children with a wide range of reading abilities	Individuals with severe and profound mental retardation, autism spectrum disorder, pervasive developmental disabilities, as well as those who demonstrate problem behaviors, such as children with emotional or behavior disorder
General characterization of methods	Provision of controlled interactions with rich sensory environments	Intensive use of software-based exercises that use language, listening, and reading content	Application of behavioral or operant teaching techniques
Nature of goals	Improvement of children's ability to process and use sensory input successfully in typical childhood activities	Enhancement of auditory processing skills and improvement of working memory, syntax, and other skills important to oral language and reading	Decreasing the frequency of problem behaviors and increasing functionally equivalent, socially acceptable communication behaviors
Intervention agents	Occupational therapist trained in SI, in collaboration with multidisciplinary team often including a speech-language pathologist (SLP)	Clinicians and teachers trained in administering Fast ForWord Language	Professional trained in FCT working in collaboration with significant others (e.g., teachers, family members, therapists)
Nature of sessions	Individual, but consultation also provided to parents and teachers to facilitate application to other settings	Individual	Individual and group sessions
Demands for technology and specialized equipment	Limited use of technology, but suspended and floor equipment used frequently	Computer-based approach with Internet access facilitating use of resources designed to help track and analyze student progress	Little use of technology, although augmentative systems may be used

the idea that SI should be used as a primary language intervention and instead focuses on the possibility that children with deficits in SI may have difficulty with the acquisition and mastery of communication and language skills. Therefore, they describe the theoretical bases for the diagnosis of SI deficits (also called sensory processing deficits) as well as techniques used in subsequent intervention. In addition, they briefly review the existing literature on the efficacy of SI interventions, focusing primarily on the extent to which there is evidence that such interventions have secondary effects on speech and language variables.

SI and its deficits were first described in the mid-1960s and 1970s (e.g., Ayres, 1965, 1969, 1971) to explain sensory differences observed in children who also demonstrated problems in academics, behavior, or motor learning. Among the diagnoses that Cermak and Mitchell list as associated with SI problems are learning disabilities, autism spectrum disorder, attention-deficit/hyperactivity disorder, and developmental disabilities, as well as speech and language disorders seen in combination with motor discoordination.

In their chapter, Cermak and Mitchell explain that diagnosis of SI disorders is accomplished primarily with one of two standardized instruments: the Sensory Profile (Brown & Dunn, 2002) or the Sensory Integration and Praxis Test (Ayres, 1989). These instruments are used to identify two major categories of SI disorders. The first of these are *disorders of sensory modulation*: sensory overresponsivity, sensory underresponsivity, sensory seeking, and combined sensory reactivity patterns. The second major category consists of *disorders of discrimination and praxis*. Cermak and Mitchell cite several studies as supporting diagnoses of SI disorders involving sensory modulation, specifically by showing patterns of physiological responding (viz., electrodermal activity) that correlates with different profiles on an SI test, the Short Sensory Profile (e.g., McIntosh, Miller, Shyu, & Hagerman, 1999; Miller, McIntosh, et al., 1999).

SI interventions are designed to alter the sensory processing abnormalities thought to cause observed limitations in function, thereby enhancing a child's participation in the social roles of childhood. Based on that view, Cermak and Mitchell suggest that improvements in speech and language development may follow from SI intervention as an indirect result of the child's improved participation in everyday, language-fostering experiences. For children with co-occurring problems in motor coordination (e.g., those who demonstrate speech as well as language difficulties), they seem to suggest more direct benefits from SI treatments designed to influence sensorimotor integration. Even for children for whom SI intervention is not recommended, however— as in the case of children with frank neurological damage such as cerebral palsy—Cermak and Mitchell propose value in SI theory to parents, and presumably others, as a means of understanding a child's response to sensation.

Research on SI intervention, especially research that examines communication outcomes, is relatively limited. Furthermore, as Cermak and Mitchell emphasize, what has been done focuses primarily on direct treatment by occupational therapists. Therefore, it may not generalize as well to treatment conducted in the classroom and when other professionals are working in concert with the occupational therapist. Cermak and Mitchell concentrate their review on three narrative reviews of the literature and two meta-analyses (Ottenbacher, 1982; Vargas & Camilli, 1999) that largely represented alternative considerations of the same limited research base. They conclude that the literature demonstrates "mixed support for sensory integration for improving motor and academic functions and does not provide support for language as an outcome measure" (p. 452). However, they go on to argue for the need for additional, more rigorous study of these questions. This need arises largely from problems in many studies that could lead one to underestimate the value of SI for children with language disorders. These problems include the use of problematic language measures as outcome variables (Griffer, 1999), small sample sizes, and poorly described and insufficiently individualized treatments. Cermak and Mitchell propose that, if it is appropriate at all, the SI treatment they describe be considered as an adjunctive treatment for children with language disorders who also show weaknesses in SI and related problems, such as poor attention and poor listening skills.

FAST FORWORD LANGUAGE (CHAPTER 18)

In Chapter 18, Agocs, Burns, De Ley, Miller, and Calhoun have described the theoretical origins, emerging empirical base, and basic aspects of the structure and implementation of Fast ForWord Language. Fast ForWord Language is implemented through a software program that incorporates exercises designed to address auditory processing, memory, and language skills underlying both oral and written language. Although originally designed to address the needs of children with specific language impairment and/or auditory processing difficulties, it has more recently been recommended and used for children and adults with a wide range of additional diagnoses, including autism spectrum disorder, developmental disabilities, and frank neurological impairments.

This intervention grew out of the basic position that children with language impairments have specific difficulty with the processing of rapidly changing aspects of speech (e.g., Stark & Tallal, 1988; Tallal & Piercy, 1974). If this is true, intensive practice with such signals might result in improvements in performance and fundamental cortical reorganization of the processing of speech stimuli (Merzenich et al., 1996). Direct gains in auditory processing are thought to lead to improvements in children's ability to access oral language and language-based aspects of reading, thus helping them avoid associated literacy and academic difficulties.

Because of these basic tenets, the earliest prototypes of Fast ForWord Language (Merzenich et al., 1996; Tallal et al., 1996) focused on children's discrimination of speech stimuli that were acoustically altered in terms of time-scale and intensity to make them easier for children to process. As the child demonstrated mastery of discrimination tasks, the extent of modification was gradually reduced until natural speech could be used. The software was later revised so that it now includes practice with aspects of the English linguistic system that are particularly affected in children with language impairments, such as closed-class morphemes (e.g., pronouns, *be* forms) and complex sentences—also based on the premise that large amounts of practice are likely to result in positive changes in neural substrates.

Agocs and her colleagues indicate that, in its current commercially available form, Fast ForWord is designed to build "perceptual, cognitive, and linguistic skills that provide the foundation for language and literacy development" and to develop "processing speed, phoneme discrimination, sound sequencing ability, sustained and focused attention, and working memory" (p. 494). Beyond the use of acoustically modified speech, key features of the intervention that are designed to achieve these numerous goals are a protocol that involves the child in activities 100 minutes per day, 5 days per week for 4–8 weeks; immediate feedback; and flexibility in item difficulty based on the child's performance. Thus, whereas dosage is likely a factor in all of the interventions described in this book, very high-intensity presentation of the auditory exercises is judged to be critical to the neural reorganization targeted in Fast ForWord. In addition, motivation is addressed through the game-like format of exercises and through the use of a token economy to reward participation. Exercises are grouped according to whether the stimuli used focus on sound-, word-, or sentence-level skills.

Tools used to identify children for whom Fast ForWord Language may prove useful are conventional standardized tests, such as the Clinical Evaluation of Language Fundamentals-3 (Semel, Wiig, & Secord, 1995) and the Comprehensive Test of Phonological Processing (Wagner, Torgesen, & Rashotte, 1999), among others. Assessment of children's progress once the intervention is under way is recorded by the program. Because of the computerized nature of Fast ForWord Language, the adult responsible for administering the treatment, termed a *monitor,* plays a considerably smaller role in this intervention than in other interventions included in this volume. Nonetheless, monitors make decisions regarding the acceptability of a child's progress and implement offline, remedial activities designed to help a child who is struggling understand task requirements.

The array of research studies conducted using this intervention is relatively large and growing. One of the initial studies (Tallal et al., 1996) made use of a control group and provided encouraging suggestions that children receiving Fast ForWord intervention improved not simply on speech perception measures, as might be expected, but also on language measures.

These studies were followed by a national field trial (http://www.scientific learning.com/results) conducted by volunteer professionals for a much larger group of children with a more heterogenous set of diagnoses (including those with pervasive developmental disorder, traumatic brain injury, attention deficit/hyperactivity disorder, and central auditory processing disorder). It is important to note that this study was not experimental and did not employ any type of controls. Although the study often is assumed to reflect efficacy, it addresses primarily the feasibility of the current version of Fast ForWord Language, which had been expanded to include exercises incorporating practice with specific language structures as well as with speech perception tasks. As with the earlier studies, significant changes in speech processing skills were also associated with significant changes in scores on standardized tests of language—both expressive and receptive.

The field trial was followed by a study (Miller, Merzenich, et al., 1999) that included a randomly selected control group and included children who were at risk for academic failure because of poor performance on a language arts curriculum, although not identified as having impaired language, as participants. The Fast ForWord Language group ($n = 288$) and the control group ($n = 164$) included a substantial number of ESL students. Both the entire group of children in the experimental group as well as the subset of ESL students in that group showed statistically significant advantages over their peers in the control group on several receptive language and phonological awareness tests. The magnitude of effects, however, was not reported. Similar studies, conducted in schools across the country and for very large numbers of participants, are continuing as a part of the Scientific Learning Corporation's ongoing data collection. Less stringent requirements regarding participation rates are used in these studies, which are seen by Agocs and colleagues as contributing to effectiveness evidence for this intervention.

In their discussion of the empirical evidence for Fast ForWord Language, Agocs and her coauthors acknowledge some of the methodological weaknesses of their studies as well as the existence of less supportive findings (e.g., Friel-Patti, DesBarres, & Thibodeau, 2001) and even contrasting findings by other researchers (e.g., Hook, Macaruso, & Jones, 2001; Porkorni, Worthington, & Jamison, 2004). We strongly encourage readers to examine these and more recent studies (e.g., Cohen et al., 2005) on Fast ForWord Language that have reported nonsignificant outcomes. However, Agocs and colleagues end their discussion of evidence with a summary of an intriguing study by Temple and colleagues (2003), which also warrants a careful examination. In that study, a small group of 20 children with dyslexia and 12 control children were studied using standardized tests as well as functional magnetic resonance imaging scans before and after intensive Fast ForWord Language intervention. Results indicated both increased activity in areas associated with phonological processing (i.e., the left temporoparietal cortex and left inferior frontal gyrus) that correlated with improvements in oral language scores. The experimental group also showed improvements on a variety of reading tasks and language and rapid naming skills; in contrast, the control group made improvements in reading comprehension but not in language scores, and they declined in scores on rapid naming. Thus, the authors include in their chapter findings that are tantalizing for the evidence base for Fast For-Word but that are also significant as yet another way in which Fast ForWord may foreshadow the future of language treatments. Perhaps language outcome measures will be used increasingly to track not just observed changes in behaviors, but the changes in brain function that are presumed to underlie language learning and development. Although such outcome measures will probably not add significantly to researchers' and clinicians' demonstrations of important functional effects, their use may advance understanding of the nature of disorders of language, with dramatic long-term effects on the treatment of these children.

FUNCTIONAL COMMUNICATION TRAINING (CHAPTER 19)

The concept of challenging, or problem, behaviors encompasses a wide range of socially disruptive actions, including physical aggression, self-injurious behavior, property destruction, and noncompliance. Because such behaviors are seen both in individuals with little functional communication as well as in those who use communication more conventionally, according to the authors the intervention described in this chapter has broad applicability. Unlike all other chapters in this book, however, functional communication training (FCT) does not have improved language functioning as its primary basic goal. Rather, improved communication behavior is seen as a means to a different end, the reduction of challenging behaviors. Thus, primary target populations include children with severe and profound mental retardation, autism spectrum disorder, and pervasive developmental delays. More recently, this list has been expanded to include children with emotional disturbance, behavior disorder, milder forms of autism spectrum disorder including Asperger syndrome, and individuals without an identified disorder who demonstrate problem behavior.

Halle, Ostrosky, and Hemmeter view as the source of problem behavior its social or communicative function; for example, a tantrum might help the child to gain attention or to escape from a disliked situation. When this happens, the behavior is reinforced despite its negative consequences for those in the child's environment. FCT, then, is based on applied behavioral analysis with theoretical roots in work on operant conditioning.

Key to this intervention are the assessment methods used in the selection of treatment targets. Usually, functional behavior assessment is used to identify the function of the problem behavior, its antecedents, and its consequences and is conducted by an individual or team trained in functional behavior assessment as well as FCT. This assessment incorporates several methods, including observation, interviews, rating scales, and record reviews. If the results of the functional behavior assessment are inconclusive, however, a functional *analysis* is conducted in which variables suspected of influencing the challenging behavior are manipulated to examine their effects as a further means of hypothesis refinement.

Once a firm hypothesis is formed about the nature of conditions affecting the challenging behavior, FCT is designed to reduce its frequency by providing the child with an alternative response that produces desired environmental outcomes more efficiently (and in more socially acceptable ways). Thus, an example offered by the authors involves a nonverbal child who acts aggressively toward children seated next to him in a group as a means of communicating his displeasure at this situation. This child could be taught to choose a preferred seat and later be taught to accept longer periods of time in the company of less preferred classmates.

Although treatment decisions are made by those trained in FCT, this intervention is implemented ideally by a team consisting of all significant adults in the child's environment so that implementation is consistent. Teaching methods that are included at the discretion of individual interventionists consist of prompting, fading of prompts, and reinforcement of correct or successively approximated forms of the target behavior. Methods used to track the progress of FCT consist of frequency or interval observational measures of the prompt, the problem or replacement behavior, and the consequence. Latency measures are also used as training progresses, when prompts are being faded and tolerance of particular antecedents is being strengthened through the use of wait-time.

The research base for FCT that is reported on in Chapter 19 consists of several exploratory studies—almost all single-subject experimental designs—in which the internal validity of the intervention's methods was demonstrated. Halle, Ostrosky, and Hemmeter also describe studies that were offered as demonstrations of treatment effectiveness (Durand & Carr, 1991, 1992; Reeve & Carr, 2000). These latter studies were selected for discussion because of their use of more naturalistic settings that are typical of effectiveness research. The authors highlight studies demonstrating the maintenance of gains made through FCT (Durand & Carr, 1991, 1992). They also call readers' attention to a study that they interpret as indicating the potential of FCT to prevent escalation of milder behavior problems into more severe problems in a small group of children with heterogeneous disorders (Reeve & Carr, 2000).

Halle, Ostrosky, and Hemmeter acknowledge widespread acceptance of FCT nationally from both research and clinical audiences but conclude their chapter with a lengthy discussion of several aspects of this intervention they believe call for additional research. They outline an ambitious program of needed research that not only could fuel several research careers, but also can guide clinicians interested in this approach. This discussion is especially valuable to clinicians because its emphasis suggests some degree of confidence in the assessment methods guiding all stages of this intervention but highlights a need for more information about especially important outcomes.

For example, Halle and his colleagues urge improvements in standardization of treatment methods used to teach replacement behaviors through increased study of the effectiveness of currently used methods (e.g., cueing, shaping), as well as through the incorporation of methods from well-studied interventions such as incidental teaching and milieu therapy (see Hancock & Kaiser, Chapter 9). For two reasons, Halle and his colleagues recommend research into the ways in which naturally occurring interaction partners actually respond to replacement behaviors. First, they see this evidence as providing information leading to improved training of such partners as team members. Second, they believe research may help identify replacement behaviors that are naturally reinforced in a wider range of contexts by a wider range of interaction partners, thus yielding greater generalization and maintenance.

It is fitting to end this book with the three diverse treatments considered in this section. Although these three interventions, as others discussed in previous sections, are used to help children with language problems, they do so using methods less directly aimed at language behaviors per se, targeting as they do sensory processing across modalities (Chapter 17, sensory integration), auditory processes (Chapter 18, Fast ForWord Language), and problem behaviors (Chapter 19, functional communication training). With this final section, then, readers have been introduced to a very rich and varied sampling of the strategies and rationales currently proposed for the treatment of children with language disorders. Despite their exposure to such salient differences across interventions, however, readers have probably detected recurring themes of equal prominence, including the ubiquitous need for additional research and the presence of emerging standards for the evaluation of competing intervention methods. Future improvements in the care of children with language disorders will depend not only on continuing research, but also on the skillful selection and implementation of treatments with the best available, if imperfect, evidence base integrated with clinical experience and family and child input. Thus, readers as well as present and future researchers face substantial challenges, but ones that promise equally substantial rewards in both intellectual and personal terms.

REFERENCES

Ayres, A.J. (1965). Patterns of perceptual-motor dysfunction in children: A factor analytic study. *Perceptual and Motor Skills, 20,* 335–368.

Ayres, A.J. (1969). Deficits in sensory integration in educationally handicapped children. *Journal of Learning Disabilities, 222,* 160–168.

Ayres, A.J. (1971). Characteristics of types of sensory integrative dysfunction. *American Journal of Occupational Therapy, 25,* 329–334.

Ayres, A.J. (1989). *Sensory Integration and Praxis Tests (SIPT).* Los Angeles: Western Psychological Services.

Brown, C., & Dunn, W. (2002). *Adolescent/Adult Sensory Profile.* San Antonio, TX: Harcourt Assessment.

Cohen, W., Hodson, A., O'Hare, A., Durrani, T., McCartney, E., Mattey, M., Naftalin, L., & Watson, J. (2005). Effects of computer-based intervention through acoustically modified speech (Fast ForWord) in severe mixed receptive-expressive language impairment: Outcomes from a randomized controlled trial. *Journal of Speech, Language, and Hearing Research, 48*(3), 715–729.

Durand, V.M., & Carr, E.G. (1991). Functional communication training to reduce challenging behavior: Maintenance and application in new settings. *Journal of Applied Behavior Analysis, 24*, 251–264.

Durand, V.M., & Carr, E.G. (1992). An analysis of maintenance following functional communication training. *Journal of Applied Behavior Analysis, 25*, 777–794.

Friel-Patti, S., DesBarres, K., & Thibodeau, L. (2001). Case studies of children using Fast ForWord. *American Journal of Speech-Language Pathology, 10*(3), 203–215.

Griffer, M.R. (1999). Is sensory integration effective for children with language-learning disorders? A critical review of the evidence. *Language, Speech, and Hearing Services in Schools, 30*, 393–400.

Hook, P.E., Macaruso, P., & Jones, S. (2001). Efficacy of Fast ForWord training on facilitating acquisition of reading skills by children with reading difficulties—A longitudinal study. *Annals of Dyslexia, 51*, 75–96.

McIntosh, D.N., Miller, L.J., Shyu, V., & Hagerman, R. (1999). Sensory-modulation disruption, electrodermal responses, and functional behaviors. *Developmental Medicine and Child Neurology, 41*, 608–615.

Merzenich, M., Wright, B., Jenkins, W., Xerri, C., Byle, N., Miller, S., & Tallal, P. (1996). Cortical plasticity underlying perceptual, motor and cognitive skill development: Implications for neurorehabilitation. *Cold Spring Harbor Symposia on Quantitative Biology, 61*, 1–8.

Miller, L.J., McIntosh, D.N., McGrath, J., Shyu, V., Lampe, M., Taylor, A.K., Tassone, F., Netizel, K., Stackhouse, T., & Hagerman, R. (1999). Electrodermal responses to sensory stimuli in individuals with Fragile X syndrome: A preliminary report. *American Journal of Medical Genetics, 83*(4), 268–279.

Miller, S.L., Merzenich, M.M., Tallal, P., DeVivo, K., LaRossa, K., Linn, N., Pycha, A., Peterson, B.E., & Jenkins, W.M. (1999). *Fast ForWord training in children with low reading performance.* Nederlandse Vereniging voor Lopopedie en Foniatrie: 1999 Jaarcongres Auditieve Vaardigheden en Spraak-taal (Proceedings of the 1999 Dutch National Speech-Language Association meeting).

Ottenbacher, J. (1982). Sensory integration therapy: Affect or effect? *American Journal of Occupational Therapy, 36*, 571–578.

Pokorni, J.L., Worthington, C.K., & Jamison, P.J. (2004). Phonological awareness intervention: Comparison of Fast ForWord, Earobics, and LIPS. *Journal of Educational Research, 97*(3), 147–157.

Reeve, C.E., & Carr, E.G. (2000). Prevention of severe behavior problems in children with developmental disorders. *Journal of Positive Behavior Interventions, 2*, 144–160.

Semel, E., Wiig, E.H., & Secord, W. (1995). *Clinical Evaluation of Language Fundamentals-3.* San Antonio, TX: Harcourt Assessment.

Stark, R.E., & Tallal, P. (1988). Children with specific language impairment. In R. McCauley (Ed.), *Language, speech, and reading disorders in children: Neuropsychological studies.* Boston: Little, Brown.

Tallal, P., Miller, S.L., Bedi, G., Byma, G., Wang, X., Nagarajan, S.S., Schreiner, C., Jenkins, W.M., & Merzenich, M.M. (1996). Language comprehension in language-learning impaired children improved with acoustically modified speech. *Science, 271*, 81–84.

Tallal, P., & Piercy, M. (1974). Developmental aphasia: Rate of auditory processing and selective impairment of consonant perception. *Neuropsychologia, 12*, 83–93.

Temple, E., Deutsch, G., Poldrac, R., Miller, S., Tallal, P., Merzenich, M., & Gabrieli, J. (2003). Neural deficits in children with dyslexia ameliorated by behavioral remediation: Evidence from functional MRI. *Proceedings of the National Academy of Sciences of the United States of America, 100,* 2860–2865.

Vargas, S., & Camilli, G. (1999). A meta-analysis of research on sensory integration treatment. *American Journal of Occupational Therapy, 53,* 189–198.

Wagner, R., Torgesen, J., & Rashotte, C. (1999). *Comprehensive Test of Phonological Processing.* Austin, TX: PRO-ED.

17

Sensory Integration

SHARON A. CERMAK AND TRACY W. MITCHELL

ABSTRACT

Sensory integration (SI) interventions consist of a variety of techniques used primarily by occupational therapists to address sensory processing disorders, or SI dysfunction. These interventions are conducted within a theoretical and assessment framework developed over the past three decades. They are relevant to children with language disorders who also demonstrate SI dysfunction, for example, children with diagnoses of attention-deficit/hyperactivity disorder, developmental disabilities, autism spectrum disorder, and learning disabilities. Rather than benefiting from any expected direct effects on language, children with language disorders and SI difficulties are thought to benefit from improvements in attention and behavior that are the more direct focus of SI interventions.

INTRODUCTION

Sensory integration (SI), described as the organization of sensation for use, was developed by A. Jean Ayres (1965, 1971) as a theory to explain how difficulties in academic and motor learning in children with certain learning disabilities relate to the ability to integrate information from the senses. Today, SI is widely used as a framework for understanding behavior and for guiding assessment and intervention with children who demonstrate functional challenges based on sensory processing disorders. By providing controlled interactions with rich sensory environments, therapists help children refine their ability to process and use sensory input successfully in typical childhood activities. Because many children with sensory processing disorders (including motor planning deficits, poor attention, and difficulties in emotional and behavioral regulation) experience coexisting language and speech impairments, speech-language pathologists (SLPs) will probably encounter children receiving SI services. Thus, it is important for practitioners to understand the key principles and components of SI.

TARGET POPULATIONS AND ASSESSMENTS FOR DETERMINING TREATMENT RELEVANCE AND GOALS

Treatment incorporating an SI approach is primarily used with children who demonstrate mild to moderate learning and/or behavior problems associated with disorders in sensory processing. SI is not designed to address primary language impairments, but children with language deficiencies frequently have co-occurring SI problems and may be receiving treatment using an SI approach. Dysfunction in SI, also referred to as a disorder of sensory processing, relates to difficulty organizing and processing sensory information for interaction in the physical and social environment.

The manifestations of dysfunction in SI are numerous. Children may be overly sensitive or underresponsive to normal sensory inputs of touch, movement, sights, and sounds. They may have difficulty with discriminating sensory information, which results in difficulty planning movements, poor coordination, and delayed acquisition of complex motor skills. These children also may have delayed speech and language skills and communication deficits. Sensory processing difficulties can also lead to more global problems such as difficulty in attention and learning, poor self-concept, psychosocial issues, and poor academic achievement (Ayres, 1972b, 1979; Dunn, 1997; Spitzer & Roley, 2001).

Diagnoses associated with dysfunction in SI include learning disabilities, autism, attention-deficit/hyperactivity disorder (ADHD), and developmental disabilities. Intervention using an SI approach is not recommended for individuals with frank neurological damage such as cerebral palsy (Bundy & Murray, 2002), although SI theory may be used to help parents better understand their child's response to sensation.

Dysfunction in SI is of particular interest to SLPs for several reasons. Research has shown a relationship between language, speech production, and motor coordination skills in children (Archer & Witelson, 1988; Crary, 1993; Dewey & Wall, 1997; Estil & Whiting, 2002; Hill, 1998; Katz, Curtiss, & Tallal, 1992; Shriberg, Aram, & Kwiatkowski, 1997; Tallal, Sainburg, & Jernigan, 1991; Tallal, Miller, & Fitch, 1995; Thal, Tobias, & Morrison, 1991; Velleman & Strand, 1994; Wolff, Michel, Ovrut, & Drake, 1990). Moreover, there is consistent support for a subgroup of children with language impairment who also have co-occurring problems in motor coordination (Dewey, 2002). Some researchers have suggested that there may be an underlying function such as sequencing or temporal processing common to language, speech production, and motor functions that may influence performance in all areas (MacKay, 1983; Rothi, Ochipa, & Heilman, 1991). For example, Tallal and colleagues have proposed that an underlying deficit in temporal processing may affect both phonological speech production and motor production skills in children with language impairments (Tallal, Merzenich, Miller, & Jenkins, 1998; Tallal et al., 1995; Tallal et al., 1991). Other researchers have suggested that a common mechanism underlying motor and speech and language functions may be the vestibular or somatosensory system (Ayres & Mailloux, 1981; Gotze, Kiese-Himmel, & Hasselhorn, 2001; Tremblay, Shiller, & Ostry, 2003). As a result, some investigators have suggested that interventions designed to influence sensorimotor processes may also influence language functions and speech production (Ayres, 1972a, 1972b; Ayres & Mailloux, 1981; Kantner, Kantner, & Clark, 1982; Oetter, Richter, & Frick, 1993; Reynolds, Nicolson, & Hambly, 2003).

Although occupational therapy using an SI approach is not focused on improving language skills directly, it has been hypothesized that improvement in SI may lead to increased language skills in general, although the mechanisms are not clear (Ayres, 1972a; Ayres & Mailloux, 1981; Kawar, 1973; Clark, Miller, Thomas, Kucherway, & Azin, 1978; Magrun, McCue, Ottenbacher, & Keefe, 1981; Parham & Mailloux, 2001). For example, Ayres (1972a) found that children whose only identified cause of academic difficulties was in the auditory-language domain (as opposed to the somatosensory and visual domains) made significant gains in reading compared with a matched control group after a program of SI. Ayres (1972a, 1972b) hypothesized that the possible effectiveness of motor activity on language function may relate to enhanced interhemispheric integration at the brain-stem level or enhanced neural integration subserving language function. Ayres's study has not been replicated, however, nor has this hypothesis been more fully explored. It is also possible that amelioration of behavioral and learning difficulties associated with SI deficits may improve the child's ability to participate in typical childhood activities and arenas with their peers and result in greater naturally occurring opportunities for language and communication skill development.

Sensory integrative abilities may relate more directly to certain aspects of communication. For example, the ability to gesture, which requires motor planning, is a fundamental tool for communication. As mentioned previously, children who experience language impairments alone are not likely to be treated using an SI approach; however, children whose communication deficits are accompanied by motor planning deficits (e.g., dyspraxia) may benefit from occupational therapy using an SI approach concurrent with speech and language services. In many settings, the occupational therapist and the SLP may co-treat children with overlapping needs.

Dysfunction in SI should be assessed by a trained occupational therapist, although a multidisciplinary team that includes an SLP may complete a holistic assessment and design an intervention plan that covers multiple treatment areas (Mauer, 1999). Two assessments are commonly used together as the gold standards to examine SI and determine the appropriateness of occupational therapy using an SI approach: the Sensory Profile (Brown & Dunn, 2002; Dunn, 1999a, 1999b, 2002) and the Sensory Integration and Praxis Tests (Ayres, 1989).

The Sensory Profile, with four age-related versions (see Table 17.1), was developed based on Ayres's theory and provides standardized informa-

Table 17.1. Versions of the Sensory Profile

Test	Ages	Number of items
Sensory Profile	3–10 years	125
Short Sensory Profile	3–10 years	38
Infant/Toddler Sensory Profile	0–6 months	36
	7–36 months	48
Adolescent/Adult Sensory Profile	11–97 years	60

tion on an individual's ability to process sensory information in the context of daily activities. The original Sensory Profile (Dunn, 1999a), designed for children ages 3–10, has 125 items that caregivers answer concerning the child's sensory processing abilities and how these abilities support or interfere with functional performance. The Sensory Profile is divided into three main sections: sensory processing, modulation, and behavioral and emotional responses. This assessment takes approximately 30 minutes to administer and 20 minutes to score. The Short Sensory Profile (Dunn, 1999b) is an abbreviated version of the Sensory Profile and focuses mainly on signs of sensory defensiveness. The Infant/Toddler Sensory Profile (Dunn, 2002) is for children ages birth to 36 months, and the Adolescent/Adult Sensory Profile (Brown & Dunn, 2002) is for individuals 11 years and older. All four versions of the Sensory Profile are questionnaire measures: the Sensory Profile, Short Sensory Profile, and Infant/Toddler Sensory Profile are caregiver questionnaires, and the Adolescent/Adult Sensory Profile is a self-report questionnaire. The information garnered from the Sensory Profile provides valuable insights into how sensory processing abilities may be affecting functional performance.

Several validity studies have shown that different clinical populations including children with autism spectrum disorders and pervasive developmental disorder (PDD), ADHD, sensory modulation disorder, and fragile X show different patterns on the Sensory Profile when compared with typically developing children or with other clinical groups (Dunn & Bennett, 2002; Dunn, Myles, & Orr, 2002; Ermer & Dunn, 1998; Johnson-Ecker & Parham, 2000; Kientz & Dunn, 1997; Watling, Deitz, & White, 2001). The relationship of sensory processing to school function was supported through a convergent and discriminant validity study with children with fragile X syndrome. Baranek and colleagues found that avoidance of sensory experience was associated with lower levels of school participation, self-care, and play as measured on the School Function Assessment, the Vineland Adaptive Behavior Scales, and a measure of play duration (Baranek et al., 2002).

In contrast to the questionnaire format of the Sensory Profile, the Sensory Integration and Praxis Tests (SIPT; Ayres, 1989) contains a performance-based group of subtests that assess the child's sensory discrimination and praxis and incorporate clinical observations of sensory modulation. The SIPT is an extensive assessment that takes approximately 2 hours to administer and an additional 30–45 minutes to score. Standard scores are determined using software from the publisher, or test forms may be sent directly to the publisher for analysis. Only professionals who have received specific training should administer, score, and interpret results of the SIPT.

The 17 tests of the SIPT assess a range of sensory integrative abilities, such as tactile and kinesthetic discrimination, vestibular-proprioceptive processing including balance, and praxis or motor planning (see Table 17.2 for a description of the tests of the SIPT). There are five tests of motor planning. Of particular interest to SLPs are the Praxis on Verbal Command and Oral Praxis tests. The Praxis on Verbal Command test examines the child's ability to translate the therapists' verbal directions into motor actions. There are 24 items on this test, such as "Put the backs of your hands together" and "Put your feet together and your hands apart." These commands tax the verbal comprehension and memory abilities of many children with language impairments. Performance on this test can be compared with performance on the other praxis tests that demand less language processing abilities as a means of attempting to separate praxis from language comprehension difficulties. The Oral Praxis test assesses the child's ability to imitate the examiner's lip, tongue, and jaw movements. This Oral Praxis test relates to an individual's ability to produce and articulate speech. However, the test also correlates highly with the child's ability to perform motor planning with the body (Ayres, 1989; Mulligan, 2002) and highlights the relationship between speech production and praxis.

Construct validity of the Southern California Sensory Integration Tests (Ayres, 1972c, 1975) and its revision, the SIPT (Ayres, 1989), has been examined through a series of factor and cluster analysis studies (Ayres, 1965, 1969, 1971, 1977, 1989; Mulligan, 1998, 2002). Studies using the SIPT will be reviewed with particular attention to the language-related tests. In a factor analysis of 125 children, ages 5–9 years, with learning disabilities (identified by the school) and/or SI deficits (identified by occupational therapists), Ayres (1989) identified several factors: bilateral integration and sequencing, somatosensory processing and oral praxis, visuopraxis, somatopraxis, and praxis on verbal command. The Praxis on Verbal Command test loaded most highly on its own factor. The other score on this factor was (prolonged) post-rotary nystagmus, which is not considered an indicator of SI dysfunction. The Praxis on Verbal Command test did not load on the somatopraxis factor, indicating that this test may be a better indicator of language than praxis. However, these findings were not confirmed in another study that included both typical children and children with learning disabilities and/or SI deficits. In this study, Praxis on Verbal Command loaded on a factor with the other praxis tests (Postural Praxis, Oral Praxis, Bilateral Motor Coordination, Sequencing Praxis; Ayres, 1989).

Using the Ward method of cluster analysis with a heterogeneous group of 139 children with typical development and 117 children with SI disorder and/or learning disabilities, Ayres (1989) identified six clusters, characterized by different patterns on the SIPT. Dyspraxia on Verbal Command was asso-

Table 17.2.   The Sensory Integration and Praxis Tests (SIPT; Ayres, 1989)

- Most comprehensive standardized assessment of sensory integration
- Normative scores for children ages 4;0 to 8;11 years

Tests of visual perception

Space Visualization (SV)	This test assesses perception of stimuli composed largely of spatial elements including, in the more advanced items, mental manipulation of objects in space.
Figure–Ground (FG)	This test requires the selection of foreground stimuli from a rival background.

Visual-motor tests (assess aspects of praxis)

Design Copying (DC)	This test is a visual-motor test and evaluates the child's ability to copy geometric designs. The accuracy as well as the child's approach to the task, such as the direction in which the child's lines are drawn and the degree to which the design is drawn in parts or as a whole, are included in the scoring system.
Constructional Praxis (CP)	This test measures the child's ability to relate objects to each other in space and construct a three-dimensional design by replicating a structure provided by the examiner. The test has two parts, one in which the child watches the structure being built and a more difficult task involving the presentation of a permanent prefabricated structure.
Motor Accuracy (MAC)	This test assesses an aspect of eye–hand coordination in which the child must draw a line on top of an existing line.

Tests of praxis

Postural Praxis (PPr)	This test evaluates the child's ability to imitate positions demonstrated by the examiner.
Bilateral Motor Coordination (BMC)	This test assesses the child's ability to coordinate use of both sides of the body. Items include upper extremities as well as lower extremities. Rhythm and smoothness of movements is emphasized.
Sequencing Praxis (SPr)	This test measures the child's ability to replicate dynamic, sequential movements of the hands and fingers following demonstration by the examiner. The ability to replicate a series of movements is emphasized rather than rhythm or smoothness of movement.
Oral Praxis (OP)	This test measures the child's ability to replicate oral and facial postures and movements based on verbal directions and demonstrations.
Praxis on Verbal Command (PVC)	This test measures the child's ability to assume various postures based on verbal directions alone. Length of response time and accuracy are recorded.

Somatosensory tests

Manual Form Perception (MFP)	This test measures stereognosis. Part I involves identifying the visual counterpart of a geometric form held in the hand. Part II involves feeling a shape with one hand and finding the matching shape among a line of blocks manipulated with the other hand without the use of vision.
Kinesthesia (KIN)	This test measures the accuracy with which a child replicates the movement of his or her finger from one point in space to another while vision is occluded. The test taps the ability to perceive joint position and movement.
Finger Identification (FI)	This test measures the child's ability to identify which finger or fingers are touched by the examiner while the child's vision is occluded.
Graphesthesia (GRA)	This is a test of tactile perception, which also evaluates the ability to translate tactile input into a motor response. It assesses integration between tactile and visual input, and fine motor planning.

Localization of Tactile Stimuli (LTS)	This test measures the child's ability to identify the location where he or she was touched.
Vestibulo-proprioceptive tests	
Standing and Walking Balance (SWB)	This test assesses the child's balancing skills with and without vision, while performing a series of standing and walking balance items.
Postrotary Nystagmus (PRN)	This test measures duration and regularity of nystagmus following rotation.

ciated with low scores on bilateral integration and sequencing tests. Ayres questioned whether the bilateral integration and sequencing problem was primarily one of bilateral integration or whether it was largely a sequencing problem which is often considered to reflect left hemisphere processing.

Evidence for construct validity of the SIPT was also provided by contrasting group analyses including children with autism spectrum disorder, learning disabilities, brain injury, mental retardation, SI dysfunction, spina bifida, reading disorder, language disorder, and cerebral palsy (Ayres, 1989), and children postinstitutionalization (Lin, Cermak, Coster, & Miller, 2005). Of particular interest to SLPs are the results for children with language disorders. In a group of 28 children with an educational diagnosis of language disorder, their lowest SIPT score was Praxis on Verbal Command (-1.74 standard deviation [SD]). Scores below -1 SD were also found on Oral Praxis, Sequencing Praxis, Bilateral Motor Coordination, and Standing and Walking Balance, as well as on four of the five somatosensory tests. These findings indicate that there is likely overlap (comorbidity) of children with language disorders and SI disorders.

For the most accurate assessment of children with suspected dysfunction in SI, results of the SIPT and/or the Sensory Profile should be examined in conjunction with developmental and cognitive abilities, diagnostic information, and clinical observations of postural movements (Bundy, 2002a), including the ability to cross the midline when manipulating objects, equilibrium or righting reactions, muscle tone, prone extension, and supine flexion. In addition, interviews, observation of the child's function in context such as on the playground, in school, or at home, and other standardized tests may also be used together with a trained therapist's clinical reasoning to determine whether the child may be an appropriate candidate for an SI approach to treatment (Parham & Mailloux, 2001).

THEORETICAL BASIS

SI describes both the complex neural processing of sensory input as well as a "frame of reference for treatment of children who have difficulty with these neural functions" (Parham & Mailloux, 2001, p. 380). Simply stated, SI describes how we organize sensory inputs from the environment and from our own bodies and process these inputs for use (Ayres, 1979). The theoretical basis of occupational therapy using an SI approach depends on four major assumptions regarding neural plasticity, neural organization, adaptive responses, and the inner drive of children (Bundy & Murray, 2002; Parham & Mailloux, 2001).

Neural plasticity describes the malleability of brain; specifically, the ability of the brain to change at the neuronal synaptic level. Ayres (1979) concentrated on the neural plasticity of the young, developing brain, but it should be noted that some degree of plasticity has been found to exist throughout the life span (Buonomano & Merzenich, 1998). As a child interacts with the appropriately challenging environment with enhanced sensory feedback that an SI environment provides, it is hypothesized that gradual changes are made to the way the brain processes information so that the child will be able to function more effectively.

In addition to neural plasticity, SI theory utilizes both the holistic/ heterarchical and hierarchical models of neural organization. The hierarchical model of neural organization assumes that the brain develops in a particular fashion such that the successful development of higher-order cortical functions depends on successful development of lower-order subcortical functions. For example, language, learning, reasoning, complex motor skills, behavior, and self-regulation are assumed to rely on somatosensory and vestibular integration. Based on this model, which was the predominant view of central nervous system (CNS) organization at the time Ayres (1965, 1972b) was formulating SI theory, intervention to enhance the functioning of the systems associated with SI would result in more optimal higher-order functioning. Although current research does not support a hierarchical model (Montgomery & Connolly, 2003; Shumway-Cook & Woollacott, 1995), some concepts pertaining to maturation of the CNS (e.g., the vestibular and tactile systems mature earlier than other sensory systems; the prefrontal lobes mature relatively later) remain relevant.

SI also takes into account a holistic model of neural organization (Bundy & Murray, 2002). The holistic model explains that the brain operates heterarchically so that different systems in the brain interact in a nonlinear manner. That is, different systems in the brain work together but do not necessarily exert higher-level to lower-level control. Within this view of organization, SI results from interaction between both cortical and subcortical systems. Therefore, if certain systems involved in SI are functioning inadequately, they cannot properly interact with the other systems and the manifestations of poor SI appear in an individual. Current researchers (Montgomery & Connolly, 2003; Shumway-Cook & Woollacott, 1995) emphasize a more holistic model of neural organization, and SI theorists believe that this model lends additional support to the importance of addressing SI for therapeutic intervention.

Most individuals develop SI abilities through a normal developmental path, and the ability to integrate more complex sensory inputs and successfully respond to the environment relies on a mastery of integrating simpler inputs. To help children who have fallen behind in this development or who have developed atypically, occupational therapy using an SI approach attempts to normalize SI by facilitating adaptive responses, another assumption of SI theory.

An adaptive response describes an appropriate reaction to sensory input. In SI theory, an adaptive response not only signifies proper sensory integrative functioning, but also contributes to increased sensory integrative abilities by providing feedback that reinforces future adaptive responses. Therefore, experiencing adaptive responses is a crucial element of enhancing development of SI. In order to experience an adaptive response, individuals must be able to interpret and organize sensory inputs from the environment and their own bodies, and act on the environment accordingly. Simply receiving sensory input (e.g., sensory stimulation) is not enough for an adaptive response to occur because an adaptive response relies on active participation from the individual and needs to be goal-directed.

The final assumption of SI theory is that individuals possess an inner drive or motivation to actively interact with the environment. For children who have dysfunction in SI, dissatisfaction with their abilities and past failures may result in a decreased inner drive that prevents them from engaging in activities that could lead to critical adaptive responses. Hence, the potential for improving SI is greater the more inner drive is promoted through therapeutic rapport and appropriate activities. For this reason, it is critical for intervention to be fun for the child.

Taken together, these assumptions provide the basic foundation for SI theory. Neural plasticity and organization support the idea of the development of SI and the potential to promote SI through facilitation of adaptive responses. When using an SI approach, the therapist sets up the sensory environment in which the child interacts not only to promote adaptive responses, but also to encourage the child's inner drive. With each adaptive response, children become better able to integrate sensory information and become more confident in their abilities. Confidence in their abilities to interact successfully with the environment, in turn, increases children's inner drive to continue to seek out new and challenging experiences and thus further enhances SI.

Types of Sensory Processing Disorders

Using a series of factor analysis and cluster analysis studies, researchers have identified different patterns of dysfunction and have categorized types of sensory integrative dysfunction in various ways (Ayres, 1965, 1969, 1977, 1989; Dunn, 1999a; Mulligan, 1998, 2002). These types have been supported by clinical work (Kimball, 1999a, 1999b). It is useful to divide disorders of sensory processing into two main categories: disorders of sensory modulation and disorders of sensory discrimination and praxis. It is important to note that these categories can overlap and that individuals with dysfunction in SI may have deficits in modulation, discrimination, or both.

Disorders of Sensory Modulation

Disorders of Sensory Modulation Sensory modulation refers to the ability to organize varying degrees of sensory input and respond in an adaptive manner that matches the intensity of the stimulus (Lane, 2002; Miller, Cermak, Lane, Anzalone, & Koomar, 2004). In other words, sensory modulation describes how an individual regulates different sensory inputs to produce an appropriately graded response. Children who demonstrate disorders of sensory modulation have impairments in the ability to regulate and organize the degree, intensity, and nature of their responses to sensory input. When an individual has an impairment in sensory modulation, functional problems often result, including impairments in daily routines, social-emotional difficulties, and behavioral and attentional problems. Although disorders of sensory modulation are prevalent in children with ADHD, learning disability, autism spectrum disorder, and other developmental disabilities, their prevalence in children with specific communication impairments has not been examined.

There are four types of disorders of sensory modulation (Miller et al., 2004).

Type 1: Sensory Overresponsivity Overresponsivity to sensory stimuli is sometimes referred to as *sensory defensiveness*. These children have responses to certain types of sensations that are more intense, quicker in onset, or longer lasting than those of children with typical sensory responsivity under the same conditions. Their responses are particularly pronounced when the stimulus is not anticipated. Sensory defensiveness can be related to all sensory systems.

Tactile defensiveness is the most familiar type of sensory modulation disorder with children showing discomfort with or adverse response (fright, flight, or fight) to light touch. In preschool, children may avoid playing with messy materials such as finger paint or glue. In school, these children have difficulty standing in line or sitting in circle time where they may be bumped or jostled by another child. Children may show difficulty with eating, avoiding textured foods or foods with lumps.

Gravitational insecurity is related to vestibular processing and describes an excessive fear of movement, particularly when the head is tipped backward. Infants may resist having their diaper changed or having their hair rinsed off because these activities involve tipping the child's head back in space.

Auditory defensiveness may also be evident. Children are especially bothered by loud or high-pitched noises such as vacuum cleaners or fans. One child reported being distracted by the sound of the pencil of the child writing next to him. Another child reported that the sound of his teacher's voice hurt his ears.

Children may demonstrate overresponsivity in only one particular sensory system—for example auditory defensiveness or tactile defensiveness—or they may demonstrate overresponsivity in multiple sensory systems. Children with sensory overresponsivity often avoid sensory experiences. Responses to sensory stimuli occur along a spectrum. Some children manage their tendency toward overresponsivity most of the time, whereas other children are overresponsive almost continuously. Their responses may appear inconsistent because overresponsivity is highly dependent on context. Sensitivities may vary throughout the day and from day to day. Because sensory input tends to have a cumulative effect, the child's efforts to control responses to sensory stimuli may build up and erupt suddenly in response to a seemingly trivial stimulus. When children overrespond to the sensory input around them, they may not be able to attend to the content of teacher or parent instructions and may be incorrectly referred for language impairments or for attention problems.

Type 2: Sensory Underresponsivity   Children who are underresponsive to sensory stimuli are often quiet and passive, disregarding or not responding to stimuli of typical intensity available in their sensory environment. They may appear withdrawn, difficult to engage, and/or self-absorbed because they have not registered the sensory input in their environment. The term *poor registration* may be used to describe their behavior because they appear to ignore incoming sensory information. They may seem to lack the inner drive that most children have for socialization and motor exploration, when, in effect, they have not yet noticed the possibilities for action that are around them. Their underresponsivity to tactile and proprioceptive inputs may lead to poorly developed body scheme, clumsiness, or poorly modulated movement. These children may fail to respond to bumps, falls, cuts, or scrapes that can present a danger, because they may not notice pain, such as injuries to the skin, and objects that are too hot or too cold.

Type 3: Sensory Seeking   Children with this pattern actively seek or crave sensory stimulation and seem to have an almost insatiable desire for sensory input. They energetically engage in activities or actions that are geared toward adding more intense "feelings" of sensation to satisfy a basic need or desire for sensory input. They tend to be constantly moving, crashing, bumping, and jumping, may play music or the TV at loud volumes, may fixate on visually stimulating objects or events, or may seek unusual olfactory or gustatory experiences that are more intense and last longer than those of children with typical sensory responsivity. Safety is often an issue. One parent described finding her 5-year-old son perched at the top of the stairs with his bicycle, ready to ride down the stairs.

Type 4: Combined Sensory Reactivity Patterns   It is quite common for children to display combined sensory modulation patterns (Miller, Lane, Cermak, Anzalone, & Osten, 2005). In fact, their atypical response patterns to sensation can vary as a function of time or day, environmental context, stress, fatigue, level of arousal, and many other factors. Fluctuation among patterns in one child is not uncommon, and various sensory domains frequently have different patterns in the same child.

Several patterns are so frequently observed that special recognition is deserved:

- *Sensory overresponsivity with sensory seeking.* It is common for children to be overresponsive in one domain (e.g., tactile or auditory) while sensory seeking in another domain (e.g., movement and proprioceptive). Intense movement and proprioceptive input may be used by some children as a method to self-regulate their aversion to other types of sensory input. For other children it is a way to feel active, excited, and engaged (i.e., it feels good).

- *Sensory underresponsivity with sensory overresponsivity.* These children are underresponsive to stimuli at first, but when stimuli are provided systematically they quickly meet their quota and become overresponders. This may be related to a narrowed band of tolerance for sensory input. It may appear as if the child is labile, swinging from one extreme of responsiveness to the other. Different sensory modalities can be differentially affected; for example, the child may remain underresponsive to olfactory stimuli (e.g., intrusively trying to smell people and objects) but show overresponsiveness to touch.

- *Sensory overresponsivity with sudden sensory underresponsivity.* Some children start out with extreme overresponsivity and suddenly appear underresponsive, appearing almost to "shut down." These children are also believed to have a narrow band of normal responsiveness. They are so overresponsive that their nervous system may be shutting down as a defensive mechanism so that no additional sensory input is registered by their nervous system. At times, they may look underresponsive but actually are having extreme defensive reactions to stimuli.

Disorders of Discrimination and Praxis   The second major category of disorders of sensory processing is disorders of discrimination and praxis. *Sensory discrimination* refers to an individual's ability to accurately interpret the temporal and spatial characteristics of stimuli from the environment and from one's body. An example of a task involving tactile-kinesthetic sensory discrimination is reaching into one's pocket to find a key among other items. Problems with discrimination can occur in any sensory system and can directly affect an individual's ability to respond to and act on the environment.

Praxis relates to the process of conceptualizing, planning, and executing nonhabitual motor tasks and relies in part on adequate sensory discrimination (Ayres, 1979; Cermak, Larkin, & Gubbay, 2002; Reeves & Cermak, 2002). An individual with dyspraxia may have difficulty with one or more of the steps of praxis, including the conceptualization of a motor response appropriate to the environment (known as *ideation*), motor planning of the response, and carrying out the planned response. Often, individuals with dyspraxia have to work harder than typical children to complete everyday activities, and yet even with additional effort, they still produce inferior results.

In factor analysis studies, Ayres (1989) identified three major types of sensory-integrative–based dyspraxia: somatodyspraxia, visuodyspraxia, and bilateral integration and sequencing disorder. *Somatodyspraxia* refers to dyspraxia (poor motor planning) that involves poor processing of somatosensory information such as tactile, vestibular and proprioceptive sensation. Children with motor planning problems have difficulty learning new motor skills such as handwriting, riding a tricycle or bicycle, cutting with scissors, or buttoning buttons. *Visuodyspraxia* is characterized by difficulties with visuomotor and constructional abilities. Children have difficulty with drawing and copying, with construction toys, and with puzzles. *Bilateral integration and sequencing disorder* describes difficulty with bilateral coordination and projected action sequences. Children have difficulty with activities involving using both sides of the body together, such as jumping rope or skipping, and have difficulty anticipating the effects of actions of their bodies and those of objects such as is needed in ball games (i.e., knowing where and how far to run to catch a ball). A later exploratory factor analysis performed by Mulligan (1998) identified similar patterns of practic dysfunction as well as a more general dyspraxia category. However, it has also been questioned whether deficits of praxis may be a single disorder that encompasses a continuum of practic function and dysfunction (Mulligan, 2002).

Although the overarching goal of occupational therapy using an SI approach is to help children better process and integrate information from their senses and enable them to participate as fully as possible in typical roles of childhood, it is important to note that occupational therapy using an SI approach targets multiple levels of functioning according to the International Classification of Functioning (ICF) terminology (WHO, 2001). Kimball (1999b) describes the sensory integrative functioning on three levels that roughly correspond with ICF levels of functioning. Sensory system modulation functions are the body structure/function components on which functional support capabilities such as sensory discrimination, balance and equilibrium, and bilateral integration rely. In turn, functional support capabilities underlie the highest level of sensory integrative functioning, end-product abilities. End-product abilities include praxis, form and space perception, behavior, academics, language and speech production, emotional tone, activity level, and environmental mastery. Although occupational therapy using an SI approach focuses on altering specific components of body processes that result in functional limitations, it also addresses these limitations more holistically in the context of activities that are pertinent to the roles of childhood. The aim of occupational therapy using an SI approach is always linked to the abilities that enable successful participation in the social and physical environments important to the individual child and his or her family.

EMPIRICAL BASIS

Evidence supporting SI can be considered on a number of levels. First is evidence for the existence of the disorder. There is now well-documented evidence that disorders of sensory processing do exist. In fact, recent research by Miller and colleagues has shown physiological correlates of behavioral responses to sensory stimuli. Children with sensory modulation disorders, fragile X, and ADHD show different profiles on the Short Sensory Profile, and these are accompanied by different patterns of electrodermal reactivity (Mangeot et al., 2001; McIntosh et al., 1999; Miller et al., 1999; Miller, Reisman, McIntosh, & Simon, 2001).

Another area to consider is intervention. The strength of the empirical basis for an SI approach to treatment has been debated since the theory was introduced, and this remains a much-discussed topic. As with many frames of rehabilitation, much of the controversy is due to the fact that there are few strong studies that consistently support or refute the efficacy of an SI approach to treatment. This is especially true as SI-based treatments are applied to children with communicative disorders. To familiarize readers with the empirical basis for SI, the best place to start is an examination of the literature reviews and meta-analyses concerning SI intervention. Due to the limited number of randomized controlled efficacy studies on SI, it is important to note that the three literature reviews and two meta-analyses that will be summarized in this section included many of the same research studies. Also, although an SI approach to treatment can be incorporated into parent/ teacher education, occupational therapy consultation, and occupational therapy in the classroom, much of the research reviewed in these articles refers to direct SI intervention provided within the context of a school clinic or private occupational therapy clinic. An exception involves some of the single-subject research conducted within the context of the child's classroom.

Polatajko, Kaplan, and Wilson (1992) reviewed the research literature from 1979 to 1992 and found seven randomized controlled trials concerning SI treatment for academic and/or motor problems in children with learning disabilities, at risk for learning disabilities, and with SI dysfunction (criteria not specified). Polatajko and colleagues did not include adults or studies with individuals with mental retardation (as did Ottenbacher [1982] in his meta-analysis). A total of 311 children, ages 4 years, 8 months to 13 years, 0 months were included in the collective sample. Each study had at least one comparison group, either a control group or an alternative treatment group.

SI treatment was described as individualized according to the child's needs, making replication or comparison across studies difficult. Both pre- and post-test measures were used to evaluate academic and/or motor functioning. The frequency and duration of treatment sessions varied widely among the studies, from one to three sessions (hours) per week and a total duration ranging from 19 to 76 hours. Details were not provided about what constituted SI treatment. All studies, except one, showed significant improvement on one or more variable, regardless of the type of intervention. In nine of 44 comparisons, SI resulted in significantly greater improvement than the control or alternative treatment; in two of the comparisons, the alternative treatment was significantly better. The remaining 33 comparisons showed no significant differences. Polatajko calculated effect sizes (d) based on the reports of authors of the seven studies. Effect sizes were small ($d = 0.10–0.25$) to medium ($d = 0.25–0.40$) (Cohen, 1988) for general motor function, visual, perceptual, and visual-motor skills and language measures. In some cases SI treatment improved certain motor and academic outcomes, but in the majority of cases it was not significantly more effective than alternative treatment methods such as perceptual-motor training and tutoring.

Based on the theoretical assumption that speech and language are end products of SI, Griffer (1999) searched the literature from 1984 to 1992 and identified only five controlled studies that investigated the effectiveness of SI therapy for academic abilities or language functioning. She reported that only two of these studies used measures specifically to assess language skills and stated that these language measures were not considered highly reliable. Based on this, Griffer suggested that SI treatment does not have a significant effect on academic performance or language functioning. However, given that the language measures were unreliable, the internal validity of the studies must be questioned. Thus, it seems that a more appropriate conclusion is that no conclusion can be drawn concerning the ability of SI to improve language skills. Griffer appropriately advised SLPs that even though an inter-relationship exists between language and motor development, deficits in these areas can occur independently of each other and, thus, treatment designed to improve abilities in one area might not have an effect on the other area.

Hoehn and Baumeister's (1994) review of the evidence takes perhaps the most critical stance regarding the effectiveness of SI. It concluded that SI is not more effective than alternate treatments on any of the outcome variables including perceptual-motor, vestibular (postrotary nystagmus), or academic domains. However, it is important to reiterate that their sample of studies greatly overlaps with the other reviews. This difference in interpretation across studies illustrates the potential bias in narrative literature reviews and highlights the value provided by true meta-analytic studies (systematic reviews) with careful statistical analysis.

Two meta-analyses have been conducted to examine the effectiveness of SI (Ottenbacher, 1982; Vargas & Camilli, 1999). Ottenbacher (1982) reviewed 49 research articles on SI treatment efficacy and found that eight met the following inclusion criteria: 1) they investigated SI as the treatment variable; 2) they included at least one operationally defined outcome measure related to one or more of the following areas: academic achievement, motor skill or reflex integration, and language function; 3) they reported a comparison between at least two groups or conditions; and 4) they included sufficient information to generate an effect size measure and other statistics used in meta-analysis. Participants in these studies included both children and adults with varying diagnoses including mental retardation (28% of participants), learning disabilities (60% of participants), aphasia (6%), and at risk for learning disabilities (reading problems) (6%). Analysis of the studies indicated that, collapsing across all diagnostic conditions and dependent variables, the average d-index was 0.79, a large effect (Cohen, 1977). The average subject receiving SI therapy performed better than 78.8% of the subjects in the control or comparison conditions not receiving SI therapy. When results were examined according to type of outcome measure, effect size was greatest for motor variables ($d = 1.03$) and lowest when the dependent variable was a measure of language function ($d = 0.43$). When results were analyzed according to diagnostic category, SI had the greatest effect on subjects diagnosed as aphasic or at risk for learning disabilities ($d = 1.20$; $SD = 0.65$) and the least effect on individuals diagnosed with mental retardation ($d = 0.52$; $SD = 0.49$). However, the authors point out that diagnostic category was confounded with age because the aphasic and at-risk group was the youngest. Based on the outcomes of both effect size and combined-probability analyses, Ottenbacher concluded, "The effect of sensory integration therapy applied to the representative population appears to have empirical support" (1982, p. 577).

In a more recent meta-analysis, Vargas and Camilli (1999) reviewed 76 articles on the efficacy of an SI approach to treatment published between 1972 and 1994 and identified 22 studies that met the following inclusion criteria: 1) a focus on the effect of SI; 2) the comparison of at least two groups (SI treatment versus no treatment, or SI treatment versus alternative treatments); 3) the reporting of results in a way that allowed for quantitative analysis; and 4) the use of outcome variables that could be classified into the broad categories of academic skills, behavior, motor function, language and speech function, and sensorimotor function. Treatment hours in these studies ranged from 13 hours (two 25-minute sessions weekly for 4 months) to 180 hours (five 45-minute sessions weekly for 12 months).

Vargas and Camilli calculated effect sizes (Cooper, 1989; Hedges & Olkin, 1985) for 16 comparisons between SI treatment and no treatment and 16 comparisons between SI and alternative treatments. Collective sample sizes for these comparisons ranged from 191 to 341, and samples included a wide variety of subjects, the majority of whom were children between the ages of 3 and 10 years with learning disabilities. Children and adults with mental retardation and psychiatric disability also participated in some studies. Vargas and Camilli also examined the quality of SI treatment, total treatment hours, quality of design of the study, sampling method, professional affiliation of the researcher, number of outcome variables, geographic location, and publication year when analyzing their results. They reported an overall average effect size of 0.29, $p < .05$ (95% confidence interval [CI] = 0.12–0.48) for SI versus no treatment, which is small but reliably greater than zero. On the other hand, the effect for SI versus alternative treatments was small and non-significant, 0.09 (95% CI = 0.11–0.28). Further analyses revealed that larger effect sizes existed in the motor (0.40) and psychoeducational (IQ, cognition, and academic performance; 0.39) categories. This is similar to findings of Ottenbacher (1982), although the observed effects are notably smaller in the more recent Vargas and Camilli study. The average effect size for language measures, however, was small, 0.13, and not reliably different from zero.

Several additional investigations published after the studies included in these reviews and meta-analyses also warrant consideration. Wilson and Kaplan (1994) carried out a follow-up study 2 years after an earlier study that compared the efficacy of SI versus tutoring for academic and motor outcomes in 5–9-year-old children with learning disabilities (Wilson, Kaplan, Fellowes, Gruchy, & Faris, 1992). They retested 22 of the original 29 children to examine longer-term effects of these two treatment approaches. The group that received SI treatment maintained significantly greater gross motor functioning than the alternate treatment, but there were no significant between-group differences in academic skills.

A number of single-subject designs examined the effectiveness of therapy using principles of SI to improve children's attention. In a study with five preschoolers with autism, Case-Smith and Bryan (1999) found that weekly occupational therapy with an SI emphasis resulted in decreased frequency of nonengaged behaviors in four subjects and increased frequency of mastery (goal-directed) play during classroom free-play in three children. Two studies examined the effectiveness of deep pressure through the use of a weighted vest (Fertel-Daly, Bedell, & Hinojosa, 2001; Vandenberg, 2001). Preliminary findings suggested that the use of a weighted vest might increase attention to task during classroom activities in children with pervasive developmental disorders (Fertel-Daly et al., 2001) and children with ADHD (Vandenberg, 2001). These findings may have implications for children with communication disorders as well, many of whom have difficulty attending. Use of a weighted vest (or perhaps other means of providing deep pressure) to enhance attention may result in children being better able to attend to and profit from speech-language therapy, although this possibility has not been examined. If SI is to have an impact on children's language knowledge and performance, it is likely to be indirect. In children with certain problems, SI may improve their ability to remain seated and attend for longer periods of time. Thus, for these children, SI coupled with speech-language pathology might be an especially powerful intervention. By the same token, the meta-analyses do not provide support for SI for language outcomes when SI is not combined with speech-language intervention.

In summary, research evidence provides mixed support for SI for improving motor and academic functions and does not provide support for language as an outcome measure. However, as with research with many clinical interventions, several limitations exist weakening any clinical conclusions based on studies on the efficacy of SI. Sample sizes for the majority of studies were small which might have caused researchers to falsely reject the null hypotheses due to the Type II error of low power, although meta-analysis should overcome this to some extent. In addition, instruments used to assess change in outcome variables may not have been sensitive enough to detect the degree of change or may not have been appropriate measures of the outcome variables. For example, Griffer (1999) recommended that measures to examine language skills should assess abilities in more naturalistic and functional contexts. Cohn and Cermak (1998) also supported the importance of having outcome data reflect the child's everyday functioning in naturalistic contexts. Outcome measures in many studies used standardized assessments that were at the body structure/function level rather than at the activity or participation level.

Constraints related to designing a study with high internal validity might also limit the effectiveness of SI in a research context. For example, despite general guidelines for intervention using an SI approach, there is great variability in actual treatment due to the importance of individualizing therapeutic activities for each child (Cermak & Henderson, 1989/1990). Standardized and controlled activities intended to limit variability within a treatment group may not be representative of typical SI intervention. No studies have examined the fidelity of treatment provided in these studies. Thus, it is not even clear that the treatments described were actually employed reliably. Similarly, individualized outcome measures would most likely detect change in abilities more accurately than standard outcome measures for all participants; however, this has not been done. Determining the appropriateness of SI for an individual child is a complex process, so although randomization is critical for well-designed research studies, it may not lead to the most precise assessment of the effectiveness of SI. Many studies of SI effectiveness have focused on children with learning disabilities, which is a heterogeneous group, with children who may or may not have disorders of sensory processing. In looking across studies, it is apparent that the criteria for sample selection varied tremendously from study to study. Moreover, because populations with which this approach is commonly used are diverse, group results may overshadow individual differences. Finally, in practice, SI is rarely the sole intervention in the treatment plan. Although discriminating between the effectiveness of specific treatment approaches is not without value, examining which combinations of treatment approaches are most effective with certain populations may be more useful clinically (Vargas & Camilli, 1999). For example, in the child with speech and language problems, combining SI intervention with strong conventional speech and language interventions may lead to outcomes much greater than those achieved by either type of intervention alone.

PRACTICAL REQUIREMENTS

Occupational therapists are the main providers of therapy using an SI approach, although SLPs will probably encounter children who demonstrate dysfunction in SI because these children may have difficulties in multiple areas including speech and language. In practice today, it is common and desirable for multidisciplinary teams to coordinate intervention plans for children with learning and behavior problems. Therefore, SLPs will benefit from an increased knowledge of how other therapists use an SI approach with children who are also receiving speech and language services.

An SI approach to intervention can take several forms, each with different demands for therapist training and for facilities and equipment. Occupational therapists can act as consultants to parents and teachers to help them understand the child's sensory needs and reframe the child's behavior, develop new strategies for helping children cope with the challenges in their daily activities, or develop a *sensory diet*—a planned and scheduled activity program designed to meet a child's specific sensory needs.

Principles of SI are commonly used by occupational therapists working in the schools (Case-Smith, 2004) and may be incorporated into activities in the classroom. Henry Occupational Therapy Services (2005) has developed excellent training materials for teachers for incorporating SI principles in the classroom with children of varying ages.

Finally, occupational therapists may provide direct SI treatment. This approach is usually a child-centered/child-directed approach, which occurs more easily with a single child–therapist dyad. However, group treatment sessions may be utilized when several individuals have reached a stage at which it would be beneficial to incorporate a more naturalistic peer play environment.

Because manipulation of sensory input is a key component for using an SI approach, equipment is designed to provide enriched vestibular, proprioceptive, and tactile sensory input in order to elicit adaptive responses (Bundy, 2002b; Bundy & Murray, 2002). An SI approach typically incorporates suspended equipment and floor equipment along with other materials that facilitate sensory experiences. It is critical to be able to rearrange the environment and combine equipment to facilitate a variety of activities and allow for generalization. Types of suspended equipment include various swings such as tire, net, bolster, helicopter, flexion, and platform swings, spandex hammocks, and trapezes. Suspended equipment may hang from one or two points of contact with the ceiling, depending on the nature of the equipment. Usually an anchor point rather than a specific piece of equipment is mounted on the ceiling, so that suspended equipment can be used interchangeably. Suspended equipment demands large open areas so that the equipment can move freely and safely. A room of 12×12 feet is considered the minimum acceptable space (Koomar & Bundy, 2002), with larger children needing more space. In addition, pieces of equipment may be suspended next to each other to create more complex tasks or to allow the therapist or another child to participate in the activity. It is recommended that an area contain at least three points of suspension or anchors, each spaced approximately 3 feet apart (Koomar & Bundy, 2002). A more complete description of how equipment is incorporated into treatment sessions can be found in the next section.

Assessing the appropriateness of occupational therapy using an SI approach for an individual, as well as implementing the treatment itself, requires extensive training. Continuing education courses (including SI theory, assessment and interpretation, and intervention) and mentorship are the primary modes of advanced training. It is recommended that providers of SI treatment complete didactic training as well as a minimum of 3 months of practice under the supervision of an experienced therapist before utilizing SI principles unaided (Bundy & Koomar, 2002).

KEY COMPONENTS

Direct treatment using an SI approach requires several interrelated components that are essential for every therapy session. A thorough understanding of the key components is necessary for the implementation of SI treatment. These components include the following (Bundy, 2002b; Bundy & Koomar, 2002):

- Opportunities for enhanced sensory input and feedback (discussed in the previous section)
- Playfulness and purposefulness
- Active participation by the child
- Child-directed activities
- A balance between structure and freedom
- The just-right challenge
- An emotionally and physically safe environment
- A positive therapist–child relationship

Occupational therapy using an SI approach is both playful and purposeful. Activities must be purposeful in terms of therapy goals but must also be purposeful to the child. If the child does not perceive a sense of purpose, then the child will not be as motivated to participate in therapy. Therapy tends to be highly playful because play is naturally purposeful for children. Treatment sessions often employ imaginative games that are developmentally appropriate and interesting for the individual child. Thus, a sense of fun is instilled in therapy sessions and encourages the inner drive of the child to interact with the environment. This active participation is critical for improving SI abilities. Passive reception of sensory input alone does not compel the child to produce and experience adaptive responses.

To further motivate children and stimulate their inner drives to actively participate, sessions are child-directed. That is, sessions are structured in such a way to enable the child to have choice. The child is actively involved in inventing imaginative games that align with the activity at hand, and he or she is permitted to influence the course of the session as much as possible. Of course, the therapist must ensure that the activities chosen by the child are appropriate and present opportunities for adaptive responses. As such, the therapist must balance freedom for the child to choose activities and lead the session with the structure necessary to guarantee that therapy goals are met. Skilled therapists are able to maintain this balance by offering carefully crafted choices of activities and quickly adapting activities as necessary based on the child's responses.

The just-right challenge refers to an activity that is neither too easy nor too hard for the child. If the task is too simple, the child will have already become competent in this area, so no new adaptive responses or learning will occur. However, therapists often start and finish sessions with activities that are easier for the child, in order to guarantee success which will, in turn, promote self-esteem. If the task is too difficult or complex, the child may be unable to produce the desired adaptive response and will experience a sense of failure, which may reduce motivation to participate both in the session and in similar activities outside the clinic. The therapist must also be aware of the child's perceptions of his or her own abilities when determining the just-right challenge. Even if the therapist considers a task to be manageable, the child may be unwilling to try because it appears too demanding. Providing the just-right challenge for a child not only enhances child's inner drive and encourages active participation, but also facilitates an appropriate adaptive response as a mechanism for change. Experienced therapists have the ability to continually modify activities to maintain the just-right challenge during treatment.

An effective therapist–child dyad is necessary for the successful implementation of all of the previous components. The therapist must engage the child actively in the process of treatment by offering relevant and interesting opportunities for success with the just-right challenge approach. Instructions, praise, and feedback from the therapist both during and after activities will assist the child in processing what he or she is doing and help to facilitate change. In addition, it is critical that the therapist also provides the child with a sense of physical and emotional safety, especially because most children with dysfunction in SI have experienced multiple failures in the past and may need confidence in the therapist to keep them safe before they are willing to engage in activities.

These key principles of SI treatment are put into practice during treatment sessions using a variety of equipment designed to provide multifaceted sensory input and elicit adaptive responses. As described in the previous section, suspended equipment is a hallmark of direct SI treatments because it provides enhanced sensory input and feedback from the child's adaptive response. Another defining feature is the use of proprioceptive and deep-touch pressure input "to enhance body awareness, improve motor coordination, help modulate arousal level, and aid in the processing of sensation through other sensory systems" (Blanche & Schaaf, 2001, p. 109). For example, proprioceptive input is used to help regulate overresponsivity to touch and movement in the child who demonstrates sensory defensiveness.

Additional materials used in SI treatments include floor equipment, materials for target games, and other sensory media. Floor equipment may include therapy balls, heavy blankets, tumbling mats, scooter boards, ramps, balance boards, air pillows, climbing structures, trampolines, inner tubes, foam blocks, and ball pits. Target games using bins, baskets, hoops, or flat targets, as well as different types of balls and beanbags to aim at the targets, are also popular in SI treatment. Sensory media such as sand, water, beans, clay, shaving cream, and putty may also be incorporated into treatment. Tools to manipulate these media and small "prize" objects hidden in these media may be used to encourage exploration. In addition, chewing gum, tart candies, and other foods and objects to increase oral sensations and proprioceptive input to oral-motor musculature may be used both in the clinic and at home and school to facilitate sensory experiences and increase organization.

Using the imagination of the therapist and the child, various pieces of SI equipment can be combined and manipulated in countless ways to create therapeutic activities that stimulate adaptive responses. Activities should be graded to facilitate the just-right challenge and continually adapted to meet the changing needs of the child as he or she progresses. Activities can be graded by gradually increasing or decreasing the frequency, duration, intensity, and/or complexity of the required adaptive response. For example, a simple target game where a child is required to toss a beanbag at a static target can be made more complex by either using a moving target, placing the child on a swing so the child is moving, or both. For a game in which the child sits on a bolster swing and kicks therapy balls being rolled toward the swing, the therapist can make the activity more difficult by putting the bolster swing in motion and increasing the speed or frequency of balls rolled. The therapist can make the activity easier by allowing the child to hold on firmly to the bolster swing and anchor the swing securely so it does not move as much when the child kicks the therapy balls. An example of adapting the intensity of the activity would be to use a flexion swing rather than a platform swing. Platform swings tend to move in a more linear fashion than flexion swings, which involve rotary motion. Incorporating a flexion swing into the activity allows for more intense vestibular input and requires greater ability to produce an adaptive response. Increasing or decreasing the difficulty of the activity may even be as simple as allowing the child more time to complete the task and take breaks or having the child play a game continually for a longer period of time.

During treatment sessions, the therapist must be able to predict the child's ability to respond to the activity, monitor the child's actual responses, and tailor the activities accordingly with as little disruption to the flow of the session as possible. Thus, the process is both dynamic and highly individualized by nature and requires the therapist to be flexible and creative. There is no "cookbook" for SI treatment; rather, good therapy demands that the therapist view SI as both an art and a science when designing treatment sessions.

The expected outcomes of using an SI approach to treatment relate to improved functional abilities at all three levels of sensory integrative functioning: sensory system modulation functions (e.g., under- or overresponsiveness), functional support capabilities (e.g., sensory discrimination, balance, equilibrium), and end-product abilities (e.g., praxis, form and space perception, behavior, academics, language and speech production). Therapy sessions work to improve the ability of the child to modulate sensory input, which in turn allows for enhanced functional support capabilities to develop. Strong functional support capabilities coupled with competence in SI lead to desired end-product abilities such as refined practic abilities, appropriate behavior and activity level, and improved scholastic achievement. Thus, successful occupational therapy using an SI approach expects improved processing of sensory information to enable the child to interact effectively with the environment and participate in the typical roles of childhood. Although this type of intervention may make it easier to learn in the classroom and benefit from speech-language intervention, there is not strong research evidence that leads one to anticipate a direct influence on language knowledge or performance.

ASSESSMENT METHODS TO SUPPORT ONGOING DECISION MAKING

To determine whether occupational therapy using an SI approach is producing a positive effect for an individual child, continual assessment of multiple factors should be incorporated into the treatment process. Observations of the child's response to a challenge in the clinic should be documented on a weekly basis. Therapists should consult with parents concerning the child's ability to transfer skills acquired during treatment sessions to outside environments to gauge the generalizability of SI treatment. For example, with a child who shows tactile defensiveness and problems with food textures, the therapist may have the parent document new items that the child is willing to try at meals. For the child who shows tactile defensiveness and has difficulty at circle time at preschool, fighting with children when he or she is bumped, the therapist may have the teacher record the length of time the child is able to stay in the circle. Progress should be reassessed at least every 3–6 months (Bundy & Koomar, 2002). The SIPT is considered a diagnostic test that provides guidance for intervention but is not typically readministered to assess progress. Goal attainment scaling has been used as a method to measure individualized goals.

Bundy and Koomar (2002) suggest that monitoring functional abilities provides a helpful guide for determining when discharge from SI intervention is appropriate. As an example, they describe how a child who is approaching discharge may begin to express the desire to play with peers rather than attend therapy sessions. This transition in the child's preference from attending therapy sessions to interacting in more typical childhood situations may signify in part the child's increasing ability to function without further support from the therapist.

CONSIDERATIONS FOR CHILDREN FROM CULTURALLY AND LINGUISTICALLY DIVERSE BACKGROUNDS

For SI practitioners to work successfully with children of various cultural and linguistic backgrounds, each of the key components of SI treatment must be considered with respect to this issue. Although cultural and linguistic factors may alter the way a therapist provides treatment to some extent, through careful planning, the therapist should be able to maintain the integrity of SI treatment while remaining sensitive to these considerations.

Although play is an almost universal activity of children of all backgrounds, therapists should be aware of different cultural preferences and acceptable play behaviors (Goncu, 1999). Although playing on the floor is acceptable in our culture, for example, it is not appropriate in many cultures. The child-directed nature of sessions in SI intervention may be hindered by language barriers as well as cultural attitudes to authority figures. Nonverbal communication such as facial expressions and gestures may be extremely valuable in ascertaining the child's feelings about an activity and establishing the just-right challenge, as long as impaired praxis resulting in the inability to gesture does not hamper these nonverbal indicators. The therapist–child relationship may also be affected when children have cultural and linguistic background and values that are different from those of the therapist.

Consultation with parents and caregivers may also be an area of special importance due to cultural and linguistic diversity. Because clear and open communication between the therapist and caregiver is essential for a comprehensive understanding of the functional difficulties the child is experiencing as well as carryover of treatment principles to more naturalistic environments outside the clinic, barriers to communication based on cultural and linguistic differences must be thoroughly considered (Odom, Hanson, Blackman, & Kaul, 2003). When speaking to the parents about the child, interpreters should be utilized even if the child is bilingual (Jezewski & Sotnik, 2001). The therapist should also be aware that in some cultures, asking questions of health care professionals is not customary, and thus care should be taken to ensure that caregivers both understand the treatment and can provide critical information about the child (Jezewski & Sotnik, 2001).

APPLICATION TO AN INDIVIDUAL CHILD

Michael was 5 years, 6 months of age and attended kindergarten when he was referred to occupational therapy for fine motor concerns. His teacher reported that he had difficulty cutting with scissors and was unable to form any of the letters to print his name. Michael refused to participate in class activities such as finger painting and sand table. He had difficulty sitting in circle time, typically only staying 5 minutes before moving away. His teacher reported that on two occasions in the last month, Michael hit the child sitting next to him and had to be removed from the group. Michael insisted that the child hit him first; however, the teacher observed that Michael had only been jostled slightly when the child next to him changed position.

Educational History

Michael was on an individualized education program and was receiving speech-language therapy two times per week. He was referred to speech-language therapy at age 3 years, 3 months. He did not use any words until he was 18 months old. At age 3 years, Michael used primarily single words and was very difficult to understand. His mother was able to understand 50% of what he said in context, but most other people could not understand him. By kindergarten, Michael spoke in short utterances but speech intelligibility was poor. His teacher was able to understand about 50% of what he said in context, but peers were, for the most part, unable to understand him.

Michael was given a comprehensive speech and language evaluation at age 4 years, 8 months and received a probable diagnosis of childhood apraxia of speech. Receptive language abilities were superior to expressive language abilities as assessed by the Test of Language Development–Primary, Second Edition (Newcomer & Hammill, 1988). Michael's receptive quotient was 92; his expressive quotient was 76. He was found to have reduced oral diadochokinetic rates. Michael had difficulty with repetition of multisyllabic real and nonsense words on a multisyllabic-word repetition task (described in Catts, 1986) and the nonsense-word repetition task (described in Kamhi & Catts, 1986). He had difficulty sequencing sounds and syllables. His consonant repertoire was greatly reduced compared with other children his age, as demonstrated by his performance at less than 1% on the Goldman-Fristoe Test of Articulation-2 (Goldman & Fristoe, 2000). In addition, in both single-word productions and in connected speech, he evidenced numerous vowel errors.

Sign language was chosen as the method of augmenting Michael's communication because two other children in his classroom were also using signs so that it had become a goal for several children in the class. However, Michael's SLP reported that Michael had difficulty forming signs correctly. Moreover, when she tried to use hand-over-hand to teach him the signs, Michael pulled away and became angry. In the 3 months since they had initiated signing, Michael only learned to use two signs consistently (*more* and *drink*).

Occupational Therapy Assessment: Sensory Integration and Praxis Test

The SIPT was administered to Michael, and his mother completed the Short Sensory Profile. Results of the SIPT are reported in *z*-scores.

Tactile Discrimination   Three of the five somatosensory test scores were significantly below average. Michael had difficulty identifying which finger was touched when vision was occluded (Finger Identification = $-1.5\,SD$), replicating designs drawn on the back of his hand (Graphesthesia = $-1.8\,SD$), and identifying the precise place on his arm where he was touched (Localization of Tactile Stimuli = $-1.6\,SD$). Michael's score on the Manual Form Perception test, which integrates vision and touch, was in the low average range ($-0.7\,SD$), as was his score on Kinesthesia ($-0.8\,SD$), which involves the ability to replicate the direction and extent of passive arm movements.

On the tactile tests, Michael showed evidence of discomfort with light touch stimuli. After the design was drawn on his hand in the Graphesthesia test, Michael rubbed and scratched his hand repeatedly. When stimuli were administered during the Localization of Tactile Stimuli test, Michael said, "Ow, that hurts" and "Stop that." He frequently asked, "Are we done?" This had not been noted on the other tests. These behaviors were suggestive of tactile defensiveness.

Vestibular-Proprioceptive Processing   This score was in the low average range on a test of static and dynamic balance (Standing and Walking Balance = $-0.8\,SD$). Duration of nystagmus following rotation was reduced (Postrotary Nystagmus = $-1.1\,SD$). Clinical observations indicated that Michael had marked difficulty assuming and maintaining the prone extension position that involved maintaining an antigravity position. Muscle tone was low.

Visual Perception and Visual-Motor Abilities   When there was not a demand for a fine motor response, visual perception was in the average range (Space Visualization = $0.3\,SD$; Figure-Ground Perception = $-0.2\,SD$). Visual-motor tests were in the low average to below average range (Design Copying $= -1.3\,SD$; Constructional Praxis $= -0.8\,SD$; Motor Accuracy $= -0.9\,SD$).

Praxis   Michael's lowest scores on the SIPT were in the praxis area. His lowest scores were in Postural Praxis ($-2.1\ SD$), which involved the ability to reproduce novel body and hand positions assumed by the examiner, and Oral Praxis ($-2.3\ SD$), which involved the ability to replicate positions and movements of the tongue, lips, and jaw. Michael scored below average on Sequencing Praxis ($-1.4\ SD$), a test involving the ability to copy arm and hand sequences, and on Bilateral Motor Coordination ($-1.3\ SD$), a test of smooth coordinated movements of the arms and legs. Michael also had difficulty carrying out therapist-directed movements on the Praxis on Verbal Command test ($-1.4\ SD$).

Michael's mother completed the Short Sensory Profile. Michael scored in the definite difference range (less than $-2\ SD$) in tactile sensitivity, a finding that confirmed observations made during behavioral testing. Michael's mother reported that as an infant, Michael was not a cuddly baby, a common report for children showing tactile defensiveness. She described bathroom routines as a "nightmare." Michael screamed when she washed his hair or cut his fingernails. In other words, the maternal report on the Short Sensory Profile confirmed the SIPT results.

Discussion with Michael's mother indicated that he struggled with learning new motor skills. She stated that he had difficulty learning to ride a tricycle and didn't master it until he was 4 years old. She said he had just learned to button buttons but was not able to even make the first knot to tie his shoelaces. She stated that she enrolled him in a beginning karate class to help him with his motor skills, but she withdrew him because he couldn't keep up with the other children. The occupational therapist observed Michael in the classroom and on the playground. On the playground, Michael tended to run around the perimeter of the playground. He did not use the slide or gym equipment. However, he loved the swing and would ask the teacher to push him "higher and higher." The teacher tried to teach Michael to pump the swing himself but Michael was unable to coordinate the movements.

Summary of Findings

Michael exhibited a profile of developmental dyspraxia, a type of SI disorder characterized by difficulty in motor planning and poor somatosensory processing. Michael "knew" what he wanted to do but was not able to make his body do what he wanted. Learning new motor skills was challenging and related to the delay in his learning to ride a tricycle, fasten buttons, use scissors, and write legibly. It was believed that Michael's difficulty learning to sign was in part related to dyspraxia and was further hindered by his sensory (tactile) defensiveness. Michael perceived the light touch of the therapist's hand as aversive. Tactile defensiveness was noted on the Sensory Profile as well as in the classroom with Michael's refusal to participate in "messy" activities, such as paint and paste. It was felt that part of Michael's difficulty sitting in circle time also related to aversive response to being touched unexpectedly by other children.

Goals and Benchmarks

The focus of occupational therapy was to reduce sensory defensiveness and improve motor planning to enable Michael to participate more fully in the school routine. Benchmarks indicating reduced sensory defensiveness included increased time sitting in circle without altercation and allowing the SLP to use hand-over-hand methods for teaching signing. Benchmarks indicating improved motor planning included improved performance in three skills that involved motor planning: pumping on the swing, writing the first two letters of his name legibly, and cutting a 6-inch straight line. It also was expected that improving motor planning skills would enhance Michael's ability to sign because imitating hand postures involves motor planning.

Projects and Scaffolding

Michael was seen twice weekly for occupational therapy incorporating an SI framework to improve motor planning and reduce sensory defensiveness. Deep touch pressure activities such as playing "hot dog" between two mats were incorporated into all therapy sessions to reduce sensory sensitivity. Motor planning activities were emphasized in the occupational therapy clinic where we provided Michael with opportunities for enhanced sensation in the context of meaningful activities. For example, in an activity involving motor planning and projected action sequences ("landing on the moon"), Michael climbed up a ramp onto a platform, held onto a trapeze and swung out over a pile of pillows. The goal was to let go over the target and land on the pillows. The activity was graded so that as Michael's skill improved, the size of the target landing area was decreased. Variations of the activity were included, such as increasing and decreasing the distance of the target area and changing the target from pillows to a large tire, to allow Michael to have many opportunities for practice developing flexible strategies. Various obstacle courses were designed. These involved climbing up ladders and inclines, crawling through tunnels, jumping into ball pits, and using arms to push and pull in swinging activities. Many of these activities utilized skill components that Michael needed for pumping a swing. The focus was on gross motor activities that demanded adaptive responses and provided enhanced sensory input, particularly vestibular and somatosensory. Specific skills were also taught within the classroom/playground environments. Three specific skills that were meaningful to Michael in the context of his daily routine at school were targeted for intervention: pumping the swing, printing his name, and cutting with scissors.

The occupational therapist and SLP met regularly to review Michael's progress. The occupational therapist saw Michael prior to his speech-language session and used a modification of the Wilbarger brushing protocol (Wilbarger & Wilbarger, 2002) to reduce sensory defensiveness so the speech-language therapist could use a hand-over-hand approach for teaching signing. Weekly consultation was provided to Michael's teacher. The occupational therapist described sensory defensiveness and its impact on daily activities. This helped to reframe Michael's behavior. Suggestions for classroom accommodations were made to reduce the impact of Michael's sensory (tactile) defensiveness to enable him to participate in the classroom. It was suggested that in circle time, Michael be seated between teacher and a "nonfidgety" child so he would be less likely to be accidentally bumped. Alternatively, it was suggested that the teacher might have several beanbag chairs placed strategically around the circle for use by the children. When seated in a beanbag chair, Michael would not get jostled by another child and, at the same time, would receive deep touch pressure from the beans. The occupational therapist also made recommendations for "sensory diet" activities and demonstrated activities such as crab walks, wheelbarrow walks, or chair push-ups that could be used with the entire class to provide deep pressure input prior to activities such as fingerpainting. Deep pressure is hypothesized to reduce sensory defensiveness.

Progress

Progress was assessed through monthly consultation with Michael's teacher, as well as monitoring Michael's skills in the three targeted tasks and a near-transfer task. Michael's teacher reported that the beanbag chair was effective, and Michael was able to stay with the group during circle time. After 3 months of therapy, Michael was also beginning to participate in craft activities within the classroom. Michael's teacher also reported that he was able to print the first two letters of his name with 80%–90% accuracy, and he could copy the individual letters in his name. Michael was beginning to pump the swing. He was now joining the other children at recess and using the slide, as well.

The SLP reported that Michael allowed hand-over-hand demonstrations and had learned 15 signs that he produced recognizably. Although it is not clear that occupational therapy contributed to improved ability to sign, it is possible that intervention designed to reduce sensory defensiveness enabled the speech-language therapist to use a hand-over-hand approach to help Michael learn to form the signs. It is also possible that enhanced motor planning ability in general resulted in an increased motor planning ability needed to imitate signs. A controlled trial would need to be implemented to examine this.

FUTURE DIRECTIONS

Since Ayres developed SI theory and treatment principles in the mid–late-1960s and early 1970s, the basis and merits of SI have been debated but have gained increasing recognition. Although research has shown a relationship between language, speech production, and motor coordination skills in children (Archer & Witelson, 1988; Crary, 1993; Dewey & Wall, 1997; Estil & Whiting, 2002; Hill, 1998; Katz et al., 1992; Shriberg et al., 1997; Tallal et al., 1991, 1995; Thal et al., 1991; Velleman & Strand, 1994; Wolff et al., 1990), and preliminary studies that examined the effectiveness of occupational therapy using an SI approach to improve language function in children with learning disabilities showed promise (Ayres, 1972a; Kantner et al., 1982; Magrun et al., 1981), the recent and overall evidence does not support the effectiveness of SI for improving language function in children. Many questions still need to be answered. As with any treatment or frame of reference based on theoretical principles, we must keep in mind that SI theory is both provisional and dynamic (Bundy & Murray, 2002). Continuing research and clinical experience will undoubtedly lead to further evolution of the theory and revised and refined guidelines for practice. As our knowledge of neurological functioning and nature of SI increases, we will be better able not only to predict which populations will benefit most from occupational therapy using an SI approach and what long-term gains they will achieve, but also to tailor this treatment for individuals. Continued exploration of the relationship between speech and language skills and dysfunction in SI will also assist us in determining the effectiveness of SI treatment for these deficits, as well as how combinations of treatment techniques can be used to facilitate improved functioning.

RECOMMENDED READINGS

Bundy, A.C., Lane, S.J., & Murray, E.A. (Eds.). (2002). *Sensory integration: Theory and practice* (2nd ed.). Philadelphia: F.A. Davis.

Kimball, J.G. (1999). Sensory integration frame of reference: Postulates regarding change and application to practice. In P. Kramer & J. Hinojosa (Eds.), *Frames of reference for pediatric occupational therapy* (2nd ed., pp. 169–204). Philadelphia: Lippincott Williams & Wilkins.

Kimball, J.G. (1999). Sensory integration frame of reference: Theoretical base, function/dysfunction continua, and guide to evaluation. In P. Kramer & J. Hinojosa (Eds.), *Frames of reference for pediatric occupational therapy* (2nd ed., pp. 119–168). Philadelphia: Lippincott Williams & Wilkins.

Roley, S.S., Blanche, E.I., & Schaaf, R.C. (Eds.). (2001). *Understanding the nature of sensory integration with diverse populations*. San Antonio, TX: Therapy Skill Builders.

REFERENCES

Archer, S., & Witelson, S. (1988). Manual motor function in developmental dysphasia. *Journal of Clinical and Experimental Neuropsychology, 10*, 47.

Ayres, A.J. (1965). Patterns of perceptual-motor dysfunction in children: A factor analytic study. *Perceptual and Motor Skills, 20*, 335–368.

Ayres, A.J. (1969). Deficits in sensory integration in educationally handicapped children. *Journal of Learning Disabilities, 2*, 160–168.

Ayres, A.J. (1971). Characteristics of types of sensory integrative dysfunction. *American Journal of Occupational Therapy, 25*, 329–334.

Ayres, A.J. (1972a). Improving academic scores through sensory integration. *Journal of Learning Disabilities, 5*, 336–343.

Ayres, A.J. (1972b). *Sensory integration and learning disorders*. Los Angeles: Western Psychological Services.

Ayres, A.J. (1972c). *The Southern California Sensory Integration Tests*. Los Angeles: Western Psychological Services.

Ayres, A.J. (1975). *Southern California Postrotary Nystagmus Test*. Los Angeles: Western Psychological Services.

Ayres, A.J. (1977). Types of sensory integration dysfunction among disabled learners. *American Journal of Occupational Therapy, 26*, 13–18.

Ayres, A.J. (1979). *Sensory integration and the child*. Los Angeles: Western Psychological Services.

Ayres, A.J. (1989). *Sensory Integration and Praxis Tests (SIPT)*. Los Angeles: Western Psychological Services.

Ayres, A.J., & Mailloux, Z. (1981). Influence of sensory integrative procedures on language development. *American Journal of Occupational Therapy, 35*, 383–390.

Baranek, G.T., Chin, Y.H., Hess, L.M., Yankee, J.G., Hatton, D.D., & Hooper, S.R. (2002). Sensory processing correlates of occupational performance in children with Fragile X syndrome: Preliminary findings. *American Journal of Occupational Therapy, 56*, 538–546.

Blanche, E., & Schaaf, R. (2001). Proprioception: A cornerstone of sensory integration intervention. In S.S. Roley, E.I. Blanche, & R.C. Schaaf (Eds.), *Understanding the nature of sensory integration with diverse populations* (pp. 109–124). San Antonio, TX: Therapy Skill Builders.

Brown, C., & Dunn, W. (2002). *Adolescent/Adult Sensory Profile*. San Antonio, TX: Harcourt Assessment.

Bundy, A.C. (2002a). Assessing sensory integrative dysfunction. In A.C. Bundy, S.J. Lane, & E.A. Murray (Eds.), *Sensory integration: Theory and practice* (2nd ed., pp. 169–198). Philadelphia: F.A. Davis.

Bundy, A.C. (2002b). The process of planning and implementing intervention. In A.C. Bundy, S.J. Lane, & E.A. Murray (Eds.), *Sensory integration: Theory and practice* (2nd ed., pp. 211–225). Philadelphia: F.A. Davis.

Bundy, A.C., & Koomar, J.A. (2002). Orchestrating intervention: The art of practice. In A.C. Bundy, S.J. Lane, & E.A. Murray (Eds.), *Sensory integration: Theory and practice* (2nd ed., pp. 241–260). Philadelphia: F.A. Davis.

Bundy, A.C., & Murray, E.A. (2002). Sensory integration: A. Jean Ayres' theory revisited. In A.C. Bundy, S.J. Lane, & E.A. Murray (Eds.), *Sensory integration: Theory and practice* (2nd ed., pp. 119–168). Philadelphia: F.A. Davis.

Buonomano, D.V., & Merzenich, M.M. (1998). Cortical plasticity: From synapses to maps. *Annual Review of Neuroscience, 21*, 149–186.

Case-Smith, J. (2004). *Occupational therapy for children* (5th ed.). St. Louis: Mosby.

Case-Smith, J., & Bryan, T. (1999). The effects of occupational therapy with sensory integration emphasis on pre-school age children with autism. *American Journal of Occupational Therapy, 53*, 489–497.

Catts, H. (1986). Speech production/phonological deficits in reading disordered children. *Journal of Learning Disabilities, 19,* 504–508.

Cermak, S.A., & Henderson, A. (1989, December/1990, March). The efficacy of sensory integration procedures. *Sensory Integration Quarterly.* Retrieved on July 28, 2004, from http://www.spdnetwork.org/research/cermak.pdf

Cermak, S.A., Larkin, D., & Gubbay, S. (2002). What is developmental coordination disorder? In S.A. Cermak & D. Larkin (Eds.), *Developmental coordination disorder* (pp. 1–58). Clifton Park, NY: Thomson Delmar.

Clark, F.A., Miller, L.R., Thomas, J.A., Kucherway, D.A., & Azin, S.P. (1978). A comparison of operant and sensory integration methods on vocalizations and other developmental parameters in profoundly retarded adults. *American Journal of Occupational Therapy, 32,* 86–93.

Cohen, J. (1977). *Statistical power analysis for the behavioral sciences* (rev. ed.). New York: Academic Press.

Cohen, J. (1988). *Statistical power analysis for the behavioral sciences* (2nd ed.). Hillsdale, NJ: Lawrence Erlbaum Associates.

Cohn, E.S., & Cermak, S.A. (1998). Including the family perspective in sensory integration research outcomes. *American Journal of Occupational Therapy, 52,* 540–546.

Cooper, H.M. (1989). *Integrating research* (2nd ed.). Newbury Park, CA: Sage.

Crary, M. (1993). *Developmental motor speech disorders.* San Diego: Singular.

Dewey, D. (2002). Subtypes of coordination disorder. In S.A. Cermak & D. Larkin (Eds.), *Developmental coordination disorder* (pp. 40–53). Clifton Park, NY: Thomson Delmar.

Dewey, D., & Wall, K. (1997). Praxis and memory deficits in language impaired children. *Developmental Neuropsychology, 10,* 265–284.

Dunn, W. (1997). The impact of sensory processing abilities on the daily lives of young children and their families: A conceptual model. *Infants and Young Children, 9*(4), 23–35.

Dunn, W. (1999a). *Sensory Profile.* San Antonio, TX: Harcourt Assessment.

Dunn, W. (1999b). *Short Sensory Profile.* San Antonio, TX: Harcourt Assessment.

Dunn, W. (2002). *Infant/Toddler Sensory Profile.* San Antonio, TX: Harcourt Assessment.

Dunn, W., & Bennett, D. (2002). Patterns of sensory processing in children with attention deficit hyperactivity disorder. *Occupational Therapy Journal of Research, 22*(1), 4–15.

Dunn, W., Myles, B., & Orr, S. (2002). Sensory processing issues associated with Asperger syndrome: A preliminary investigation. *American Journal of Occupational Therapy, 56,* 97–102.

Ermer, J., & Dunn, W. (1998). The Sensory Profile: A discriminant analysis of children with and without disabilities. *American Journal of Occupational Therapy, 52,* 283–290.

Estil, L., & Whiting, H.T.A. (2002). Motor/language impairment syndromes: Direct or indirect foundations? In S.A. Cermak & D. Larkin (Eds.), *Developmental coordination disorder* (pp. 54–68). Clifton Park, NY: Thomson Delmar.

Fertel-Daly, D., Bedell, G., & Hinojosa, J. (2001). Effects of a weighted vest on attention to task and self-stimulatory behaviors in preschoolers with pervasive developmental disorders. *American Journal of Occupational Therapy, 55*(6), 629–940.

Goldman, R., & Fristoe, M. (2000). *Goldman-Fristoe Test of Articulation-2.* Circle Pines, MN: American Guidance Service.

Goncu, A. (Ed). (1999). *Children's engagement in the world: Sociocultural perspectives.* New York: Cambridge University Press.

Gotze, B., Kiese-Himmel, C., & Hasselhorn, M. (2001). Haptic perception and language development assessment in kindergarten and preschool children [Abstract]. Praxis der *Kinderpsychologie und Kinderpsychiatrie, 50,* 640–648.

Griffer, M.R. (1999). Is sensory integration effective for children with language-learning disorders? A critical review of the evidence. *Language, Speech, and Hearing Services in Schools, 30,* 393–400.

Hedges, L.V., & Olkin, L. (1985). *Statistical methods for meta-analysis*. Orlando, FL: Academic Press.

Henry Occupational Therapy Services. (2005). A teach about.com: Henry occupational therapy materials. Retrieved on July 28, 2005, from http://shop.henryot.com/pk4/store .pl?sub_section=1

Hill, E. (1998). A dyspraxic deficit in specific language impairment and developmental co-ordination disorder? Evidence from hand and arm movements. *Developmental Medicine and Child Neurology, 40*, 388–395.

Hoehn, T.P., & Baumeister, A.A. (1994). A critique of the application of sensory integration therapy to children with learning disabilities. *Journal of Learning Disabilities, 27*(6), 338–350.

Jezewski, M.A., & Sotnik, P. (2001). *The rehabilitation service provider as culture broker: Providing culturally competent services to foreign-born persons.* Buffalo, NY: Center for International Rehabilitation Research and Information Exchange (CIRRIE). Retrieved on July 29, 2004, from http://cirrie.buffalo.edu/monographs/cb.pdf

Johnson-Ecker, C.L., & Parham, L.D. (2000). The evaluation of sensory processing: A validity study using contrasting groups. *American Journal of Occupational Therapy, 54*, 454–503.

Kamhi, A.G., & Catts, H.W. (1986). Toward an understanding of developmental language and reading disorders. *Journal of Speech and Hearing Disorders, 51*, 337–347.

Kanter, R.M., Kantner, B., & Clark, F. (1982). Vestibular stimulation effect on language development in mentally retarded children. *American Journal of Occupational Therapy, 36*, 36–41.

Katz, W., Curtiss, S., & Tallal, P. (1992). Rapid automatized naming and gesture by normal and language-impaired children. *Brain and Language, 43*, 623–641.

Kawar, M. (1973). The effects of sensorimotor therapy on dichotic listening in children with learning disabilities. *American Journal of Occupational Therapy, 27*, 226–231.

Kientz, M., & Dunn, W. (1997). A comparison of the performance of children with and without autism on the Sensory Profile. *American Journal of Occupational Therapy, 51*, 530–537.

Kimball, J.G. (1999a). Sensory integration frame of reference: Postulates regarding change and application to practice. In P. Kramer & J. Hinojosa (Eds.), *Frames of reference for pediatric occupational therapy* (2nd ed., pp. 169–204). Philadelphia: Lippincott Williams & Wilkins.

Kimball, J.G. (1999b). Sensory integration frame of reference: Theoretical base, function/dysfunction continua, and guide to evaluation. In P. Kramer & J. Hinojosa (Eds.), *Frames of reference for pediatric occupational therapy* (2nd ed., pp. 119–168). Philadelphia: Lippincott Williams & Wilkins.

Koomar, J.A., & Bundy, A.C. (2002). Creating direct intervention from theory. In A.C. Bundy, S.J. Lane, & E.A. Murray (Eds.), *Sensory integration: Theory and practice* (2nd ed., pp. 261–308). Philadelphia: F.A. Davis.

Lane, S.J. (2002). Sensory modulation. In A.C. Bundy, S.J. Lane, & E.A. Murray (Eds.), *Sensory integration: Theory and practice* (2nd ed., pp. 101–122). Philadelphia: F.A. Davis.

Lin, S., Cermak, S., Coster, W., & Miller, L. (2005). The relation between length of institutionalization and sensory integration in children adopted from Eastern Europe. *American Journal of Occupational Therapy, 59*, 139–147.

MacKay, D. (1983). A theory of the representation and enactment of intentions. In R. Magill (Ed.), *Advances in psychology, Vol. 12. Memory and control of action* (pp. 217–229). New York: North Holland.

Magrun, W.M., McCue, S., Ottenbacher, K., & Keefe, R. (1981). Effects of vestibular stimulation on spontaneous use of verbal language in developmentally delayed children. *American Journal of Occupational Therapy, 35*, 101–104.

Mangeot, S.D., Miller, L.J., McIntosh, D.N., McGrath-Clarke, J., Simon, J., Hagerman, R.J., & Goldson, E. (2001). Sensory modulation dysfunction in children with attention deficit hyperactivity disorder. *Developmental Medicine and Child Neurology, 43*, 399–406.

Mauer, D.M. (1999). Issues and application of sensory integration theory and treatment with children with language disorders. *Language, Speech, and Hearing Services in Schools, 30*, 383–392.

McIntosh, D.N., Miller, L.J., Shyu, V., & Hagerman, R. (1999). Sensory-modulation disruption, electrodermal responses, and functional behaviors. *Developmental Medicine and Child Neurology, 41*, 608–615.

Miller, L.J., Lane, S.J., Cermak, S.A., Anzalone, A., & Koomar, J.A. (2004, Summer). Position statement on terminology related to sensory integration dysfunction. *In-Focus*, 6–8.

Miller, L., Lane, S., Cermak, S., Anzalone, M., & Osten, B. (2005). Regulatory-sensory processing disorders in children. In *Interdisciplinary Council on Developmental and Learning Disorders (ICDL) Diagnostic manual or infancy and early childhood (ICDL-DMIC)*. Bethesda, MD: Interdisciplinary Council on Developmental and Learning Disorders.

Miller, L.J., McIntosh, D.N., McGrath, J., Shyu, V., Lampe, M., Taylor, A.K., Tassone, F., Neitzel, K., Stackhouse, T., & Hagerman, R. (1999). Electrodermal responses to sensory stimuli in individuals with Fragile X syndrome: A preliminary report. *American Journal of Medical Genetics, 83*(4), 268–279.

Miller, L.J., Reisman, J.E., McIntosh, D.N., & Simon, J. (2001). An ecological model of sensory modulation: Performance of children with Fragile X syndrome, autism, attention-deficit/hyperactivity disorder, and sensory modulation dysfunction. In S.S. Roley, E.I. Blanche, & R.C. Schaaf (Eds.), *Understanding the nature of sensory integration with diverse populations* (pp. 57–88). San Antonio, TX: Therapy Skill Builders.

Montgomery, P.C., & Connelly, B.H. (2003). *Clinical applications for motor control*. Thorofare, NJ: Slack.

Mulligan, S. (1998). Patterns of sensory integrative dysfunction: A confirmatory factor analysis. *American Journal of Occupational Therapy, 52*(10), 819–828.

Mulligan, S. (2002). Advances in sensory integration research. In A.C. Bundy, S.J. Lane, & E.A. Murray (Eds.), *Sensory integration: Theory and practice* (2nd ed., pp. 397–411). Philadelphia: F.A. Davis.

Newcomer, P., & Hammill, D. (1988). *Test of Language Development-2: Primary*. Austin, TX: PRO-ED.

Ochipa, C., Rothi, L., & Heilman, K. (1997). Conceptual apraxia in Alzheimer's disease. *Brain, 115*, 1061–1071.

Odom, S.L., Hanson, M.J., Blackman, J.A., & Kaul, S. (2003). *Early intervention practices around the world*. Baltimore: Paul H. Brookes Publishing Co.

Oetter, P., Richter, E., & Frick, S. (1993). *MORE: Integrating the mouth with sensory and postural functions*. Hugo, MN: PDP Press.

Ottenbacher, K. (1982). Sensory integration therapy: Affect or effect. *American Journal of Occupational Therapy, 36*, 571–578.

Parham, L.D., & Mailloux, Z. (2001). Sensory integration. In J. Case-Smith (Ed.), *Occupational therapy for children* (4th ed., pp. 329–381). St. Louis: Mosby.

Polatajko, H.J., Kaplan, B.J., & Wilson, B.N. (1992). Sensory integration treatment for children with learning disabilities: Its status 20 years later. *Occupational Therapy Journal of Research, 12*(6), 323–341.

Reeves, G.D., & Cermak, S.A. (2002). Disorders of praxis. In A.C. Bundy, S.J. Lane, & E.A. Murray (Eds.), *Sensory integration: Theory and practice* (2nd ed., pp. 71–100). Philadelphia: F.A. Davis.

Reynolds, D., Nicolson, R.I., & Hambly, H. (2003). Evaluation of an exercise-based treatment for children with reading difficulties. *Dyslexia, 9*, 48–71.

Rothi, L.G.J., Ochipa, C., & Heilman, K.M. (1991). A cognitive neuropsychological model of limb praxis. *Cognitive Neuropsychology, 8*, 443–458.

Shriberg, L., Aram, D., & Kwiatkowski, J. (1997). Developmental apraxia of speech: I. Description and theoretical perspectives. *Journal of Speech, Language, and Hearing Research, 40*, 273–285.

Shumway-Cook, A., & Woollacott, M. (1995). *Motor control: Theory and practical application.* Baltimore: Lippincott Williams & Wilkins.

Spitzer, S., & Roley, S.S. (2001). Sensory integration revisited: A philosophy of practice. In S.S. Roley, E.I. Blanche, & R.C. Schaaf (Eds.), *Understanding the nature of sensory integration with diverse populations* (pp. 1–28). San Antonio, TX: Therapy Skill Builders.

Tallal, P., Merzenich, M., Miller, S., & Jenkins, W. (1998). Language learning impairments: Integrating basic science, technology and remediation. *Experimental Brain Research, 123*, 210–219.

Tallal, P., Miller, S., & Fitch, R. (1995). Neurobiological basis of speech: A case for the preeminence of temporal processing. *Irish Journal of Psychology, 16*, 194–219.

Tallal, P., Sainburg, R., & Jernigan, T. (1991). The neuropathology of developmental dysphasia: Behavioral, morphological, and physiological evidence for a pervasive temporal processing disorder. *Reading and Writing: An Interdisciplinary Journal, 3*, 363–377.

Thal, D., Tobias, S., & Morrison, D. (1991). Language and gesture in late talkers: A 1-year follow-up. *Journal of Speech and Hearing Research, 34*, 604–612.

Tremblay, S., Shiller, D.M., & Ostry, D. (2003). Somatosensory basis of speech production. *Nature, 423*, 866–869.

Vandenberg, N.L. (2001). The use of a weighted vest to increase on-task behavior in children with attention difficulties. *American Journal of Occupational Therapy, 55*(6), 621–628.

Vargas, S., & Camilli, G. (1999). A meta-analysis of research on sensory integration treatment. *American Journal of Occupational Therapy, 53*, 189–198.

Velleman, S., & Strand, K. (1994). Developmental verbal dyspraxia. In J.E. Bernthal & N.W. Bankson (Eds.), *Child phonology: Characteristics, assessment, and intervention with special populations* (pp. 110–139). New York: Thieme.

Watling, R., Deitz, J., & White, O. (2001). Comparison of sensory profile scores of young children with and without autism spectrum disorders. *American Journal of Occupational Therapy, 55*, 416–423.

Wilbarger, J.L., & Wilbarger, P.L. (2002). Wilbarger approach to treating sensory defensiveness and clinical application of the sensory diet. In A.C. Bundy, E.A. Murray, & S.J. Lane (Eds.), *Sensory integration: Theory and practice* (2nd ed., pp. 333–341). Philadelphia: F.A. Davis.

Wilson, B.N., & Kaplan, B.J. (1994). Follow-up assessment of children receiving sensory integration treatment. *Occupational Therapy Journal of Research, 14*(4), 244–266.

Wilson, B.N., Kaplan, B.J., Fellowes, S., Gruchy, C., & Faris, P. (1992). The efficacy of sensory integration treatment compared to tutoring. *Physical & Occupational Therapy in Pediatrics, 12*(1), 1.

Wolff, P., Michel, G., Ovrut, M., & Drake, C. (1990). Rate and timing precision of motor coordination in developmental dyslexia. *Developmental Psychology, 26*, 349–359.

World Health Organization (WHO). (2001). *International classification of functioning, disability, and health (ICF).* Geneva: Author.

18

Fast ForWord Language

MELISSA M. AGOCS, MARTHA S. BURNS,
LOGAN E. DE LEY, STEVEN L. MILLER, AND BARBARA M. CALHOUN

ABSTRACT

Fast ForWord Language software was first developed to address oral language skills in children with specific language impairment and auditory processing deficits, but it has been broadened to address skills underlying oral and written language for use with individuals from 4 years to adulthood. Its use is advocated both for individuals with language-related diagnoses and typical development. The intervention provides computer-based practice with auditory tasks and specific language forms that is intensive (e.g., 100 minutes per day), extensive (5 days per week for 4–8 weeks), and adaptive, in that stimulus difficulty is modified based on the child's performance. Outcomes from a variety of research methodologies and for a variety of populations are described by the authors as evidence supporting the use of this intervention. Some recent nonsupportive results also are acknowledged.

INTRODUCTION

Fast ForWord Language software engages the user in a series of cognitive exercises using language and listening designed to build the language-based skills necessary to improve reading ability. Based on more than 30 years of research on learning, brain plasticity, and the auditory skills of children with language-learning problems, patented technologies behind the software adapt to each student's progress and continually build critical skills to improve thinking, listening, speaking, and reading. Since the first exploratory studies on components of Fast ForWord Language, evidence has accumulated demonstrating that the approach may produce improvements in critical skill areas in participants of various ages (4 years to adulthood), developmental levels, backgrounds, and disabilities, including subjects with specific language impairment, pervasive developmental disorder, auditory processing disorder, dyslexia, and attention-deficit/hyperactivity disorder. To help ensure success

---

Chapter 18 does not have a video clip on the accompanying DVD.

with the approach, available services allow participants' progression on the software to be closely monitored and recommended activities are given to help participants understand the tasks and stay motivated.

TARGET POPULATIONS AND ASSESSMENTS FOR DETERMINING TREATMENT RELEVANCE AND GOALS

Auditory processing skills, adequate working memory, syntax, and other skills are vital to oral language and reading. Although these skills are important for all children, weakness (or deficits) in these areas can be especially devastating to children whose language skills substantially lag behind their other skills. Fast ForWord Language was initially designed for two populations: children with specific language impairment (SLI) and children with temporal auditory processing disorders. Many children share these two problems. That is, many children with SLI have problems perceiving and manipulating the rapidly changing acoustic elements within speech sounds which we believe contribute to their core developmental language problems. In addition to these two populations, evidence indicates that Fast ForWord Language can be beneficial for children with a wide range of reading abilities, including students considered average or gifted (Scientific Learning, 2004a–2004e).

Target Populations

Two early publications in the journal *Science* described an intensive language-learning product that targeted language and processing fundamentals in a group of children with SLI (Merzenich, Jenkins, et al., 1996; Tallal et al., 1996). The children all tested within the normal range on measures of nonverbal intelligence prior to using Fast ForWord Language. These children, 7–11 years of age, showed marked increases in standard measures of speed of processing, phonological discrimination, and language comprehension after 4 weeks of using the software for 100 minutes per day, 5 days per week.

The tests that were used to select children for this and a follow-up field study included the Clinical Evaluation of Language Fundamentals–Third Edition (CELF-3; Semel, Wiig, & Secord, 1995), the Goldman-Fristoe-Woodcock Test of Auditory Discrimination (GFW; Goldman, Fristoe, & Woodcock, 1970), the Token Test for Children (DiSimoni, 1978), and the Test of Language Development–Primary, Third Edition (TOLD-I:2, TOLD-P:2; Hammill & Newcomer, 1988). Results from the initial lab study (Merzenich, Jenkins, et al., 1996; Tallal et al., 1996) and a follow-up field investigation (Bedi et al., 1995) confirmed that children ages 7–11 who performed at least 1 standard deviation (*SD*) below the mean on at least one of these tests at pretest were likely to show significant gains after using the software.

Subsequent to the initial lab and field trials with Fast ForWord Language, audiologists Battin, Young, and Burns (2000) demonstrated that children with auditory processing disorders, but without obvious language problems, also show marked improvements after using the software. They provided data on a group of 15 children who improved significantly in Figure–Ground Discrimination and Competing Stimuli subtests of the Screening Test for Auditory Processing Disorders (SCAN; Keith, 1986) as well as on the Staggered Spondee Word Test (Katz, 1962, 1968, 1985; Katz & Smith, 1991) delivered through a calibrated audiometer. These results were subsequently corroborated in a study showing that children who exhibit a set of auditory processing disorders related to temporal processing benefit from Fast ForWord Language (Morlet, Norman, Ray, & Berlin, 2003). Many children who exhibit these auditory processing disorders do not exhibit SLI, but they show problems with listening skills, especially listening in noise. They also show problems with auditory working memory and other skills that affect academic performance. In addition, many of these children have histories of chronic or recurring otitis media with effusion during their early development.

Other populations for which preliminary evidence of benefit from Fast ForWord has been obtained include children on the autism spectrum or with developmental disabilities, and children and adults with neurological impairments. Merzenich and colleagues (1999) report data on 29 children with pervasive developmental disorder (PDD): 10 with PDD-autistic (PDD-A) and 19 with PDD-not otherwise specified (PDD-NOS). The children ranged in age from 5 to 14 years and were selected by therapists who believed they could undergo reliable standardized language assessments prior to participation, and had the behavioral or conceptual competencies believed necessary for participating in the exercises. Behavioral and conceptual competencies included the ability to manipulate a computer mouse and to demonstrate an understanding of the concept of same-different, and they had to have completed an age-appropriate standardized language battery within 6 months of the study. In addition to the 29 children who completed participation and for whom data are available, 11 children did not complete participation due to behavioral problems. Not all children were evaluated on all tests. On average, the children achieved significant improvements on assessments administered, including the Token Test, GFW, TOLD, and CELF-3, as well as subtests of the assessments. There was not a significant difference between the performance of the children with PDD-A and the children with PDD-NOS. Melzer and Poglitsch (1998) presented results on 77 children on the autism spectrum. Many of the children in their study required one-on-one training on Fast ForWord exercises with a speech-language pathologist (SLP) for longer periods than are customarily needed by children with SLI. In some cases, the children on the autism spectrum also required special adaptations to maintain their focus and attention to the tasks, as well as to ensure their continued motivation. The children who responded the best to the intensive intervention were those for whom language limitations were more pronounced than visual or motor impairments.

Although currently unpublished, studies of children with Down syndrome and other developmental disorders have been completed, and anecdotal evidence indicates the possibility of excellent responses to the approach. Anecdotally, those who appear to have the best responses have receptive language ages of 3 years or older, although this still requires empirical verification. These children may or may not exhibit fundamental temporal processing disorders, although there is evidence that their language and memory disorders are similar to those of children with SLI in many ways (Eadie, Fey, Douglas, & Parsons, 2002; Lawa & Bishop, 2003). These children appear to respond positively to the intense demands of the auditory tasks, the working memory load required for success on several of the components, and the intensive language instruction.

Focusing on adults with receptive aphasia, Dronkers and colleagues (1999) reported that adults with receptive aphasia show significant improvements in receptive language measures on the Western Aphasia Battery (Kertesz, 1982) after 6 weeks of participation on Fast ForWord Language. Studies are currently under way to test whether younger adults with traumatic brain injury show the same positive results. From Dronkers's study and smaller clinical studies (Dronkers et al., 1999), it appears that brain injury in the left temporal lobe impairs phonemic perceptual abilities crucial to language comprehension and auditory verbal working memory. Fast ForWord Language appears to have a positive impact on these neurological processing fundamentals in adults, just as it does in children with language impairments.

ASSESSMENTS FOR DETERMINING TREATMENT RELEVANCE AND GOALS

The assessment tests that seem most powerful for selecting children and adults who will benefit from the Fast ForWord Language exercises are included in Table 18.1. Generally, individuals ages 4 years to adulthood who fall 1–2 *SD* below the mean on any of these tests are excellent candidates for Fast ForWord Language.

In addition to the individuals who score below average on the assessments discussed previously, it should be noted that average and above-average children and adults can benefit from the exercises, especially when there is a significant gap between their language or processing skills and their IQs. Although the exercises were initially targeted at children with SLI, empirical studies have shown that Fast ForWord Language can help a broader population improve the specific language and cognitive skills addressed in this software (Marion, 2004; Miller et al., 1999; Schopmeyer, Mellon, Dobaj, Grant, & Niparko, 2000; Scientific Learning Corporation, 2003, 2004a, 2004b, 2004c, 2004d, 2004e; Slattery, 2003; Tallal et al., 1996; Troia & Whitney, 2003).

Table 18.1.   Assessment tests for selecting children and adults who will benefit from Fast ForWord Language

Test	Brief description
Clinical Evaluation of Language Fundamentals–3 (CELF-3; Semel, Wiig, & Secord, 1995)	A comprehensive language test widely used to measure a student's ability to understand words and sentences, follow directions, recall and formulate sentences, and understand relationships between words and categories
Comprehensive Test of Phonological Processing (CTOPP; Wagner, Torgesen, & Rashotte, 1999)	Assesses phonological awareness. The Phonological Awareness Composite, comprising the Elision and Blending Words subtests, measures an individual's awareness of and access to the phonological structure of oral language.
Goldman-Fristoe-Woodcock Test of Auditory Discrimination (GFW; Goldman, Fristoe, & Woodcock, 1970)	A screening measure of speech sound discrimination ability for students in quiet and noisy environments
Lindamood Auditory Conceptualization Test (LAC; Lindamood & Lindamood, 1971/1979)	Designed to measure auditory perception and conceptualization of speech sounds and assess a student's ability to perform encoding tasks similar to those required in reading and spelling
A Screening Test for Auditory Processing Disorders (SCAN; Keith, 1986)	A screening test for auditory processing disorders. It consists of three subtests, each of which is presented via audiocassette and requires the student to report the words that are heard under various listening conditions.
Staggered Spondee Word Test (SSWT; Katz, 1962, 1968, 1985; Katz & Smith, 1991)	A dichotic test of binaural separation. The stimuli represent both competing and noncompeting words presented to each ear simultaneously.
Token Test for Children (DiSimoni, 1978)	Measures a child's ability to follow spoken directions. The test uses plastic tokens of different shapes, colors, and sizes, which the child manipulates according to the tester's directions. The directions range from simple commands ("Touch the red circle") to more complex procedures involving multiple steps ("Put the white square behind the yellow circle").
The Test of Phonological Awareness (TOPA; Torgesen & Bryant, 1994)	Designed to diagnose deficits in phonological processing and phoneme–grapheme correspondence
Western Aphasia Battery (WAB; Kertesz, 1982)	Evaluates clinical aspects of language function and nonverbal skills, as well as the ability to read, write, and calculate. The battery is used to identify aphasia syndromes and determine the degree of their severity.

THEORETICAL BASIS

Models of language and reading development can be characterized as bottom up, top down, or interactive (Rayner & Pollatsek, 1989). Bottom-up models typically focus on information flow that is based primarily on the inputs to the information processing system. Top-down models typically focus on prior information that is stored in the system (e.g., memory) and how this information facilitates information processing and decision making. Interactive models allow for various forms of communication between bottom-up and top-down processes. We believe that there is not sufficient evidence to justify a purely bottom-up or top-down processing model. Fast ForWord Language software is based on an interactive model with a developmental perspective. Fast ForWord exercises include activities that build rapid tone processing (the ability to discriminate between frequency-modulated tones of various durations), phoneme perception, word discrimination, and the comprehension of various grammatical forms.

Decades of research on learning and the brain have led to the development of a set of core principles for building cognitive skills: repetition, intensity, immediate feedback, adaptivity, and motivation. Correctly applied, these principles hold great promise for remediating learning disorders and for improving the educational outcomes of all students. Fast ForWord Language represents such an application, with a focus on building skills that are characteristically low among children with language, literacy, and learning disorders. The original focus on perceptual skill training aspects of Fast ForWord Language is founded on two distinct theories. The first theory states that many children with language-based learning impairments have significant deficits in their ability to represent and manipulate the spectrotemporal fine structure of speech (Leonard, 1998; Leonard, McGregor, & Allen, 1992; Liberman, Shankweiler, Fisher, & Carter, 1974; Tallal & Piercy, 1974, 1975). The second asserts that the ability to discriminate and recognize rapid successive sensory inputs can be improved through intensive training (Karni & Sagi, 1991, 1993; Merzenich & deCharms, 1996).

Fast ForWord Language exercises build both cognitive and perceptual skills believed to be deficient in at least a subset of individuals with SLI and/or other learning problems. If signal perception problems for complex auditory signals such as speech contribute to the phenotype of SLI, then improvements in fast and accurate signal perception would be expected to help students benefit more from classroom instruction, traditional communication therapy, and other language-rich environments. Support for this hypothesis is evident when, despite the absence of text-related activities in the Fast ForWord Language software, students with some preexisting reading ability have shown improvements in reading comprehension following the use of the software.

SLI continues to be one of the most controversial topics in speech-language pathology. There are various competing theories about its nature and origin, along with many different approaches to its diagnosis and treatment. Meanwhile, children with SLI continue to represent a large part of the clinical population treated by SLPs. Regardless of their theoretical perspective, clinicians widely recognize that the population of children with SLI is not homogeneous. Unfortunately, the functional consequences of SLI, including poor literacy development and academic failure, are all too consistent (Catts, Fey, Tomblin, & Zhang, 2002). Numerous studies have documented the negative impact of SLI on children's literacy, academic success, social development, and behavioral adjustment (Aram, Ekelman, & Nation, 1984; Catts, 1993; Catts et al., 2002; Leonard, 1998; Tallal, Allard, Miller, & Curtiss, 1997). In a 14-year longitudinal study, Johnson and her colleagues (1999) found that children identified with SLI at 5 years of age continued to show language deficits as young adults, along with deficits on measures of reading, spelling, and math. Researchers have also documented higher rates of learning disability among students with SLI, as well as a range of deficits in more basic cognitive processes such as digit-naming speed, verbal working memory, and executive function (Young et al., 2002). Children with SLI are at especially high risk for developing reading disorders (Catts, 1993; Catts et al., 2002; Leonard, 1998). In his 1993 study, Catts found that weaknesses in phonological awareness and rapid naming are predictive of difficulty in early word reading, whereas weak expressive and receptive language skills are predictive of problems in reading comprehension.

In the long search for the cause of SLI, researchers have identified a number of lower-level perceptual, cognitive, and motor disorders that are prevalent in the SLI population. These include deficits in working memory (Gathercole & Baddeley, 1990; Gillam, Cowan, & Marler, 1998; Montgomery, 2000), general processing speed (Miller, Kail, Leonard, & Tomblin, 2001; Windsor & Hwang, 1999), rapid auditory processing (Merzenich, Jenkins, et al., 1996; Tallal et al., 1996; Wright et al., 1997), attention (Stark & Tallal, 1988), and sequencing (Merzenich, Jenkins, et al., 1996; Tallal et al., 1996). Children with SLI have even been found to have difficulties in such nonverbal realms as mental imagery (Leonard, 1998) and in coordination, balance, and motor functions (Noterdaeme, Mildenberger, Minow, & Amorosa, 2002). Although no single disorder has been shown to affect every child diagnosed with SLI, there is good reason to believe that one or more of these disorders cause (or exacerbate) the condition.

Although SLI has been found to have an impact on virtually every aspect of language use, morphosyntactic skill deficits are especially characteristic of children with SLI (in English-speaking communities). These children have difficulty with bound morphemes and other closed-class morphemes such as pronouns and auxiliary *be* forms. They also have trouble understanding and producing sentences that are long or complex (see Leonard, 1998, for a review of linguistic deficits in SLI). Traditional language therapy addresses these deficits with focused language stimulation designed to help children build stronger linguistic representations. Therapeutic activities generally strive to provide extensive experience with selected forms and to support success and learning through such modifications as simplified vocabulary and visual cues. Unfortunately, it is challenging to provide extensive practice using conventional therapy activities. Furthermore, unless the stimuli are carefully selected, children may rely on semantics or common sense to respond, rather than focusing on grammatical structure.

It is well understood that language disorders often arise secondary to other disorders such as hearing loss. Likewise, disorders in cognitive or perceptual processes may cause or contribute to SLI by degrading the linguistic input a child receives. For example, a child with limited verbal working memory may not have the resources to both retain a sentence's meaning and process its structure completely. This kind of limitation would especially affect knowledge of the complex syntactic structures and low-frequency vocabulary that typically occur in longer sentences. Likewise, a child with auditory processing problems may have a hard time discerning the subtle acoustic profile of certain morphemes (e.g., "She walk*ed* to the store"), leading to deficiencies in morphological representations (Fellbaum, Miller, Curtiss, & Tallal, 1995). We hypothesize that even if a particular disorder only disrupts linguistic processing in a narrow way, the ultimate effect on a child's developing language system may be substantial—including dysfunctional compensations or disengagement from the language environment (Merzenich, Spengler, et al., 1996).

Although it is reasonable to hypothesize that the various cognitive, perceptual, and/or linguistic deficits that co-occur in children with SLI either cause or contribute to their language disorder, the true relationship among these deficits has yet to be determined conclusively. For this reason, the selection of the specific cognitive, perceptual, and linguistic processes to target in the Fast ForWord Language exercises was guided by empirical evidence as well as the theoretical reasons outlined above. Early studies with prototypes of Fast ForWord Language confirmed that this kind of protocol, which focuses on lower-level processes and basic subskills as well as focused language stimulation, can improve students' performance on measures of language skill (Merzenich, Jenkins, et al., 1996; Tallal et al., 1996).

Fast ForWord Language addresses SLI by attempting to remediate underlying cognitive and perceptual disorders and providing focused language stimulation. Use of the product builds skills at three levels within the verbal/receptive modality. At the lowest level, auditory perception skills are targeted—including sensitivity to rapid, subtle changes in the sound stream that are critical for phoneme discrimination. At higher levels, the exercises are designed to build skills in speech perception and listening comprehension. In addition, the product develops primary cognitive skills critical to language and learning, including working memory capacity and the ability to focus and sustain attention.

Because morphosyntactic skills are so important for children with SLI, Fast ForWord Language software incorporates listening comprehension exercises that target these skills. The stimuli are carefully constructed so that participants must attend to word order, affixes, articles, prepositions, and other morphosyntactic features. The listening comprehension exercises also have features that eliminate some of the limitations found in conventional language therapy activities. For example, computer-based delivery and engaging exercises support high response rates, and the recommended schedule guarantees that participants get frequent practice.

It is important to note that although it is especially beneficial for children with SLI to work on building their auditory processing and language skills, it may be that most children can benefit from these exercises. Therefore, while the exercises were initially targeted at children with SLI, there is some evidence that Fast ForWord Language can help many children improve linguistic and cognitive skills, even those with typically developing language.

The Fast ForWord Language exercises incorporate two neuroscience-based innovations: speech stimuli that are acoustically modified to be more intelligible to children with SLI, and a participation protocol designed to drive cortical reorganization. A study conducted by Tallal and colleagues (1996) during the development of the Fast ForWord Language product indicated that the modified speech stimuli and the participation protocol each made unique contributions to the children's language improvements.

Children with SLI have special difficulty discriminating speech sounds that are differentiated by rapid frequency transitions of the second and third formants (such as /b/ and /d/). However, they can successfully discriminate these sounds when the speech stimuli are modified to slow the critical frequency transitions (Tallal & Piercy, 1974). By using temporally modified speech stimuli, the exercises allow children with SLI to achieve success early on. To further heighten sensitivity to the rapid transitions in phonemes, these components are selectively amplified. This serves both to increase the salience of these transitions and to reduce masking effects. (For a technical description of the speech modification algorithms used, see Nagarajan et al., 1998.) As an individual progresses through the product, the time-scale and intensity modifications are reduced in successive approximations. Finally, at the highest level, natural speech stimuli are presented. The use of acoustically modified speech is a feature of the listening comprehension exercises in the product that set them apart from conventional language therapy activities. With acoustically modified speech, participants can be more successful, and they can build more accurate representations of the linguistic stimuli.

The Fast ForWord Language schedule is based on the principles of learning: repetition, intensity, immediate feedback, adaptivity, and motivation (Merzenich & Jenkins, 1995; Merzenich, Wright, et al., 1996). These principles will sound familiar to most speech-language clinicians and educators, because learning theory has long recognized the importance of such factors. However, contemporary neuroscience is providing a more complete understanding of how they can be harnessed to produce specific changes in the brain and in performance.

Neuroscientists have demonstrated that intensive training can improve skilled movements and sharpen perceptual skills in the visual, auditory, and tactile domains (Karni & Sagi, 1991; Merzenich & Jenkins, 1995). During skill acquisition, systematic changes take place in the cortical regions dedicated to sensory processing and/or motor control. While a skill is being learned, relevant cortical areas will expand, annexing neurons in neighboring regions to support the demands of increased sensitivity and/or refined motor control.

The dynamic processes at work in cortical reorganization can drive improved perceptual or motor skills, given appropriate learning experiences. However, these same mechanisms can also lead to degraded skills. For example, learning a task that requires repeatedly moving two fingers in tandem can lead to a merging of the cortical regions representing those fingers until eventually the fingers may be incapable of independent movement (Merzenich, Spengler, Byl, Wang, & Jenkins, 1996). Set in the wrong direction early on by factors such as fluctuating hearing loss, the normally adaptive processes of brain plasticity may be responsible for establishing and maintaining deficient linguistic representations in children with SLI.

Repetition is critical to stimulating cortical reorganization, and this requires a learning schedule that is both intensive (hundreds of trials per day) and extensive (lasting many weeks). To ensure that the individual is not practicing incorrect responses, immediate feedback is critical. Likewise, the adaptivity of the task to the individual's error level ensures that the individual is working at a level at which most responses are correct. Adaptivity also functions to progressively move the individual toward higher skill levels. Finally, motivation also plays an essential role. The desired cortical changes only take place when an individual is attending to the task at hand; passive exposure to a stimulus is not enough. Maintaining attention through intensive practice sessions depends on high levels of motivation. This is another reason to ensure that the individual is working at a level at which a high degree of success is experienced. Other forms of reinforcement are also helpful for bolstering motivation, especially with young children.

Fast ForWord Language incorporates these principles through the combination of a prescribed schedule, computer-based delivery, and provider education. The schedule provides the necessary intensity and duration for sufficient practice and repetition. Computer-based delivery permits immediate feedback to be provided on each trial, and feedback about errors—because it comes from the computer—is perceived as a natural consequence rather than a criticism. The computer tracks each response and adapts to the individual's current level of performance, keeping the appropriate balance of success and challenge. The exercises have a game-like format and use rewards such as humorous animated sequences and the accumulation of points, to help maintain attention and motivation. Provider education helps the clinicians and teachers who administer the product maintain optimal learning conditions, keep levels of participation and motivation high, intervene when appropriate, and utilize information on each child's progress to guide curriculum or therapy decisions. For more information on the scheduled use of the Fast ForWord Language exercises, see Key Components.

EMPIRICAL BASIS

Early Studies at Rutgers University and
the University of California at San Francisco

Having considered the theoretical basis of SLI and approaches for improving sensory perception from a theoretical perspective, this section looks at the empirical results of studies investigating these theories and demonstrates that regardless of the validity of the theoretical assumptions on which they are based, the Fast ForWord Language exercises have produced significant effects for a variety of populations.

Early exploratory studies for Fast ForWord Language products looked at the effects of using temporally modified speech with children who have language-learning impairments. The first study, by Merzenich, Jenkins, et al. (1996), conducted in the summer of 1994, used early versions of the two audiovisual exercises now known within the Fast ForWord Language product as Circus Sequence and Phoneme Identification. At this point in the evolution of the software, components related to specific language forms challenging to English-speaking children with SLI were not yet included. (See the Key Components for a brief description of these exercises.) In the study, both exercises started with stimuli that children with SLI could easily identify (e.g., with relatively longer interstimulus intervals and longer stimulus durations). As a child answered accurately, the adaptive variables slowly progressed toward more difficult settings while maintaining a level of accuracy of approximately 80% for the child.

This exploratory study included seven children with SLI. They ranged in age from 5.8 to 9.1 years (mean age = 7.3 years, SD = 1.5 years), with mean nonverbal intelligence scores of 106 (SD = 18.25). All seven children demonstrated a severe delay in receptive and expressive language development, with mean language ages equal to 4.8 years. The children used the exercises for 4 consecutive weeks, approximately 5 days per week, 2 hours per day. Results of the study are described below.

- The Tallal Repetition Test was given to the children before and after they used the exercises. (The Tallal Repetition Test is a test of temporal processing ability. To determine whether a subject has difficulty processing rapid temporal auditory stimuli, the test finds 1) an interstimulus interval threshold for the subject with 75% probability, and 2) the minimum duration of stimuli that can be correctly sequenced. At this level, two tones spaced by the interstimulus interval, would be accurately identified 75% of the time.) The study's results indicated that the children made statistically significant improvements in their pre- to post-interstimulus interval thresholds $F(1, 6) = 36.7$, $p < 0.001$) and their ability to sequence sounds of shorter durations ($F(1, 6) = 7.3, p < 0.05$). Please note that caution is suggested when interpreting results from relatively small numbers of subjects (fewer than 30).

- Within the exercise of Phoneme Identification, all of the seven children made substantial improvements in their ability to identify consonants presented at brief transitions, a very difficult task for many children with SLI.

For six of the seven children, this progression in the Phoneme Identification exercise translated to statistically significant gains in identifying phonetic elements as measured by the GFW (Goldman, Fristoe, & Woodcock, 1970). Their average improvement on the GFW converted to a gain of approximately 1.5 years in language development age.

The same group of researchers later conducted a small-scale efficacy study in the summer of 1995 to reproduce the results of the previous study while using a treatment control group (Tallal et al., 1996). In total, 22 children with SLI and deficits in temporal processing participated in this study. They ranged in age from 5.2 to 10.0 years (mean age = 7.4 years, SD = 1.4 years) and exhibited a mean language age of 4.9 years. The mean nonverbal intelligence score of the group was 96.4 SD = 9.7). The children were divided into two matched groups based on receptive language abilities and measures of nonverbal intelligence. The groups participated simultaneously to ensure that they received equal encouragement and reinforcement throughout the 4-week participation period. The treatment control group received classical, intensive language training but used exercises that did not have adaptive, temporally modified speech.

This study used revised prototype versions of two components of Fast ForWord Language (Circus Sequence and Phoneme Identification) to better maintain the attention of the children and to improve performance consistency. In addition, two supplemental exercises were designed to aid speech perception generalization: Old MacDonald's Flying Farm and Phonic Match. (See the Key Components for a brief description of these exercises.)

As seen in the earlier exploratory study, substantial gains were achieved on various assessments:

- All children in the treatment group improved on the Tallal Repetition Test. After working with the temporally modified sounds, children could distinguish the sequence order of almost immediately successive tonal stimuli that were, on average, 18 milliseconds in duration. This duration was approximately one-fifth of the duration required by the children for accurate discrimination before participation. In comparison, after the 4-week time period, the performance of the majority of the treatment control group did not improve.

- In addition to the Tallal Repetition Test, the children also received the GFW, the Token Test, and the Curtiss-Yamada Comprehensive Language Evaluation–Receptive (Curtiss & Yamada, 1987). A repeated-measures analysis of variance concluded that the experimental group made significantly greater gains on these measures than the treatment control group ($F(1, 20) = 5.44, p = 0.02$).

- Follow-up testing was conducted 3 months after the study and again at 6 months after the study. At both time points, the experimental group performed significantly better on the assessments than the treatment control group.

Interestingly, in both Study 1 and Study 2, the amount the modified speech exercises were used directly correlated with language outcomes, as measured by the Token Test for Children (Study 1: $n = 7$, correlation coefficient = 0.85, $p < 0.01$; Study 2: $n = 11$, correlation coefficient = 0.73, $p < 0.01$). In general, the longer the children worked on the exercises with modified speech, the more gains they made in their ability to follow spoken commands.

The National Field Trial

After the positive results of the first small-scale efficacy study, we believed it was necessary to investigate whether the exercises could yield the same substantial results in the nonideal conditions of clinics and classrooms. That is, we wished to determine the effectiveness of the approach. To determine this, a new company named Scientific Learning Corporation was formed. The company conducted a large-scale National Field Trial across 35 sites in the United States and Canada (Scientific Learning Corporation, n.d.). Fifty-eight volunteer professionals, who were not employed by the company, helped collect data for the field trial. These professionals included psychologists, SLPs, special education teachers, audiologists, and physicians.

The company enhanced the existing four exercises and created three additional language exercises, resulting in the seven exercises that comprise the version of Fast ForWord Language available today. The three new exercises introduced in the study were Block Commander, Phonic Word, and Language Comprehension Builder. (See the Key Components for a brief description of these exercises.) Scientific Learning Corporation developed a data collection system to track the performance of each participant. Exercise data were uploaded and saved on a database server located at the company's headquarters. These exercise data, including the tasks that were presented and the skills that were measured, were then summarized and sent back to the professionals at their sites via the Internet, enabling the professionals to recognize when a participant was having difficulty on an exercise or to track when a participant was not practicing the desired number of exercises each day. Unlike in the earlier studies, the number of weeks the children participated was allowed to vary. To be a part of the study, however, the children were required to use five of the seven exercises each day, spending a total of at least 75 minutes per day. In the previous studies the participation period was strictly held to 4 weeks, whereas the children in the National Field Trial were able to continue using the product until mastery, regardless of the time needed. Some children benefited from this flexibility and finally reached mastery after up to 21 weeks of use.

The 409 children in this field trial were receiving clinical services and ranged in age from 4 to 14 (mean age = 8.4 years, *SD* = 2.0 years). They used the exercises to completion. Some pre- and postexercise test data were received for 269 of these children (for a copy of this report, see http://www .scilearn.com/results/science/main=papers). These children used the exercises for an average of 96 minutes per day over an average of 31 days. Twenty-six of these participants were identified with PDD, 17 had a history of traumatic brain injury and/or epilepsy, 64 were classified as co-morbid for attention deficit disorder, and 76 were identified with a central auditory processing disorder (CAPD).

As a requirement of the National Field Trial, professionals administered several standardized assessments to the Fast ForWord Language participants. Statistically significant gains were demonstrated postintervention on the various assessments, which included tests of speech discrimination, receptive and expressive language, and language processing. It should be noted that no stimulus sets included in the Fast ForWord Language exercises directly exposed participants to any of the specific test items. Following are some of the specific findings of the study. Please note that without the use of a control group, the contribution of spurious factors, statistical or methodological, that may have contributed to these results cannot be accurately estimated, and, therefore, caution should be taken in evaluating the magnitude of the effects.

- Before using Fast ForWord Language, 61% of the children who took the Quiet subtest of the GFW scored more than 1 *SD* below the normal median. After using the exercises, only 11% remained more than 1 *SD* below the median. Likewise, before participation, 53% who took the Noise subtest scored more than 1 *SD* below the normal mean; only 10% remained this low after using the exercises. On the GFW Noise subtest, considered the more difficult of the two, 61% of the participants met or surpassed the normal mean after participation.

- The Lindamood Auditory Conceptualization Test (Lindamood & Lindamood, 1971, 1979) was given to 116 of the participants before and after they worked with the product. Eighty-nine of the 116 children made positive gains on the test, with their average gains translating to approximately two grade levels (average grade change of 1.8).

- Statistically significant improvements were made on all subtests of the CELF-3 and all six TOLD-P:2 (Hammill & Newcomer, 1988) battery subtests and quotients ($p < 0.05$) (see Figure 18.1). These tests evaluate various receptive and expressive abilities. Ninety-three percent of the 97

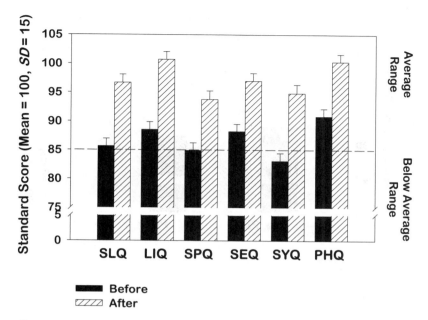

Figure 18.1. Improvements on the Test of Language Development–Primary, Second Edition (TOLD-P:2; Newcomer & Hammill, 1991). After using the Fast ForWord Language exercises, 77 participants exhibited statistically significant improvements on all TOLD P:2 tests. Quotients measured were SLQ, Spoken Language; LIQ, Listening; SPQ, Speaking; SEQ, Sequencing; SYQ, Syntax; PHQ, Phonology.

children who took the TOLD before and after using Fast ForWord Language made gains in their Spoken Language Quotients.

- For the 65 participants who took the CELF-3 Receptive subtests, average gains were approximately 1 *SD*.

- Before using the exercises, 150 of the 255 participants who took the Token Test scored more than 1 *SD* below the normal median. Ninety-one percent of the children in this group improved; the subset of children who showed improvement made average gains of 1.7 *SD*.

- Participants with a diagnosis of PDD, CAPD, or ADD made gains nearly equivalent to those of children without these diagnoses. For example, children classified as PDD-A or PDD-NOS achieved significant gains that were no different from children without PDD on the GFW (see below). Overall, preparticipation versus postparticipation results on the GFW subtests showed statistically significant gains (on the Quiet subtest: $F(1, 128) = 71.54$, $p < 0.0001$; on the Noise subtest: $F(1, 103) = 54.0$, $p < 0.0001$). Figure 18.2 shows a comparison of the gains of the children with PDD to the gains of children without PDD—there is no significant difference between their improvements on the GFW (on the Quiet subtest: $F(1, 128) = 3.22$, $p > 0.05$; on the Noise subtest: $F(1, 103) = 0.53$, $p > 0.05$).

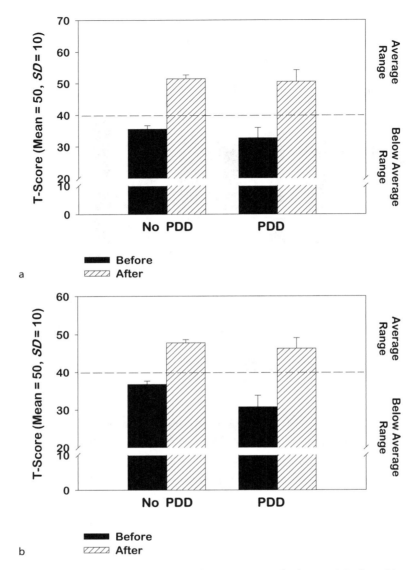

Figure 18.2. Improvements on the Goldman-Fristoe-Woodcock Test of Auditory Discrimination (GFW; Goldman, Fristoe, & Woodcock, 1970). Children with pervasive developmental disorder (PDD) participated in the National Field Trial and achieved significant gains on the GFW. There was no significant difference between their improvements on the GFW and the gains of the children without PDD in either (a) Noise or (b) Quiet.

- In addition to being independent of the above-mentioned diagnoses, positive results were independent of age and gender.

The National Field Trial was a feasibility study without a control group. After an average of 6 weeks of participation, the group of children made statistically significant gains in all areas tested. Unlike earlier studies in which only selected children with language impairments were included, children identified with a variety of diagnoses were a part of this study. Observing their results, it became evident that the benefits of the Fast ForWord Language exercises could reach a wider range of children with language impairments than the selective range originally tested. Furthermore, the National Field Trial showed that children with various deficits are capable of improving the skills in which they are deficient. More information about the National Field Trial is available in the Results section of the Scientific Learning web site (http://www.scientificlearning.com/results).

The School Pilot Study

The next large investigation by Scientific Learning was an effectiveness study designed to demonstrate that the exercises work in a school environment with students identified as "at-risk for academic failure" (Miller et al., 1999; see Robey & Schultz, 1998, for a discussion of efficacy versus effectiveness). Teachers from nine districts across the United States identified students who had weak skills and were performing in the lowest quartile of their language arts curriculum. These children were representative of a large population of students in the United States who are not classified as having language or learning impairments, yet are considered to be at risk for academic failure. The students ranged from kindergarten to fifth grade, although the majority fell into the range between kindergarten and third grade, inclusive. A stratified randomization within grade and gender was used to assign students to one of two groups in a fixed ratio of 1.74:1: The two groups were the Fast ForWord Language group ($n = 288$), and the control group ($n = 164$). The random assignment ensured that the groups were chosen without bias. Fifty-three experimental children and 32 control children spoke English as a Second Language (ESL). Seventy-six percent of these ESL children spoke Spanish as their native language.

The Fast ForWord Language group used the exercises in their school classrooms or laboratories under the supervision of a professional. The study design expected the participants to use the exercises for 100 minutes per day, 5 days per week. The students used the exercises for an average of 39 participation days. The number of participation days ranged from 15 days to 116 days because of various typical factors: the variability of the group was due to each individual's ability to reach completion, lack of motivation, or poor access to the computer facilities. The control group remained in their regular classrooms and continued receiving their standard curriculum.

Before and after participation, three standardized measures were given to the subjects in this school study: 1) the Test of Auditory Comprehension of Language–Revised (TACL-R; Carrow-Woolfolk, 1985), 2) the Isolation and Deletion subtests of the Phonological Awareness Test (PAT; Robertson & Salter, 1997), and 3) the Letter-Word Identification subtest of the Woodcock-

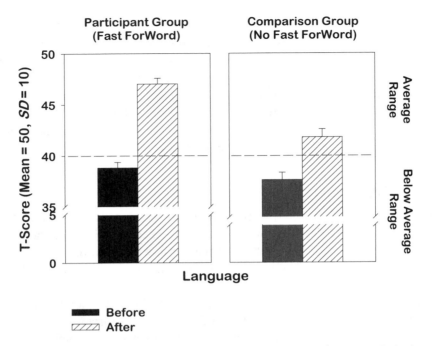

Figure 18.3. Performance on the Test of Auditory Comprehension of Language–Revised (TACL-R; Carrow-Woolfolk, 1985). Students who used the intensive Fast ForWord Language exercises performed significantly better than the students who remained in the regular classroom while receiving the standard curriculum.

Johnson Psycho-Educational Battery–Revised (WJR-R; Woodcock & Johnson, 1989, 1990). Statistical results are shown below.

- When comparing gains on these assessments, the group that received the intensive instruction with the Fast ForWord Language exercises for an average of 6 weeks made statistically greater improvements than the control group on the TACL-R language comprehension tasks ($F(1, 386) = 26.3$, $p < 0.0001$) (see Figure 18.3).

- To further express the differences in performance on the TACL-R assessment, average pretest performances for the Fast ForWord Language group and the control group were approximately equivalent to the 12th percentile, well below the population mean. At posttesting, the experimental group improved their performance to approximately the 38th percentile, making an average improvement of 1.8 years, whereas the control students improved their performance to the 21st percentile.

- The Fast ForWord Language group also made statistically greater improvements than the control group on the PAT Isolation subtest ($F(1, 383) = 4.9$, $p < 0.05$).

- On the TACL-R, average improvement for the experimental ESL students was significantly greater than the improvements made by the control ESL students ($F(1, 79) = 4.63$, $p < 0.05$) (see Figure 18.4).

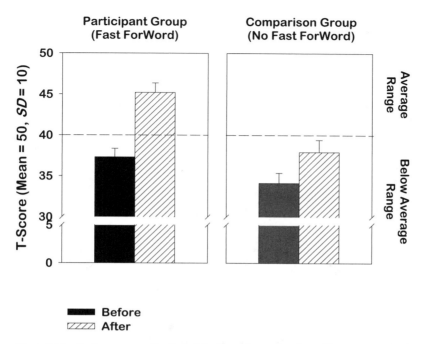

Figure 18.4. Performance on the Test of Auditory Comprehension of Language–Revised (TACL-R; Carrow-Woolfolk, 1985). ESL students who used the Fast ForWord Language exercises performed significantly better than the ESL students who remained in the regular classroom while receiving the standard curriculum.

More Recent Research from Scientific Learning Corporation

In the studies mentioned previously, the children used the exercises fairly consistently and were monitored by professionals. In other words, they closely followed the suggested Fast ForWord Language participation schedule. This resulted in statistically significant gains on language assessments. However, substantial language gains have also been found for participants who do not follow the schedule as closely, as depicted in Figure 18.5. A measure is made of the minutes a participant actually uses the product compared with the minutes of suggested use. It ranges from 0% to 100%. It is important to note that a low percentage of participation does not necessarily indicate that a participant is not working on the exercises. By participating intermittently or by only using a few exercises each day (instead of the suggested five), it is possible to have very low percentage of participation and eventually master all the content in the exercises. Figure 18.5 depicts the mean percentage of participation versus the mean difference in language score (as measured by either the CELF-3 or the TOLD) for nearly 3,000 Fast ForWord Language participants.

As of the winter of 2001, the mean percentage of participation of Fast ForWord Language participants nationwide was 76%, and the mean improvement in language scores (as measured by the CELF-3 or TOLD) was 11

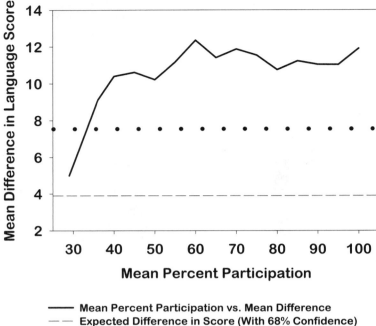

Figure 18.5. Performance based on participation. Using the Clinical Evaluation of Language Fundamentals–Third Edition (CELF-3; Semel, Wiig, & Secord, 1995) total language score standard error of the measure for the test-retest sample (*SEM* = 3.9), with 68% confidence, subjects will retest with a total language score within 3.9 points of the original standard score. With 95% confidence, subjects will retest with a total language score within 7.8 points of the original standard score (Semel, Wiig, & Secord, 1995).

standard score points (both tests have a mean of 100, $SD = 15$). Figure 18.5 shows that the language skills of the participants who have participation levels below the national average are still benefiting. These high improvements with low participation levels support the use of the Fast ForWord Language exercises in a variety of settings. For example, schools and clinicians who need to use a flexible schedule often have low participation levels, yet many students may still attain substantial benefits from such limited use.

As Fast ForWord Language has slowly shifted its target population from clinics to schools, ongoing studies continue to evaluate its effectiveness. Figure 18.6 shows the results from pilot studies in three large, urban school districts that assessed the language skills of students before and after they used Fast ForWord products. These students, with a mean age of 9.4 years ($SD = 1.6$ years), were selected for Fast ForWord Language participation by their teachers and used the product under everyday conditions in their schools. The CELF-3 and/or TOLD tests were administered to the students by school personnel before and after using the exercises. In all, 153 students were assessed. On average, after using the software, the students demonstrated sig-

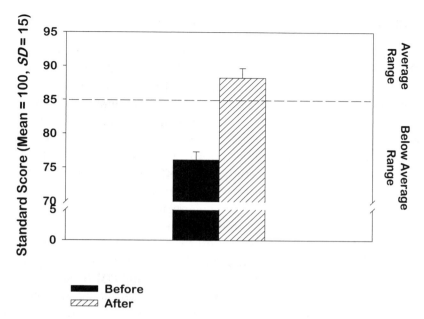

Figure 18.6. Improvements in language skills. Scores from students from three large, urban school districts are shown. Before participation, on average, the students were performing in the below-average range. After using Fast ForWord Language, the group made statistically significant gains, with the mean language standard score moving into the average range.

nificant gains ($t(152) = 15.6, p < 0.0001$) in language fundamentals, as measured by one of the two tests. Students differed in various ways such as ethnicity, age, and language ability, yet still showed, on average, statistically significant gains.

A Different Perspective

Many of the studies cited in this section report positive outcomes following use of Fast ForWord products. In each case, while the studies found positive benefits for the children using Fast ForWord software, the effects were limited in some way compared with the investigators' expectations or prior research findings. For example, Fast ForWord use only appeared to have effects for a small subset of the groups studied by several researchers (Friel-Patti, DesBarres, & Thibodeau, 2001; Loeb, Stoke, & Fey, 2001; Troia, 2004; Troia & Whitney, 2003). In other studies, effects may have been observed on auditory or phonological awareness tasks but not on oral language or reading (Agnew, Dorn, & Eden, 2004; Beattie, 2001; Gillingham, 2001; Hook, Macaruso, & Jones, 2001; Pokorni, Worthington, & Jamison, 2004). Examination of these articles, which vary greatly in the number of subjects being reported, the nature of the subjects' difficulties, and the methods of implementation, may give the reader a broader perspective on our current understanding of the effects of Fast ForWord software.

Brain Function and Fast ForWord Language

Recent studies have shown that individuals with developmental dyslexia typically have difficulty with language processing (Snow, Burns, & Griffin, 1998). In addition to this, studies have suggested that individuals with developmental dyslexia have a neural deficit affecting phonological processing of written material (Temple, 2002). More specifically, individuals with dyslexia have lower brain activity in the left temporoparietal cortex when trying to identify the sounds that make up written words. Temple and colleagues (2003) recently completed a study on the effects of Fast ForWord Language on the brain function of children with dyslexia.

Twenty children with dyslexia (general intelligence in the average range and a reading measure below the 16th percentile), ages 8–12 years, used Fast ForWord Language for 100 minutes per day, 5 days per week, for an average of 28 days. Before and after their intensive language instruction, they underwent functional magnetic resonance imaging (fMRI) scans while performing a phonological processing task of determining whether letters rhymed (e.g., *t* and *d* rhyme, *g* and *k* do not) and were assessed with various language and reading standardized tests. A control group of 12 children with typical reading was matched by age, gender, handedness, and nonverbal IQ. Results from the recent study are summarized below.

- Prior to using the exercises, the children with dyslexia showed less brain activity (compared with the typical controls) in regions involved in phonological processing; namely, the left temporoparietal cortex and the left inferior frontal gyrus. After using Fast ForWord Language, the children with dyslexia showed increased activity in these critical brain areas, resulting in brain function that more closely resembled the typically reading controls.

- The analyses showed a significant positive correlation between oral language improvement (on the CELF-3) and increased activity in the left temporoparietal cortex, suggesting that improved oral language skills, typically achieved through the Fast ForWord Language exercises, have a direct relationship with increased brain activity in regions used during reading ($r = 0.58, p = 0.01$).

- On average, the Fast ForWord Language group made significant improvements in word identification, word attack, and passage comprehension skills, as measured by the Woodcock Reading Mastery Tests–Revised (Woodcock, 1987) ($p < 0.01$). The control children made significant improvements in passage comprehension skills ($p < 0.05$).

- Using the CELF-3 to measure oral language, the children with dyslexia made statistically significant gains in Receptive and Expressive Language scores ($p < 0.01$), and the control children did not.

- The children who used Fast ForWord Language made statistically significant improvements on the Rapid Naming subtest of the Comprehensive Test of Phonological Processing (CTOPP; Wagner, Torgesen, & Rashotte, 1999) ($p < 0.01$), whereas the control group decreased in their overall performance on this subtest.

This study provides evidence of brain plasticity and the ability of intense instruction to change brain activity and related language functioning, the underlying theories of Fast ForWord Language. After working with the exercises, the brain images of children with dyslexia showed physiological changes, resulting in brain function closer to that seen in children with typical reading skills. The Fast ForWord Language participants also exhibited significant improvements in six subtests that measure critical areas in oral language, reading, and rapid naming. In comparison, the control children did not make significant gains on any subtests.

Summary

Children with SLI generally have deficits in their auditory processing abilities. The Fast ForWord Language exercises are designed to develop phoneme identification and speech reception skills. In many studies, following an average of 4–6 weeks of use, statistically significant improvements were made on various standardized assessments, including measurements of expressive and receptive language, auditory discrimination, phonological awareness, and critical reading skills. In addition to these gains on standardized assessments, children who have used the product have been shown to have increased neurological activity in the areas of the brain necessary for reading effectiveness. These studies, done with varying populations and constraints, show that through the intensive instruction of the Fast ForWord Language exercises, children with language-learning deficits can be helped greatly.

PRACTICAL REQUIREMENTS

Fast ForWord Language is a computer-based product that offers the user the option of using the Internet to track and analyze student progress. To learn how to implement the Fast ForWord Language product, users typically attend a 2-day training session held by Scientific Learning. A small-scale implementation, such as that for a clinician, can be undertaken after a 1-day training or sometimes after just a self-paced tutorial called Fast ForWord Getting Started that is provided via the Internet. The training covers the science behind the product, how to choose appropriate participants, proper settings, and how to achieve an overall effective implementation.

The studies described here all use the Fast ForWord Language 100-Minute Protocol that has children work on the exercises for 100 minutes per day, 5 days per week, for 4–8 weeks, Scientific Learning has also evaluated alternative protocols that allow users more flexibility in the daily regimen: fewer minutes per day, more total days. For both protocols, the number of days the participant uses the product depends on how rapidly the child progresses through the material. Clinicians may have children use a computer in the clinic, either under the direct supervision of a professional or under the supervision of another trained individual whom Scientific Learning refers to as a *monitor*. Clinicians may also set up home sites, or other special sites, to accommodate a child's needs. Educators may have students use computers within the classroom or in a special lab or center. The number of children who can simultaneously use the product under the supervision of one person depends on the ages and abilities of the children. Young children and others who may have difficulty staying on-task for the full 100 minutes per day (e.g., children with autism spectrum disorder or ADHD diagnoses) may need one-on-one attention, whereas for many older children a group administration is appropriate. The monitor must be able to keep the children motivated and on-task. The monitor must also recognize when a child has stopped progressing, as intervention may be appropriate (e.g., ensuring that the child understands the task, or determining which language constructs are causing the child the most difficulty and working offline on those particular constructs). After each day's participation, the child's data can be sent via the Internet to Scientific Learning for analysis. The analyzed results can then be downloaded to the monitor's computer for review. Using monitoring tools available from Scientific Learning Corporation, such as Progress Viewer and Progress Tracker, it is possible to ensure that the child is making steady progress and to determine which components (e.g., language structures, phoneme discriminations, memory tasks) are particularly difficult for the child. This knowledge allows the clinician or educator to provide additional individualized support to the child, as appropriate. Fast ForWord Language can be run on either PC or Macintosh computers. For specific technical requirements, visit the Scientific Learning Corporation web site at http://www.scilearn.com. Because high-fidelity sound is necessary, it is important for children to wear headphones with ear cups. It is useful for the headphones to be connected by way of y-connectors that allow the monitor to listen to the stimuli the child is hearing—a most helpful aid when working with a child who has difficulties with the tasks.

KEY COMPONENTS

Nature of the Goals Addressed by the Intervention

The goal of the Fast ForWord Language exercises is to build perceptual, cognitive, and linguistic skills that provide the foundation for language and literacy development. Processing speed, phoneme discrimination, sound sequencing ability, sustained and focused attention, and working memory are all developed across the product's suite of exercises. In addition, some exercises directly address the language skills of auditory word recognition, language comprehension, and morphosyntax.

The central goal of improving listening skills is seen in all seven exercises. Other targeted skills, including working memory and syntax, are developed in two or more exercises. Having exercises overlap in the goals they address enhances generalization of skills. For instance, three of the tasks in Fast ForWord Language improve phoneme discrimination, but each task presents a different context and focuses on different phoneme combinations. Thus, all exercises work in tandem, and improvements on one will feed into improvements on another.

Procedural or Operational Description of Activities

The seven exercises comprising Fast ForWord Language can be categorized into sound, word, or sentence exercises, depending on their primary focus. During the initial orientation week, students gradually increase their attention span until they can attend to five exercises per day. After this initial period, students rotate through the exercises seeing each exercise at least 2 days each week. Key components of these exercises include repetition, motivation, and adaptive levels that match the difficulty of the task to the child's performance.

Repetition   The current recommended participation protocols are 100 minutes per day, 5 days per week, for 4–8 weeks or 50 minutes per day, 5 days per week for 8–12 weeks. These schedules allow students to use five exercises each day. Exercises that participants often take longer to master, such as sequencing frequency sweeps, are presented daily. The exercises that students often progress through rapidly are presented on a rotating schedule of 2 out of 4 days, or 3 out of 6 days. Although all of the exercises target a specific skill set, they also reinforce skills taught by the other exercises. As a child starts to work on an exercise that uses speech, for example, the speech is processed such that fast transitions are elongated and high frequencies are emphasized. This processing facilitates the ability of the child to distinguish between similar syllables, such as /ba/ and /da/. In another exercise (Circus Sequence), the child is being exposed to pairs of frequency sweeps and is asked to identify the order and direction of the sweeps. As the child correctly identifies the sweeps, the interstimulus interval (the time between the two sweeps) decreases from 500 to 0 milliseconds. This task directly addresses the child's rapid auditory processing skills, which are reinforced by the processed speech in the exercises that use speech. Additional protocols, including those that allow shorter periods of daily use or fewer days per week, are currently being evaluated.

Motivation   Motivation and attention are important components of the learning process. A child who is not engaged will not attend and will have difficulty mastering the material. Rewards, in the form of animations, are used to keep the children eagerly and actively participating in the exercises. In addition, the Fast ForWord Language exercises are based around a token economy. As students participate in the various exercises, they earn points. Because the exercises adjust to the level of the individual students, the numbers of points students earn are fairly similar. In an effort to keep students working to the full extent of their abilities, schools or clinicians are encouraged to help students set goals and also reward them for their activity. It can be useful to involve the family in this particular aspect. For example, giving the child a favorite meal when a goal is reached can be rewarding.

Adaptive Level   The difficulty level of the exercises is continually adapted to an appropriate level for the child. For example, children initially are presented with short sequences of instructions and sounds that vary slowly. Once they have mastered these stimuli, they are presented with longer sequences of instructions and the presentation rate of the sounds increases. If the child has difficulty with the sequences, the stimuli stay the same, or become easier, until the child is able to respond correctly. The result is that the child is working at a level at which he or she is achieving success—correctly responding to over 80% of the stimuli—but is constantly being exposed to stimuli that are near the limits of his or her ability. Across all the exercises that include words or sentences, Fast ForWord processing stretches fast transitions and enhances high frequencies, thus enhancing the differences between similar syllables and words. All speech to which children are exposed is initially altered to reduce perceptual difficulty to the greatest extent possible. As the children are able to correctly perform tasks and respond to instructions, the processing is reduced until the speech is unprocessed.

Sound Exercises   *Circus Sequence* improves working memory, sound processing speed, and sequencing skills. Participants hear a series of short, nonverbal tones. Each tone represents a different fragment of the frequency spectrum used in spoken language. Participants are then asked to differentiate between these tones and reproduce the sequence by clicking on two buttons in the correct order.

Old MacDonald's Flying Farm improves auditory processing, develops phoneme discrimination, and increases sustained and focused attention. Participants use the computer mouse to catch and hold a flying animal. When they do this, the animal begins repeating a single syllable. Participants must release the mouse when they detect a change in the syllable. The syllables are synthesized, and the changes in syllable relate to voice onset time; for example, /kɪ/ versus /gɪ/ or /doʊ/ ("doy") versus /toʊ/ ("toy").

Phoneme Identification is designed to improve auditory discrimination skills, increase rate of processing, improve working memory, and help students identify a specific phoneme. At the start of each trial, a target syllable or pseudoword is presented. Next, a pair of animal characters appears and each utters either the target or something similar. To respond correctly, participants must click on the animal that reproduced the target.

Word Exercises   *Phonic Match* develops auditory word recognition and phoneme discrimination, improves working memory, and strengthens rate of auditory processing. Participants choose a square on a grid and hear a syllable or word. Each syllable or word has a match somewhere within the grid. Every time the participant selects a matching pair, those squares disappear, until the grid has been cleared. Stimuli sets include combinations of *big, bit, dig, dip,* or other easily confused syllables or words.

Phonic Words was created to improve sound processing speed and phoneme and word recognition, and to help participants gain an understanding of word meaning. Participants see pairs of pictures representing words that differ only by one or two sounds. When they hear a word, participants must click the picture that matches it. Word pairs typically differ only by initial or final consonant (e.g., *tack* versus *tag*, *vase* versus *face*, *me* versus *knee*, *path* versus *pat*).

Sentence Exercises   *Language Comprehension Builder* is intended to develop oral language and listening comprehension, improve understanding of syntax and morphology, and increase rate of auditory processing. Participants listen to sentences depicting action and complex relational themes, selecting a picture that matches each sentence. Each correct picture is presented along with one, two, or three foils. The foil images are carefully constructed so that the correct selection cannot be made on the basis of content words alone. Rather, the participant must grasp the meaning conveyed by the sentence structure to make the correct selection.

The sentence stimuli are divided into seven comprehension levels, based on syntactic complexity. As participants successfully progress across levels, they will encounter more sophisticated syntactic structures. Within all comprehension levels, sentences are presented at all processing levels.

Block Commander is designed to increase listening comprehension and the ability to follow directions, improve syntax, develop working memory, and improve sound processing speed. A three-dimensional game board is filled with familiar shapes that participants select and manipulate, following verbal directions. These directions become increasingly complex across five difficulty levels.

At each Block Commander level, the participant is given instructions to be followed.

Level 1: The participant selects 1 of 8 objects based on color and shape.

Level 2: The participant selects 1 of 16 objects based on size, color, and shape.

Level 3: The participant selects 2 of 8 objects based on color and shape.

Level 4: The participant selects 2 of 16 objects based on size, color, and shape.

Level 5: The participant selects 2 or more of 8 objects and manipulates them based on syntactically complex directions involving time and space.

ASSESSMENT METHODS TO SUPPORT ONGOING DECISION MAKING

Various options are available to review children's performances and determine how they are progressing to completion. Progress History, one component of Progress Viewer and Progress Tracker, consists of a series of line graphs that depict the percent mastery for each exercise since the child began. By examining the graphs, the monitor can determine whether children are making gains in the exercises. If plateaus occur, the monitor should consider the number of days the child has worked with the product and the specific exercises on which the plateaus are occurring. Plateaus that develop after at least 20 participation days and continue for 4–5 participation days in several exercises could indicate that the child has reached a point of diminishing returns and should stop using the product.

When assessing a child's percent completion to help determine whether participation is complete, it is helpful to remember that 100% completion is not necessarily the goal during participation. Instead, it is important to consider whether the child is making gains in the exercises. It is also important to consider the reasons the child is seeking the services of a clinician. For example, a child with an auditory processing disorder may make especially slow progress on Circus Sequence, an exercise that focuses on auditory processing. To progress on this exercise, the child will need to understand sequencing and association. To help the child progress on Circus Sequence, the monitor can use visual, tactile, and auditory activities to help the child gain an understanding of the task.

If a child has been using the Fast ForWord Language exercises for fewer than 20 days and has reached at least 90% mastery on all the exercises, or has been using the product for more than 20 days and has reached a sufficiently high level on all exercises, the child may be considered finished with the program. Progress Viewer and Progress Tracker have flags that give guidance when a child has finished the product, or is not making satisfactory progress on an exercise. The guidance is based on the number of days a child has participated, the protocol the child is using, and the percentage complete in each of the individual exercises. As the number of participation days increases, the necessary percent complete decreases. After 25 days of participation on the 100-Minute Protocol, Progress Viewer and Progress Tracker check whether the participant has reached a plateau (remained at the same level in the exercises for at least 4 or 5 days). If this occurs, and the monitor has already tried the suggested interventions, the participant may also be considered finished with the exercises. At this point, the clinician may be interested in reassessing the child's language or phonological awareness skills.

CONSIDERATIONS FOR CHILDREN FROM CULTURALLY AND LINGUISTICALLY DIVERSE BACKGROUNDS

Children who are from culturally or linguistically diverse backgrounds often present special challenges to the SLP. Evidence collected to date suggests that Fast ForWord Language can be effective with children from a wide range of cultural and linguistic backgrounds (see Figure 18.7). Based on results from all students who have shared language assessment scores, it has been determined that, on average, these children improve their language skills following use. Before and after using Fast ForWord products, the students' language skills were assessed using the CELF-3, TOLD, or TACL-R. These comprehensive language tests measure a student's ability to understand words and sentences, follow directions, recall and formulate sentences, make generalizations, and understand relationships between words and categories. On average, students in each demographic group were well below the average range prior to using Fast ForWord products. After use, all demographic groups showed significant improvements in their language skills, with mean scores for the groups moving into the low-average to average range ($p < 0.0001$). In a study using random assignment to either Fast ForWord Language or the standard classroom curriculum, English language learners (ELLs) who used the product made significantly greater improvements on the TACL-R following product use than ELLs who did not use the product ($F(1, 79) = 4.63, p < 0.05$).

Depending on a child's background, some words or specific language structures used in the exercises may pose difficulty. The professional can use data gathered by the software as the child works on the exercises to guide them in providing extra instruction on those words or structures. In Language Comprehension Builder, for example, some of the tasks require the participant to focus on the verb to determine whether the subject is singular or plural. If a child makes no progress, or suddenly stops making progress, the clinician can use Progress Tracker to determine the linguistic structure causing the difficulty. The monitor may then instruct the participant on the word(s) or structure(s) causing the difficulty either before the session be-

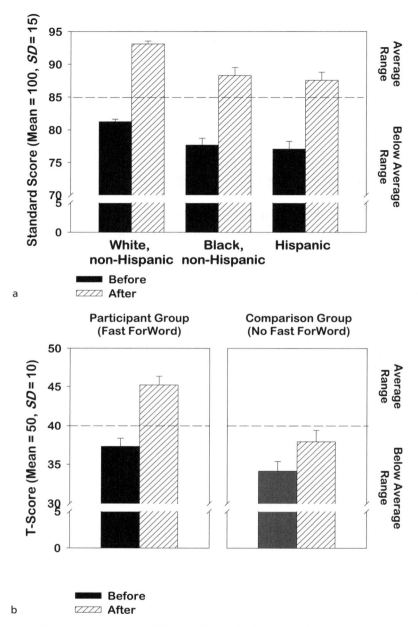

Figure 18.7. Improvements in children of different backgrounds. (a) Standard scores from the Clinical Evaluation of Language Fundamentals–Third Edition (CELF-3; Semel, Wiig, & Secord, 1995), Test of Language Development–Primary, Second Edition (TOLD-P:2; Hammill & Newcomer, 1988), or Test of Auditory Comprehension of Language–Revised (TACL-R; Carrow-Woolfolk, 1985) from different ethnic groups are shown. Before participation, on average, the students were performing in the below-average range. After using Fast ForWord Language, the groups made statistically significant gains, with the mean language scores moving into the average range. (b) ESL students who used Fast ForWord Language exercises performed significantly better on the TACL-R than the ESL students who remained in the regular classroom while receiving the standard curriculum.

gins or by drawing attention to the word or structure the child needs to focus on during the exercise.

APPLICATION TO AN INDIVIDUAL CHILD

A typical case is Christopher, a 7-year-old boy who received 1 year of speech and language intervention when he was 4 years old. At that time, he was speaking in short sentences but his speech was unintelligible.

History

Christopher was the third child in a family of four boys. Christopher's mother reported that Christopher started talking late, at about 16 months. He had had several ear infections during his first year of life, but they cleared after standard antibiotic therapy. Myringotomy tubes were not recommended. Christopher's pediatrician had reportedly told the parents at his 1-year checkup that Christopher might start talking a little later because of the ear infections and because he was a middle child. The doctor suggested that if Christopher did not begin speaking by 18 months, a professional SLP should be consulted. Christopher did begin saying "mama" and a few other words around age 16 months, so his parents no longer saw a need to worry. However, as Christopher began talking more, others could not understand him. At first, his mother thought it was typical baby talk. His mother noted that he called Mickey Mouse [humama], for example. But unlike her older children, these "baby words" did not change. Her friends and family constantly commented on how hard it was to understand Christopher. Many of his words did not resemble what he was trying to say at all. Christopher's mother said she usually knew what he was saying, but even her husband could not understand him most of the time.

Initial Speech and Language Intervention

At Christopher's 3-year checkup a pure-tone audiological screening and tympanography were ordered and found to be normal. Christopher began talking more during the next year, but as his sentences became longer they were harder and harder to understand. Finally, his parents and physician decided it was time for speech-language therapy. The therapist targeted phonological processes (e.g., Hodson & Paden, 1991) with Christopher. After about 1 year, his speech was considered within normal limits and he was discharged.

Recent Academic Problems

When Christopher entered kindergarten, at 5.5 years of age, he seemed to do well in some areas. He was very social and energetic. He had good physical coordination for sports. His kindergarten teacher was somewhat concerned that he had trouble learning the alphabet, but his father noted that he, too, had had the same problems when he was young, so no intervention was recommended. Christopher was rated as an average student in first grade, but by the middle of second grade his teacher noticed he had trouble "sounding out" new words. She also was concerned because Christopher seemed to "tune out" during story time, appeared to daydream a lot, and did not follow instructions well. The teacher recommended that Christopher's parents read more with him at home.

At the end of the second grade, the standardized testing performed at school indicated a marked drop in Christopher's reading score. He had scored at the 5th stanine after first grade but was now testing at the 2nd stanine. He also had started to exhibit some behavioral problems in school. He often "acted out" during reading lessons and was disruptive during the day, especially when the teacher was giving lessons. The teacher again recommended that his parents spend more time with Christopher on his homework and read to him.

Christopher's parents decided to revisit the speech clinic to see if there could be residuals of his speech problem that could explain the problems in school. The SLP noted on retesting that Christopher fell 1–2 *SD* below the norm on several CELF-3 subtests: Formulated Sentences, Recalling Sentences, and Concepts and Directions. On the Phonological Awareness Test. Christopher showed marked impairments in isolation of phonemes, segmentation, and decoding nonsense words. The SLP felt that the combination of the history of a phonological disorder, significant delays in some language areas, and a marked phonological awareness disorder represented a pattern of disturbance that would respond very well to Fast ForWord Language. She immediately enrolled Christopher in the intensive instruction.

Fast ForWord Intervention

Christopher did very well on some of the components such as Phonic Words and Language Comprehension Builder. However, he struggled with Circus Sequence, Phoneme Identification, and Block Commander. It was not surprising that these exercises posed particular difficulty for Christopher because these are the same areas (i.e., rapid auditory processing, phonemic discrimination, and following directions) that often led to problems with acquisition of phonology, language processing, and phonological awareness.

Christopher successfully completed the Fast ForWord Language exercises after 8 weeks during the summer before third grade. The SLP retested him and found that the following scores had increased: CELF-3 Receptive Language standard score increased from 84 to 99 and CELF-3 Expressive Language standard score increased from 74 to 89. The Receptive Language standard score increase was due primarily to changes in the Concepts and Directions subtest, for which standard score increased from 5 to 8. The Expressive Language standard score improvement was due to changes in the Formulated Sentences and Recalling Sentences subtests, for which his standard scores increased from 4 to 8, and from 6 to 9, respectively. Christopher also improved on the Phonological Awareness Test, for which his major gains were made on the Isolation and Deletion subtests.

Christopher's parents were pleased with the new confidence he seemed to exhibit when he entered the third grade. They noticed he seemed to be listening better at home as well, and entered into conversations with his family more freely. The SLP advised that although he performed better on the standardized tests, the Fast ForWord Language product addresses language fundamentals but does not teach reading per se. She continued work on phonological awareness and phonological decoding to support his early months in the third grade and help him quickly catch up to his peers in reading skills. Christopher's parents enrolled him in a phonics-based reading tutoring program at a nearby center.

In the third grade, Christopher had a new teacher, and his parents were anxious to see if she would notice the same problems with decoding and listening. At Christopher's fall conference, the teacher said he was a good student in many areas. She said he seemed to be a little behind in reading vocabulary but was learning quickly. By the spring conference, Christopher's teacher stated he was a "solid reader" and a "good classroom citizen."

FUTURE DIRECTIONS

Scientific Learning continues to engage in research on the learning conditions under which students can derive the greatest benefit from using Fast ForWord Language. Factors currently under examination include participant selection, product implementation, monitor activities, and protocols.

When the Fast ForWord Language product is used with Progress Tracker, participant performance data can regularly be uploaded to Scientific Learning. Participants also have the opportunity to share background information (e.g., ethnicity, ELL, gifted classes). With more than 100,000 students having used the Fast ForWord Language exercises, we have accrued a unique database of usage information. Currently, we are making a detailed analysis of daily exercise results from various groups of students to investigate how they progress and to identify how and when progress is impaired.

Some participants also have their language skills assessed before and after using the product. When participants are willing to share their results with us, we can take a closer look at the relationship between product use and benefits. This information is currently being applied to studies investigating the benefits found with alternate protocols.

REFERENCES

Agnew, J.A., Dorn, C., & Eden, G.F. (2004). Effect of intensive training on auditory processing and reading skills. *Brain and Language, 88*(1), 21–25.

Aram, D.M., Ekelman, B.L., & Nation, J.E. (1984). Preschoolers with language disorders: 10 years later. *Journal of Speech and Hearing Research, 27*, 232–244.

Battin, R.R., Young, M., & Burns, M. (2000). Use of Fast ForWord in remediation of Central Auditory Processing Disorders. *The Bulletin of the American Academy of Audiology, Audiology Today, 12*(2), 13–15.

Beattie, K.K. (2001). *The effects of intensive computer-based language intervention on language functioning and reading achievement in language-impaired adolescents. Dissertation Abstracts International, 61* (08), 3116A.

Bedi, G.C., Tallal, P., Miller, S.L., Byma, G., Merzenich, M.M., & Jenkins, W.M. (1995). Efficacy of temporal-based training for receptive language and auditory discrimination deficits in language-learning impaired children: A follow-up study. *Journal of Cognitive Neuroscience Supplement*, April, 55.

Catts, H.W. (1993). The relationship between speech-language impairments and reading disabilities. *Journal of Speech and Hearing Research, 36,* 948–958.

Catts, H.W., Fey, M.E., Tomblin, J.B., & Zhang, X. (2002). A longitudinal investigation of reading outcomes in children with language impairments. *Journal of Speech, Language, and Hearing Research, 45,* 1142–1157.

Carrow-Woolfolk, E. (1985). *Test of Auditory Comprehension of Language–Revised Edition*. Austin, TX: PRO-ED.

Curtiss, S., & Yamada, J. (1987). *The Curtiss-Yamada Comprehensive Language Evaluation*. Irvine, CA: CYCLE, Inc.

DiSimoni, F. (1978). *The Token Test for Children*. Austin, TX: PRO-ED.

Dronkers, N.F., Husted, D.A., Deutsch, G., Tayler, M.K., Saunders, G., & Merzenich, M.M. (1999). Lesion site as a predictor of improvement after "Fast ForWord" treatment in adult aphasic patients. *Brain & Language, 69,* 450–452.

Eadie, P.A., Fey, M.E., Douglas, J.M., & Parsons, C.L. (2002). Profiles of grammatical morphology and sentence imitation in children with specific language impairment and Down syndrome. *Journal of Speech, Language, and Hearing Research, 45,* 720–732.

Fellbaum, C., Miller, S., Curtiss, S., & Tallal, P. (1995). An auditory processing deficit as a possible source of SLI. In D. MacLaughlin & S. McEwen (Eds.), *Proceedings of the 19th annual Boston University Conference on Language Development* (pp. 1204–1215). Somerville, MA: Cascadilla Press.

Friel-Patti, S., DesBarres, K., & Thibodeau, L. (2001). Case studies of children using Fast ForWord. *American Journal of Speech-Language Pathology, 10*(3), 203–215.

Gathercole, S.E., & Baddeley, A.D. (1990). Phonological memory deficits in language disordered children: Is there a causal connection? *Journal of Memory and Language, 29,* 336–360.

Gillam, R.B., Cowan, N., & Marler, J.A. (1998). Information processing by school-age children with specific language impairment: Evidence from a modality effect paradigm. *Journal of Speech, Language, and Hearing Research, 41,* 913–926.

Gillingham, G.G. (2001). Differential diagnosis and treatment of attention deficit hyperactivity disorder and central auditory processing disorders. *Dissertation Abstracts International, 62* (04), 2057B.

Goldman, R., Fristoe, M., & Woodcock, R.W. (1970). *Goldman-Fristoe-Woodcock Test of Auditory Discrimination*. Circle Pines, MN: American Guidance Service.

Hammill, D.D., & Newcomer, P.L. (1988). *Test of Language Development–Intermediate, Second Edition (TOLD-I:2)*. Austin, TX: PRO-ED.

Hammill, D.D., & Newcomer, P.L. (1988). *Test of Language Development–Primary, Second Edition (TOLD-P:2)*. Austin, TX: PRO-ED.

Hodson, B., & Paden, E. (1991). *Targeting intelligible speech: A phonological approach to remediation* (2nd ed.). Austin, TX: PRO-ED.

Hook, P.E., Macaruso, P., & Jones, S. (2001). Efficacy of Fast ForWord training on facilitating acquisition of reading skills by children with reading difficulties: A longitudinal study. *Annals of Dyslexia, 51,* 75–96.

Johnson, C.J., Beitchman, J.H., Young, A., Escobar, M., Atkinson, L., Wilson, B., Brownlie, E.B., Douglas, L., Taback, N., Lam, I., & Wang, M. (1999). Fourteen-year follow-up of children with and without speech/language impairments: Speech/language stability and outcomes. *Journal of Speech, Language, and Hearing Research, 42,* 744–760.

Karni, A., & Sagi, D. (1991). Where practice makes perfect in texture discrimination: Evidence for primary visual cortex plasticity. *Proceedings of the National Academy of Sciences of the United States of America, 88,* 4966–4970.

Karni, A., & Sagi, D. (1993). The time course of learning a visual skill. *Nature, 365,* 250–253.

Katz, J. (1962). The use of staggered spondaic words for assessing the integrity of the central auditory nervous system. *Journal of Auditory Research, 2,* 327–337.

Katz, J. (1968). The SSW test: An interim report. *Journal of Speech and Hearing Disorders, 33,* 132–145.

Katz, J. (1985). Combined national sample—1985 norms: Ages 5 to 60 years. *SSW Report, 7,* 1–6.

Katz, J., & Smith, P.S. (1991). The Staggered Spondaic Word Test: A ten-minute look at the central nervous system through the ears. *Annals of the New York Academy of Sciences, 620,* 233–251.

Keith, R.W. (1986). *SCAN: A screening test for auditory processing disorders.* San Antonio, TX: Harcourt Assessment.

Kertesz, A. (1982). *The Western Aphasia Battery.* London: Grune & Stratton.

Lawa, G., & Bishop, D.V.M. (2003). A comparison of language abilities in adolescents with Down syndrome and children with specific language impairment. *Journal of Speech, Language, and Hearing Research, 46,* 1324–1339.

Leonard, L. (1998). *Children with specific language impairments.* Cambridge, MA: The MIT Press.

Leonard, L., McGregor, K., & Allen, G. (1992). Grammatical morphology and speech perception in children with specific language impairment. *Journal of Speech and Hearing Research, 35,* 1076–1085.

Liberman, I.Y., Shankweiler, D., Fisher, R.W., & Carter, B. (1974). Explicit syllable and phoneme segmentation in the young child. *Journal of Experimental Child Psychology, 18,* 201–212.

Lindamood, C., & Lindamood, P. (1971, 1979). *Lindamood Auditory Conceptualization Test.* Austin, TX: PRO-ED.

Loeb, D.F., Stoke, C., & Fey, M.E. (2001). Language changes associated with Fast ForWord Language: Evidence from case studies. *American Journal of Speech-Language Pathology, 10*(3), 216–230.

Marion, G.G. (2004). An examination of the relationship between students' use of the Fast ForWord reading program and their performance on standardized assessments in elementary schools. *Dissertation Abstracts International, 65*(01), 106A.

Melzer, M., & Poglitch, G. (1998, November). *Functional changes reported after Fast ForWord training for 100 children with autism spectrum disorders.* Paper presented at the annual meeting of the American Speech-Language-Hearing Association, San Antonio, TX.

Merzenich, M., & deCharms, R.C. (1996). Neural representation, experience and change. In R. Llinas & P. Churchland (Eds.), *The mind-brain continuum.* Cambridge, MA: The MIT Press.

Merzenich, M.M., & Jenkins, W.M (1995). Cortical plasticity, learning, and learning dysfunction. In B. Julesz & I. Kovacs (Eds.), *Maturational windows and adult cortical plasticity* (pp. 247–272). Santa Fe, NM: Addison-Wesley.

Merzenich, M.M., Jenkins, W.M., Johnston, P., Schriener, C.E., Miller, S.L., & Tallal, P. (1996). Temporal processing deficits of language-learning impaired children ameliorated by training. *Science, 271,* 77–80.

Merzenich, M.M., Saunders, G., Jenkins, W.M., Miller, S., Peterson, B., & Tallal, P. (1999). Pervasive developmental disorders: Listening training and language abilities. In S. Broman & J. Fletcher (Eds.), *The changing nervous system: Neurobehavioral consequences of early brain disorders* (pp. 365–385). New York: Oxford University Press.

Merzenich, M., Spengler, F., Byl, N., Wang, X., & Jenkins, W. (1996). Representational plasticity underlying learning: Contributions to the origins and expressions of neurobehavioral disabilities. In T. Ono, B.L. McNaughton, S. Molotchnikoff, E.T. Rolls, & H. Nishijo (Eds.), *Perception, memory and emotion: Frontiers in neuroscience.* Oxford, England: Elsevier.

Merzenich, M., Wright, B., Jenkins, W., Xerri, C., Byl, N., Miller, S., & Tallal, P. (1996). Cortical plasticity underlying perceptual, motor, and cognitive skill development: Implications for neurorehabilitation. *Cold Spring Harbor Symposia on Quantitative Biology, 61,* 1–8.

Miller, C.A., Kail, R., Leonard, L.B., & Tomblin, J.B. (2001). Speed of processing in children with specific language impairment. *Journal of Speech, Language, and Hearing Research, 44,* 416–433.

Miller, S.L., Merzenich, M.M., Tallal, P., DeVivo, K., LaRossa, K., Linn, N., Pycha, A., Peterson, B.E., & Jenkins, W.M. (1999). *Fast ForWord training in children with low reading performance.* Nederlandse Vereniging voor Lopopedie en Foniatrie: 1999 Jaarcongres Auditieve Vaardigheden en Spraak-taal (Proceedings of the 1999 Dutch National Speech-Language Association meeting).

Montgomery, J.W. (2000). Verbal working memory and sentence comprehension in children with specific language impairment. *Journal of Speech, Language, and Hearing Research, 43,* 293–308.

Morlet, T., Norman, M., Ray, B., & Berlin, C.I. (2003). Fast ForWord: Its scientific basis and treatment effects on the human efferent auditory system. In C.I. Berlin & T.G. Weyand (Eds.), *The brain and sensory plasticity: Language acquisition and hearing* (pp. 129–148). Clifton Park, NY: Thomson Delmar Learning.

Nagarajan, S.S., Wang, X., Merzenich, M.M., Schreiner, C.E., Johnston, P., Jenkins, W., Miller, S., & Tallal, P. (1998). Speech modifications algorithms used for training language-learning impaired children. *IEEE Transactions on Rehabilitation Engineering, 6,* 257–268.

Newcomer, P.L., & Hammill, D.D. (1991). *Test of Language Development–Primary, Second Edition.* Austin, TX: PRO-ED.

Noterdaeme, M., Mildenberger, K., Minow, F., & Amorosa, H. (2002). Quantitative and qualitative evaluation of neuromotor behavior in children with a specific speech and language disorder. *Infant and Child Development, 11,* 3–15.

Pokorni, J.L., Worthington, C.K., & Jamison, P.J. (2004). Phonological awareness intervention: Comparison of Fast ForWord, Earobics, and LIPS. *Journal of Educational Research, 97*(3), 147–157.

Rayner, K., & Pollatsek, A. (1989). *The psychology of reading.* Englewood Cliffs, NJ: Prentice Hall.

Robertson, C., & Salter, W. (1997). *The Phonological Awareness Test.* East Moline, IL: LinguiSystems.

Robey, R.R., & Schultz, M.C. (1998). A model for conducting clinical-outcome research: An adaptation of the standard protocol for use in aphasiology. *Aphasiology, 12,* 787–810.

Schopmeyer, B., Mellon, N., Dobaj, H., Grant, G., & Niparko, J.K. (2000). Use of Fast ForWord to enhance language development in children with cochlear implants. *Annals of Otology, Rhinology, and Laryngology, 109*(12), 95–98.

Scientific Learning Corporation. (n.d.). *National field trials.* Retrieved April 15, 2003, from http://www.scilearn.com/scie/index.php3?main=nft/scienational

Scientific Learning Corporation. (2003). Improved listening comprehension by middle school students in the Waupun School District who used Fast ForWord Middle & High School. *MAPS for Learning: Educator Reports, 7*(2), 1–4.

Scientific Learning Corporation. (2004a). Improved language and early reading skills by students at Cherry Hill Public School District in New Jersey who used Fast ForWord Language. *MAPS for Learning: Educator Reports, 8*(4), 1–5.

Scientific Learning Corporation. (2004b). Improved language skills by students at Mora School District who used Fast ForWord Language. *MAPS for Learning: Educator Reports, 8*(19), 1–4.

Scientific Learning Corporation. (2004c). Improved Ohio Reading Proficiency Test Scores by students in the Springfield City School District who used Fast ForWord products. *MAPS for Learning: Educator Reports, 8*(8), 1–5.

Scientific Learning Corporation. (2004d). Improved reading achievement by students in the Pawhuska and Harlandale School Districts who used Fast ForWord to Reading 3. *MAPS for Learning: Educator Reports, 8*(13), 1–3.

Scientific Learning Corporation. (2004e). Improved reading skills by students at the Cobb County School District in Georgia who used Fast ForWord products. *MAPS for Learning: Educator Reports, 8*(5), 1–5.

Semel, E., Wiig, E.H., & Secord, W. (1995). *Clinical evaluation of language fundamentals* (3rd ed.). San Antonio, TX: Harcourt Assessment.

Slattery, C. (2003). *The impact of a computer-based training system on strengthening phonemic awareness and increasing reading ability level.* Ann Arbor, MI: ProQuest Information and Learning Company.

Snow, C.E., Burns, M.S., & Griffin, P. (1998). *Preventing reading difficulties in young children.* National Academy Press, Washington DC.

Stark, R., & Tallal, P. (1988). *Language, speech, and reading disorders in children: Neuropsychological studies.* Boston: Little, Brown.

Tallal, P., Allard, L., Miller, S.L., & Curtiss, S. (1997). Academic outcomes of language impaired children. In C. Hulme & M. Snowling (Eds.), *Dyslexia: Biology, cognition and intervention* (pp. 167–181). London: Whurr Publishers/British Dyslexia Association.

Tallal, P., Miller, S.L., Bedi, G., Byma, G., Wang, X., Nagarajan, S.S., Schreiner, C., Jenkins, W.M., & Merzenich, M.M. (1996). Language comprehension in language-learning impaired children improved with acoustically modified speech. *Science, 271*, 81–84.

Tallal, P., & Piercy, M. (1974). Developmental aphasia: Rate of auditory processing and selective impairment of consonant perception. *Neuropsychologia, 12*, 83–93.

Tallal, P., & Piercy, M. (1975). Developmental aphasia: The perception of brief vowels and extended stop consonants. *Neuropsychologia, 13*, 69–74.

Temple, E. (2002). Brain mechanisms in normal and dyslexic readers. *Current Opinions in Neurobiology, 12*, 178–183.

Temple, E., Deutsch, G., Poldrack, R., Miller, S., Tallal, P., Merzenich, M., & Gabrieli, J. (2003). Neural deficits in children with dyslexia ameliorated by behavioral remediation: Evidence from functional MRI. *Proceedings of the National Academy of Sciences of the United States of America, 100*, 2860–2865.

Torgesen, J.K., & Bryant, B.R. (1994). *Test of Phonological Awareness.* Austin, TX: PRO-ED.

Troia, G.A. (2004). Migrant students with limited English proficiency: Can Fast ForWord Language™ make a difference in their language skills and academic achievement? *Remedial and Special Education, 25*(6), 353–366.

Troia, G.A., & Whitney, S.D. (2003). A close look at the efficacy of Fast ForWord Language for children with academic weaknesses. *Contemporary Educational Psychology, 28*, 464–495.

Wagner, R., Torgesen, J.K., & Rashotte, C. (1999). *Comprehensive Test of Phonological Processing (CTOPP).* Austin, TX: PRO-ED.

Windsor, J., & Hwang, M. (1999). Testing the generalized slowing hypothesis in specific language impairment. *Journal of Speech, Language, and Hearing Research, 42*, 1205–1218.

Woodcock, R. (1987). *Woodcock Reading Mastery Tests–Revised.* Circle Pines, MN: American Guidance Service.

Woodcock, R.W., & Johnson, M.B. (1989, 1990). *Woodcock-Johnson Psycho-Educational Battery–Revised.* Itasca, IL: Riverside.

Wright, B.A., Lombardino, L.J., Wayne, M.K., Puranik, C.S., Leonard, C.M., & Merzenich, M.M. (1997). Deficits in auditory temporal and spectral resolution in language-impaired children. *Nature, 387,* 176–178.

Young, A.R., Beitchman, J.H., Johnson, C., Douglas, L., Atkinson, L., Escobar, M., & Wilson, B. (2002). Young adult academic outcomes in a longitudinal sample of early identified language impaired and control children. *Journal of Child Psychology and Psychiatry, 43,* 635–645.

19

Functional Communication Training

A Strategy for Ameliorating Challenging Behavior

JAMES W. HALLE, MICHAELENE M. OSTROSKY, AND MARY LOUISE HEMMETER

ABSTRACT

This chapter is devoted to a relatively new communication- or language-based strategy for addressing problem behavior of individuals with and without labeled disabilities. It is referred to as *functional communication training* (FCT) and is based on the notion that problem behavior may function as a means of communication. FCT involves assessing the function that a problem behavior serves for the individual, then teaching a new response that serves the same function. Viewing behavior other than words as communicative is a necessity when working with individuals who have little, if any, functional language. For this group, problem behavior may play an especially significant role, enabling them to influence others in their environment. Even for those with more sophisticated language, problem behavior may be the most efficient means to produce intended outcomes.

INTRODUCTION

The conceptual framework on which functional communication training (FCT) is based is logical and compelling: If challenging behavior has a particular communicative function, and we can teach a socially acceptable means of achieving the same function, then the latter might replace the former. Such an approach has at least two beneficial outcomes: First, the challenging behavior is no longer needed; thus, its frequency may be reduced. Second, a new skill (i.e., form of communication) is acquired. Although this process may sound simple, teaching a functional replacement skill that is used in a vari-

This chapter was supported in part by Grants H324C020098, H324Z010001, and H325D010009 from the Office of Special Education Programs of the U.S. Department of Education and by Grant 90YD0119 from the Public Health Service. Opinions expressed herein are those of the authors and do not necessarily reflect the position of the U.S. Department of Education or the Public Health Service.

ety of situations and is durable over time is anything but simple. A recent and burgeoning literature has revealed multiple methods for assessing problem behavior and multiple strategies for intervention, based on the assessment results. However, even with federal support and a very active group of talented researchers focusing on the topic, many issues remain to be resolved. These include the determination of optimal occasions for implementing FCT, teaching *multiple* socially adaptive options, and ensuring the generalized use of newly taught options over time and across varied situations (Carr et al., 1994; Durand, 1990; Meyer & Evans, 1989; Wacker, Peck, Derby, Berg, & Harding, 1996). All of these issues and more will be addressed in this chapter.

Before beginning our discussion of FCT, we need to clarify three issues. The first concerns the nature of FCT research. The majority of experimental research on FCT can be found in the *Journal of Applied Behavior Analysis* spanning the years 1990–2004. Most of these are efficacy investigations that are limited to 10–30-minute sessions or samples of behavior in situations intentionally structured to trigger problem behavior and then teach replacement responses. In a series of efficacy studies, researchers have investigated variations in FCT or associated features in an effort to refine the procedure and to isolate its functional elements (e.g., Hanley, Iwata, & Thompson, 2001; Perry & Fisher, 2001; Winborn, Wacker, Richman, Asmus, & Geier, 2002). We purposely have omitted many of these analogue studies from our review and, instead, have chosen to focus on those with greater ecological validity (i.e., conducted in settings that more closely approximate natural routines and contexts) and, thus, may be considered to be effectiveness studies (Fey, 2002).

The second and third issues relate to our use of wording to describe two key concepts. One pertains to the type of behavior that is a primary focus of this chapter. We will use two adjectives interchangeably: *challenging* and *problem*. Both refer to behavior of targeted individuals that has been identified by teachers, parents, and/or others or others who inhabit the same settings as dangerous, disruptive, or disturbing. The third issue deals with the concept of *behavior,* another primary focus. Most often we will use synonymously the nouns *behavior* or *response*. Occasionally, we may use the nouns *form* or *signal,* especially when referring to behavior that may be communicative.

TARGET POPULATIONS AND ASSESSMENTS FOR DETERMINING TREATMENT RELEVANCE AND GOALS

The primary target population for FCT includes individuals who have severe and profound mental retardation, autism spectrum disorders, pervasive developmental disorder (PDD), or other syndromes and who present profiles of challenging behavior. Originally, FCT was designed for individuals who had not acquired language or had very rudimentary communicative repertoires and who engaged in problem behavior (Carr & Durand, 1985a; Durand, 1982, 1990). In fact, these two characteristics were not viewed as independent of one another. Carr and Durand (1985b) reviewed literature that supports the existence of an inverse relationship between the development of language and the development of problem behavior. This inverse relationship is evident among typically developing infants around 10–18 months of age who demonstrate reductions in levels of crying as words are acquired. It is easy to imagine that if an individual does not acquire language to convey wants and needs to others, then alternative means of communication will emerge. Whether these alternatives are socially adaptive depends to a large extent on their effect on the social partners with whom that individual interacts. Over time, challenging forms of behavior may produce desired outcomes more immediately and more consistently than more conventional forms (Baer, 1982; Halle & Drasgow, 2003).

More recently, however, FCT has been applied to a second group of individuals. Unlike the original group targeted, this new group possesses age-appropriate language (in many cases, sophisticated language), but they still engage in problem behavior; not because they do not have the requisite repertoire of language forms, but perhaps due to efficiency considerations (discussed later in this chapter). The labels given to this new group might include emotional or severe emotional disturbance, behavior disorder, and autism spectrum disorder, including Asperger syndrome.

It is noteworthy that the common denominator for both groups who have been the focus of FCT is problem behavior. Problem behavior is the trigger that sets into motion consideration of FCT and its associated battery of assessments. The assessments used to determine the appropriateness of FCT for individual children are well established and carefully delineated in the developmental disabilities literature (Carr et al., 1994; Durand, 1990; O'Neill et al., 1997). Later in this chapter, we discuss in some detail functional behavior assessment (FBA) as a key component of FCT. FBA encompasses a comprehensive set of strategies that isolate not only the function of challenging behavior, but also its triggering antecedents and maintaining consequences.

Although we have provided specific descriptors or labels for target populations that have benefited from FCT, we believe that the approach is generic. That is, its effectiveness is not limited to those with particular diagnoses, even though its empirical support may be limited at this time to individuals with specific labels. Its wide-scale application to anyone, inclusive of the authors of this chapter as well as its readers, is supported by a conceptual logic that is simultaneously compelling and intuitive (but still requires empirical support). We all find ourselves in situations in which our behavior could have been more effective and efficient at producing the intended outcome we seek. When this occurs, some form of FCT could be invoked. As we will discuss later in the chapter, such changes in behavior depend in large part on how others respond to our behavior, both immediately and over time.

THEORETICAL BASIS

In this section, we will trace the conceptual underpinnings of FCT by reviewing B.F. Skinner's contributions and by providing an overview of the functional approach to behavior.

Skinner's Contributions

The theoretical perspective most closely aligned with FCT is operant, or instrumental, conditioning. This approach can be traced most directly to Skinner, who made two major contributions to present-day FCT, one methodological and the other substantive. First, his methodological approach to experimentation, referred to as the *experimental analysis of behavior*, is still the most common methodology in studies providing the evidence base for FCT. It now is referred to as *single-subject research*, and most of the literature cited in this chapter reflects this methodology. It is characterized by at least five features: 1) a focus on behavior and its objective measurement; 2) small numbers (e.g., 1–5) of participants; 3) repeated measures of the dependent variable gathered within and across conditions; 4) subjects serving as their own controls, so varying conditions are introduced to the same subject over time; and 5) demonstration of experimental control through replication of effect across conditions within an individual (cf. Horner et al., 2005; Kazdin, 1982; McReynolds & Kearns, 1983).

Skinner's second major contribution to FCT was his theory of human behavior, referred to as *operant conditioning*. As part of this theory, Skinner elucidated principles that explain behavior as a function of the consequences produced by the behavior. People *operate* on their environment to produce intended consequences or outcomes. The behavioral or operant approach includes the following primary features: 1) environmental influence is prominent; 2) behavior can be understood by referring to current conditions (see ABC framework, in the next paragraph) with less emphasis on past events as explanatory; and 3) the principles of behavior describing relationships between behavior and the environment are ubiquitous, influencing behavior whether or not we realize it. For example, the principle of reinforcement refers to a relationship whereby a behavior is followed by a consequence that strengthens the future probability of the behavior. Consider an example of a child pointing to and vocalizing a request for potato chips at the supermarket. Her dad says, "No," which results in the child screaming and crying. When her dad immediately gives her the chips, screaming and crying have been reinforced by gaining access to the chips. Technically, we could say potato chips were a reinforcer only if the child's screaming and crying at the supermarket increased in the future. Incidentally, another behavior principle was operating in this example: extinction of the child's pointing and vocalizing because her father did not respond to these signals. According to the principle of extinction, these request forms would become less probable in the future at the supermarket.

In highlighting the primacy of environmental determination, Skinner described a three-term contingency, also referred to as the ABCs (Antecedents–Behavior–Consequences) of behavioral influence. As will become apparent below, the contingency between behavior and its consequences empowers antecedents such that they too influence the likelihood of behavior. The *A* represents antecedent events that "set the occasion" for or cue behavior. Behavior becomes more probable in the presence of particular antecedent events or contextual stimuli because, in the past, such stimuli have been present when the behavior has been reinforced. Therefore, reinforcement strengthens or increases the probability not just of a response, but a response *in a particular situation.* If we were to teach a child to greet others by reinforcing the greeting response only when an individual looks at the child and is in proximity, the child likely would learn to initiate greetings *when another is close by and establishes eye contact* and would withhold greetings at other times. Proximity and eye contact become functional cues that signal that a greeting likely will be reinforced.

The *B* in the ABCs of behavioral influence represents the behavior under study. It must be operationally defined such that an observer could measure reliably its occurrence and lack of occurrence. Although the systematic or intentional use of the principles of behavior are codified as applied behavior analysis and target specific behavioral deficits or excesses, their unsystematic or unintentional operation affects behavior all of the time. In other words, it is assumed in this approach that even when we are not systematically analyzing behavior and its determinants, the principles are still operating and influencing behavior.

C stands for the consequences of a behavior. Consequences are those environmental events that occur after the behavior and have one of three functions. They either increase, decrease, or have no effect on future probability of a behavior. If an increase occurs, the consequence is *reinforcing;* if a decrease occurs, it is *punishing;* if no change occurs, the consequence was irrelevant in relation to the behavior. The principles of behavior are defined, in large part, by the effect of consequences on behavior (i.e., increase or decrease in future probability).

In recent years, a fourth term, *setting events,* has been added to this early framework. Setting events, closely associated with *establishing operations* (Michael, 1982), are a relatively new addition to the analysis of environmental influence. Behavior analysts posit that events occurring earlier in time (often much earlier) that either have ended or are ongoing predispose learners to behave in particular ways. Unlike antecedents, which directly trigger problem behavior, setting events strengthen the reinforcing value of particular consequences and weaken the value of others, producing a change in the probability of behavior options. Thus, after a poor night's sleep, a boy with autism may scream and hit his teacher the next morning in school when she instructs him to put his backpack in his locker, even though he complies readily on most mornings (those when he has slept well). As a consequence of his screaming and hitting, the child is placed in an isolated corner of the classroom by himself where he closes his eyes and rests. Due to his sleep deficit, the reinforcing value of consequences associated with complying with the teacher's instruction (i.e., teacher approval) is weakened and the reinforcing value of consequences associated with challenging behavior (i.e., being left alone to rest) is enhanced.

Although Skinner's two contributions have been a major impetus to present-day behavioral applications, it was the early experimental applications of operant conditioning to human behavior of social significance in the late 1950s and early 1960s (e.g., Allyon & Michael, 1959; Bijou, 1955, 1957; Ferster, 1961; Staats, Staats, Schultz, & Wolf, 1962) that permitted a direct link to present-day FCT. Baer, Wolf, and Risley (1968) coined the term *applied behavior analysis* to refer to these experimental applications.

Functional Approach to Behavior

Operant conditioning is an example of a functional approach to human behavior. It emanates from the conceptual explanation that environmental variables determine behavior. The mechanisms by which consequences influence the future probability of behavior are defined by the principles of behavior: people will behave in ways that maximize positive consequences and minimize negative consequences. Thus, behavior that in the past produced reinforcing consequences or outcomes will be emitted. The following six concepts are fundamental to understanding the underpinnings of FCT.

Behavior serves a function for the person engaging in it (Carr et al., 1994; Durand, 1990; O'Neill et al., 1997). Behavior is not a random event; it occurs for a reason. Therefore, if children repeatedly engage in problem behavior, they benefit in some way. They are reinforced either by accessing/ obtaining or by escaping/avoiding an object, an event, an activity, or another's attention. Problem behaviors are not viewed as the result of abnormal processes in this framework. "Instead, these responses are reasonable behavioral adaptations necessitated by the abilities of our students and the limitations of their environments" (Durand, 1990, p. 6).

Behavior can be categorized by function. Typically these functions have been divided into two primary categories: 1) access/obtain and 2) escape/ avoid. Often each primary category is subdivided into three additional categories: 1) tangible, 2) social, and 3) sensory (see Figure 19.1). A child might engage in problem behavior to obtain a preferred tangible item (e.g., a toy

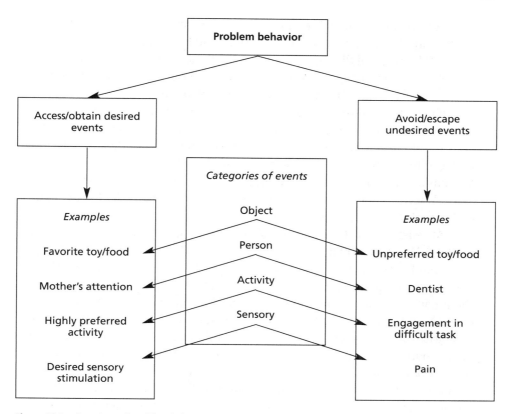

Figure 19.1. Functions of problem behavior with examples.

truck), to access a favorite peer's attention, or to obtain a form of pleasant self-stimulation (e.g., rocking). Conversely, the same child might engage in problem behavior to avoid a distasteful item (e.g., Brussels sprouts), to escape an aversive activity (e.g., having to write numbers) or person (e.g., the dentist), or to avoid unpleasant auditory stimulation (e.g., hum loudly to avoid a noisy classroom).

In recent years, another concept borrowed from operant conditioning has been applied to FCT as a heuristic for understanding the mechanisms by which it operates. The notion of *response class* has been invoked to describe a situation in which varying topographies of behavior share the same behavioral function. That is, the varying behaviors that serve a specific function (e.g., obtain attention) are said to form a response class. By definition, when a group of behaviors produces the same outcome in the environment (i.e., has the same function), we refer to the group as a response class. Each response, or behavior, is a member of the class and is said to be *functionally equivalent* to all other members. Functionally equivalent responses can be substituted for one another. Thus, when a child vocalizes, taps an adult on the arm, raises her hand, asks, "Can you come here?" or screams, each of these five responses may function as a request for attention and, in the presence of another person, may produce the same functional outcome (see Figure 19.2 for a visual display of an obtain-attention response class).

When functionally equivalent responses exist, there is potential for *response competition* (Horner & Billingsley, 1988). If a number of responses in a child's repertoire all produce the same environmental outcome, then what mechanisms determine which response will occur? The notion of *response efficiency* has heuristic value. It is hypothesized that the response that produces the reinforcer most efficiently will prevail. Both conceptual and empirical work appear to support this hypothesis (e.g., Horner & Day, 1991; Mace & Roberts, 1993; Neef, Mace, & Shade, 1993; Neef, Mace, Shea, & Shade, 1992; Sprague & Horner, 1992).

At least five factors determine the efficiency of competing responses (Halle & Drasgow, 2003; Horner & Billingsley, 1988), in which efficiency can be defined as the degree to which a response class member optimizes the desired outcome and minimizes other potential outcomes. *Response effort* is the amount of effort (sometimes measured in calories expended or level of cognitive effort) required to produce the response. For a child just beginning to learn words, screaming to obtain attention may be easier than saying, "Come here" and thus, all other factors being equal, would be more efficient. *Immediacy* of obtaining the desired outcome is the second factor. If screaming produces attention more quickly than vocalizing, then screaming is more efficient. The third factor, *consistency* of obtaining the desired outcome, refers to how often the response produces the outcome. If a child has to raise his or her hand or tap an adult four times before the adult attends, then these behaviors are less efficient than screaming which is attended to each and every time it occurs.

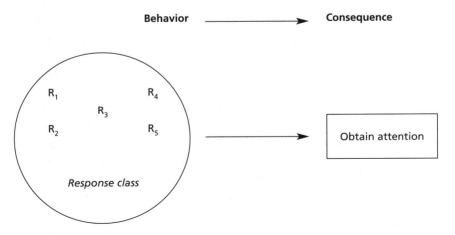

Figure 19.2. Visual illustration of a response class or a group of topographically different behaviors that produce the same effect on the environment or have the same consequence (e.g., obtain attention). R_1, vocalizes; R_2, taps an adult's arm; R_3, raises hand; R_4, asks, "Can you come here?"; R_5, screams.

Quality or *magnitude* of outcome produced is the fourth factor determining efficiency. If a child receives 3 minutes of a favored adult's attention by screaming and only 20 seconds by tapping the adult on the arm, then screaming once again is considered more efficient than tapping, based on magnitude of outcome. The fifth factor, *probability of punishment,* has not been widely recognized as a determinant of efficiency and, therefore, has not yet been demonstrated empirically (Halle & Drasgow, 2003). We have included it here because we believe it influences which response in a class will occur. Thus, if screaming is punished 1 out of 5 times it is used to gain attention, and vocalizing is punished 1 out of 50 times, all other factors being equal, vocalizing is more efficient because it minimizes the probability of punishment. Here, punishment is defined as any consequence that reduces the likelihood of the response. At least four caveats warrant mention in this discussion of response efficiency. First, all five factors affecting efficiency are highly dependent on the behavior of the social partners with whom a child interacts. It is these partners who decide to which request for attention they will respond and the immediacy, magnitude, and form of their response. Later, in the Key Components section of this chapter, we will revisit this issue by describing in more detail the role that partners must assume to ensure the efficiency of desired responses and the inefficiency of problem responses. Second, none of these five factors operates alone or independent of the other four. That is, the value of all five combined is what determines which member of the class of *requesting attention* will occur in any particular situation. So all five must be considered when selecting responses 1) to teach the child and 2) to which the social partners will be taught to be responsive.

The third caveat is that our entire discussion of response efficiency has been restricted to requesting attention. Efficiency factors are equally applicable to communicative functions other than requesting. For example, commenting may depend on the most efficient response for producing joint attention, or rejecting may depend on the most efficient response that produces the removal of the aversive event or material or release from an aversive activity. The fourth and final caveat encompasses the impact of varying environmental conditions (e.g., identity of the social partner, proximity of the partner, whether or not the partner is attending) on communicative options. These conditions may affect efficiency factors such that one adult may respond more immediately, consistently, and with greater quality to words, whereas another adult may produce these same outcomes (and never punish) in response to screams. Or, if a favored adult is nearby, then arm-tapping might become more efficient than words. Or if an adult already is looking at the child, then raising one's hand may become more efficient than words or screams. Varying responses become more or less efficient depending on a combination of contextual conditions. These ever-changing contextual conditions render one or another member of the response class most efficient. When a response is triggered by a combination of contextual conditions or stimuli, the phenomenon is referred to as a *conditional discrimination* (Reichle & Johnston, 1999; Sigafoos & Drasgow, 2001).

A practical example can help illustrate the concepts of response class, functional equivalence, response competition, and response efficiency. It has been reported for years in the language intervention literature that newly taught responses often fail to generalize to novel situations (Halle, 1987; Hart & Rogers-Warren, 1978; Warren, Rogers-Warren, Baer, & Guess, 1980). Recent research has documented that at least some of these generalization failures are not truly failures to generalize, but rather situations in which the newly taught response has become a member of a larger response class; however, it is not the most efficient member and, therefore, is not displayed. That is, when a new functionally equivalent response is acquired, it cannot be assumed that it will occur in all appropriate contexts because it competes with existing responses that have the same function and have been reinforced repeatedly in the past. Only after the newly acquired member is made most efficient (in terms of the five factors) and the previously most efficient member is rendered less efficient (with extinction or mild punishment) can the new response "generalize."

After determining the communicative function of unconventional behavior, for example, Drasgow, Halle, and Ostrosky (1998) taught functionally equivalent and socially acceptable responses to replace the problem responses of three young children with autism. In one example, a child was taught to use a modified American Sign Language (ASL) gesture for *please* instead of grabbing or screaming to request materials he wanted. An initial barrier to the successful generalization of the gesture was response competition (i.e., the ASL gesture, grabbing, and screaming were now members of the same response class). Even after the gesture (a new response) was acquired as demonstrated by its use in the treatment context, it was not emitted on generalization occasions in which the child requested materials in his everyday routines at home; rather, grabbing and screaming (existing functionally equivalent responses) occurred until they were extinguished by partners' lack of response. When grabbing and screaming were no longer effective at obtaining materials, the ASL gesture presumably became the most efficient member of the response class and was displayed in the generalization situations (i.e., generalization occurred).

EMPIRICAL BASIS

In recent years, FCT has become a common intervention approach, particularly for students with persistent challenging behavior (Carr et al., 1994; Durand, 1990; O'Neill et al., 1997). In this section, we provide an overview of the research to date on FCT including 1) the experimental methodology that has been used to establish internal validity; 2) the populations and settings that have been studied; 3) a description of two historic papers that set the stage for FCT; and 4) a review of five key studies that focused on the effectiveness and efficiency of FCT in terms of acquisition, maintenance, and generalization. The *Journal of Applied Behavior Analysis* and the *Journal of Positive Behavior Interventions* are the two primary repositories of research devoted to FCT and other operant strategies addressing problem behavior. They provide experimental exemplars of the many variations in FCT research.

Experimental Methodology

FCT research has relied almost exclusively on the use of single-subject designs and methodology. Single-subject methodology is particularly useful when examining the effects of an intervention on one or a small number of individuals. The generality of the intervention's effect with other individuals is established or limited through replication with individuals who vary in age, gender, diagnoses, and other demographic characteristics. The designs most often employed in FCT research have been ABAB (or reversal), multiple baseline, and alternating treatments (or multielement) (see Kazdin, 1982, or McReynolds and Kearns, 1983, for detailed descriptions of these designs). Typically, either an ABAB or an alternating-treatments design is used to conduct a functional analysis to identify behavioral function. Then either an ABAB or multiple-baseline design provides the framework for the examination of the effects of FCT. Occasionally, variants of other designs are introduced to accommodate differing perspectives and questions following from each (see Durand & Carr, 1992, or Reeve & Carr, 2000, below).

Populations and Settings

Research on FCT has been conducted with individuals with a range of disabilities and problem behaviors. The research has involved students of all ages from toddlers (Galensky, Miltenberger, Stricker, & Garlinghouse, 2001) to adults with a range of diagnoses including developmental disabilities, autism, hearing impairments, communication disorders, attention deficit disorders, and developmental delays as well as individuals without disabilities who exhibit varying levels of problem behavior (Sugai et al., 2000). The research has been conducted in a variety of venues including vocational settings, residential settings (Iwata, Dorsey, Slifer, Bauman, & Richman, 1982/1994), schools (Northup et al., 1994), homes (Arndorfer, Miltenberger, Woster, Rortvedt, & Gaffaney, 1994), and early childhood/early intervention settings (Reeve & Carr, 2000). Research has demonstrated the efficacy of FCT at decreasing a range of problem behaviors including aggression toward peers and adults, property destruction, self-injurious behavior, and tantrums. The variety of forms that problem behaviors can assume is infinite; the focus of this approach is on the function, not the form, of such behavior. FCT has been implemented effectively by both teachers and parents and has resulted in increases in functional communication skills and other pro-social behaviors (Derby et al., 1997).

Two Historic Papers

An early seminal work that characterized the functional approach and served as a precursor to FCT was a conceptual paper by Carr (1977) in which he delineated five motivational hypotheses for self-injurious behavior (SIB). This paper marked the beginning of the notion that challenging behavior might be triggered and maintained by events in a child's social and physical environment. It also led to what Carr and Durand (1985b) called the *communication hypothesis,* suggesting that challenging behavior may function as a form of communication, conveying a purpose to which listeners are responsive. Following Carr's (1977) work on motivational hypotheses of self-injury, Iwata et al. (1982/1994) published an influential paper in which they developed an assessment methodology for identifying the function of SIB. This methodology, a variant of what has been referred to as functional analysis, has been emulated in much of the empirical research on FCT. That is, the first step in FCT studies is to identify the function of the problem behavior, and this typically is accomplished with some variation of the assessment methodology pioneered by Iwata et al. (1982/1994). Although SIB was the focus of these two early influential works, many variations of problem behavior in addition to SIB have been the subject of FCT (see below).

Key Studies Examining Functional Communication Training

In a seminal study on FCT, Carr and Durand (1985a) used functional analysis for determining the function of challenging behaviors, then investigated the effects of an FCT intervention for teaching a communication replacement identified through that analysis. Four students (ages 7–14 years) with significant disabilities including autism, brain damage, and severe hearing impairment exhibited a variety of problem behaviors characterized by aggression, tantrums, SIB, and noncompliance. Functional analyses revealed that escaping difficult tasks and accessing adult attention were the functions maintaining the problem behaviors. During the intervention, these two variables were manipulated (e.g., difficult tasks were presented and adult attention was withheld) to ensure motivation for student responding. All four students were taught to solicit attention and to request assistance from adults using replacement behaviors that had been identified through the functional assessment process.

The findings demonstrated that the replacement behavior increased and problem behavior decreased only when the replacement matched the function of the problem behavior (i.e., requesting attention or assistance). Thus, when students' problem behavior was motivated by accessing adult attention, and the replacement taught was requesting assistance, the students' behavior did not improve (i.e., there was no reduction in problem behavior and no increase in the replacement response); however, improvement was obvious when the replacement that was taught served to access attention. Similar findings occurred for other students whose problem behavior was motivated by escape from difficult tasks: as requests for assistance increased, the level of problem behavior decreased.

This investigation encompassed two experiments, which often is the approach of choice in FCT research. In the first experiment, the researchers conducted a functional analysis that isolated the function of the problem behaviors displayed by each student. A reversal design was used. Likewise, another reversal design was used in the second experiment, to demonstrate the primacy of functional equivalence. Thus, in repeated conditions, the replacement that matched the function of the problem behavior was interspersed with the nonmatching replacement to demonstrate experimental control of the finding.

The findings of the Carr and Durand study (1985a) supported the hypothesis that communication skills and challenging behavior can be functionally equivalent and that an increase in one can lead to a decrease in the other. A unique feature was the comparison of effect when children were taught two replacement responses: one that had the same function as the problem behavior and one that did not. An increase in the replacement form and decrease in the challenging form was observed only when the children used the functionally equivalent replacement. This study was a demonstration of the primacy of functional equivalence and served as a foundation for more recent effectiveness research on FCT that has explored questions of maintenance and generalization in naturally occurring settings—outcomes that have received scant attention in the FCT literature. Although the research on FCT is promising in its effects on problem behavior, there is some evidence that when the components of the FCT intervention are removed, problem behavior may reemerge (Carr et al., 1994; Durand, 1990).

Durand and Carr (1991, 1992) provided exceptions to this finding in two single-subject research studies demonstrating the efficacy of FCT as well as addressing the generalization and maintenance of observed changes. The first study (1991) involved three boys who had chronic challenging behavior (i.e., screaming, slapping others, head-banging, and face-slapping) that was frequent and severe. The boys ranged from 9 to 12 years of age and had mental retardation, autism, or a more general PDD. Based on the functional analysis data, undergraduate trainers taught two boys to request assistance and the third boy was taught to request assistance and attention during brief routines in their regular classrooms. Training time was an average of 130 minutes for the three boys. Although personnel associated with the research conducted the training, the data reported were based exclusively on 60-minute observations conducted during regular classroom activities in the absence of trainers. FCT was effective in terms of teaching the requesting behaviors. Specifically, although none of the boys demonstrated the socially acceptable replacement requests during baseline, rates ranging from 5.8% to 9.1% of the sampled intervals were observed during intervention in Year 1. Similar rates of requesting were observed with new teachers and in new classrooms in the subsequent two school years during which the children were monitored (means varied from 3.6% to 9% during Year 2 and from 3.5% to 8% in Year 3). It is noteworthy that the new teachers in Years 2 and 3 were not informed about the students' participation in the research.

In addition to the enduring use of the replacement requests, reductions in problem behavior were observed. During baseline, mean rates of problem behaviors ranged from 9.5% to 22.9% of the intervals, whereas mean rates during intervention in the first year were reduced to a range of 0.3% to 4.8%. Although the occurrences of problem behavior in the subsequent 2 years remained stable for two students, the third student's rate returned to baseline levels in Year 2, apparently due to his poor articulation when requesting assistance which his new teacher did not understand. When booster intervention sessions were delivered (without his teacher's knowledge of their purpose), his problem behavior decreased from 25.7% to 6.8% in Year 2 and remained low ($M = 5.5\%$) during Year 3.

By providing children with functionally equivalent alternatives to problem behavior, in this case verbal requests for assistance or attention, it appears that use of these alternatives generalized to different conditions (i.e., new teachers in new classrooms) and maintained for up to 2 years. Importantly, associated reductions in problem behavior were correlated with the increased use of socially acceptable requests. The generalization and maintenance of requesting found in this study likely are attributable to the targeting of verbal requests that were easily understood by a wide range of audiences and were functional in multiple contexts. Thus, their probability of being honored in naturally occurring situations was high. This notion of programming for generalization has been referred to as *natural maintaining contingencies* (Baer & Wolf, 1970; Stokes & Baer, 1977).

In a second study, Durand and Carr (1992) conducted another analysis of maintenance following FCT. This study involved 12 children who exhibited challenging behavior that functioned to obtain adult attention. This was established in a functional analysis that constituted Experiment 1. These behaviors included aggression, opposition, tantrums, and property destruction. The children's diagnoses included autism, attention deficit disorder, and developmental language disorders. The children were matched on a set of variables (i.e., mental age, chronological age, and language age) and were assigned to two groups. Each group included five boys and one girl with mean ages of 53.5 and 53.2 months with a range of 40–62 months. Both groups were exposed to an easy match-to-sample task during 10-minute sessions, divided into 10-second intervals for recording purposes. One group received FCT and the other group received time-out as an intervention for problem behavior. Durand and Carr (1992) employed a multiple-baseline design across the six participants in each group to examine the effects of FCT and time-out (Experiment 2). Both interventions were effective in terms of reducing the problem behavior. The mean for challenging behavior for the time-out group was 49.1% of the intervals during baseline and 8% after intervention. The mean for the FCT group was 59.6% during baseline and 5.2% after intervention. As anticipated, there was no increase in unprompted communication for the time-out group, whereas the FCT group increased their use of unprompted communication (i.e., the replacement response) from 0% during baseline to 13.9% of the intervals after intervention.

In Experiment 3, when the two groups were subsequently exposed to naïve teachers (ones who did not know about the previous interventions), differences in challenging behavior were observed across the two groups. Using a reversal design in which they alternated naïve teachers with prior trainers, the researchers found no changes in problem behavior across adults for the FCT group, whereas the time-out group participants resumed engaging in problem behavior at baseline levels in the presence of the naïve teachers. Notably, their levels of problem behavior remained low in the presence of trainers who implemented the time-out procedure. The implication of this study is that providing children with an adaptive communicative response that serves the same function as challenging behavior enables them to influence others in desired ways without having to resort to challenging behavior because they have an alternative means of achieving their outcome. Furthermore, in this study the children maintained their use of the newly acquired, socially adaptive response with naive adult social partners. Response efficiency might be the reason that children continued to use the new response. For the time-out group, no alternative response was taught, so when the children encountered novel adult partners, they resorted to challenging behavior, the only response in their repertoires that had effectively recruited teacher attention—at least occasionally—in the past. They had no alternative available to use to produce their desired outcome.

An obvious question when examining the generalization of the effects of FCT across settings and social partners is to ask precisely which responses generalize (i.e., occur under nontraining conditions). Although this question may seem obvious, its implications are not clear until one considers that a successful application of FCT requires two outcomes: 1) increased occurrence of a new communicative response under conditions that triggered problem behavior in the past, and 2) decreased occurrence of the problem behavior under these same conditions. Thus, generalization may be apparent in both the presence of the newly acquired functionally equivalent response and the absence of the problem behavior; both outcomes need to be monitored to assess their generality. This conceptualization, described by Reed Schindler and Horner (2005), draws heavily on the notions of response class and response efficiency described earlier.

In their investigation, Reed Schindler and Horner (2005) examined the interaction effects of interventions requiring high and low effort by caregivers on generalized use of newly acquired communication and the generalized reduction of problem behavior with three 4–5-year-old children with autism who were referred because of their problem behavior. The children's behavior was assessed in the intervention (primary) setting and in three generalization (secondary) settings that were part of their everyday routines. Prior to the introduction of the high-effort intervention in the primary setting, low-effort interventions were implemented in the generalization settings by those indigenous to the setting (parents, teachers), and the low-effort interventions proved to be ineffective. Although high-effort interventions incorporating FCT effectively reduced problem behavior in the primary setting in which they were treated, such interventions did not produce generalized effects in the secondary settings until low-effort interventions were reintroduced in these settings. These results suggest that the newly acquired communicative response replaced the problem behavior (i.e., the former increased in frequency and the latter decreased). The implications of this research suggest that a model for producing generalized effects of FCT in ordinary, everyday settings may require a two-tier approach: an intense intervention by those who possess expertise in FCT, and a much less intense level of follow-through by those interacting regularly with the child. Results of effectiveness studies such as the Reed Schindler and Horner study are highly relevant because they take into account feasibility of implementation or contextual fit between procedures and those charged with implementing them.

Most of the research on FCT has been reactive, focusing on decreasing problem behavior and increasing a functionally equivalent, socially acceptable communication replacement after problem behavior has been well established. Reeve and Carr (2000) have extended this program of research by investigating whether FCT can be used to prevent the escalation of problem behavior from minor to serious levels. Their study included eight target children with labels of multiple physical disabilities, speech impairment, PDD, emotional disturbances, and mental retardation. Their ages varied from 33 to 60 months, and they exhibited minor problem behaviors such as crying and whining to gain attention from adults. The eight children were assigned randomly, four to an FCT group and four to an expressive language teaching (ELT) group. The two groups were homogeneous in age, gender, and intensity of problem behaviors. The ELT group had a higher mean IQ and a higher mean baseline level of problem behavior. Each of the eight target children was paired with a nontarget child and an adult. The nontarget children were included to make the teaching situation similar to the small-group instruction that was typical in the early intervention classrooms that were the setting for this research. The design combined features of group and single-subject methods: Children from each group were assigned to matched pairs to permit analysis through pairwise comparisons (group) and, when members of the ELT group met an established intensity of problem behavior, they received FCT in a second phase replicating the results of the original application of FCT with the first group (approximating a multiple-baseline design).

The results of this study provided initial evidence that FCT can prevent the escalation of problem behaviors in terms of intensity and frequency. Both target groups engaged in similar intensities of problem behavior ($M = 1.3$) during baseline. During the intervention probe sessions, three of the four children in the FCT group showed no increase in the intensity of problem behavior, whereas all four children in the ELT group intensified their problem behavior ($M = 4.1$). Similar changes were observed for frequency of problem behavior. The duration of intervention required to produce these results varied across children from 12 to 48 eight-minute sessions or from approximately 1.5 to 6.5 hours. In multiple-baseline fashion, FCT was later introduced to the ELT group, producing a reduction in problem behavior intensity. These results are not surprising considering the different goals of FCT and ELT. Although both target expressive communication skills, FCT focuses directly on teaching forms that are functionally equivalent to the problem behavior displayed. ELT lacks such a focus.

In addition to observational data, the researchers provided evidence of social validity by asking 12 special-education professionals to provide global ratings of two randomly sequenced video clips of one child from the FCT group and one from the ELT group before and after each received the named intervention. According to their ratings, problem behavior intensity and frequency increased for the child in the ELT group and decreased for the child in the FCT group. Communication requests increased for both children, but more clearly for the child in the FCT group.

The authors identified a number of limitations of their study that should be considered when interpreting the results. One of the most salient pertains to the equivalence of the two groups at baseline. Although intensity levels of problem behavior (the primary dependent measure) were very similar at baseline, the frequency of these behaviors was greater in the ELT group. While this limitation is not insignificant, the study still provides initial evidence that FCT may be an effective strategy to prevent the escalation of problem behavior. Although no data are available on effect size, the social validity data suggest that changes in requesting and problem behavior intensity and frequency were apparent to those who worked daily with the participating children.

In summarizing the empirical bases for FCT, we have endeavored to provide a "tour" rather than a comprehensive review. This tour has included a brief description of the experimental methodology employed, the populations studied, the settings in which the research was conducted, and five key studies that reflect the scope of empirical inquiry into FCT.

PRACTICAL REQUIREMENTS

This section of the chapter is devoted to time and personnel demands for implementing FCT, as well as training required of personnel. Precise and objective guidelines about these practical requirements are impossible because such requirements vary substantially from one individual to another, and few data exist from which to draw generalities that would apply to each. However, we can provide considerations in the form of questions that, depending on the response to them, will determine time and personnel demands and training needs. First, what goal or outcome is sought? If the goal is limited to replacement of a single problem behavior in one specific context, then fewer resources would be required than if the problem behavior is pervasive and occurs across multiple settings and partners. Likewise, if the goal is short-term change with little concern about durability of effect, a less intensive intervention might suffice. Second, is someone involved in the case knowledgeable about the conceptual underpinnings of FCT (described above) and experienced in applied behavior analysis? If such a person is available as a team member, then the requisite expertise already exists and the training requirements would depend on the availability of this person and those who will be delivering the assessments and intervention. If such a person is not available, then someone will have to be hired or trained (this will require an initial outlay of time and financial resources to ensure a sufficient level of skill to teach others about FCT).

Third, what are the relevant social and physical conditions operating in a child's most frequent environments (Durand & Merges, 2002)? Considerations include the following: 1) responsiveness of social partners to the child's communication efforts; 2) activities and routines that ensure a structure within which the child can readily acquire new skills; 3) degree of control or choice enabling the child to influence his or her environment; 4) level of support in the form of resources for staff training, consulting services, and the flexibility of organizational restructuring; and finally, 5) if in a school setting, presence of heterogeneous groupings of students to permit staff the time and flexibility to implement FCT while some students can engage in tasks or activities independently. We are certain that numerous other considerations could be broached that would assist in determining the necessary practical requirements to ensure the viability of FCT, but we have little empirical data that permit a careful accounting for any of the requisite resources.

KEY COMPONENTS

As described previously, FCT involves assessing the function of a challenging behavior and teaching a new response that serves the same communicative function (e.g., Carr & Durand, 1985a; Durand & Carr, 1991; Wacker et al., 1990). FCT includes at least five major components, each of which is described in detail in the following section along with examples to support the descriptions: 1) conducting a functional behavioral assessment, 2) matching a communicative response to a behavioral function, 3) selecting a communicative form to teach, 4) determining how to teach the new form, and 5) deciding how to respond to both the challenging behavior and the replacement behavior. Although these five components are primary, many additional variations of FCT are possible; some will be mentioned in this section, and others in the Future Directions section. However, our coverage is not exhaustive and some less definitive features may be omitted.

Conducting a Functional Behavioral Assessment

A hallmark of FCT is functional behavioral assessments (FBAs), which are conducted to identify variables that influence challenging behavior. An FBA helps identify environmental influences that consistently trigger or maintain a child's challenging behavior (see Figure 19.1 for examples of potential functions). An FBA can be conducted by an individual or team and involves gathering information through a variety of methods described below. Once all the information is collected, it is analyzed to determine the function of the problem behavior from the child's perspective (e.g., to obtain an object or someone's attention or to escape a difficult demand or a person). The FBA process is complete when enough information has been gathered to form a confident hypothesis regarding the function of the challenging behavior. The hypothesis statement includes 1) an operational definition of the challenging behavior, 2) events that trigger it, 3) its maintaining consequences, and 4) its likely function. The hypothesis statement leads directly to interventions designed either to prevent challenging behavior by manipulating the triggering events (i.e., antecedent interventions) or to teach the child new skills to replace the challenging behavior (i.e., FCT). A key to designing effective interventions is the link to and logic derived from the FBA data. The amount of time required to conduct an FBA will vary across children and situations, depending on the clarity of patterns revealed from data gathered through interviews, rating scales, record reviews, and observations (see O'Neill et al., 1997; O'Neill & Sweetland-Baker, 2001, for more details on FBAs).

If the results of the FBAs do not yield confident hypotheses about function, often *functional analyses* are undertaken. In functional analyses, variables believed to influence challenging behavior are manipulated to confirm or disconfirm potential hypotheses. For example, consider the case of Cameron, a first grader with developmental delays who frequently screams and hits peers during small-group activities. If an FBA does not provide data that permit a confident hypothesis about function, then manipulating variables that appear to be influential, such as the seating arrangement, tasks presented, length of activity, or consequences for screaming and hitting, might provide support for the function of these frequent episodes of challenging behavior.

Functional Behavioral Assessment Strategies   At least five distinct
strategies have been identified for conducting FBAs, including interviews,
rating scales, record reviews, observations, and direct manipulation of variables (i.e., functional analysis). The purpose or expected outcomes of these
FBA strategies is to gather information about 1) the nature of the behavior
(e.g., exactly what the child does, its frequency); 2) events that may predict
the behavior (e.g., pervasive setting events, such as sleep or health problems, as well as more immediate and discrete antecedents, such as engaging
in unpleasant activities or requests to share toys); 3) events that reinforce or
maintain the challenging behavior (e.g., adult provides desired object contingent on challenging behavior); 4) function of the challenging behavior
(i.e., what the child may access or avoid); 5) efficiency of challenging behavior (i.e., how well it produces the child's intended outcome); and 6) events
or circumstances, such as free play or one-on-one instruction with an adult,
that are almost never associated with the challenging behavior. Although
these latter events may not inform FCT, they are important to consider when
designing intervention strategies because they may be programmed to occur
more often, reducing the likelihood of problem behavior (Carr et al., 1994;
O'Neill et al., 1997).

O'Neill et al. (1997) combined interviews and rating scales into a single
category that they labeled as *informant* strategies. Both are conducted to
gather information about challenging behavior from teachers, therapists, and
family members who are intimately familiar with the child. They are a relatively easy and efficient means of gathering information about children's challenging behavior across multiple settings and from the perspective of multiple
people. Due to their familiarity with the child, parents and teachers are excellent resources for describing a child's communicative behavior (Bornstein,
Painter, & Park, 2002). Research across a number of fields of inquiry has documented that observers' interpretation of an event is a powerful determinant
of the way in which they respond to that event (McCubbin & Patterson,
1983). Thus, the subjective and personal view of families and significant others is essential. The Functional Assessment Interview (O'Neill et al., 1997)
and the Motivational Assessment Scale (Durand & Crimmins, 1988) are exemplary models of an interview and a rating scale, respectively, that could be
used for this purpose.

Conducting a *record review* includes analyzing prior testing, developmental assessments, medical reports, and other written records to determine whether patterns exist in relation to the challenging behavior. These
records are an additional source of information that might provide evidence
about the function of the challenging behavior.

As hypotheses begin to emerge regarding variables thought to influence
the challenging behavior, most researchers recommend conducting observations to evaluate the hypotheses derived from informant strategies and
record review. As with the other strategies, observations provide data on fac-

tors that predict and maintain challenging behavior; however, they provide a *primary* measure of behavior because it is observed directly, whereas the other strategies are secondary measures because others who are interacting with the child are reporting about the behavior. Trained observers conduct an ABC analysis by carefully watching the child and documenting events that immediately precede (antecedents) and follow (consequences) an occurrence of problem behavior and by describing the challenging behavior in operational terms. Observations are conducted to identify patterns in the antecedents and consequences that provide evidence for their relationship to the challenging behavior.

Observations offer at least two unique benefits to the FBA process: they yield data that can be triangulated with data obtained from interviews, rating scales, and records (permitting further scrutiny when inconsistencies arise), and, because they are primary data, they are not subject to the same biases that can characterize informant reports (Skinner, 1959; Wolf, 1978). These benefits notwithstanding, specific costs are associated with observations, the most prominent one being time. Observations are not nearly as efficient as informant methods because the observer must travel to the natural settings that the focal children inhabit and, once the observation begins, await natural occurrences of the challenging behavior.

The FBA process is complete when enough information has been gathered to generate a confident hypothesis describing antecedents for, consequences of, and the purpose of the challenging behavior. If FCT is the intervention of choice or is one part of a multicomponent intervention package, then the next step for the team is to begin the process of identifying the function of the problem behavior so a functionally equivalent alternative can be selected.

Matching a Communicative Response to a Behavioral Function

Determining which communicative response to teach necessitates analyzing the FBA data and selecting a communicative response that appears to reflect the primary function of the child's challenging behavior. The replacement response needs to serve the same communicative function as the problem behavior. Returning to our example of Cameron, at least two responses might be targeted for his FCT: one might be requesting a break from the small-group activity, and the other might be requesting a different seat near a preferred peer. The former response would release Cameron from an undesirable activity contingent on a socially acceptable request for leave-taking. The latter response has the advantage of increasing Cameron's engagement in small-group activities with the rest of the children as well as reducing the problem behavior.

A key to designing an optimal FCT intervention is detailed assessment data. If the hypothesis derived from the FBA stated that Cameron screamed and hit during small-group activities to escape these situations, then teaching him a socially acceptable signal for requesting a break would seem to be an appropriate target. However, if the assessment data provided a more detailed look at the precise feature(s) of the small-group activity that triggered problem behaviors (in this case, a particular peer who was seated next to Cameron), then a functionally equivalent target might be to request a different seat. This latter option would be preferable because it would maintain Cameron's participation in small-group activities with his peers.

When selecting the communicative response, the goal is to teach a functionally equivalent behavior that is more *efficient* than the challenging behavior. To ensure efficiency, it is important to pinpoint a response that meets the child's needs and is acceptable to the intended audience. The educational relevance and social or ecological validity of the target response is important to the success of FCT. In the previous example, if the first-grade teacher were unwilling to allow Cameron to select a different seat during small-group activities, then this communicative response (i.e., requesting a certain seat location near a preferred classmate) may not be an appropriate target. The response must reflect a close contextual fit (Carr et al., 1994; O'Neill et al., 1997) with the goals and perspectives of those implementing the intervention, just as it must share the same communicative function as the challenging behavior. For example, Cameron's teacher initially might not be enthusiastic about allowing him to select his own seat, until she understands that his choice making is a temporary solution as she teaches Cameron to tolerate close proximity to varying peers for longer periods of engagement in small-group activities (teaching tolerance is described later).

Selecting a Communicative Form to Teach

Whether the decision is to teach Cameron to request a break or to sit next to a peer, the precise form of the response to be taught remains unspecified. Identifying which communicative form to teach necessitates careful consideration of skills within the child's repertoire and, if possible, building upon these preexisting skills. Sometimes, existing forms are lacking and a new form must be acquired. Possible communicative modes include verbal, sign, gesture, picture, or an augmented system. Selecting a more desirable or acceptable form of communication as a replacement for challenging behavior should include consideration of 1) behavior the child already produces, 2) behavior that can be taught easily, 3) behavior that will be readily noticed and acknowledged when the child produces it, and 4) behavior that produces an immediate response and competes successfully with the challenging form (refer to Carr et al., 1994; Durand, 1990; Meyer & Evans, 1989; Reichle, Halle, & Johnston, 1993, for an extended discussion of these considerations).

Selecting a replacement form also warrants consideration of the child's developmental level. Teaching complex signs or choosing a sophisticated communication system for a child with limited motor and cognitive skills is not likely to be efficient. In the example above, if Cameron were already using a picture system to communicate some basic wants and needs, then creating picture cards using photographs of his classmates might be a starting point when teaching him to select a seatmate during small-group activities.

Teaching the Replacement Behavior

Many considerations must be taken into account when designing an intervention program to teach a replacement behavior, including 1) a determination of when and where to teach, 2) a step-by-step plan for teaching the new skill, and 3) teaching tolerance for delays in reinforcement.

When and Where to Teach   This consideration depends on how readily the child can acquire the replacement response. Regardless of the form of the response, a key is frequent opportunities to practice it in context. If the response is already in the child's repertoire, then teaching can begin in situations that simulate those that occur naturally and are likely to trigger problem behavior. By prompting the replacement response in the presence of the antecedents that previously triggered problem behavior and then reinforcing its occurrence, the team can capitalize on these simulated or analogue occasions to provide repeated training opportunities. If the replacement form is new to the child and will require multiple practice trials to acquire, then massed-trial or discrete-trial (Bambara & Warren, 1993; Lovaas, 2003) training is warranted prior to teaching the form in context. Such training often occurs in a setting that is structured to minimize distractions and maximize efficiency of trials (i.e., a therapy room or a section of a classroom separated by a divider). Depending on the difficulty of the response to be acquired, researchers have recommended combining massed-trial training with in-context teaching (Bambara & Warren, 1993). In our example, Cameron often uses picture cards to augment his communication. Thus we might choose to conduct massed trials to teach him the correspondence between pointing to pictures of classmates and then having the opportunity to sit next to or play with them for a brief time. We would quickly transfer these peer-selection occasions to natural routines in the classroom.

How to Teach   A range of strategies is available for teaching functionally equivalent communicative alternatives to problem behavior. These strategies are not unique to FCT or even to communication training; rather, they are generic teaching strategies that can be used to teach any new behavior or concept or to encourage the emission of an existing behavior under different conditions or in a new situation. Prominent among these are prompting, prompt-fading, and reinforcement of accurate responding or of successive approximations toward target forms. These strategies have been combined in effective intervention packages with sound empirical support such as incidental or milieu teaching (see Chapter 9 in this volume; Halle, 1982; Hart, 1985). Strategies reflecting these interventions include arranging the environment, prompting with mands and models, delaying prompts systematically, ensuring motivation to respond by capitalizing on children's interests and preferences (and in some cases dislikes), and reinforcing differentially target forms with naturally occurring consequences.

To teach Cameron to point to pictures of preferred classmates, his teacher, Ms. Robinson, arranged a teaching trial in the morning immediately before a small-group activity by placing three pictures in front of Cameron and saying, "Who do you want to sit with during small group?" while simultaneously pointing to Rod's picture. Cameron imitated the model prompt by pointing to Rod's picture and Ms. Robinson immediately escorted Cameron to his place next to Rod (the natural consequence and probable reinforcer). In the afternoon, another small-group opportunity arose and Ms. Robinson repeated the trial; however, this time when she asked the question, she waited 3 seconds before pointing to the picture (prompting), permitting an opportunity for Cameron to make an independent response. If he initiated by pointing or waited for her prompt and then pointed, Ms. Robinson immediately escorted him to the child whose picture he chose. An important feature of this scenario was Ms. Robinson's choice of pictures; she intentionally chose Cameron's most preferred peer and two other children whom Cameron was not likely to choose as a seatmate to assess whether he was discriminating among three pictures.

Teaching Tolerance for Delay in Reinforcement As mentioned previously, challenging behavior often can be prevented by modifying antecedent conditions, rendering the function of the problem behavior unnecessary. For example, Cameron's teacher, Ms. Robinson, could anticipate the situation at small-group time and place Cameron's chair next to his favorite peer and across the table from the unpreferred peer. Antecedent strategies, however, are not always available or appropriate. In some situations, children cannot immediately access a preferred object or event and must learn to wait. Or they cannot immediately escape an aversive activity and must learn to tolerate it. These situations occur daily for all of us. If Cameron wants Ms. Robinson's attention, and she is helping another child in a different group, he must wait. If he doesn't like counting, but counting his classmates and delivering the attendance list to the office is a relevant individualized education program goal, he must tolerate the instruction to acquire the skill. After children acquire the replacement response through FCT and discover that it consistently produces the desired outcome, they are likely to use the new response frequently. This is an anticipated outcome of successful FCT. Thus, a natural next step in the FCT process is to teach tolerance for delays in reinforcement. Note that immediately reinforcing requests, when feasible, is still good practice and occurs for all of us on occasion.

Carr et al. (1994) provide an exemplary protocol for teaching tolerance. Their protocol includes a sequence of four primary steps: 1) the child makes a request; 2) the adult acknowledges the request and asks the child to engage in some constructive activity with a promise that reinforcement (i.e., the object of the request) will be forthcoming upon completion of the activity; 3) when the activity is completed, the child makes (or is prompted to make) the request again; and 4) the adult confirms that the activity is complete and provides the requested object, attention, or break.

To conduct this protocol successfully, many substeps are required; only the most salient are described here (refer to Carr et al., 1994, for a more complete description). When the adult asks the child to engage in an activity, the choice of activity and its duration often are determined for *that* child in *that* context. So, for example, when Cameron requests a seat next to his favorite peer, Ms. Robinson might ask him to sit next to a less preferred peer for 30 seconds after which he may request a seat next to his friend. As soon as the 30 seconds elapse, Ms. Robinson would approach Cameron, provide an expectant look and wait for another request (an indirect prompt), or she could say, "Do you want to ask me something?" (a more direct prompt). Alternatively, she could model the response. If Cameron now repeats his request by pointing to the picture of his friend, she would immediately honor it. The rate at which the duration of the activity (i.e., sitting next to the less preferred peer) can be increased depends on the child's behavior. Adults will receive immediate feedback on the success of their fading procedure by children's responses: they either will engage in the activity for the established duration or they will revert to problem behavior. If the latter occurs, the adult would ignore it (rendering it less efficient) and would recycle to a shorter activity duration and fade more gradually.

The example above pertains to accessing proximity to a peer as the communicative function. In a similar manner, tolerance for delay in reinforcement can be taught for escape and avoidance functions. Suppose we assume that Cameron engages in problem behavior during music because he doesn't like the music teacher or the highly structured format of the class, and he has recently been taught to request a break from music with FCT. Ms. Robinson may want to introduce tolerance training by asking Cameron to remain in music class until the teacher plays one song on the piano. At that time, if he requests (or is prompted to request) a break by pointing to the break picture, he can leave for 10 minutes. Then she would walk him back to music for one more song, at which time he could request a break and it would be honored immediately. Once again, gradual fading into longer durations (number of songs) of music class and gradual fading of shorter break durations would be the goal.

Responding to the Replacement Behavior and Challenging Behavior

An important principle in FCT is that the replacement behavior must be more efficient than its functionally equivalent challenging alternative in terms of children obtaining what they want (Horner & Day, 1991; Neef et al., 1993). Therefore, the replacement behavior should be easily produced by the child and readily understood and consistently honored by staff, parents, and other caregivers. When first acquiring the new replacement, each response should be reinforced (referred to as a continuous schedule of reinforcement in behavior analysis) to teach the child the contingent relationship between the response and the desired outcome. If the challenging behavior works better than the replacement behavior (e.g., the child gets what he wants quicker or more consistently by screaming or hitting), the child is more likely to revert to the challenging behavior. However, if the new replacement is more efficient, then the child is more likely to produce this response. Once the replacement response is acquired, social partners need not respond immediately or every time (a strategy referred to as intermittent reinforcement in behavior analysis) to enhance tolerance for delay and persistence in responding.

It also is important to take advantage of natural opportunities to encourage and acknowledge the replacement behavior. Creating occasions within typical routines and activities for the child to use the replacement behavior increases its proficiency. Careful and consistent observation of the child enables adults to prompt the replacement form at critical teachable moments as well as to acknowledge the child's use of appropriate communicative responses. A proactive rather than a reactive stance is assumed. For example, it is important to attend closely to the child and prompt the replacement when the triggering event arises, rather than waiting until the child begins to hit a classmate and then prompt the new form.

An important consideration is to ensure that all significant others (e.g., teachers, family members, therapists) who interact with the individual with challenging behavior are prepared to implement FCT. This team effort will help guarantee that an adequate number of communication teaching episodes are provided and will assist with generalization and maintenance of intervention effects. Also, once a team learns how to teach FCT, there is a higher likelihood that they might use these strategies with other students. Persistence with and commitment to FCT by the team is necessary. Initially, increases in challenging behavior might be observed, as the child encounters changes in consequences for problem and replacement responses. It is critical to maintain consistency because it is those who interact often with the child who determine the efficiency of the new replacement behavior. Consistent implementation of FCT by team members is not restricted to their response to the new replacement; if it is to compete successfully with the functionally equivalent challenging behavior, the consequences for the latter also require consideration. If Cameron hits and screams to avoid the small-group activity and Ms. Robinson places him in timeout in a corner of the room, then she has reinforced these problem forms of communication by providing the very outcome he sought. Cameron will engage in either pointing to a picture of a peer or hitting and screaming, depending on the efficiency factors (ease of response, immediacy, magnitude and consistency of desired outcomes, and probability of punishment).

Therefore, team members should strive not only to ensure greater efficiency of the replacement response, but also to ensure diminished efficiency of the problem behavior. This can be accomplished by extinction or withdrawing reinforcement that previously was delivered (i.e., time-out for hitting and screaming permitted escape) and requiring Cameron to go to small-group regardless of hitting and screaming, and prompting him to point to the picture of a preferred peer to sit next to. In addition to the use of extinction to reduce the efficiency of the problem behavior, researchers (Fischer et al., 1993; Hagopian, Fisher, Sullivan, Acquisto, & LeBlanc, 1998) also have recommended mild punishment that, depending on the child, might assume forms such as reprimands, removing privileges, or frowning. Remember that efficiency is not determined in an absolute sense, but rather is relative to other members of the response class, so it can be enhanced for one member (i.e., the replacement) by optimizing the efficiency factors for that member and/or by reducing the efficiency factors for other members (i.e., challenging behavior).

ASSESSMENT METHODS TO SUPPORT ONGOING DECISION MAKING

The importance of monitoring progress cannot be overstated; ongoing assessment enables adults to continually evaluate if the intervention is viable and, when it breaks down, how to adapt the procedure to repair the breakdown. Additionally, while the adult might need to provide frequent prompting and continuous reinforcement when initially teaching a replacement behavior, this support should be faded over time so that the child becomes less dependent on adult signaling and begins to rely on cues that are natural in everyday routines. Adults should provide the minimal amount of prompting needed to enable the child to complete a task, ask for assistance, or gain attention. Careful monitoring will inform caregiver decisions about when to fade support, and monitoring the level of adult support will provide evidence about the child's success in producing the replacement behavior independently. In those situations in which tolerance needs to be taught and assessment data reveal that children are demonstrating consistent use of the replacement behavior, the time is right for adults to initiate delays prior to honoring the child's replacement request. This is a first step in teaching tolerance or waiting that is so critical if a successful outcome is to be secured, because not every request in our everyday routines can be honored immediately. Continual assessment of FCT effects will signal when problems arise, and careful scrutiny of the assessment data will provide direction for how to modify the original FCT plan.

The assessment methods employed in FCT research typically have assumed the form of either frequency or interval observational measures. The observational recording sessions often are from 5 to 30 minutes in duration. *Frequency recording* refers to a count or tally of each event (e.g., prompt, challenging and replacement behavior, consequence) as it occurs. *Interval recording* is time-based and requires observers to decide whether any of the behaviors targeted occur within consecutive intervals that vary across studies from 6 to 15 seconds. Prompting, prompt-fading, and waiting (duration of tolerance) often are recorded with latency measures which refer to the elapsed time between the signaling event and the initiation of a target behavior. For example, when first teaching Cameron to point to a picture of a favorite peer, Ms. Robinson delivered a model prompt immediately after she asked, "Who do you want to sit with during small group," but across consecutive opportunities she delayed the prompt for progressively longer latencies to transfer control of Cameron's pointing to his favorite peer from her prompt to the question. The most often used methods for gathering observational recording data are paper and pencil (with the aid of audiotapes, dubbed with designated intervals that provide cues for recording) and handheld computers with programmed intervals or real-time recording capability.

CONSIDERATIONS FOR CHILDREN FROM CULTURALLY AND LINGUISTICALLY DIVERSE BACKGROUNDS

We hope it is apparent already that FCT as described above is a uniquely individualized intervention. Assessments are conducted to identify the function of the problem behavior for each individual child. Often the same behavior may have more than one function for a particular child. An additional goal of the assessment is to determine the precise events in the environment that precipitate and maintain the problem behavior. Clearly, these will vary from child to child and from behavior to behavior. As with the emphasis on individualization of assessment, intervention packages are crafted based on the data resulting from the assessment; thus, these, too, are uniquely individualized (or they should be).

We do not mean to imply that cultural and linguistic influences have little effect on children's behavior—they clearly do! However, these influences are accounted for in the individual analyses that already are fundamental to the FCT endeavor. Thus, for example, assume that Cameron is from a culture in which establishing eye contact with an adult is considered inappropriate. His teacher, Ms. Robinson, often insists that he "look at her" when she's talking to him. The FBA reveals that these are the exact times when Cameron engages in challenging behavior by either hitting or screaming. When Ms. Robinson talks to Cameron's father about what she has discovered as the triggering antecedent event, he explains to her that Cameron has been taught not to look at adults when they are talking to him. The FBA brought to light the cultural practice and allowed Ms. Robinson to abandon her insistence on having Cameron look at her when she talked with him.

APPLICATION TO AN INDIVIDUAL CHILD

Throughout the latter half of this chapter, we have discussed varying features of FCT in the context of Cameron, a young child with developmental delays who engaged in challenging behavior. Our intent was to make concepts more concrete, meaningful, and usable by applying them to his case. A few additional details and discussion points are needed to provide a more encompassing picture of this application.

Leading up to the decision to use FCT with Cameron, his teacher and other caregivers had attempted myriad intervention strategies without much success. Numerous administrative and support staff (e.g., social worker, speech and language therapist, principal) had worked with Ms. Robinson and Cameron's parents to design and implement multiple interventions. Behavior change was slow, inconsistent, and did not maintain although all caregivers reported consistently implementing the interventions across settings. As Cameron's problem behavior escalated, the team realized that they needed to explore other options. His substantial delays in expressive language development and his frequent outbursts and aggressive behavior made him an ideal candidate for FCT. Following the key components described in this chapter, FCT was implemented, beginning with a functional behavioral assessment. The team carefully monitored Cameron's progress over the course of several months, meeting frequently to review data and adapt procedures as necessary. They developed data sheets on which to document adult and child behavior, as well as to note environmental influences such as activities, materials, peers and adults present, and time of day. Periodically, the team needed to remind each other of important components of the intervention such as implementing the intervention consistently across settings and team members, honoring Cameron's new communicative requests immediately and often, and being vigilant so that challenging behavior either did not result in reinforcement or resulted in delayed reinforcement (reducing its efficiency relative to the replacement).

As the team observed increases in Cameron's use of the replacement and corresponding decreases in problem behavior, supported by their data, they began to teach tolerance for delays in reinforcement. These delays were gradually increased until he was engaging in activities for as much as 25 minutes, the typical duration of activity periods in his classroom. These were the same activities that previously triggered problem behavior. As the team experienced success with Cameron's program, they began to consider other children within the school who might benefit from their newly learned skills in applying FCT interventions. Although the team started FCT with other children in Cameron's class, they continued to monitor his behavior on a regular basis and encountered new problems twice during the school year. Booster FBAs revealed the functions of these new behaviors and their environmental correlates, permitting the design of FCT that required adapting the prior intervention to accommodate the ever-changing school environment. As they experienced further successes, the team developed confidence in their skills related to assessment and the design of effective FCT interventions.

FUTURE DIRECTIONS

FCT remains an extremely active area of research and practice. Since its introduction in the mid-1980s, the strategies that define FCT have been comprehensively described and continuously refined. Thus, issues pertaining to evidence-based teaching strategies, response efficiency, maintenance, generalization, and social validity, all of which have been the focus of prior research, will continue to chart the future course of FCT endeavors. A brief preview of how each of these issues might be addressed is offered in this final section.

Evidence-Based Teaching Strategies

The instructional strategies used in FCT vary from investigator to investigator and from interventionist to interventionist. A potential future direction of research might entail standardizing the instructional strategies by adopting evidence-based teaching practices or packages, instead of allowing this critical feature to vary from one FCT application to another. As mentioned previously, incidental teaching and milieu teaching packages (Halle, 1982; Hart, 1985; Kaiser, Yoder, & Keetz, 1992) could be adapted for this purpose. It is noteworthy that features of these packages often have been employed in FCT applications.

Response Efficiency

Although much research has been conducted to delineate the factors that determine efficiency, future efforts might include demonstrations pertinent to probability of punishment as a factor that would diminish response efficiency. Punishment here refers to any consequence for behavior that renders that behavior less probable in the future (e.g., a frown, a reprimand, the unwanted attention of an adult). Unlike the other efficiency factors, this one does not yet have empirical support, even though its intuitive appeal is compelling. Another future direction related to efficiency is an appreciation of its influence and impact by parents and practitioners. Response efficiency is a concept that is not yet well understood by many who have embraced FCT; yet without ensuring that the factors of efficiency are in place, successful application will be elusive. Related to this latter point is the fundamental role that parents and practitioners play in determining the efficiency and functional equivalence of a replacement response. How these social partners respond (in terms of immediacy, consistency, magnitude) to children's communication determines its function and efficiency. Thus, one cannot talk about the function or efficiency of a response without considering the listener's response to it. Currently, as a component of FCT, we refer to identifying a response that is functionally equivalent (to the problem behavior) and socially appropriate; however, responses are only functionally equivalent to the extent that social partners respond in the same way to the replacement (i.e., produce the same outcomes for the child) as they do to the problem behavior.

Maintenance and Generalization

Durand and his colleagues have made inroads into an understanding of the variables that produce maintenance of FCT effects, including the teaching of replacement forms that are recognizable to future social partners who were not involved in the original FCT (Durand & Carr, 1991) and that are relevant and effective in settings in addition to those in which training occurred (Durand, 1999; Durand & Carr, 1992). Future researchers will need to replicate and elaborate on these findings to illuminate the variables that produce wide-scale maintenance if this technology is to be available for application. Features of Durand's work on maintenance spill over to stimulus generality in that responses taught using FCT occurred on future occasions when FCT was no longer in effect (i.e., maintenance), and they occurred with listeners and in settings that varied from those involved in training (stimulus generalization). Perhaps the greatest need, and the most critical future direction, for FCT is related to stimulus generalization. If FCT is to be viable, the responses that are taught need to be relevant and functional across many situations and settings (at home, in school, and in the community with parents, siblings, peers, teachers, neighbors, and store clerks). In addition to Durand's work, Reed Schindler and Horner (2005) have provided a model for future efforts to promote stimulus generalization. Horner and his colleagues also pioneered an intervention package with strong empirical support, termed *general-case instruction,* that focuses on promoting the generalization of newly acquired behavior *during the training itself* instead of post-training as is typical. The package is too comprehensive to describe in detail here; however, thorough summaries and reviews are available (Chadsey-Rusch & Halle, 1992; Halle, Chadsey-Rusch, & Collet-Klingenberg, 1993; Horner, Sprague, & Wilcox, 1982; O'Neill, 1990). We believe that the application of general-case programming, an evidence-based teaching package, in concert with FCT offers a fruitful direction for future investigation.

Establishing resilience in children is a special case of generalization programming. This future direction focuses on an elaboration of FCT that would provide the child with more than one functionally equivalent replacement response. (Almost all, if not all, of the FCT research is based on teaching *only one* replacement response for problem behavior.) The rationale for this idea is that in life not all environments will be responsive to the same communicative act. Thus, even if a child learns a replacement response that is easily recognized by a wide audience, we cannot depend on the responsiveness of every future setting to the newly acquired response. Therefore, equipping children with more than one replacement response may enhance their resilience to environments that are less responsive to any particular communicative act and provide them with the means to repair a communicative interaction by employing another socially adaptive response instead of resorting to challenging forms to produce desired outcomes (Halle, Brady, & Drasgow, 2004).

Social Validity

Very few studies have addressed the social validity of intervention procedures and intervention outcomes. The social validity of the procedures encompasses questions such as

- How easily can the procedures be implemented in terms of cost, time required, and convenience?

- What skills are prerequisite for those who implement?

- Do the procedures reflect a close contextual fit (e.g., norms of setting, values of implementers) with the setting in which they are to be implemented?

Social validity of outcome is established by addressing questions such as

- How important are these effects for these participants?

- Is a clear change in problem behavior evident in everyday settings?

- Can children participate in more typical settings (e.g., neighborhood, school, community, recreation, employment) as a result of the FCT intervention?

Some researchers (e.g., Kennedy, 2002) have identified maintenance as a primary measure of the social validity of intervention outcomes. This argument follows a logic that if the behavior acquired through FCT is maintained over time, then it must be reinforced by a variety of communication partners who are a part of the future environments in which the children reside. Behavior that endures has fallen victim to what Baer and Wolf (1970) referred to as a *behavioral trap;* a newly acquired behavior maintains because it contacts "natural communities of reinforcement" and no longer requires systematic reinforcement, external to the natural environment.

Summary

FCT has been exemplary in its almost seamless transition from research to practice. It is one of very few strategies for managing behavior that moved rapidly from a research context to wide-scale practice by teachers, parents, and others in direct-care positions. FBA is now embedded in federal law (IDEA, 1997), and although implementation varies across the country, it is applied on a broad scale. Its use has increased so rapidly that the implementation has been uneven, occasionally compromising its fidelity and, thereby, its effectiveness. We believe that FCT implementation will continue to grow at impressive rates, and as research and practice refine the associated procedures (and as dissemination efforts improve), the implementation will become even more effective. In large part, the growth is due to the intuitive appeal of teaching replacement behavior that serves the same purpose as the challenging behavior; punishment is not required, and new, socially appropriate behavior is being acquired. Furthermore, most behavior management strategies advocated in the past are generic in that their use is not tied to prior assessment and, therefore, they are employed without regard to contextual factors. FCT requires the identification of behavioral function prior to implementation; this assessment process alone probably enhances the likelihood of intervention success.

RECOMMENDED READINGS

Carr, E.G., & Durand, V.M. (1985). Reducing behavior problems through functional communication training. *Journal of Applied Behavior Analysis, 18,* 111–126.

Carr, E.G., Levin, L., McConnachie, G., Carlson, J.I., Kemp, D.C., & Smith, C.E. (1994). *Communication-based intervention for problem behavior: A user's guide for producing positive change.* Baltimore: Paul H. Brookes Publishing Co.

Durand, V.M. (1990). *Severe behavior problems: A functional communication training approach.* New York: Guilford Press.

Durand, V.M., & Merges, E. (2002). Functional communication training: A contemporary behavior analytic intervention for problem behaviors. *Focus on Autism and Other Developmental Disorders, 16,* 110–121.

O'Neill, R.E., Horner, R.H., Albin, R.W., Sprague, J.R., Storey, K., & Newton, J.S. (1997). *Functional assessment and program development for problem behavior: A practical handbook.* Pacific Grove, CA: Brooks/Cole Thomson Learning.

REFERENCES

Allyon, T., & Michael, J. (1959). The psychiatric nurse as a behavioral engineer. *Journal of the Experimental Analysis of Behavior, 2,* 323–334.

Arndorfer, R.E., Miltenberger, R.G., Woster, S.H., Rortvedt, A.K., & Gaffaney, T. (1994). Home-based descriptive and experimental analysis of problem behaviors in children. *Topics in Early Childhood Special Education, 14,* 64–87.

Baer, D.M. (1982). The imposition of structure on behavior and the demolition of behavioral structures In H.E. Howe (Ed.), *Nebraska Symposium on Motivation, Vol. 29* (pp. 217–254). Lincoln: University of Nebraska Press.

Baer, D.M., & Wolf, M.M. (1970). The entry into natural communities of reinforcement. In R. Ulrich, T. Stachnik, & J. Mabry (Eds.), *Control of human behavior, Vol. 2* (pp. 319–324). Glenview, IL: Scott Foresman.

Baer, D.M., Wolf, M.M., & Risley, T.R. (1968). Some current dimensions of applied behavioral analysis. *Journal of Applied Behavior Analysis, 1,* 91–97.

Bambara, L.M., & Warren, S.F. (1993). Massed trials revisited: Appropriate applications in functional skill training. In R.A. Gable & S.F. Warren (Eds.), *Advances in mental retardation and developmental disabilities* (pp. 165–190). Philadelphia: Jessica Kingsley Publishers.

Bijou, S.W. (1955). A systematic approach to an experimental analysis of young children. *Child Development, 26,* 161–168.

Bijou, S.W. (1957). Patterns of reinforcement and resistance to extinction in young children. *Child Development, 28,* 4–54.

Bornstein, M.H., Painter, K.M., & Park, J. (2002). Naturalistic language sampling in typically developing children. *Journal of Child Language, 29,* 687–699.

Carr, E.G. (1977). The motivation of self-injurious behavior: A review of some hypotheses. *Psychological Bulletin, 84,* 800–816.

Carr, E.G., & Durand, V.M. (1985a). Reducing behavior problems through functional communication training. *Journal of Applied Behavior Analysis, 18,* 111–126.

Carr, E.G., & Durand, V.M. (1985b). The social communicative basis of severe behavior problems in children In S. Reiss & R. Bootzin (Eds.), *Theoretical issues in behavior therapy* (pp. 219–254). New York: Academic Press.

Carr, E.G., Levin, L., McConnachie, G., Carlson, J.I., Kemp, D.C., & Smith, C.E. (1994). *Communication-based intervention for problem behavior: A user's guide for producing positive change.* Baltimore: Paul H. Brookes Publishing Co.

Chadsey-Rusch, J., & Halle, J. (1992). The application of general-case instruction to the requesting repertoires of learners with severe disabilities. *Journal of the Association for Persons with Severe Handicaps, 17,* 121–132.

Derby, K.M., Wacker, D.P., Berg, W., DeRaad, A., Ulrich, S., Asmus, J., Harding, J., Prouty, A., Laffey, P., & Stoner, E.A. (1997). The long-term effects of functional communication training in home settings. *Journal of Applied Behavior Analysis, 3,* 507–532.

Drasgow, E., Halle, J.W., & Ostrosky, M.M. (1998). Effects of differential reinforcement on the generalization of a replacement mand in three children with severe language delays. *Journal of Applied Behavior Analysis, 31,* 357–374.

Durand, V.M. (1982). Analysis and intervention of self-injurious behavior. *Journal of the Association for Persons with Severe Handicaps, 7,* 44–53.

Durand, V.M. (1990). *Severe behavior problems: A functional communication training approach.* New York: Guilford Press.

Durand, V.M. (1999). Functional communication training using assistive devices: Recruiting natural communities of reinforcement. *Journal of Applied Behavior Analysis, 32,* 247–267.

Durand, V.M., & Carr, E.G. (1991). Functional communication training to reduce challenging behavior: Maintenance and application in new settings. *Journal of Applied Behavior Analysis, 24,* 251–264.

Durand, V.M., & Carr, E.G. (1992). An analysis of maintenance following functional communication training. *Journal of Applied Behavior Analysis, 25,* 777–794.

Durand, V.M., & Crimmins, D.B. (1988). Identifying the variables maintaining self-injurious behavior. *Journal of Autism and Developmental Disabilities, 18,* 99–117.

Durand, V.M., & Merges, E. (2002). Functional communication training: A contemporary behavior analytic intervention for problem behaviors. *Focus on Autism and Other Developmental Disorders, 16,* 110–121.

Ferster, C.B. (1961). Positive reinforcement and behavioral deficits of autistic children. *Child Development, 32,* 437–456.

Fey, M. (2002, February/March). *Intervention research in child language disorders: Some problems and solutions.* 32nd Annual Mid-South Conference on Communicative Disorders. Memphis, TN.

Fischer, W., Piazza, C., Cataldo, M., Harrell, R., Jefferson, G., & Conner, R. (1993). Functional communication training with and without extinction and punishment. *Journal of Applied Behavior Analysis, 26,* 23–36.

Galensky, T.L., Miltenberger, R.G., Stricker, J.M., & Garlinghouse, M.A. (2001). Functional assessment and treatment of mealtime behavior problems. *Journal of Positive Behavior Interventions, 3,* 211–224.

Hagopian, L.P., Fisher, W.W., Sullivan, M.T., Acquisto, J., & LeBlanc, L.A. (1998). Effectiveness of functional communication training with and without extinction and punishment: A summary of 21 inpatient cases. *Journal of Applied Behavior Analysis, 31,* 211–235.

Halle, J.W. (1982). Teaching functional language to the handicapped: An integrative model of natural environment teaching techniques. *Journal of the Association for Persons with Severe Handicaps, 7,* 29–37.

Halle, J.W. (1987). Teaching language in the natural environment to individuals with severe handicaps: An analysis of spontaneity. *Journal of the Association for Persons with Severe Handicaps, 12,* 28–37.

Halle, J., Brady, N.C., & Drasgow, E. (2004). Enhancing socially adaptive communicative repairs of beginning communicators with disabilities. *American Journal of Speech-Language Pathology, 13,* 43–54.

Halle, J.W., Chadsey-Rusch, J., & Collet-Klingenberg, L. (1993). Applying contextual features of general-case instruction and interactive routines to enhance communication skills. In R. Gable & S.F. Warren (Eds.), *Advances in mental retardation and developmental disabilities, Vol. 5* (pp. 231–267). London: Jessica Kingsley Publishers.

Halle, J.W., & Drasgow, E. (2003). Response classes: Don Baer's contribution to understanding their structure and function. In K.S. Budd & T. Stokes (Eds.), *A small matter of proof: The legacy of Donald M. Baer* (pp. 113–124). Reno, NV: Context Press.

Hanley, G.P., Iwata, B.A., & Thompson, R.H. (2001). Reinforcement schedule thinning following treatment with functional communication training. *Journal of Applied Behavior Analysis, 34,* 17–38.

Hart, B. (1985). Naturalistic language training techniques. In S.F. Warren & A.K. Rogers-Warren (Eds.), *Teaching functional language* (pp. 63–88). Austin, TX: PRO-ED.

Hart, B., & Rogers-Warren, A. (1978). A milieu approach to teaching language. In R.L. Schiefelbusch (Ed.), *Language intervention strategies* (pp. 193–235). Baltimore: University Park Press.

Horner, R.H., & Billingsley, F.F. (1988). The effect of competing behavior on the generalization and maintenance of adaptive behavior in applied settings. In R.H. Horner, G. Dunlap, & R.I. Koegel (Eds.), *Generalization and maintenance: Lifestyle changes in applied settings* (pp. 197–220). Baltimore: Paul H. Brookes Publishing Co.

Horner, R.H., Carr, E.G., Halle, J., McGee, G., Odom, S., & Wolery, M. (2005). The use of single subject research to identify evidence-based practice in special education. *Exceptional Children, 71,* 165–179.

Horner, R.H., & Day, H.M. (1991). The effects of response efficiency on functionally equivalent competing behaviors. *Journal of Applied Behavior Analysis, 24,* 719–732.

Horner, R.H., Sprague, J.R., & Wilcox, B. (1982). General case programming for community activities. In B. Wilcox & G.T. Bellamy (Eds.), *Design of high school programs for severely handicapped students* (pp. 61–98). Baltimore: Paul H. Brookes Publishing Co.

Individuals with Disabilities Education Act (IDEA) of 1997, 20 U.S.C. 1400 *et seq.* Retrieved Fall, 2004, from http://www.ed.gov/offices/OSERS/Policy/IDEA/the_law.html

Iwata, B.A., Dorsey, M.F., Slifer, K.J., Bauman, K.D., & Richman, G.S. (1994). Toward a functional analysis of self-injury. *Journal of Applied Behavior Analysis, 27,* 197–209.

(Reprinted from *Analysis and Intervention in Developmental Disabilities, 2,* 3–20, 1982.)

Journal of Applied Behavior Analysis. (1990–present). Lawrence, KS: Allen Press.

Journal of Positive Behavior Interventions. (1999–present). Austin, TX: PRO-ED.

Kaiser, A.P., Yoder, P.J., & Keetz, A. (1992). Evaluating milieu teaching. In S.F. Warren & J. Reichle (Series & Vol. Eds.), *Communication and language intervention series: Vol. 1. Causes and effects in communication and language intervention* (pp. 9–47). Baltimore: Paul H. Brookes Publishing Co.

Kazdin, A.E. (1982). *Single-case research designs: Methods for clinical and applied settings.* New York: Oxford University Press.

Kennedy, C.H. (2002). The maintenance of behavior change as an indication of social validity. *Behavior Modification, 26,* 594–604.

Lovaas, O.I. (2003). *Teaching individuals with developmental delays: Basic intervention techniques.* Austin, TX: PRO-ED.

Mace, F.C., & Roberts, M.L. (1993). Factors affecting selection of behavioral interventions. In S.F. Warren & J. Reichle (Series Eds.) & J. Reichle & D.P. Wacker (Vol. Eds.), *Communication and language intervention series: Vol. 3. Communication alternatives to challenging behavior: Integrating functional assessment and intervention strategies* (pp. 113–133). Baltimore: Paul H. Brookes Publishing Co.

McCubbin, H.I., & Patterson, J.M. (1983). Family transitions: Adaptations to stress. In H. McCubbin & C. Figley (Eds.), *Stress and the family: Vol. 1. Coping with normative transitions* (pp. 5–25). New York: Brunner/Mazel.

McReynolds, L.V., & Kearns, K.P. (1983). *Single-subject experimental designs in communicative disorders.* Baltimore: University Park Press.

Meyer, L.H., & Evans, I.M. (1989). *Nonaversive intervention for behavior problems: A manual for home and community.* Baltimore: Paul H. Brookes Publishing Co.

Michael, J. (1982). Distinguishing between discriminative and motivational functions of stimuli. *Journal of the Experimental Analysis of Behavior, 37,* 149–155.

Neef, N.A., Mace, F.C., & Shade, D. (1993). Impulsivity in students with severe emotional disturbance: The interactive effects of reinforcer rate, delay, and quality. *Journal of Applied Behavior Analysis, 26,* 37–52.

Neef, N.A., Mace, F.C., Shea, M.C., & Shade, D. (1992). Effects of reinforcer rate and reinforcer quality on time allocation: Extensions of matching theory to educational settings. *Journal of Applied Behavior Analysis, 25,* 691–699.

Northup, J., Wacker, D.P., Berg, W.K., Kelly, L., Sasso, G., & DeRaad, A. (1994). The treatment of severe behavior problems in school settings using a technical assistance model. *Journal of Applied Behavior Analysis, 27,* 33–47.

O'Neill, R.E. (1990). Establishing verbal repertoires: Toward the application of general case analysis and programming. *The Analysis of Verbal Behavior, 8,* 113–126.

O'Neill, R.E., Horner, R.H., Albin, R.W., Sprague, J.R., Storey, K., & Newton, J.S. (1997). *Functional assessment and program development for problem behavior: A practical handbook.* Pacific Grove, CA: Brooks/Cole Thomson Learning.

O'Neill, R.E., & Sweetland-Baker, M. (2001). Brief report: An assessment of stimulus generalization and contingency effects in functional communication training with two students with autism. *Journal of Autism and Developmental Disorders, 31,* 235–240.

Perry, A.C., & Fisher, W.W. (2001). Behavioral economic influences on treatments designed to decrease problem behavior. *Journal of Applied Behavior Analysis, 34,* 211–215.

Reed Schindler, H.K., & Horner, R.H. (2005). Generalized reduction of problem behavior of young children with autism: Building trans-situational interventions. *American Journal of Mental Retardation, 110,* 36–47.

Reeve, C.E., & Carr, E.G. (2000). Prevention of severe behavior problems in children with developmental disorders. *Journal of Positive Behavioral Interventions, 2,* 144–160.

Reichle, J., Halle, J., & Johnston, S. (1993). Developing an initial communicative repertoire: Applications and issues for persons with severe disabilities. In S.F. Warren & J. Reichle (Series Eds.) & A.P. Kaiser & D. Gray (Vol. Eds.), *Communication and language intervention series: Vol. 2. Enhancing children's communication: Research foundations for early language intervention* (pp. 105–135). Baltimore: Paul H. Brookes Publishing Co.

Reichle, J., & Johnston, S.S. (1999). Teaching the conditional use of communicative requests to two school-age children with severe developmental disabilities. *Language, Speech, and Hearing Services in Schools, 30,* 324–334.

Sigafoos, J., & Drasgow, E. (2001). Conditional use of aided and unaided AAC: A review and clinical case demonstration. *Focus on Autism and Other Developmental Disabilities, 16,* 152–161.

Skinner, B.F. (1959). *Cumulative record.* New York: Appleton-Century-Crofts.

Sprague, J.R., & Horner, R.H. (1992). Covariation within functional response classes: Implications for treatment of severe problem behavior. *Journal of Applied Behavior Analysis, 25,* 735–745.

Staats, A.W., Staats, C.K., Schultz, R.E., & Wolf, M.M. (1962). The conditioning of textual responses using "extrinsic" reinforcers. *Journal of the Experimental Analysis of Behavior, 5,* 33–40.

Stokes, T.F., & Baer, D.M. (1977). An implicit technology of generalization. *Journal of Applied Behavior Analysis, 10,* 349–367.

Sugai, G., Horner, R.H., Dunlap, G., Hieneman, M., Lewis, T.J., Nelson, C.M., et al. (2000). Applying positive behavior support and functional behavioral assessment in schools. *Journal of Positive Behavior Interventions, 2,* 131–143.

Wacker, D.P., Peck, S., Derby, K.M., Berg, W., & Harding, J. (1996). Developing long-term reciprocal interactions between parents and their young children with problematic behavior. In L.K. Koegel, R.L. Koegel, & G. Dunlap (Eds.), *Positive behavioral support: Including people with difficult behavior in the community* (pp. 51–80). Baltimore: Paul H. Brookes Publishing Co.

Wacker, D.P., Steege, M.W., Northup, J., Sasso, G., Berg, W., Reimers, T., et al. (1990). A component analysis of functional communication training across three topographies of severe behavior problems. *Journal of Applied Behavior Analysis, 23,* 417–429.

Warren, S.F., Rogers-Warren, A., Baer, D.M., & Guess, D. (1980). Assessment and facilitation of language generalization. In W. Sailor, B. Wilcox, & L. Brown (Eds.), *Methods of instruction for severely handicapped students* (pp. 227–258). Baltimore: Paul H. Brookes Publishing Co.

Winborn, L., Wacker, D.P., Richman, D.M., Asmus, J., & Geier, D. (2002). Assessment of mand selection for functional communication training packages. *Journal of Applied Behavior Analysis, 24,* 719–732.

Wolf, M.M. (1978). Social validity: The case for subjective measurement or how applied behavior analysis is finding its heart. *Journal of Applied Behavior Analysis, 35,* 295–298.

Afterword

REBECCA J. MCCAULEY AND MARC E. FEY

In closing, we want to leave readers with a few thoughts inspired by a well-worn phrase: *Caveat emptor!* Buyer beware! An odd inspiration, perhaps, but we hope that readers interested in learning about interventions for their clinical application recognize how it is reflected in the components we included in the contributing authors' template and in the tone of our own chapters in this book. Given the individual needs of each child with significant difficulties in communication and language development and the practical limitations of practice settings, any parent or clinician considering a treatment for a given child must examine that treatment scrupulously for its fit to the child and the available resources. Critical questions abound for professionals who are committed to evidence-based practice. First, these clinicians must consider the quantity and level of evidence supporting a candidate intervention. *Is there sufficient evidence of efficacy for children similar in important respects to the target child to justify a significant investment of time, resources, and hope in this treatment?* The chapters in this book make clear that although a great deal of evidence is available to support intervention practices for children with language impairment, the evidence base is rarely, if ever, of sufficient quantity and quality to provide a simple answer to this question.

Even if the answer to this question concerning the external evidence base is a resounding *Yes,* selection of the intervention for a specific child requires the integration of this external evidence with information concerning the child and the child's family and the clinician's expertise, experience, and institutional resources. This integration must be performed on a case-by-case basis, and our book provides only a limited illustration of how clinicians might proceed in this process. For example, consider some of the crucial questions that must be raised for each candidate child and family:

Do the goals and procedures of the treatment make sense for this child?

Are the activities utilized likely to engage this child's attention and imagination?

Is the intervention consistent with the personal attitudes and values of the parents/family?

In addition, note how answers to questions that relate to clinician expertise and institutional resources and support might influence attempts to implement an evidence-based decision:

Can other possible intervention agents, such as parents, child care workers, and even trained speech-language pathologists, readily learn the procedures required to implement the intervention?

Can the intervention be implemented at the frequency and with the supporting resources that research indicates may be important to its efficacy?

If the intervention must be modified to suit a clinician's and client's limited resources or institutional support, how reasonable is it to expect client change like that observed in reported studies?

By the same token, an equally discerning eye is required for researchers interested in understanding and contributing to the quality and breadth of language treatments in children through study and research:

What level of evidence currently exists to support an intervention of interest?

What questions concerning the intervention remain to be addressed?

What methodologies are needed to provide answers to these questions?

Is funding available for such studies, and, if so, how should the researcher proceed to obtain it?

The chapters in this book can assist researchers in their efforts to address such questions, but this book cannot substitute for the comprehensive search for peer-reviewed evidence and the critical appraisal of published reports characteristic of systematic reviews and meta-analyses. Furthermore, the chapters cannot be assumed to be fully up to date, even immediately after publication.

In sum, there are many challenges facing professionals who believe that children with language impairments and their families will best be served when the intervention decisions they make are grounded in evidence. The evidence base must be carefully evaluated and improved, and professionals must gain experience in how best to integrate that evidence with their knowledge of the children and families they serve and their own expertise and resource limitations. We believe that with this book, we have taken a step toward the implementation of evidence-based practice for children with developmental language impairments. That step may be small, but it is definitely a step in the right direction.

Glossary

CHAPTER 3 Responsivity Education/Prelinguistic Milieu Teaching

canonical vocalization The production of a syllable composed of both a true consonant and a vowel (e.g., [da], [fa])

contingent vocal imitation A partial, exact, or modified vocal imitation by an adult following the child's nonverbal vocalization that is not part of an intentional communication act

coordinated eye gaze Alternating attention between an object or event of interest and a communication partner (i.e., coordinated attention)

enabling contexts Optimal teaching situations that create or support frequent opportunities for the child to communicate and the communication partner to respond. The procedures that create enabling contexts are 1) arranging the environment, 2) following the child's lead, and 3) building social routines.

linguistic mapping Adult verbal responses that reflect the core meaning of an immediately preceding child communication act (e.g., a child holds up a ball and the adult says, "Ball")

noncanonical vocalization The production of only vowel-like sounds or only consonants or glides (e.g., [I], [m:], [ha])

prelinguistic intentional communication Acts composed of gestures and/or vocalizations directed toward a communication partner. These acts clearly send a message, such as proto-imperatives and proto-declaratives, to a communication partner.

prelinguistic milieu teaching An intervention approach that teaches early intentional communication acts comprising combinations of gestures, coordinated eye gaze, and canonical vocalizations in the context of child-directed social routines

proto-declarative A communicative act that is social in nature and directs another person's attention to an object, entity, or event of interest (i.e., comment)

proto-imperative A communicative act intended to direct another person to carry out an action (i.e., request)

responsive interaction training A training technique that is designed to help parents recognize and respond to their child's nonlinguistic or linguistic communication bids

time delay   A type of nonverbal prompt used to encourage more frequent and/or complex communication. Time delay functions as an interruption of a routine and serves as a cue for the child to communicate.

CHAPTER 4   It Takes Two to Talk—The Hanen Program for Parents

language intervention   Any activity that is consciously designed to promote language development in children at risk of or with confirmed language disorders

focused stimulation   A therapy technique that provides a high frequency of a target goal within a naturalistic interaction (e.g., three to five repetitions) with no attempt to elicit the goal expressively

parent–child interaction   All verbal and nonverbal communication between a parent and a child

responsive language   Utterances that reflect 1) the semantic content of the partner's preceding verbal or nonverbal communication or 2) the partner's play or focus of interest

synchronicity   An interaction that is mutually responsive

CHAPTER 5   The Picture Exchange Communication System

AAC   *see* **Augmentative and alternative communication**

auditory-transient modality   Communication modality in which information is presented auditorily and is not long lasting, such as speech

augmentative and alternative communication (AAC)   Use of multiple components or modes of communication for individuals who are partially verbal or nonverbal

discrimination   Telling the difference between two or more stimuli based on specific attributes. For example, when the item *juice* is presented to the child who has three PECS cards available to him or her, the child selects the card with the picture of the juice (discriminates the "juice card" from other cards).

experimental   When methodologically controlled data are collected to demonstrate a phenomenon in a scientific manner to decrease the likelihood that other factors aside from the treatment being used are responsible for the findings. The general types of experimental designs when studying Picture Exchange Communication System (PECS) are group design and single-subject designs, which include multiple-baseline designs and ABA Reversal design.

mands   Words or phases that specify a desired item (i.e., *I want juice*); requests

PECS   *see* **Picture Exchange Communication System**

Picture Exchange Communication System (PECS)   An augmentative/ alternative communication (AAC) program for children with autism and other severe social-communication deficits which uses a pictorial system

reinforcer   An item, activity, or person that is pleasurable or liked by the child and is likely to increase behavior when provided contingent on occurrence of behavior.

spontaneous speech   Speech that occurs in the absence of a verbal cue or prompt to speak

tact   Words or phrases that make a statement or describe a situation (i.e., "It is juice"); comments, labels

visual-constant modality   Communication information is presented visually and is maintained in the environment, such as PECS, orthography

visual-transient modality   Communication information is presented visually but is not long lasting, such as manual sign language

CHAPTER 6   The System for Augmenting Language

augmented language input   Incoming communication/language from an individual's communicative partner that includes speech and is supplemented by AAC symbols, the speech output produced by the AAC device when the symbol is activated, and the environmental context. Serves several functions for the listener or participant including 1) provision of a model for how AAC can be used, in what contexts, and for what purposes; 2) reinforces the effectiveness of using the system; and 3) makes an implicit statement to the participant that AAC provides an acceptable vehicle for communicating

communication   Any means, symbolic (e.g., spoken or written language, sign language) or nonsymbolic (e.g., gestures, eye pointing, crying, behaviors), by which an individual relates or exchanges experiences, ideas, preferences, knowledge, and feelings. All people throughout the lifespan communicate, whether it be conventional or unconventional, intentional or unintentional (National Joint Committee for the Communication Needs of Persons with Severe Disabilities. [1992]. Guidelines for meeting the communication needs of persons with severe disabilities. *Asha, 34*[Suppl. 7], 2–3).

SAL   *see* **The System for Augmenting Language**

speech comprehension skills   The ability to understand what is said so that one can function as a listener in communicative exchanges; provides an essential foundation on which individuals can build productive language (definition from information in chapter and Sevcik & Romski [2002]. The role of language comprehension in establishing early augmented conversations. In J. Reichle, D.R. Beukelman, & J.C. Light [Eds.], *Exemplary practices for beginning communicators: Implications for AAC* [pp. 453–474]. Baltimore: Paul H. Brookes Publishing Co.)

The System for Augmenting Language (SAL)   An AAC intervention approach consisting of five integrated components: 1) a speech-generating device; 2) individually chosen visual-graphic symbols; 3) use in natural everyday environments that encourage, but do not require, the individual to produce symbols; 4) models of symbol use by communicative partners; and 5) an ongoing resource and feedback mechanism. The SAL is implemented using a collaborative service delivery model in home, school, and community environments and can be beneficial for a broad range of children and adults with congenital disabilities who are at the beginning stages of language and communication development, regardless of their chronological age

CHAPTER 7   Language is the Key

bilingual   Able to use two languages with equal or nearly equal fluency

book reading   Adult–child interaction around books where, traditionally, the majority of utterances were from the adult and consisted of reading of text

dialogic reading   Adult–child interaction around books that consists primarily of conversation about the book, in contrast to reading of text. Specific strategies are used by the adult to elicit and extend child utterances and model language use.

early language   Typical language development from birth through 4 years of age.

emergent literacy   Reading and writing concepts and skills of young children that precede and contribute to conventional literacy, including general book awareness, letter recognition, pretend writing, understanding of symbols, and other skills

English as a Second Language (ESL)   Learning English after proficiency or partial proficiency has been gained in a first language.

English language learner   An individual who is learning English after proficiency or partial proficiency has been gained in a first language

ESL   *see* **English as a Second Language**

literacy   At the most basic level, the ability to read and write effectively. Literacy also encompasses the broad ability to make and share meaning, including complex skills such as metacognition, prediction, and interpretation.

multicultural   A social model that promotes interest in and valuing of many cultures rather than only a mainstream culture

parent involvement   Encouraging parent participation in the child's education and other formal services. This may include planning, implementation, and evaluation.

parent training Sharing of information and resources with parents, and also listening to and learning from parents, with the goal of facilitating everyone's ability to promote children's development

picture books Books that are developmentally appropriate for young children and consist primarily of drawings or photographs depicting objects and actions, usually with only a few sentences or less of text per page

play To participate in primarily self-directed and/or self-selected activity that is intrinsically motivating and usually involves objects and/or other individuals

CHAPTER 8   Focused Stimulation

concentrated models Multiple exemplars of linguistic targets that are naturally available in the social milieu from which typically developing children learn to extract and process information. Concentrated models are typically associated with social learning theories.

developmental disabilities Disruption or delay in one or more of the major developmental domains that have an impact on an individual's life activities such as language, mobility, learning, self-help, and independent living. Developmental disabilities are manifested during the developmental period (generally birth through adolescence) and are considered to be life-long.

focused stimulation Treatment technique in which the child is provided with concentrated exposures of specific linguistic forms/functions/uses within naturalistic communicative contexts. Attempts to evoke production of the target from the child are not a required component of this technique.

information processing models Various related theories of human learning that study the way information moves through the cognitive system. Most models include components related to attention, discrimination, organization, memory, recall, and transfer of information.

language intervention Treatment designed to facilitate development or rehabilitation of receptive and/or expressive communication skills

late talkers Toddlers who demonstrate a substantial delay in the onset of language despite typical development in nonlinguistic domains

linguistic input Information received by the human cognitive system related to language, such as phonemes, words, phrases, or sentences

negative social spiral Phenomenon whereby children with constrained linguistic skills are provided with fewer and less idealized linguistic models through routine social interactions than are typically provided to a more verbally responsive child. This often leads to a reduced pattern of social interaction and continuing decrease in the child's linguistic skills.

social learning theory Various related theories of human learning that posit bi-directional interactions among the cognitive characteristics of the learner, the environment, and the people within that environment. In contrast to behavioristic principles of learning, individuals are viewed as cognitively active in the learning process.

specific language impairment   A language disorder characterized by a marked deficiency in expressive and/or receptive language skills in the absence of similar delays in related domains

treatment effectiveness   The usefulness of a treatment under the conditions of everyday practice. Often includes broader measures of language gains and functional outcome measures in related areas such as social skills, school readiness, or perceptions of quality of life

treatment efficacy   The effects of a treatment under ideal, controlled conditions and typically focus is on specific, short-term language outcomes

CHAPTER 9   Enhanced Milieu Teaching

enhanced milieu teaching   A third generation of naturalistic teaching strategies, building on the principles of milieu teaching and systematically adding principles for responsive conversational skills in everyday communication contexts

environmental arrangement   Specific procedures for organizing and managing the natural environment to increase children's requesting behavior, which in turn provides the adult with language prompting and scaffolding opportunities

language interventions   Specific procedures for facilitating language skills

mand model   A specific milieu teaching prompting procedure that supports a child's communication response by either instructing the child to make a response or asking the child a question

milieu teaching   A naturalistic approach to teaching communication skills in everyday communication contexts, which uses environmental arrangement, specific natural prompts for language, and functional consequences to increase the frequency and complexity of children's communication

naturalistic language interventions   Embedded language instruction in children's ongoing interactions and everyday activities providing functional opportunities and consequences for language use

parent-based interventions   Parents and other primary caregivers are provided with specific knowledge and skills with the goal of promoting the development of their children

responsive interaction   A set of strategic behaviors including following the child's lead, responding to initiations, providing meaningful semantic feedback, and expanding the child's utterances, which maintains child interest in conversations and provides linguistic models slightly in advance of the child's current language

CHAPTER 10   Conversational Recast Intervention

autism   A form of pervasive developmental disorder (PDD) characterized by severely reduced motivation for social communication. It is also characterized by extreme adherence to routines, disruptive behavior, stereotypic or ritualistic behavior, severe language disorder, and often includes mental retardation.

conversational recast   A response to a child's verbal or nonverbal initiation that includes an adult model of linguistic structures in addition to those used by the child. For example, a conversational recast of a child's production of "Elmo kiss" could be the adult response "Elmo is kissing Cookie Monster."

language disorders   Clinically significant reductions in expressive or expressive and receptive syntactic, grammatical, lexical, and/or pragmatic abilities. A language disorder can occur in isolation or can co-occur with a broader clinical condition (e.g., autism, hearing impairment).

language intervention   Validated methods for increasing expressive or expressive and receptive abilities in syntax, grammar, vocabulary, phonology, and/or the social use of these forms.

preschool language treatment   Validated methods for increasing expressive or expressive and receptive abilities in syntax, grammar, vocabulary, phonology, and/or the social use of these forms in children between the ages of 2 and 6 years

speech disorders   Clinically significant reductions in oral intelligibility or in the ability to correctly articulate speech sounds

CHAPTER 12   Phonological Awareness Intervention

complex phoneme awareness tasks   Tasks that require demonstration of multiple phonological awareness skills (e.g., both phoneme segmentation and phoneme blending ability) to complete the tasks successfully

irregular words   Words that cannot be completely decoded using knowledge of how letters relate to speech sounds. For example, in *sword* the letter *w* is not pronounced when articulated.

letter-name knowledge   The ability to name letters of the alphabet

literacy difficulties   Difficulties with written language such as reading, writing, and spelling difficulties

onset-rime awareness   Awareness that a syllable can be segmented into an onset (consonant/s that proceed a vowel) and a rime unit (the vowel plus following consonant/s). For example: in the word *stop, st* is the onset and *op* is the rime unit.

phoneme awareness   Awareness that words comprise individual speech sounds or phonemes. For example, awareness that the word *cat* can be segmented into /k/ /æ/ /t/.

phoneme blending   Blending phonemes together to form a word

phoneme deletion   Deleting a phoneme from a word

phoneme identity   Identifying phonemes in words. For example, identifying that the word *dog* starts with a /d/ sound

phoneme manipulation   Manipulating phonemes in words. For example, changing *cat* to *cap*

phoneme segmentation   Segmenting a word into individual phonemes

phoneme–grapheme relationships   The relationship between a phoneme (individual speech sound) and its grapheme (alphabet letter or letters). For example, understanding the relationship between /f/ and the letter *f* or the letters *ph*

phonological awareness intervention   Structured activities that specifically target developing an individual's awareness that words are comprised of speech sound units

phonological awareness   Explicit awareness of the sound structure of spoken words

preventive intervention   Intervention that aims to reduce or alleviate known risks for a target population. For example, intervention to reduce or prevent reading and spelling difficulties during the school years

regular words   Words that can be decoded or spelled using knowledge of how letters relate to speech sounds (phonemes) in words. For example, *sheep*

syllable awareness   Awareness that words are composed of syllables. For example, the word *baby* can be divided into two syllables: *ba-by*

word decoding   Reading a printed word through relating the letters in the word to corresponding speech sounds

word recognition   The ability to recognize a printed word

CHAPTER 13   Balanced Reading Intervention

augmentative and alternative communication   Aided or unaided modes of communication that supplement or serve as an alternative to oral language. Modes can include gestures, sign language, picture symbols, the alphabet, and computers and other dedicated devices with digitized and synthetic speech.

automatic word recognition   The ability to identify familiar words without conscious attention to the process

decoding   Using knowledge of letter–sound relationships to pronounce unfamiliar words vocally or subvocally

eye movements   A cognitively controlled process of systematically moving the eyes in rapid, intermittent jumps (i.e., saccades) with split-fixations and metacognitively controlled regressions

inner speech   Subvocal, linguistic thinking that supports readers in holding words in working memory and projecting prosody during silent reading

integration   The ability to orchestrate all the subprocesses of silent reading so that they work together simultaneously to achieve comprehension of the text

language comprehension   The ability that oral reading comprehension, silent reading comprehension, and listening comprehension all require and share in common

listening comprehension   The ability to listen to and understand connected text

literacy   Reading, writing, and communicating

mediated word identification   The ability to consciously apply knowledge of spelling–sound relationships to pronounce a printed word vocally or subvocally. A synonym of **decoding**; the opposite of **automatic word recognition**

phonics   An approach to mediated word identification instruction that emphasizes letter–sound relationships and the spelling–sound relationship within and between words

print-to-meaning links   The ability to use spelling, capitalization, and punctuation to determine the meaning of words and phrases that would be ambiguous if you only listened to them. For example, "Her brother is rich" versus "Her brother is Rich"

projecting prosody   Reading words orally or in inner speech in phrases with pitch, stress, and pauses that reflect a good interpretation of the meaning of the sentence

silent reading comprehension   The process of reading for meaning that requires the integration of word identification, language comprehension, and whole-text print processing

whole-text print processing   Everything that is required to read silently with comprehension that is not word identification or language comprehension. At a minimum, whole-text print processing involves eye movements, inner speech, projection of prosody, print-to-meaning links, and the integration of all of the subprocesses of silent reading.

word identification   The ability to translate familiar and unfamiliar printed words into pronunciations, whether vocally or subvocally. There are two forms of word identification, both of which lead to a vocal or subvocal phonological representation of the printed word: **automatic word recognition** and **mediated word identification.**

CHAPTER 14   Visual Strategies to Facilitate Written Language Development

auditory learning style   Learning that predominantly relies upon analysis of auditory features, verbal symbols, combinations, and patterns

canonical processing   Processing that organizes combinations of categories including syllable structures

categorical processing   Processing that results in the creation of categories of perceptual features such as phonemes and letters

connotative processing   Processing that creates and interprets implied, inferred, and figurative meaning

denotative processing   Processing that relates grammatical structures with action elements of event structures

iconic words   Printed words with added visual cues to word meaning

macrostructure processing   Processing that creates knowledge of the structure of events and verbal discourse

perceptual processing   Processing that results in the detection and recognition of relationships among features of sensory input

Phonic Faces alphabet   A teaching alphabet that adds visual clues to speech sound production to letters

picture sentences   Sentences divided into meaningful units with visual cues related to meaning and punctuation

prior knowledge processor   Processing that creates hierarchically arrangements of information

reading inventory   Informal reading tests that assess oral reading of words, passages, and passage comprehension

reading miscue   An aspect of oral reading that varies from the printed text

referential processing   Processing that constructs concepts and relates them to language units

storyboard   A visual representation of the components of story structure

visual learning style   Learning that predominantly relies on analysis, recombination, and reordering of visual patterns

CHAPTER 15   The Writing Lab Approach

author notebooks   Binders that students can consult as they write, which are organized into sections to hold writing lab schedules, works in progress, minilesson handouts, personal dictionary

author's chair   Routine event in writing lab classrooms in which students take turns reading a portion of a work in progress to peers; then call on one or two fellow students to make comments about a specific feature they liked or ask a question about an area in which they would like to know more

backdrop principles   Acronym for guiding principles of the writing lab approach, including **b**alance, **a**uthentic audience, **c**onstructive learning, **k**eep it simple, **d**ynamic, **r**esearch-based/reflective, **o**wnership, and **p**atience

baseline   Level of ability as measured prior to beginning a series of treatment sessions

benchmark   An observable behavior that is used as a specific indicator of progress toward an objective

developing edge of competence The learning threshold just beyond a student's level of independent functioning where the child can be successful, but only with scaffolding (i.e., within the zone of proximal development)

dialogic mediation A synonym for scaffolding, emphasizing the use of clinical discourse (what a teacher or clinician says to help a student learn) for mediating (i.e., scaffolding) learning experiences and building higher-level understandings

discourse Higher-level language units, in which sentences are organized into such structures as stories, reports, conversations, or poetry (examples of discourse types)

dynamic assessment Assessment approach that begins by testing a student's independent abilities, then introducing instructional scaffolding, and later withdrawing it to measure how easily a learner acquires a new concept or skill

executive control Goal-oriented, purposeful activity on the part of a learner to direct attention and take a strategic approach to problem solving

homophones Words with different meanings that sound alike, but are spelled differently (e.g., *their, there*)

inclusive instructional practices Language intervention provided in classrooms in such a manner as to bring students with disabilities closer to meeting the demands of the general education curriculum

meta-analysis A statistical analysis of the results of existing published studies meeting established standards in such a manner as to permit their results to be compared and compiled

minilesson A brief whole-group lesson (10–15 minutes) to introduce a concept or skill in the writing lab approach, often including questions that invite multiple answers, opportunities to practice new skills, and a handout to place in the student's author notebook for later review and use.

morphological-orthographic Associations between meaning units (i.e., morphemes, word roots, verb endings, derivational affixes such as *pre-* or *-tion*) and the letter patterns (i.e., orthographic patterns) that represent them

phonological-graphemic Associations between speech sounds (phonemes) and the letters (i.e., graphemes) that represent them

scaffolding Things a clinician or instructor says or does to frame and focus cues and to provide feedback strategically to guide a learner to construct new understandings of relationships and higher level abilities that can then be maintained without scaffolding

transcription Handwriting and spelling of words in written modality

writing lab approach The use of writing process instruction as an inclusive approach for helping children with special needs develop higher-level language and literacy abilities along with their peers

writing processes   The planning, organizing, drafting, revising, editing, publishing, and presenting activities that authors use when preparing a written product for an audience

zone of proximal development   The difference between the level of skill a learner can demonstrate with independence and the higher level of skill possible with the support of dialogic mediation (i.e., scaffolding)

CHAPTER 17   Sensory Integration

adaptive response   A successful response to an environmental challenge (Ayres, 1979)

bilateral integration and sequencing deficits   A sensory integration problem characterized by poor bilateral coordination and difficulty with projected action sequences; hypothesized to have its basis in poor processing of vestibular and proprioceptive information (Bundy, Lane, & Murray, 2002)

dyspraxia   A developmental condition in which the ability to plan new unfamiliar motor tasks is impaired (Cermak, Larkin, & Gubbay, 2002; Reeves & Cermak, 2002). An impairment in the ability to conceptualize, organize, and execute nonhabitual motor tasks (Ayres, 1979; Ayres & Mailloux, 1981)

sensory overresponsivity   A type of sensory modulation disorder, also known as *sensory defensiveness,* in which individuals have responses to sensations that are more intense, quicker in onset, or longer lasting than those of individuals with typical sensory responsivity. Responses are often with strong negative emotion and are particularly pronounced when the stimulus is not anticipated (Miller et al., 2004; Parham & Mailloux, 2001)

sensory underresponsivity   A disorder of sensory modulation in which the individual tends to ignore or be relatively unaffected by sensory stimuli to which most people respond. Individuals who are underresponsive to sensory stimuli are often quiet and passive, not responding to stimuli of typical intensity available in their sensory environment (Miller et al., 2004; Parham & Mailloux, 2001).

inner drive/internal motivation   When used in sensory integration, it refers to the motivation to engage in sensorimotor activities and master one's physical environment.

just-right challenge   The appropriate match between the individual's capabilities, the task, and the environmental supports

neural plasticity   The ability of a structure and concomitant function to be changed gradually by its own ongoing activity (Ayres, 1972).

proprioceptive   Sensations derived from position and movement of the muscles and joints (i.e., speed, rate, sequencing, timing, and force) (Bundy, Lane & Murray, 2002)

sensory defensiveness   Fight-or-flight reaction to sensation that most others would consider non-noxious (Bundy et al., 2002). A condition characterized by overresponsivity in one or more sensory systems (Parham & Mailloux, 2001)

sensory discrimination   The ability to recognize and interpret the temporal and spatial characteristics of sensory stimuli

sensory integration   The neurological process that organizes sensation from one's own body and from the environment and makes it possible to use the body effectively within the environment (Bundy et al., 2002). This term is also used to refer to a frame of reference for treatment of children who have difficulty with these neural functions (Parham & Mailloux, 2001).

sensory integrative dysfunction   Difficulty with central nervous system (CNS) processing of sensation, especially vestibular, tactile, or proprioceptive, which is manifested as poor praxis, poor modulation, or both (Bundy et al., 2002). The diagnostic term used is *disorder of sensory processing* (Miller et al., 2004).

sensory modulation   The ability to regulate and organize reactions to sensory input in a graded (neither underresponding nor overresponding) and adaptive manner (behavioral definition). The balancing of excitatory and inhibitory inputs, and adapting to environmental changes (neurophysiological definition) (Lane, 2002; Parham & Mailloux, 2001)

sensory processing   CNS functions that include reception, modulation, integration, and organization of sensory stimuli; also includes the behavioral responses to sensory input (Bundy et al., 2002; Parham & Mailloux, 2001)

somatodyspraxia   A type of impairment in motor planning characterized by difficulty processing tactile-kinesthetic and likely vestibular and proprioceptive sensations (Ayres, 1989; Reeves & Cermak, 2002)

somatosensory   Pertaining to the tactile, kinesthetic and proprioceptive systems (Parham & Mailloux, 2001)

vestibular   Sensation derived from stimulation to the vestibular mechanism in the inner ear (semicircular canals and otolith organs) which occurs through movement and position of the head; contributes to posture and the maintenance of a stable visual field (Bundy et al., 2002). Detects head position and movement as well as gravity (Parham & Mailloux, 2001)

visuodyspraxia   A type of practic disorder characterized by difficulties with visuomotor and constructional abilities

CHAPTER 18   Fast ForWord Language

dyslexia   A language-based learning disability that limits an individual's ability to learn to read in the absence of obvious accompanying conditions, such as a frank neurological, sensorimotor, nonverbal cognitive, or social-emotional deficits.

learning disability   Disorders of the basic psychological processes that affect the way a child learns. Many children with learning disabilities have average or above average intelligence. Learning disabilities may cause difficulties in listening, thinking, talking, reading, writing, spelling, or arithmetic. Included are perceptual handicaps, dyslexia, and developmental aphasia. Excluded are learning difficulties caused by visual, hearing, or motor handicaps, mental retardation, emotional disturbances, or environmental disadvantage.

neuroscience   The area of science that studies the nervous system, the brain, and its functions

oral language skills   The verbal communication skills needed to understand (listen) and to use (speak) language

phonological awareness skills   The skills necessary to identify, blend, segment, rhyme, or in other ways manipulate the sounds of language

reading skills   The skills necessary to examine and recognize the meaning of written characters, words, or sentences

CHAPTER 19   Functional Communication Training

applied behavior analysis   The systematic application of behavior principles to change socially important behavior in meaningful ways. It encompasses a research methodology that permits a determination about the relationship between an intervention program changes in the behavior that is the focus of the program.

challenging or problem behavior   Any behavior that interferes with the students' learning or the learning of other students, impedes positive social interactions and relationships, or harms the student, peers, or adults

communicative replacement   A socially acceptable or adaptive behavior that shares the same function or purpose as a challenging behavior

evidence-based practice   Interventions and supports that have empirical research documenting their effectiveness. Practices that are considered evidence-based are ones that have been demonstrated as effective across multiple experimental studies by multiple investigators.

functional analysis   The systematic manipulation of variables thought to trigger or maintain problem behavior in order to confirm or disconfirm a hypothesis about a behavior

functional behavior assessment   A process for determining the function or purpose of problem behavior as well as the antecedents and consequences associated with it. Such assessment typically entails interviews and direct observation.

functional equivalence   Behaviors that have a common function or purpose and produce the same outcome

generalization   The display of a newly acquired behavior across different situations including people, places, times, materials, and activities (referred to as *stimulus generalization*). Also when only one behavior is targeted for training, the display or emergence of novel, untrained behaviors (referred to as *response generalization*)

hypothesis generation and testing Implementing functional assessments to identify the purpose problem behavior is serving for the individual as well as the antecedent events that trigger it and the consequences that maintain it. Once a hypothesis about the purpose, the antecedents, and the consequences is formed, it can be tested by intentionally manipulating these antecedent and consequent events to determine whether predictions based on the hypothesis are confirmed.

maintenance The continuation of a behavior change after the program that produced the change is terminated. Often referred to as *response durability* or *behavioral persistence*

operant conditioning A type of learning in which behavior is influenced by the consequences that follow it. The probability of behavior increases or decreases depending on the consequences. Events that occur prior to the behavior also influence learning by their association with consequences; antecedent events signal the probability of reinforcement being available.

response class A group of topographically different behaviors that produce the same effect on the environment or produce the same consequence. The behaviors are said to be functionally equivalent or substitutable for one another.

response competition When different behaviors are functionally equivalent (i.e., members of the same class), they compete with one another for expression. Their success depends on their efficiency on any particular occasion.

social validity The extent to which the goals, procedures, or outcomes of an intervention are judged to be acceptable to or meaningful by relevant consumers. The methods used to assess social validity are *subjective evaluation* (i.e., asking consumers their opinion) and *social comparison* (i.e., gathering normative data on others who are similar in demographic variables but vary with regard to the target behavior).

Index

Page numbers followed by *f* indicate figures; those followed by *t* indicate tables.